Oxford Higher Specialty Training: Advanced Training in Anaesthesia

Oxford Higher Specialty Training: Advanced Training in Anaesthesia

The Essential Curriculum

Edited by

Jeremy Prout BSc MB BS MRCP(UK) FRCA FRCS(Eng)

Consultant Anaesthetist, Royal Free London NHS Foundation Trust
Honorary Senior Clinical Lecturer, University College London

Tanya Jones MB ChB MRCP(UK) FRCA

Consultant Anaesthetist, Royal Free London NHS Foundation Trust

Daniel Martin BSc MB ChB FRCA FFICM PhD

Senior Lecturer and Honorary Consultant, Critical Care and Anaesthesia,
University College London Division of Surgery and Interventional Science
and Royal Free London NHS Foundation Trust

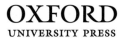

OXFORD
UNIVERSITY PRESS

OXFORD
UNIVERSITY PRESS

Great Clarendon Street, Oxford, OX2 6DP,
United Kingdom

Oxford University Press is a department of the University of Oxford.
It furthers the University's objective of excellence in research, scholarship,
and education by publishing worldwide. Oxford is a registered trade mark of
Oxford University Press in the UK and in certain other countries

© Oxford University Press, 2014

First Edition published 2014

Impression: 1

Published in the United States of America by Oxford University Press
198 Madison Avenue, New York, NY 10016, United States of America

British Library Cataloguing in Publication Data
Data available

Library of Congress Control Number: 2013944919

ISBN 978–0–19–960995–6

Printed and bound by
Bell & Bain Ltd, Glasgow

JP

To Maryam and Oscar, and to my parents, Joan and the late Colin.

TJ

A huge thank you to Nick Stephenson, for all the reading, patience, and support.

DM

To Georgina, and my long-suffering family and friends.

All

Also to the late Dr John Ruston, FRCA (1955–2013), Consultant Anaesthetist to the Royal Free Hospital.
We miss the benefits of his wisdom and experience.

Foreword

Drs Prout, Jones, and Martin have endeavoured to provide a comprehensive reference text for all those involved in the practice and safe delivery of anaesthesia, with the direct aim of following the Royal College of Anaesthetists published syllabus for the final FRCA examination. Succinct and clearly laid out, it enables readers to build on their knowledge of basic science, and provides fresh insight into the applications of basic science applied to clinical anaesthesia. Modern anaesthesia encompasses vast topics, and although a relatively young medical specialty, change is inevitable. The wealth of knowledge in medicine and how this impacts on the safe delivery of anaesthesia expands exponentially. The FRCA syllabus for examinations in anaesthesia is now clearly defined, but this is just the beginning. Interpretation and emphasis is always going to need guidance, and the authors have aspired to provide that guidance.

The book is divided into two main categories: the first is dedicated to applied basic science, and is followed by the application of basic science into clinical anaesthesia. This is exactly the stance taken by the Royal College of Anaesthetists with the final FRCA examination. The book is thoughtfully laid out, with very clear subject headings, in which information on clinical topics is easily available. It provides practical advice, based on sound physiology and pathophysiology to provide guidance for the safe delivery of modern anaesthesia, in the context of patients with much co-morbid disease. Appropriate references are provided at the end of each chapter for further in depth reading.

With the ageing population, anaesthesia will be required for an increasing number of individuals, with an ever expanding array of inherited and acquired conditions. Preoperative risk analysis features prominently in the chapters, with a commitment to optimising the medical conditions of the patient prior to anaesthesia and surgery. Recommendations for levels of monitoring go hand in hand with the choice of anaesthetic techniques for delivering safe anaesthesia, in order to ensure the best possible outcome for patients.

This is a concise reference text for revision purposes. It enables readers to build on their academic knowledge, and provides fresh insight into the applications of basic science relevant to safe clinical anaesthesia. The inclusion of over seventy enthusiastic young authors has ensured modern interpretation, and brought both great diversity and lateral thought to the book.

The book will be indispensable for candidates involved in sitting the final FRCA examination. Interestingly, it will also be of great value to those of us who sat the examination some time ago. Access to information in the 21st century is instant, but appropriate emphasis is always going to need guidance.

We have come a long way since W.T.G. Morton, William Squire, John Snow, and Joseph Clover began giving ether and chloroform to allow surgical intervention without time constraint. I am sure that they would all be amazed by the increasingly sophisticated and precise administrations of the modern speciality, particularly as it is delivered to so many people with such diverse conditions of ill-health.

Advanced Training in Anaesthesia will successfully complement other key medical texts as a reference guide that will be indispensable to those involved in the safe delivery of anaesthesia to an increasingly aged and co-morbid population.

Dr Wynne Davies
MB BCh, DRCOG, DCH, FRCA, FFICM
Consultant Anaesthetist, UCLH

Preface

The principal aim of this book is to assist candidates preparing for final examinations in anaesthesia, both in the UK and elsewhere.

We very much hope, however, that the book will find a place beyond the requirements of exam preparation. We have tried to produce a stand-alone account of the essentials of our specialty and its subspecialties that will provide a ready source of reference in most situations.

The Final FRCA (Fellowship of the Royal College of Anaesthetists) examination in the UK is a major hurdle in anaesthetic training, representing the highest professional qualification in the specialty and the gateway to specialist training at an advanced level.

The book attempts to follow closely the recently revised college syllabus, published in August 2010.[1] The syllabus is extensive, comprising both applied basic sciences, and the clinical practice of anaesthesia, intensive care, and pain management. Any subject listed in the syllabus may appear in the examination: we have, therefore, adhered to it closely and attempted to be comprehensive in our presentation of topics.

This book aims to cover the required knowledge in the necessary detail, and is designed as a companion volume to *Training in Anaesthesia: The Essential Curriculum*, published by Oxford University Press in 2010 and which is aimed at the Primary FRCA. Knowledge of the Primary syllabus is assumed by the Final examiners and is often a stumbling block in the Final examination.

It cannot be stressed too highly that pure basic science topics are frequently examined in the Final FRCA, and candidates would be most unwise not to take account of this during their revision. Together, the two volumes are intended to be a comprehensive guide to the FRCA examination.

In this volume, topics in applied basic science are presented in a systems-based format as laid out in the college syllabus. The sections that follow cover all the major clinical subspecialties. The double-page spread is intended to provide a succinct format for learning, yet containing all the important detail.

References and suggestions for further reading from the recent literature are included for readers who wish to explore subjects in more depth.

The editors have been fortunate to recruit both distinguished contributors who are leaders in their field, but also trainees—who have made an important contribution to ensure that the resulting information meets their needs.

We are hugely grateful to everyone at Oxford University Press, most especially to Christopher Reid who offered such encouragement after our initial approach, to Fiona Richardson and Geraldine Jeffers who displayed powers of extreme patience (sorely tested!) whilst awaiting the manuscript, and to Abigail Stanley and Jane Williams for seeing the project through to publication and beyond.

We hope that this will be the first of many editions and look forward to your feedback such that future editions can evolve according to the needs and wishes of the readership we seek to serve.

Jeremy Prout
Tanya Jones
Daniel Martin
London 2013

---

[1] www.rcoa.ac.uk/system/files/TRG-CCT-ANNEXC.pdf

Contents

Abbreviations

6MWT	Six-minute walk test
AAA	Abdominal aortic aneurysm
AAGBI	Association of Anaesthetists of Great Britain and Ireland
AASM	American Academy of Sleep Medicine
ABG	Arterial blood gas
ABPM	Ambulatory blood pressure monitoring
ACC	American College of Cardiology
ACEI	Angiotensin converting enzyme inhibitor
ACT	Activated clotting time
ACTH	Adrenocorticotrophic hormone
ADH	Anti-diuretic hormone
ADP	Adenosine diphosphate
ADQI	Acute dialysis quality initiative
AED	Antiepileptic drug
AEP	Auditory evoked potential
AF	Atrial fibrillation
AFOI	Awake fibreoptic intubation
AG	Anion gap
AHA	American Heart Association
AHI	Apnoea-hypopnoea index
AKI	Acute kidney injury
ALA	Aminolaevulinic acid
ALS	Advanced Life Support
cAMP	cyclic adenosine monophosphate
ANP	Atrial natriuretic peptide
ANS	Autonomic nervous system
AP	Anteroposterior
APACHE	Acute Physiology and Chronic Health Evaluation
APC	Activated protein C
APH	Antepartum haemorrhage
APTT	Activated partial thromboplastin time
AR	Absolute risk
ARR	Absolute risk reduction
ARA	Angiotensin receptor antagonist
ARDS	Acute respiratory distress syndrome
ARVD	Arrhythmogenic right ventricular dysplasia
ASA	American Society of Anesthesiologists
ASD	Atrial septal defect
AT	Anaerobic threshold *or* antithrombin *or* angiotesin
ATLS	Advanced Trauma Life Support
ATN	Acute tubular necrosis
ATP	Adenosine triphosphate
AV	Atrioventricular
AVN	AV node/nodal
AVNRT	AV nodal re-entrant tachycardia
BiPAP	Bi-level positive airways pressure
BMR	Basal metabolic rate
BNP	Brain natriuretic peptide
BP	Blood pressure
BPEG	British Pacing and Electrophysiology Group
BPF	Bronchopleural fistula
BTS	British Thoracic Society
CABG	Coronary artery bypass grafting
CAC	Coronary artery calcium
CAD	Coronary artery disease
CARP	Coronary Artery Revascularisation Prophylaxis
CATS	Childrens' Acute Transport Service (UK)
CCB	Calcium channel blocker
CCF	Congestive cardiac failure
CCO	Critical care outreach
CCOM	Continuous cardiac output monitoring
CCTA	Coronary CT angiography
CHD	Congenital heart disease
CI	Confidence interval
CICV	Can't intubate, can't ventilate
CIN	Contrast-induced nephropathy
CMAP	Compound muscle action potential
CMRI	Coronary MRI
$CMRO_2$	Cerebral metabolic rate of oxygen consumption
CMV	Cytomegalovirus
CNS	Central nervous system
CO	Cardiac output *or* carbon monoxide
CO_2	Carbon dioxide
COPD	Chronic obstructive pulmonary disease
COX	Cyclo-oxygenase
CPAP	Continuous positive airways pressure
CPB	Cardiopulmonary bypass
CPET	Cardiopulmonary exercise testing
CPP	Cerebral perfusion pressure
CRBSI	Catheter-related bloodstream infection
CRMD	Cardiac rhythm management device
CRP	C-reactive protein
CRT	Cardiac resynchronization therapy

CSE	Combined spinal epidural
CSF	Cerebrospinal fluid
CT	Computed tomography
CTPA	Computed tomography pulmonary angiography
CVC	Central venous catheter
CVP	Central venous pressure
CVS	Cardiovascular system
CW	Continuous wave
CXR	Chest X-ray
DAS	Difficult Airway Society
DASI	Duke Activity Status Index
DC	Direct current
DCM	Dilated cardiomyopathy
DHCA	Deep hypothermic circulatory arrest
DI	Diabetes insipidus
DIC	Disseminated intravascular coagulation
DNA	Deoxyribonucleic acid or Did not attend
DPP	Dipeptidyl peptidase
DPPC	Dipalmitoyl phosphatidylcholine
DSE	Dobutamine stress echocardiography
DVT	Deep vein thrombosis
EACA	Epsilon-aminocaproic acid
EBV	Epstein–Barr virus
ECF	Extracellular fluid
ECG	Electrocardiogram
ECHO	Echocardiography
ECT	Electroconvulsive therapy
EDV	End-diastolic volume
EEG	Electroencephalogram
ELISA	Enzyme-linked immunosorbent assay
EMG	Electromyogram
EMI	Electromagnetic interference
ENT	Ear, nose, and throat
ERCP	Endoscopic retrograde cholangiopancreatography
ERPC	Evacuation of retained products of conception
ESA	European Society of Anaesthesiology
ESC	European Society of Cardiology
ESLD	End-stage liver disease
ESRD	End-stage renal disease
ETT	Endotracheal tube
EVAR	Endovascular aneurysm repair
EVD	External ventricular drain
EVLW	Extravascular lung water
EWS	Early warning score
FBC	Full blood count
FEV_1	Forced expiratory volume in one second
FFP	Fresh frozen plasma
FMV	Facemask ventilation
FNA	Fine needle aspiration
FRC	Functional residual capacity
FT	Flow time
FVC	Forced vital capacity
GA	General anaesthesia
GABA	γ-aminobutyric acid
GCS	Glasgow Coma Scale
GEDV	Global end-diastolic volume
GFR	Glomerular filtration rate
GI	Gastrointestinal
GIFTASUP	Guidelines on intravenous fluid therapy in adult surgical patients
GLP	Glucagon-like peptide
cGMP	cyclic guanosine monophosphate
GORD	Gastro-oesophageal reflux disease
Gp	Glycoprotein
G6PD	Glucose-6-phosphate dehydrogenase
GCSE	Generalised convulsive status epilepticus
GTN	Glyceryl trinitrate
GTP	Guanosine triphosphate
GUCH	Grown-up congenital heart disease
HAPE	High altitude pulmonary oedema
Hb	Haemoglobin
HCM	Hypertrophic (obstructive) cardiomyopathy
HDL	High density lipoprotein
HDU	High dependency unit
HES	Hydroxyethyl starch
HFO	High-frequency oscillation
HFPEF	Heart failure with preserved ejection fraction
HFREF	Heart failure with reduced ejection fraction
HIT	Heparin-induced thrombocytopenia
HOPE	Heart Outcomes Prevention Evaluation
HPA	Hypothalamic–pituitary–adrenal (axis)
HR	Heart rate
HRT	Hormone replacement therapy
5-HT	5-hydroxytryptamine
IABP	Intra-aortic balloon pump
IAP	Intra-abdominal pressure
ICD	Implantable cardioverter defibrillator
ICF	Intracellular fluid
ICP	Intracranial pressure
ICRP	International Commission on Radiological Protection
ICS	Intraoperative cell salvage or Intensive Care Society
IHD	Ischaemic heart disease
IL	Interleukin
INR	International normalized ratio
IOP	Intraocular pressure
IPPV	Intermittent positive pressure ventilation
ISWT	Incremental shuttle walk test
ITU	Intensive therapy unit
IV	Intravenous
IVC	Inferior vena cava
LA	Local anaesthetic
LAD	Left anterior descending (coronary artery)
LAP	Left atrial pressure
LASER	Light amplification by stimulated emission of radiation
LAUP	Laser-assisted uvuloplasty
LBBB	Left bundle branch block
LDL	Low density lipoprotein

LED	Light-emitting diode
LFTs	Liver function tests
LiDCO	Lithium dilution cardiac output
LIMA	Left internal mammary artery
LMWH	Low-molecular-weight heparin
LODS	Logistic Organ Dysfunction Score
LOS	Lower oesophageal sphincter
LV	Left ventricular
LVAD	Left ventricular assist device
LVEDP	Left ventricular end-diastolic pressure
LVEDV	Left ventricular end-diastolic volume
LVEF	Left ventricular ejection fraction
LVH	Left ventricular hypertrophy
LVOT	Left ventricular outflow tract
MAP	Mean arterial pressure
MA	Mean acceleration
MAP	Mean arterial pressure
MELD	Model for end-stage liver disease
MEP	Motor evoked potential
MET	Metabolic equivalent (of task)
MEWS	Modified early warning system
MI	Myocardial infarction
MIBG	Meta-iodobenzylguanidine
MILS	Manual in-line stabilization
MODS	Multiple Organ Dysfunction Score
MOF	Multiple organ failure
MPAP	Mean pulmonary artery pressure
MPI	Myocardial perfusion imaging
MPM	Mortality Prediction Model
MRI	Magnetic resonance imaging
NAP	National Audit Project
NASPE	North American Society of Pacing and Electrophysiology
NBM	Nil by mouth
NCEPOD	National Confidential Enquiry into Patient Outcome and Death
NGT	Nasogastric tube
NICE	National Institute for Health and Clinical Excellence
NIV	Non-invasive ventilation
NHS	National Health Service (UK)
NMBA	Neuromuscular blocking agent
NMDA	N-methyl-D-aspartic acid
NNT	Number needed to treat
NO	Nitric oxide
NOD	Nucleotide oligomerization domain
NOS	Nitric oxide synthetase
NPSA	National Patient Safety Agency
NREM	Non-rapid eye movement
NS	Normal saline
NSAID	Non-steroidal anti-inflammatory drug
NSTEMI	Non ST-elevation myocardial infarction
NSVT	Non-sustained ventricular tachycardia
NTS	Nucleus (of) tractus solitarius
NYHA	New York Heart Association
ODM	Oesophageal Doppler monitor
OLV	One lung ventilation
OPCAB	Off-pump coronary artery bypass
OR	Odds ratio
OSA	Obstructive sleep apnoea
PA	Pulmonary artery
PAC	Pulmonary artery catheter
PAO_2	Alveolar partial pressure of oxygen
PaO_2	Arterial partial pressure of oxygen
PAP	Pulmonary artery pressure
PAH	Pulmonary arterial hypertension
PAOP	Pulmonary artery occlusion pressure
PCA	Patient-controlled analgesia
PCEA	Patient-controlled epidural analgesia
PCI	Percutaneous coronary intervention
PDA	Patent ductus arteriosus or posterior descending (coronary) artery
PDEI	Phosphodiesterase inhibitor
PDPH	Post-dural puncture headache
PE	Pulmonary embolism
PEA	Pulseless electrical activity
PEEP	Positive end-expiratory pressure
PFO	Patent foramen ovale
PHT	Pulmonary hypertension
PICC	Peripherally-inserted central catheter
PiCCO	Pulse contour cardiac output
PICU	Paediatric intensive care unit
PMN	Polymorphonuclear neutrophil
PMP	Pain management programme
PND	Paroxysmal nocturnal dyspnoea
PNI	Peripheral nerve injury
PNS	Parasympathetic nervous system
POCT	Point of care testing
POISE	PeriOperative Ischaemia Study Evaluation
POMS	Postoperative Morbidity Survey
PONV	Postoperative nausea and vomiting
POSSUM	Physiological and Operative Severity Score for Enumeration of Mortality and Morbidity
PPCM	Peripartum cardiomyopathy
PPHN	Persistent pulmonary hypertension of the newborn
PPV	Pulse pressure variation
PRCs	Packed red cells
PRES	Posterior reversible encephalopathy syndrome
PRR	Pattern recognition receptor
PT	Prothrombin time
PTFE	Polytetrafluoroethylene
PV	Peak velocity
PVR	Pulmonary vascular resistance
PVB	Paravertebral block
PVR	Pulmonary vascular resistance
PW	Pulsed wave
RAAA	Ruptured abdominal aortic aneurysm
RAAS	Renin–angiotensin–aldosterone system
RCoA	Royal College of Anaesthetists (UK)
RCM	Restrictive cardiomyopathy

RCT	Randomized controlled trial
RCV	Red cell volume
REM	Rapid eye movement
RFTs	Respiratory function tests
RIFLE	Risk-Injury-Failure-Loss-Endstage
RIG-1	Retinoic acid-inducible gene-1
RIJV	Right internal jugular vein
ROC	Receiver operating curve
ROS	Reactive oxygen species
ROTEM®	Rotational thromboelastometry
RR	Relative risk
RRR	Relative risk reduction
RRT	Renal replacement therapy *or* rapid response team
RS	Respiratory system
RSI	Rapid sequence induction
RV	Right ventricular
RVOT	Right ventricular outflow tract
SAH	Subarachnoid haemorrhage
SAM	Systolic anterior motion
SAPS	Simplified Acute Physiology Score
SBP	Systolic blood pressure
SCD	Sudden cardiac death
SCI	Spinal cord injury
SIADH	Syndrome of inappropriate antidiuretic hormone (secretion)
SID	Strong ion difference
SIRS	Systemic inflammatory response syndrome
SLE	Systemic lupus erythematosus
SNS	Sympathetic nervous system
SR	Systematic review
SSRI	Selective serotonin reuptake inhibitor
SOB	Shortness of breath
SOFA	Sequential Organ Failure (score)
SSEP	Somatosensory evoked potential
SSRI	Selective serotonin reuptake inhibitor
STEMI	ST-elevation myocardial infarction
SvO_2	Mixed venous oxygen saturation
SV	Stroke volume
SVR	Systemic vascular resistance
SVV	Stroke volume variation
TBI	Traumatic brain injury

TBSA	Total body surface area
TCA	Tricyclic antidepressant
TCI	Target controlled infusion
TEBI	Thoracic electrical bioimpedance
TEBR	Thoracic electrical bioreactance
TEG®	Thromboelastography
TF	Tissue factor
TFPI	Tissue factor pathway inhibitor
TGA	Transposition of the great arteries
TIA	Transient ischaemic attack
TIPS	Transjugular intrahepatic portosystemic shunt
TIVA	Total intravenous anaesthesia
TLC	Total lung capacity
TLR	Toll-like receptor
TNF	Tumour necrosis factor
TOE	Transoesophageal echocardiography
ToF	Train of four
tPA	Tissue plasminogen activator
TPN	Total parenteral nutrition
TPDT	Transpulmonary dilutional technique
TPN	Total parenteral nutrition
TSH	Thyroid-stimulating hormone
TTE	Transthoracic echocardiography
TUR	Transurethral resection
UA	Unstable angina
UFH	Unfractionated heparin
UPPP	Uvulo-palato-pharyngoplasty
VAD	Ventricular assist device
VATS	Video-assisted thoracoscopic surgery
VF	Ventricular fibrillation
VKA	Vitamin K antagonist
VMA	Vannilyl mandelic acid
VOTO	Ventricular outflow obstruction
VRII	Variable rate insulin infusion
VSD	Ventricular septal defect
VT	Ventricular tachycardia *or* ventilatory threshold
VTE	Venous thromboembolism
vWF	Von Willebrand's factor
WHO	World Health Organization

Contributors

Ray Ackwerh
Specialist Trainee, Anaesthesia
Great Ormond Hospital for Children NHS
Foundation Trust, UK
Section 25.7

Lee Adams
Fellow in Ophthalmic Anaesthesia
Moorfields Eye Hospital NHS Foundation
Trust, UK
Sections 27.1–27.6

Rachel Baumber
Specialist Trainee, Anaesthesia and Intensive Care
Medicine
Central London School of Anaesthesia, UK
Sections 22.9 and 22.10

Philip Bearfield
Consultant in ITU and Anaesthesia
Royal Free London NHS Foundation Trust, UK
Sections 23.1–23.6

Jon Bramall
Specialist Trainee, Anaesthesia and Intensive Care
Medicine
Central London School of Anaesthesia, UK
Sections 3.1–3.6

George Collee
Consultant Anaesthetist
Royal Free London NHS Foundation Trust, UK
Sections 22.3 and 22.6

Roger Cordery
Consultant in Cardiothoracic Anaesthesia and
Critical Care
University College London Hospitals NHS
Foundation Trust, UK
Sections 14.1–14.9 and 15.1–15.6

Dominic Cox
Clinical Scientist, Critical Care Unit
Royal Free London NHS Foundation Trust, UK
Sections 10.1–10.2

Karen Darragh
Fellow in Heart Failure
Royal Brompton and Harefield NHS Trust, UK
Section 1.11

Tim Dawes
Specialist Trainee, Anaesthesia and Intensive Care
Medicine
Central London School of Anaesthesia, UK
Sections 1.6 and 1.8

Kulwant Dhadwal
Consultant in ITU and Anaesthesia
Royal Free London NHS Foundation Trust, UK
Sections 13.1–13.3

Marie-Clare Elder
Head of Legal Services
Royal Free London NHS Foundation Trust, UK
Section 20.6

Adrian England
Consultant Anaesthetist
Royal Free London NHS Foundation Trust, UK
Sections 6.7 and 6.8

Priti Gandre
Specialist Trainee, Anaesthesia
Barts and The London NHS Trust, UK
Section 13.1–13.3

Edward Gilbert-Kawai
Specialist Trainee, Anaesthesia and Intensive Care
Medicine
Central London School of Anaesthesia, UK
Research Leader, Centre for Altitude, Space and
Extreme Environment Medicine,
University College London, UK
Sections 2.1–2.9

Michael Grocott
Professor of Anaesthesia and Critical Care,
University of Southampton, UK
Honorary Consultant in Critical Care Medicine,
Southampton University Hospitals, NHS Trust, UK
Director of NIAA Health Services Research Centre, UK
Sections 9.1–9.3

Paul Gunning
Consultant Anaesthetist
Royal National Orthopaedic Hospital NHS
Trust, UK
(formerly Consultant Vascular Anaesthetist,
Imperial College Healthcare NHS Trust)
Sections 16.1–16.3

Matt Henley
Specialist Trainee, Anaesthesia
Central London School of Anaesthesia, UK
Sections 18.1–18.4

Lucy Hepburn
Consultant Anaesthetist
Great Ormond Street Hospital for Children NHS
Foundation Trust, UK
Sections 25.1–25.5

Barrie Higgs
Consultant Anaesthetist
Royal Free London NHS Foundation Trust, UK
Section 22.2

Dan Horner
Consultant Vascular Anaesthetist
Imperial College Healthcare NHS Trust, UK
Section 16.4

Julian Howard
Consultant in ITU and Anaesthesia
Royal Free London NHS Foundation Trust, UK
Section 20.5

Helen Hume-Smith
Consultant Anaesthetist
Great Ormond Street Hospital for Children NHS Foundation
Trust, UK
Sections 25.3, 25.6, 25.8, and 25.9

Annie Hunningher
Consultant Anaesthetist
Barts and The London NHS Trust, UK
Sections 5.4, 11.7–11.9, and 22.8

Tom Hurst
Consultant in ITU and Trauma Anaesthesia
King's College Hospital NHS Foundation Trust, UK
Consultant at East Anglian Air Ambulance, UK
Sections 22.1–22.7

Nicholas Jenkins
Specialist Trainee, Anaesthesia
Central London School of Anaesthesia, UK
Sections 1.15 and 1.16

Jasmeet Kaur
Consultant Anaesthetist
Royal National Orthopaedic Hospital NHS Trust, UK
Sections 18.1–18.4

Carlos Kidel
Specialist Trainee, Anaesthesia
Central London School of Anaesthesia, UK
Section 13.8

Stephanie King
Specialist Trainee, Anaesthesia
Great Ormond Hospital for Children NHS Foundation
Trust, UK
Sections 25.8 and 25.9

Emma Knaggs
Chronic Pain Physiotherapist
Royal Free London NHS Foundation Trust, UK
Section 26.10

Dominik Krzanicki
Specialist Trainee, Anaesthesia
Central London School of Anaesthesia, UK
Sections 1.4, 1.14 and 1.17

Gautam Kumar
Specialist Trainee, Anaesthesia
Central London School of Anaesthesia, UK
Section 7.7

Mark Lambert
Specialist Trainee, Anaesthesia
Central London School of Anaesthesia, UK
Sections 6.1–6.6

Christopher Leech
Regional Anaesthesia Fellow
Royal Free London NHS Foundation NHS Trust, UK
Sections 19.1–19.3

Suresh Loganathan
Locum Consultant Anaesthetist
Royal Free London NHS Foundation Trust, UK
Sections 1.5 and 7.4

Jonathan Mathers
Specialist Trainee, Anaesthesia
Central London School of Anaesthesia, UK
Sections 14.1–14.9 and 15.1–15.6

Katherine Mitchell
Consultant Anaesthetist
Royal Free London NHS Foundation Trust, UK
Sections 1.18 and 16.7

Alastair Mulcahy
Consultant Anaesthetist
Barts and The London NHS Trust, UK
Section 11.10

Steve Oakey
Consultant in Anaesthesia and Burns Intensive Care
Broomfield Hospital, Mid Essex Hospital Services NHS Trust, UK
Sections 28.1–28.4

Dilip Patel
Consultant Anaesthetist
Royal Free London NHS Foundation Trust, UK
Sections 19.1–19.4

Tom Pickworth
Consultant Anaesthetist
Royal Brompton and Harefield NHS Trust, UK
Section 16.3

Susanna Price
Consultant Cardiologist and Intensivist
Royal Brompton and Harefield NHS Trust, UK
Sections 1.6–1.8, 1.11, 1.12 and 1.19

Rajkumar Rajendram
Regional Anaesthesia Fellow
Royal Free London NHS Foundation Trust, UK
Sections 19.4 and 23.1–23.6

Manish Raval
Consultant Anaesthetist
Moorfields Eye Hospital NHS Foundation Trust, UK
Sections 27.1–27.6

Jon Read
Consultant Anaesthetist
Royal Free London NHS Foundation Trust, UK
Section 22.4

Danielle Reddi
Specialist Trainee, Anaesthesia
Central London School of Anaesthesia, UK
Sections 26.1–26.4

Jim Roberts
Consultant Anaesthetist
Royal National Throat, Nose and Ear Hospital, London, UK
Sections 11.7–11.9

Alex Sell
Consultant Anaesthetist
Royal National Orthopaedic Hospital NHS Trust, UK
Section 16.5

Steve Shaw
Consultant in ITU and Anaesthesia
Royal Free London NHS Foundation Trust, UK
Section 20.6

Peter Sherren
Specialist Trainee, Anaesthesia
Barts and The London NHS Trust, UK
Section 22.8

Manpreet Singh
Fellow in Cardiothoracic Anaesthesia
The Heart Hospital, London, UK
Sections 15.1–15.6

Imrat Sohanpal
Chronic Pain Fellow and Specialist Trainee in Anaesthesia
Royal Free London NHS Foundation Trust, UK
Section 26.6–26.7

Tony Sousalis
Specialist Trainee, Anaesthesia
Central London School of Anaesthesia, UK
Section 13.6

Mike Spiro
Specialist Trainee, Anaesthesia
Central London School of Anaesthesia, UK
Sections 6.1–6.6

Justin Stebbing
Professor of Cancer Medicine and Consultant Oncologist
Imperial College and Imperial College Healthcare NHS
Trust, UK
Section 13.2

Anita Sugavanam
Specialist Trainee, Anaesthesia
Central London School of Anaesthesia, UK
Sections 11.1–11.4, 11.6, and 13.7

Sonali Thakrar
Specialist Trainee, Anaesthesia
Central London School of Anaesthesia, UK
Section 1.20

Shahana Uddin
Consultant in Critical Care, Anaesthesia and Major Trauma
King's College Hospital NHS Foundation Trust, UK
Sections 1.7 and 1.12

Ali Vazir
Consultant Cardiologist
Royal Brompton and Harefield NHS Trust, UK
Section 1.11

Andre Vercueil
Consultant in ITU and Trauma Anaesthesia
King's College Hospital NHS Foundation Trust, UK
Sections 21.1–21.7

Liesl Wandrag
NIHR Clinical Doctorate Research Fellow
Imperial College Healthcare NHS Trust, UK
Sections 8.1–8.4

Lucy Ward
Consultant in Chronic Pain and Anaesthesia
Royal Free London NHS Foundation Trust, UK
Section 26.10

Hugo Wellesley
Consultant Anaesthetist
Great Ormond Street Hospital for Children NHS Foundation
Trust, UK
Section 25.10

Mary White
Senior Fellow in ITU
Royal Brompton and Harefield NHS Trust, UK
Section 1.19

Abigail Whiteman
Specialist Trainee, Anaesthesia
Central London School of Anaesthesia, UK
Sections 22.3 and 22.6

Jeremy Windsor
Specialist Trainee, Anaesthesia
Central London School of Anaesthesia, UK
Sections 7.5 and 7.6

Marc Wittenberg
Specialist Trainee, Anaesthesia
Central London School of Anaesthesia, UK
Sections 17.1–17.3

Reshma Woograsingh
Specialist Trainee, Anaesthesia
Central London School of Anaesthesia, UK
Section 17.4

Sandi Wylie
Consultant Anaesthetist
Royal Free London NHS Foundation Trust, UK
Sections 11.1–11.6

Jonathan Yen
Specialist Trainee, Anaesthesia and Pain Medicine
Central London School of Anaesthesia, UK
Sections 26.8 and 26.9

Part 1

Applied Basic Science

Chapter 1

Cardiovascular system

1.1 An approach to cardiovascular risk assessment

Perioperative risk

Patients undergoing surgery may suffer complications that result in life-altering morbidity or even mortality. Assessment of perioperative risk involves consideration both of the premorbid state of the patient along with the nature, extent, and urgency of the surgery to be performed.

Risk may be modified by optimization of the patient's underlying medical conditions and appropriate management intra- and postoperatively.

Whilst no surgical intervention is without risk, a thorough knowledge of how to identify and manage those patients identified as 'high risk' may lead to improved outcomes.

Perioperative cardiovascular complications are a major source of mortality and morbidity with an overall incidence of cardiac death in the region of 0.5–1.5%. Tissue injury secondary to surgery triggers a stress response that can detrimentally affect the cardiovascular system. Myocardial oxygen demand may rise and lead to ischaemia, arrhythmia, infarction, and heart failure. In addition, inter-compartmental fluid shifts, haemodynamic stresses, altered coagulation and disruption of regular medications can significantly exacerbate cardiovascular pathology.

Cardiac risk index

The first widely used cardiac risk index was proposed by Goldman et al. in 1977 with the aim of evaluating cardiac risk in non-cardiac surgery. Nine criteria were identified by multivariable analysis that independently predicted increased risk (see Box 1.1).

Box 1.1 Goldman risk criteria

- Preoperative 3rd heart sound and/or raised jugular venous pressure
- Myocardial infarction (MI) in the preceding 6 months
- >5 premature ventricular contractions per minute
- A cardiac rhythm other than sinus rhythm or the presence of premature atrial contractions on preoperative electrocardiogram (ECG)
- Age >70 years
- Intraperitoneal, intrathoracic, or aortic surgery
- An emergency operation
- Significant aortic stenosis
- Poor general medical condition.

From *The New England Journal of Medicine*, Goldman et al., 'Multifactorial Index of Cardiac Risk in Noncardiac Surgical Procedures', 297, 16, Copyright © 1977, Massachusetts Medical Society. Reprinted with permission from Massachusetts Medical Society.

The Goldman criteria were modified in 1986 by Detsky et al. to form the Modified Cardiac Risk Index, and again in 1999 by Lee et al, resulting in the Revised Cardiac Risk Index. In the latter, patients are categorized according to the presence of 0, 1, 2, or ≥3 risk factors (see Box 1.2).

A number of taskforce guidelines have been published by the American College of Cardiology (ACC)/American Heart Association (AHA) and European Society of Cardiology (ESC)/European Society of Anaesthesiology (ESA). These contain a series of consecutive suggestions which create a framework for perioperative cardiovascular evaluation in non-cardiac surgery.

Box 1.2 Revised Cardiac Risk Index criteria

- High-risk surgical procedure
- History of ischaemic heart disease
- History of congestive heart failure
- History of cerebrovascular disease
- Preoperative insulin therapy for diabetes
- Preoperative serum creatinine >177μmol/L.

With kind permission from Springer Science+Business Media: *Journal of General Internal Medicine*, 'Predicting cardiac complications in patients undergoing non-cardiac surgery', 1, 4, 1986, pp. 211–19, AS Detsky et al.

The 2007 ACC/AHA guidelines stratify cardiac conditions into those that require immediate investigation, those that may be associated with increased risk, and those that are not (see Box 1.3). The 2009 ESC/ESA guidelines outline a stepwise approach to evaluating a patient, with the aim of creating an individualized cardiac risk assessment. They make suggestions regarding optimization prior to surgery, and emphasize the lack of evidence to support preoperative coronary revascularization as a risk reduction strategy (see section 1.5 and Box 1.4).

Box 1.3 Guidelines for preoperative cardiac evaluation

Active cardiac conditions requiring further evaluation:
- Unstable coronary syndromes
- Decompensated heart failure
- Significant arrhythmias
- Severe valvular disease.

Clinical risk factors that may impact upon outcome:
- History of ischaemic heart disease
- History of compensated or prior heart failure
- History of cerebrovascular disease
- Diabetes mellitus
- Renal insufficiency.

Factors not proven to increase perioperative risk:
- Advanced age
- Abnormal ECG
- Rhythm other than sinus
- Uncontrolled systemic hypertension.

Reprinted from Journal of American College of Cardiology, 50, 17, Fleisher et al., 'ACC/AHA 2007 Guidelines on Perioperative Cardiovascular Evaluation and Care for Noncardiac Surgery: A Report of the American College of Cardiology/American Heart Association Task Force on Practice Guidelines (Writing Committee to Revise the 2002 Guidelines on Perioperative Cardiovascular Evaluation for Noncardiac Surgery), pp. e159–e242, Copyright 2007, with permission from Elsevier and American College of Cardiology, Foundation of the American Heart Association Inc.

Box 1.4 A stepwise approach to cardiac risk assessment

1. Assess the urgency of the surgical procedure.
2. Does the patient have an unstable cardiac condition (for example, unstable angina or acute heart failure)? If so, assess and treat.
3. Assess the risk of the surgical procedure.
4. Consider the patient's functional capacity.
5. Review (and aim to continue) chronic aspirin therapy.
6. Consider pharmacological interventions ± non-invasive testing in patients found to have reduced functional capacity.
7. Review the results of non-invasive tests to determine whether or not intervention is appropriate (for example, revascularization).

The risk attached to the surgical procedure itself is categorized according to the 30-day incidence of adverse cardiac events (cardiac death or MI). Three categories of surgical risk are identified (Table 1.1).

Table 1.1	Risk of cardiac death or myocardial infarction within 30 days of surgery	
Low risk: <1%	Intermediate risk: 1–5%	High risk: >5%
Breast	Abdominal	Aortic and major vascular surgery
Dental	Carotid	Peripheral vascular surgery
Endocrine	Peripheral arterial angioplasty	
Eye	Endovascular aneurysm repair	
Gynaecology	Head and neck surgery	
Reconstructive	Neurological	
Minor orthopaedic	Major orthopaedic	
Minor urology	Major urology	

Referral for preoperative investigations

An ECG should be performed in all patients who have cardiac risk factors, and should be considered in those without risk factors who are scheduled for intermediate or high-risk surgery. Non-invasive investigations must be specifically aimed at identifying and quantifying underlying left ventricular dysfunction, myocardial ischaemia, and valvular dysfunction. These include the exercise ECG (stress test) and echocardiography (ECHO). The rationale for these tests should be similar to that applied to patients with symptoms of cardiovascular disease in the non-surgical setting. An investigation should be ordered only when the results of the test would lead to a clear change in the perioperative management strategy (see section 1.4). In the case of emergency surgery, investigations are limited by the timeframe in which the operation must be performed.

Patient age

The chronological age of a patient accounts for only a small increase in overall perioperative risk, and in isolation is, therefore, a poor predictor of complications. However, increasing age is associated with accumulating comorbidities, each of which requires careful consideration preoperatively and may contribute to increased risk. The prevalence of cardiovascular disease increases with age along with a decline in respiratory and renal function.

Measures of functional capacity

Functional capacity is the ability to perform physical exercise and can be assessed by questioning or formal testing. Physical fitness correlates with the ability to increase systemic oxygen delivery in order to match the rise in oxygen consumption (VO_2) in the perioperative period that accompanies major surgery.

The Duke Activity Status Index (DASI)

Simple questioning about perceived maximal activity can provide an insight into limitations during daily life. The DASI is a questionnaire that requires the patient to indicate whether he or she can perform specific tasks and assigns scores accordingly. The scores from the DASI are known as a metabolic equivalent of task (MET), where 1 MET (see Box 1.5) is equivalent to basal metabolic rate (a VO_2 of approximately 3.5mL/kg/min).

Box 1.5 Metabolic equivalents of task (METs)	
1 MET:	Eating, washing.
3 METs:	Walking 100m on flat ground.
4 METs:	Walking up one flight of stairs.
10 METs:	Strenuous sporting activities.

The sum of METs from the DASI (maximum is 58.2) can then be used to estimate an individual's peak oxygen uptake:

$$\text{Estimated peak VO}_2 \text{ (mL/kg/min)} = (0.43) \times \text{DASI} + 9.6$$

The DASI has been shown to correlate well with perioperative outcome. The inability to perform exercise at less than 4 METs is associated with an increased incidence of postoperative complications. This form of assessment is, however, liable to bias if the patient's completion of the questionnaire is inaccurate.

The incremental shuttle walk test (ISWT)

During an ISWT, the patient must walk back and forth between two markers placed 10m apart on flat ground. The pace is to the sound of a tone that begins at 30m per minute and increases by 10m per minute each minute after that. The subject must continue walking until exhausted or unable to complete the 10m distance within the time of two tones. The outcome measured is the total distance walked. There is a linear relationship between systemic VO_2 and walking distance and when compared to treadmill testing, peak VO_2 can be accurately predicted from the ISWT distance.

Cardiopulmonary exercise testing (CPET)

CPET can provide detailed information that may allude to underlying cardiopulmonary limitations and disease. It is a non-invasive test with minimal associated risks. It requires the patient to exercise until exhaustion on a bicycle ergometer whilst respiratory gas exchange is measured at the mouth. Oxygen uptake and carbon dioxide production is calculated and along with heart rate, these data can be used to calculate a number of variables that may assist perioperative risk stratification (see section 1.2).

Further reading

Detsky AS, Abrams HB, McLaughlin JR, et al. (1986). Predicting cardiac complications in patients undergoing non-cardiac surgery. Journal of General Internal Med, 1(4):211–19.

Fleisher LA, Beckman JA, Brown KA, et al. (2007). ACC/AHA 2007 guidelines on perioperative cardiovascular evaluation and care for noncardiac surgery. J Am. Coll. Cardiol, 50:159–241.

Goldman, L, Caldera, DL, Nussbaum, SR, et al. (1977). Multifactorial index of cardiac risk in noncardiac surgical procedures. NEJM, 297(16):845–50. doi: 10.1056/NEJM197710202971601.

Lee TH, Marcantonio ER, Mangione CM, et al. (1999). Derivation and prospective validation of a simple index for prediction of cardiac risk of major noncardiac surgery. Circulation, 100:1043–9.

Older P, Hall A, & Hader R. (1999). Cardiopulmonary exercise testing as a screening test for perioperative management of major surgery in the elderly. Chest, 116:355–62.

Task Force for Preoperative Cardiac Risk Assessment and Perioperative Cardiac Management in Non-cardiac Surgery, European Society of Cardiology (ESC), Poldermans D, Bax JJ, et al. (2009). Guidelines for pre-operative cardiac risk assessment and perioperative cardiac management in non-cardiac surgery. European Heart J, 30:2769–2812. doi:10.1093/eurheartj/ehp337.

1.2 Cardiopulmonary exercise testing

A cardiopulmonary exercise test (CPET) provides objective measures of cardiovascular, respiratory, and circulatory physiology that are related to physical fitness, pathophysiology, and perioperative survival. This is in contrast to many alternative assessment modalities, which are only able to summarize resting single organ function. CPET is a dynamic measure of functional capacity and is used widely in the field of sports and exercise medicine.

The physiology of exercise

The primary measure of the CPET is oxygen uptake (VO_2), which is expressed in either mL/min or normalized for the patient's weight as mL/kg/min. Oxygen uptake increases linearly during progressively more strenuous exercise and two points of significance during this increase are the ventilatory threshold (VT), commonly referred to as the anaerobic threshold (AT), and maximal oxygen uptake (VO_2max). The latter is a plateau in VO_2 that is reached at maximal exercise capacity and is a reliable measure of physical fitness. If no plateau is achieved, the maximum VO_2 attained is referred to as VO_2 peak. VO_2max is determined by factors that govern oxygen delivery such as respiratory, cardiovascular, and circulatory function and influenced by gender, age, level of physical fitness, and a degree of genetic inheritability. Consideration of the Fick equation emphasizes the importance of oxygen delivery in determining VO_2 max and highlights the mathematical coupling between VO_2 and oxygen delivery (see Box 1.6).

Box 1.6 The Fick equation for oxygen consumption

$$VO_2 = (HR \times SV) \times (CaO_2 - CvO_2)$$

CaO_2 = arterial oxygen content; CvO_2 = mixed venous oxygen content; HR = heart rate; SV = stroke volume

---

AT is the VO_2 during an increasing exercise load at which metabolism switches to a predominantly anaerobic source of energy rather than an aerobic one. It coincides with the point at which there is a sharp upwards inflection in the serum lactate concentration and production of additional carbon dioxide.

Practical considerations

To perform a CPET requires an exercise stimulus, a means of measuring gas exchange at the nose or mouth, and a system to collate the data. Exercise on an electronically braked bicycle ergometer produces the most repeatable data and is preferable to a treadmill in a clinical setting. For patients with lower limb incapacity it is possible to perform a CPET using a hand-crank system.

Breath-by-breath gas analysis provides the most reliable means of data collection and can be achieved via a tight fitting mask or mouthpiece. The concentration of oxygen and carbon dioxide is measured along with gas flow; computer software then calculates the volume of each gas inspired and expired per minute. Many other respiratory values can also be calculated. Additional physiological measurements are collected during the test, including heart rate, ECG, and non-invasive blood pressure.

The commonest exercise protocol is one of a continuous 'ramped' workload based upon predictions of the patient's VO_2

max. According to age, gender, weight, and level of physical fitness a ramp gradient is selected that will result in a test lasting 10–12min. Perioperative patients commonly require a ramp of 10 to 15 watts per minute.

The CPET has a reported mortality of 2–4 per 100 000 tests and is conducted in the presence of an exercise physiologist and physician. A variety of contraindications to CPET exist (see Box 1.7).

Box 1.7 Contraindications to CPET

Absolute

Acute MI	Aortic dissection
Unstable angina	Uncontrolled asthma
Unstable arrhythmias	Pulmonary oedema
Syncope	Resting SaO_2 ≤85%
Endocarditis or myocarditis	Respiratory failure
Severe aortic stenosis	Other medical disorders affecting performance
Uncontrolled heart failure	Inability to cooperate.
Acute pulmonary embolism	

Relative

Left main stem disease	Hypertrophic cardiomyopathy
Moderate valvular stenosis	
Severe untreated hypertension	Pulmonary hypertension
Arrhythmias	Advanced pregnancy
High-degree AV block	Electrolyte abnormalities.

Patients are asked to pedal on the bicycle ergometer for as long as possible, stopping only when exhausted. A clinician may halt a test if concerned with the patient's condition or data.

Data presentation

Data are traditionally presented in a 'nine-panel plot' that consists of nine graphs of different physiological measurement collected during the CPET (Fig. 1.1). Salient values such as VT, VO_2 max (or peak), the ventilatory equivalents for oxygen (Ve/VO_2) and carbon dioxide (Ve/VCO_2) will be highlighted and accompanied by a description of the nine-panel plot and of the patient's performance during exercise. From this information clinicians should be able to derive an indication of perioperative risk.

Determination of anaerobic threshold

For perioperative patients the most frequently reported measurement from the CPET is AT. Cardiopulmonary disease that limits systemic oxygen delivery will reduce both AT and VO_2 max.

The commonest method of determining AT from the nine-panel plot is by the 'V-slope' method. At a cellular level, anaerobic metabolism generates lactate and hydrogen ions. The latter combine with bicarbonate and lead to increased carbon dioxide production:

$$H^+ + HCO_3^- \rightarrow H_2CO_3 \rightarrow H_2O + CO_2$$

This increase in carbon dioxide production can be detected at the mouth during exercise. After the test, in a plot of VO_2 against VCO_2 there will be a marked change in the slope of the line, and the VO_2 at which this occurs is the AT (Fig. 1.2).

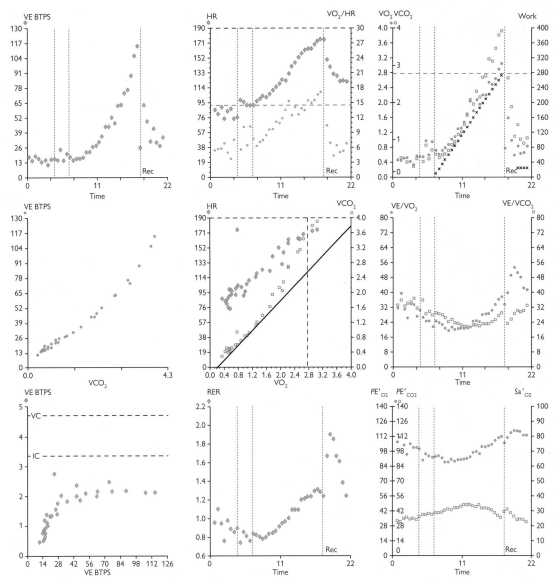

Fig. 1.1 Cardiopulmonary exercise testing: a nine-panel plot. Reproduced from Neil Agnew, 'Preoperative cardiopulmonary exercise testing', *Continuing Education in Anaesthesia, Critical Care, and Pain*, 2010, 10, 2, pp. 33–37, by permission of Oxford University Press and the *British Journal of Anaesthesia*. doi:10.1093/bjaceaccp/mkq001.

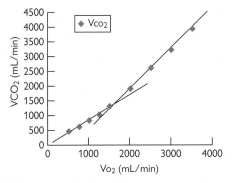

Fig. 1.2 V-slope method for determining ventilator threshold. Reproduced from *Postgraduate Medical Journal*, Albouaini et al., 83, 985, pp. 675–682, copyright 2007, with permission from BMJ Publishing Group Ltd. doi:10.1136/hrt.2007.121558.

It can be estimated by placing a line with a slope of 1 against the VO_2: VCO_2 plot and marking the point of inflection. A number of other changes occur at AT that can be used to verify its presence:

- The respiratory exchange ratio (RER) is the ratio of carbon dioxide output and oxygen uptake (VCO_2/VO_2). It is roughly equivalent to the respiratory quotient (RQ) during strict steady state resting conditions and rises to >1.0 at AT.

- The ventilatory equivalents for oxygen and carbon dioxide are calculated by dividing minute volume (Ve) by the expired volume of the desired gas (Ve/VO_2). This dimensionless value can be considered as a measure of ventilatory efficiency, indicating the magnitude of minute volume required to expire a litre of oxygen (or carbon dioxide). Both Ve/VO_2 and Ve/VCO_2 rise after AT, the latter occurring slightly later than the former.

- End-tidal oxygen rises at AT.

Clinical significance of CPET results

Physicians have used CPET for many years to determine the cause of dyspnoea in patients and to investigate respiratory and cardiovascular disorders. Only recently has CPET gained popularity for the preoperative assessment of high-risk surgical patients.

A low AT is associated with poor outcome postoperatively, and high risk is suggested when the AT is <11mL/kg/min. Knowledge of a patient's AT can facilitate postoperative triage to a specific level of care. In this way, patient outcome may be improved, length of hospital stay reduced, and resources saved.

Studies have confirmed the usefulness of CPET in specific cohorts of patients including those undergoing aortic aneurysm repair, oesophagectomy, and liver transplantation.

The ventilatory equivalent for oxygen (Ve/VO_2) is also a useful indicator of functional capacity. The ability to train patients and improve physical fitness prior to surgery is an interesting prospect as part of preoperative optimization.

Oxygen pulse is a term that describes the oxygen uptake per heartbeat. It is calculated as VO_2/heart rate. Rearrangement of the Fick equation shows that it is equal to SV × ($CaO_2 - CvO_2$) that is, the product of stroke volume and oxygen extraction. Oxygen pulse is depicted on the nine-panel plot and generally increases during exercise. A flattening off of this upwards trajectory is a strong indicator of cardiac limitation and usually a sign of ischaemic heart disease.

Further reading

Albouaini K, Egred M, Alahmar A, *et al*. (2007). Cardiopulmonary exercise testing and its application. *Postgraduate Medical J*, 83(985):675–82. doi:10.1136/hrt.2007.121558.

Gibbons RJ, Balady GJ, Bricker JT, *et al*. (2002). ACC/AHA 2002 guideline update for exercise testing: summary article: a report of the American College of Cardiology/American Heart Association Task Force on Practice Guidelines (Committee to Update the 1997 Exercise Testing Guidelines). *Circulation*, 106:1883–92.

Older P, Smith R, Hall A, et al. (2000). Preoperative cardiopulmonary risk assessment by cardiopulmonary exercise testing. *Crit Care Resusc*, 2(3):198–208.

1.3 Special investigations in the assessment of cardiac disease

The initial approach to assessing cardiac risk (cardiac death or non-fatal MI) in patients undergoing non-cardiac surgery is described in section 1.1. In summary, *three* components contribute to this risk:

- Patient-specific variables
- Exercise capacity
- Surgery-specific risk.

Patients at low risk generally require no further evaluation before surgery.

Patients at high risk (e.g. those with symptoms of unstable coronary disease) frequently undergo coronary angiography.

Patients who are judged to be at intermediate risk on clinical criteria are essentially a heterogeneous group in whom non-invasive testing seeks to identify a subgroup with significant cardiac disease (Fig. 1.3).

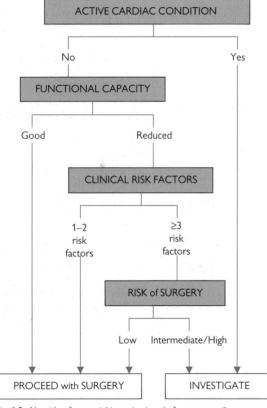

Fig. 1.3 Algorithm for special investigations before non-cardiac surgery.

Non-invasive testing

Non-invasive testing should be seen as more than simply a screening tool for potential revascularization. The aim of non-invasive tests (ECG, ECHO and stress imaging) is to identify patients with myocardial ischaemia or those with valvular or left ventricular (LV) dysfunction. The results may underpin perioperative management decisions such as choice of anaesthetic technique or the type of surgery undertaken. Non-invasive testing generally has a high *negative* predictive value but a low *positive* predictive value in terms of the likelihood of adverse perioperative cardiac events.

Resting ECG

In patients with established ischaemic heart disease (IHD), changes on the 12-lead ECG may be of prognostic significance. Current guidelines suggest an ECG should be performed in patients with one or more risk factors who are undergoing intermediate- or high-risk surgery. The ECG may of course be normal or non-specific even in the presence of active ischaemia or infarction.

Resting echocardiography

Resting ECHO is of only limited value in terms of assessing perioperative risk. This probably relates to a failure to detect even severe underlying ischaemic heart disease. The main indications for preoperative ECHO are as in the non-surgical population:

- To evaluate valve function in patients with a murmur.
- To assess LV function in patients with heart failure or dyspnoea of unknown origin.

Stress testing

Stress tests (exercise ECG, stress ECHO, and stress radionuclide myocardial perfusion imaging) have a high negative predictive value (>90%) for postoperative cardiovascular events—that is, a negative test is associated with a very low incidence of adverse events and predicts a safe procedure. The positive predictive value (see section 10.1) is, however, low (about 20%). By its nature, stress testing primarily detects flow-limiting lesions rather than non-flow-limiting plaques. The latter may often be the source of perioperative MI through plaque rupture. The positive predictive value will be further reduced if a positive result is the impetus for a change in management, for example, revascularization, initiation of drug therapy, or selection of a different surgical procedure.

Current recommendations in respect of preoperative stress testing may be summarized as shown in Box 1.8.

> ### Box 1.8 Indications for preoperative stress testing
>
> - *Recommended* for patients with ≥3 cardiac risk factors undergoing high-risk surgery.
> - *Not recommended* for patients undergoing low-risk surgery.
> - *May be considered* in patients undergoing intermediate-risk surgery or in patients with ≤2 risk factors undergoing high-risk surgery.

A variety of stress testing modalities is available. They can be classified according to:

- Type of stress: exercise, vasodilatation (dipyridamole/adenosine) or dobutamine.
- Measure of induced ischaemia: ECG changes, myocardial perfusion defects (rMPI), or wall motion abnormalities (ECHO).

Exercise ECG

Exercise ECG testing without myocardial imaging has long been used to detect myocardial ischaemia. In respect of assessing perioperative risk, *exercise tolerance* is more important than ECG changes. A patient who is unable to perform moderate exercise and/or reach 85% of maximal heart rate is at higher risk of a postoperative cardiac event—even in the absence of diagnostic ECG changes.

Limitations to exercise stress testing include:

- The presence of other conditions which may prevent many patients from exercising and/or achieving target heart rate, e.g. lung disease, arthritis, peripheral vascular disease.
- The presence of resting ECG abnormalities (e.g. bundle branch block, digoxin therapy, female sex) may prevent detection of ischaemia.

Stress radionuclide myocardial perfusion imaging (rMPI)

The use of dipyridamole-thallium imaging in patients undergoing major non-cardiac surgery has been widely investigated. The negative predictive value is high (98%) but the positive predictive value is low (only 18%). Thus a positive test result is only a weak predictor of a perioperative cardiac event.

The presence of reversible ischaemic defects in >1 segment of the myocardium may be a stronger predictor of an adverse outcome, especially if in the presence of other risk factors (age, diabetes, etc.).

Stress echocardiography

Stress (either exercise-induced or pharmacological) two-dimensional transthoracic echocardiography (TTE) combines information on resting LV function, valvular abnormalities, and on the presence and extent of inducible ischaemia.

It has a number of clinical applications:

- Diagnosis of coronary artery disease (CAD): by showing inducible wall motion abnormalities).
- Assessment of myocardial viability prior to revascularization.
- To identify a 'culprit' lesion in a patient with known coronary artery stenosis.
- Risk stratification of patients with known or suspected cardiac disease (including prior to non-cardiac surgery).

Dobutamine stress echocardiography (DSE) has become increasingly popular, especially for patients unable to perform an exercise-based stress test. Dobutamine increases heart rate and myocardial contractility. In the presence of significant coronary stenosis, regional ischaemia can therefore be expected in response to dobutamine, manifesting as area(s) of reduced contractility. DSE has a good safety profile, but may provoke arrhythmias and/or hypotension in susceptible patients. Minor arrhythmias (e.g. atrial or ventricular premature beats) occur in up to a third of patients. DSE should be avoided in patients with significant hypertension or arrhythmia. The presence of an abdominal aortic aneurysm has previously been cited as a relative contraindication to DSE—but evidence suggests stress testing in this population is safe and that the risk of rupture is very small.

Other non-invasive tests

Stress testing remains the preferred non-invasive approach to the detection of coronary disease. Sometimes, however, an equivocal result will suggest a need for an anatomical assessment of the coronary arteries in order to confirm or refute the clinical suspicion. Cardiac catheterization is expensive and carries a small but significant risk of serious complications. Novel coronary imaging techniques (computed tomography (CT) and magnetic resonance imaging (MRI)) are emerging, with the hope of improvements in both cost and safety.

Computed tomography and magnetic resonance imaging

Coronary artery calcium (CAC) can be detected by CT. The presence of CAC is highly sensitive (but less specific) for the presence of significant coronary artery stenosis. There is, at present, no evidence of benefit in respect of using a CAC score in routine screening of asymptomatic patients, but the technique has been widely marketed in this regard.

Both CT and MRI have recently emerged as potentially exciting non-invasive techniques to actually visualize both native coronary arteries and bypass grafts. The current limitations of coronary CT angiography (CCTA) and coronary MRI (CMRI) are likely to be overcome as the technology improves. MRI is likely to be preferred in younger patients due to concerns about the radiation doses associated with CCTA. There are as yet no data in respect of either technique in the setting of preoperative risk stratification.

Cardiopulmonary exercise testing

This provides a global assessment of exercise capacity, especially in relation to cardiovascular and respiratory function. The underlying physiology of CPET and its potential applications are discussed in section 1.2.

Coronary angiography

Coronary angiography remains the definitive means by which to confirm the presence of CAD. It is, however, an invasive procedure that carries with it the potential for life-threatening complications.

The indications for preoperative coronary angiography are highly limited, and are essentially identical to those that apply in the non-operative setting (see Box 1.9). This reflects the lack of evidence that preoperative coronary revascularization improves outcome (see section 1.5).

Box 1.9 Indications for preoperative coronary angiography
Recommended for:
• Acute ST elevation MI (STEMI)
• Non-STEMI and unstable angina
• Refractory angina unresponsive to medical therapy.
May be considered for:
• Stable patients undergoing high- or intermediate-risk surgery.

Before a preoperative angiogram is performed, it should be established that the patient is a candidate for *preoperative* revascularization—in addition to an acceptance that this may have implications in respect of potential postponement of surgery and/or introduction of antiplatelet therapy. Should an angiogram confirm an indication for revascularization, then a wide discussion (between patient, cardiologist, surgeon, and anaesthetist) should inform the decision as to the most appropriate therapy (see section 1.5).

Further reading

Priebe H-J (2011). Preoperative cardiac management of the patient for non-cardiac surgery: an individualized and evidence-based approach. *Br J Anaesth*, 107:83–96.

1.4 Scoring systems for outcome in anaesthesia, surgery, and critical care

The 'ideal scoring system' to predict individual outcome following anaesthesia or admission to intensive care does not exist. There are, however, many systems that seek to predict likely outcome within a population or group of patients.

The scores variously account for past medical history, physiology, and concurrent illness. Similarly, they may be based on single time points or on repeated evaluation. The predictive value of the scores varies from population to population and indeed should be only applied to those groups of patients in which they have undergone validation. Predicted outcomes include mortality and morbidity.

A classification of scoring systems is difficult. Simple classifications might be based on predicted outcome, method of scoring (e.g. anatomical, physiological, organ system, intervention based) or pathology (trauma, general surgical, neurosurgical, and so on). As classification is non-standard, it is important for the anaesthetist to be able to consider the different range of scores available, their components, and applicable population(s).

Critical care scoring systems

Acute Physiology and Chronic Health Evaluation (APACHE) score

The APACHE score was introduced in 1981. It combined 34 patient variables (on admission to ICU) and a chronic health evaluation to produce a severity score, which correlated with mortality.

APACHE II was published in 1985 and was a simpler version with only 12 variables and altered weighting. The score continued to be a single measure based on admission physiology and correlated well with in-hospital mortality across a number of populations. The score was widely adopted.

APACHE III was introduced in 1991 and was intended to predict individual patient mortality. The score is more complex and the software for calculation was held under copyright. It has not been as widely adopted as APACHE II despite potentially better accuracy.

Simplified Acute Physiology Score (SAPS)

The SAPS was introduced in 1984 as a 14-variable alternative to the physiology component of APACHE. It was superseded by SAPS II in 1993 (and subsequently SAPS III), which expanded the variables to 17 and incorporated regression calculations. It reflects scores calculated within the first 24h of critical care admission and is an alternative to the APACHE score.

Mortality Prediction Model (MPM)

The MPM and its successor MPM II are designed to predict mortality on ICU admission and at 24h. There are also variations on the model that allow prediction at 48h and 72h. The models assess multiple physiological and chronic health parameters and predict mortality following complex logistic regression.

Sequential Organ Failure (SOFA) score

Originally the Sepsis-Related Organ Failure Score, this was subsequently validated in non-sepsis organ dysfunction and is now interchangeably known as the SOFA. The score was developed by a working group of the European Society of Intensive Care Medicine (1996). Six systems are analysed: respiratory, cardiovascular, central nervous, hepatic, renal, and coagulation. This score allows repeated measures over time to assess improvement or deterioration and the rate of such change. Mean and highest SOFA scores have been shown to be useful predictors of outcome comparable with SAPS II.

Multiple Organ Dysfunction Score (MODS)

Similar to SOFA, the MODS examines six organ systems (cardiovascular, renal, respiratory, hepatic, haematological, neurological) and produces a weighted score depending on degrees of dysfunction. The score can be repeated on a daily basis to monitor progression. The score uses a unique variable (pressure-adjusted heart rate, a product of HR and the ratio of central venous pressure (CVP): mean arterial pressure (MAP)) to assess cardiovascular function. It correlates well with mortality, although some evidence suggests that the SOFA cardiovascular component is a better predictor than that of MODS.

Logistic Organ Dysfunction Score (LODS)

The LODS is broadly similar to the MODS and SOFA scores but less widely used. A more complex calculation is involved but claims to take into account both the relative severity among organ systems and the degree of severity within an organ system.

Scoring systems used in perioperative care

American Society of Anesthesiologists Physical Status (ASA-PS)

The ASA-PS has been in use in a form similar to that used today since 1963. It encompasses six categories, 1–6 (originally five), to describe the underlying fitness of patients. The addition of the 'E' suffix allows distinction of emergency operations and the 'P' suffix has been proposed for pregnancy. It is a simple system that is quick and easy to use (Table 1.2). This very simplicity, however, means that there can be significant inter-observer variation in ASA grading.

Table 1.2 The ASA-PS

ASA score	
1	Healthy individual
2	Mild systemic disease
3	Severe systemic disease
4	Severe systemic disease—a constant threat to life
5	Moribund—not expected to survive 24h
6	Brain-stem dead—organ donation

The ASA Physical Status Classification System is reproduced from http://www.asahq.org/Home/For-Members/Clinical-Information/ASA-Physical-Status-Classification-System, with permission from the American Society of Anesthesiologists, copyright 2011.

Physiological and Operative Severity Score for Enumeration of Mortality and Morbidity (POSSUM)

The POSSUM was originally conceived for surgical audit. The system combines 12 physiological and six operative parameters to give an estimated morbidity and mortality. The scoring system tends to overestimate risk in low-risk patients and at the extremes of age. The scores have been adapted since introduction. P-POSSUM uses a different equation to produce more accurate mortality data. V-, Cr-, and O-POSSUM have been introduced for vascular, colorectal, and oesophagogastric surgical groups respectively. The scoring systems have been widely validated, although nevertheless can over- or underestimate risk depending on cohort.

The score is, however, difficult to use for preoperative risk prediction, since the operative data (e.g. peritoneal soiling or blood loss) are at that point unknown.

Postoperative Morbidity Survey (POMS)

The POMS was described in the late 1990s. The nine-point enquiry into different organ systems allows quantification of patient morbidity. Postoperative morbidity of any kind can have significant bearing on outcomes such as length of stay. Although, given its nature, not useful as a predictive score, it can be used to assess therapy and compare units or techniques.

Postoperative Nausea and Vomiting (PONV) scores

A number of scoring systems exist for PONV. The Apfel score assigns 1 point each to certain risk factors: female sex, previous PONV, non-smoker, and postoperative opioid use. The total score allows a prediction of PONV risk.

An alternative is the Koivuranta score that uses a 5-point scale adding motion sickness and surgery length whilst omitting opioid use.

Surgical scoring systems

Numerous scores exist within the various surgical subspecialities. Indeed some (e.g. the POSSUM score) are widely used by both anaesthetists and surgeons.

Trauma scores

Multiple trauma scores exist and are either physiological (Revised Trauma Score), anatomical (Injury Severity Score, Abbreviated Injury Score), or a combination of the two (Trauma Injury Severity Score). They are variably able to predict outcome for multiply injured patients.

Neurosurgery

The Glasgow Coma Scale (GCS) is widely used throughout medicine although originally was (and remains) a tool for assessing conscious level following traumatic brain injury. The scale assesses motor, verbal, and eye opening function with a maximum score of 15 and a minimum of 3 (see Table 6.3). The T suffix can be appended for intubated patients, replacing the verbal component and altering the range to 2T–10T.

Subarachnoid haemorrhage is graded by the World Federation of Neurosurgical Societies (WFNS) on a 5-point scale with mortality for grade V haemorrhage approaching 90%.

Hepatobiliary

The Child–Turcotte–Pugh score (see Table 4.4) was originally conceived to predict operative mortality for patients with liver disease. A 5-point physiological score stratifies patients into one of three categories (A, B, and C). Child's C liver disease has been associated with high mortality. The MELD (Model for End-stage Liver Disease) score is often used to classify patients with liver disease prior to transplantation.

Several scores have been used to assess the severity of acute pancreatitis including Glasgow and Ranson's criteria, although the APACHE score has also been used in patients admitted to the intensive care unit.

Further reading

Barnett S & Moonesinghe SR (2011). Clinical risk scores to guide perioperative management. *Postgrad Med J*, 87(1030):535–41. doi:10.1136/pgmj.2010.107169.

Bouch DC & Thompson JP (2008). Severity scoring systems in the critically ill. *CEACCP*, 8(5):181–5. doi:10.1093/bjaceaccp/mkn033.

13

1.5 Perioperative management of the cardiac patient requiring non-cardiac surgery

Sections 1.1–1.3 dealt with cardiac risk assessment in respect of patients undergoing non-cardiac surgery. This initial approach encompasses an appraisal of clinical predictors of risk (presence of angina, heart failure, diabetes, renal insufficiency, etc.), together, most importantly, with a consideration of the patient's functional status and the perceived risk attached to the proposed surgical procedure.

This section deals with certain important management strategies aimed at reducing perioperative risk. These include:

- Drug therapy: β-blockers, statins, and management of antiplatelet therapy.
- Revascularization: percutaneous coronary intervention (PCI) vs coronary artery bypass grafting (CABG).

Drug therapy

Pre-optimization of a patient's *medical* therapy aims to confer protection through plaque stabilization and reduction of ischaemia.

β-blockers

β-blockers have long been suggested to reduce cardiovascular risk in patients undergoing non-cardiac surgery, although studies have yielded conflicting results.

Mangano et al. (1996) demonstrated an improved outcome 2 years after acute β-blockade (atenolol for 1 week post-operatively) in non-cardiac surgical patients. Other studies produced less convincing results, but it was suggested that atenolol be given preoperatively to all patients with actual coronary disease or those at risk.

A large, multinational randomized study, the POISE (PeriOperative Ischaemia Study Evaluation) trial was set up aiming to clarify the situation. Patients receiving metoprolol had a reduced 30-day incidence both fatal and non-fatal of MI and cardiac arrest, but all-cause mortality was *increased*, with an excess of hypotension, bradycardia, and stroke. The findings therefore ran contrary to the practice of advocating β-blocker therapy in all patients perceived to be at risk.

Potential limitations of the POISE trial include:

- Arguably a high dose of metoprolol (100mg twice a day) was used, and it was unadjusted for heart rate within the inclusion criteria.
- Therapy was initiated only 2–4h before surgery, which may have increased the risk of perioperative hypotension and bradycardia, whilst perhaps not allowing sufficient time for other benefits (e.g. anti-inflammatory effects) to develop.

Nonetheless, the POISE trial cast doubt upon the benefit of widespread prophylactic β-blockade, and suggested that benefit was likely to reside in a smaller percentage of high-risk patients.

A reasonable consensus of the current understanding would be:

- High-risk patients may still derive benefit from perioperative β-blockade: the POISE study showed evidence of cardiac protection.
- In patients scheduled for high-risk (major vascular) surgery who have known CAD, documented myocardial ischaemia or a high Revised Cardiac Risk Index, β-blocker therapy should be initiated perioperatively.

- If β-blocker therapy is initiated, in high-risk patients or for high-risk surgery, this should begin preferably 1 month before surgery, with careful dose titration, and pre- and perioperative monitoring of heart rate (target 60–80 beats per minute) and blood pressure (systolic >100mmHg). HDU admission may be indicated postoperatively. The benefits and risks should be discussed carefully with the patient, in particular, the increased risk of stroke.
- If β-blockers are used, long-acting β-1 cardioselective agents (atenolol or bisoprolol) may be most effective.
- If the risks appear to outweigh benefits (e.g. in patients with a history of previous stroke), initiation of β-blocker therapy may reasonably be withheld, even in high-risk cases.
- In patients already receiving chronic β-blocker therapy, this should be continued.

Statins

Statins (3-hydroxy-3-methylglutaryl coenzyme-A reductase inhibitors) are, of course, widely used clinically to reduce elevated levels of cholesterol and so decrease the risk of atherosclerosis.

They may, however, significantly reduce cardiovascular mortality and morbidity irrespective of an individual's cholesterol status.

In addition to being highly efficacious in lowering LDL (low-density lipoprotein) and cholesterol, and raising HDL (high-density lipoprotein), they also have a variety of so-called *pleiotropic* effects (see Box 1.10).

Box 1.10 Lipid-lowering and pleiotropic effects of statins

Lipid-lowering effects:
- Decreased cholesterol and LDL
- Increased HDL.

Pleiotropic effects:
- Increased endothelial production of NO synthetase
- Decreased endothelin-1 production
- Improved thrombogenic profile
- Decreased inflammation and C-reactive protein (CRP) levels
- Plaque stabilization
- Reduced atherosclerosis.

There is growing evidence to support the use of statins perioperatively, with improvements in both short- and long-term outcomes after cardiac and non-cardiac surgery.

Several randomized controlled trials (RCTs) and observational studies have demonstrated improved outcome in the perioperative period, probably related to the pleiotropic effects of statins, including plaque stabilization and reduced thrombogenesis.

In the DECREASE III trial, for example, elective vascular surgical patients were randomized to receive fluvastatin 80mg once a day or placebo for 30 days pre- and post-op. The incidence of detectable ischaemia (troponin rises or ECG changes) and of cardiovascular mortality in the treatment group was roughly halved.

The current evidence would suggest that statin therapy should be initiated in all high-risk patients who are not already receiving them, and that chronic therapy should, wherever possible, not be discontinued in the perioperative period.

Management of antiplatelet therapy during the perioperative period

The management of antiplatelet therapy in patients requiring non-cardiac surgery is an important and increasing clinical problem, most especially in patients who have undergone previous PCI. About 5–10% of patients with coronary stents undergo non-cardiac surgery within a year of stent implantation. The essential factors to consider are:

- Risk of stent thrombosis or acute coronary syndrome if antiplatelet therapy is discontinued.
- Risk of bleeding if therapy is continued.

Coronary artery *angioplasty* was first reported in 1977. *Bare metal stents* were introduced a decade later in response to high restenosis rates after angioplasty alone. However, the incidence of restenosis following intimal hyperplasia remains up to 30%.

Stent insertion causes damage to the endothelial surface, and the result of interactions between stent, blood, and the vessel wall is neointimal hyperplasia and increased thrombogenicity.

In 2003, *drug-eluting stents* (typically releasing sirolimus or paclitaxel) emerged as a solution to restenosis, although a 5–10% risk of stent thrombosis remains.

Three classes of antiplatelet drugs (see section 1.20) are available to prevent stent thrombosis:

- Aspirin
- Thienopyridines (clopidogrel and prasugrel)
- GP IIb/IIIa inhibitors (tirofiban and abciximab).

Typically, aspirin and clopidogrel are used in combination ('dual anti-platelet therapy') following stent implantation to reduce platelet activation.

Stent thrombosis is a serious complication, carrying a 20% mortality. Premature discontinuation of dual antiplatelet therapy is the most powerful independent predictor of stent thrombosis.

The greatest risk to the patient undergoing non-cardiac surgery with a stent *in situ* is from interruption of dual anti-platelet therapy, particularly if this occurs during the first 12 months following insertion (Box 1.11; see also section 1.20).

> **Box 1.11 Summary of guideline recommendations for patients with stents undergoing non-cardiac surgery**
>
> - Defer elective surgery for 6 weeks following bare metal stent insertion and 6–12 months following drug-eluting stent insertion.
> - If surgery cannot be deferred:
>   - Continue dual antiplatelet therapy perioperatively where possible.
>   - If not, continue aspirin and stop clopidogrel 5–7 days preoperatively.
>   - Restart clopidogrel as soon as possible postoperatively.

Premature discontinuation of antiplatelet therapy for minor procedures is rarely justified. Most surgical procedures can in fact be safely performed in the presence of dual platelet therapy, or at least with aspirin alone.

The role of 'bridging therapy' in high-risk individuals who stop dual antiplatelet therapy remains unclear. Unfortunately, heparins have minimal antiplatelet effect, rendering them theoretically unsuitable as bridging therapy. Tirofiban has a short half-life (2h), and may be a more attractive agent. Bleeding time returns to normal 4h after cessation of a tirofiban infusion.

Revascularization

In patients with stable coronary disease, the indications for revascularization include left main stem or severe triple-vessel disease.

Most patients with stable coronary disease who are scheduled for non-cardiac surgery do not benefit from prophylactic revascularization. In addition, any reduction in risk from revascularization must be balanced against the risks of the revascularization procedure itself, coupled with the risks of interrupting clopidogrel therapy in patients with recently inserted stents.

The Coronary Artery Revascularization Prophylaxis (CARP) trial compared preoperative revascularization (PCI or CABG) with medical therapy in patients with stable coronary disease scheduled for major vascular surgery. No significant differences in outcome were identified.

The decision to revascularize is usually based on the results of non-invasive testing, the indications for which are discussed in section 1.3. Angiography should be performed in patients with high-risk features on non-invasive testing (e.g. a reversible large anterior wall defect), and in patients with high-risk unstable angina.

CABG should be undertaken in patients with established indications for the procedure, typically significant left main stem disease, or triple vessel disease with impaired LV function.

If the disease is amenable to PCI, then consideration should be given to bare metal stent insertion, deferring surgery for 4–6 weeks if possible following the procedure.

Further reading

Barash P & Akhtar S (2010). Coronary stents: factors contributing to perioperative major adverse cardiovascular events. *Br J Anaesth*, 105(Suppl 1,):i3–15. doi:10.1093/bja/aeq318.

Chan YC, Cheng SW, & Irwin MG (2008). Perioperative use of statins in noncardiac surgery. *Vasc Health Risk Manage*, 4(1):75–81.

Devereaux PJ, Yang H, Yusuf S, et al. (2008). Effects of extended-release metoprolol succinate in patients undergoing non-cardiac surgery (POISE trial): a randomised controlled trial. *Lancet*, 371(9627):1839–47. doi:10.1016/S0140.

Dweck MR & Cruden NL (2012). Noncardiac surgery in patients with coronary artery stents. *Arch Intern Med*, 172(14):1054–5. doi:10.1001/archinternmed.2012.3025.

Mangano DT, Layug EL, Wallace A, et al. (1996). Effect of atenolol on mortality and cardiovascular morbidity after noncardiac surgery. *NEJM*, 335(23):1713–21.

Sear JW, Giles JW, Howard-Alpe G, et al. (2007). Perioperative beta-blockade, 2008: What does POISE tell us, and was our earlier caution justified? *Br J Anaesth*, 101(2):135–8.

1.6 Dynamic pressure measurements

Pressure monitoring is a core component of anaesthesia practice. Common methods of measuring dynamic pressure changes in theatre or in the critical care unit include *direct* techniques (cannulation of systemic and/or pulmonary arteries and central veins), but also *indirect* techniques including echocardiography (see section 1.8).

Physical principles: pressure versus flow

Vascular cannulation allows *pressure* measurement, whilst other measures of cardiac function, such as cardiac output and oxygen delivery, reflect *flow*. The relationship between pressure and flow is described using familiar equations (see Box 1.12) according to whether the flow is assumed to be laminar or non-laminar.

Box 1.12 Pressure: flow relationships

Laminar flow (the Hagen–Poiseuille equation):

$$\text{Flow} = \frac{\text{Pressure gradient} \times \text{radius}^4 \times \text{pi}}{\text{Tube length} \times \text{viscosity} \times 8}$$

Non-laminar/turbulent flow:

$$\text{Flow} \propto \frac{\text{Radius}^2 \times \sqrt{\text{pressure gradient}}}{\text{Length} \times \text{density}}$$

At the organ level, a pressure gradient is required to maintain flow. If the organ is contained in a non-distensible structure, a rise in pressure within the organ may lead to parenchymal injury with reduction in flow. This is seen in a variety of circulations including cerebral (raised intracranial pressure), cardiac and coronary (tamponade), hepatic (capsular swelling), and pulmonary (hyperinflation).

Arterial lines

There are numerous indications for inserting an arterial line, both for haemodynamic monitoring, and to facilitate blood sampling (see Box 1.13).

The anatomical site is chosen according to a variety of factors including:

- Anticipated ease of cannulation
- Risk of distal ischaemia (perceived higher risk with proximal insertion site)
- Patient positioning and intraoperative access
- Risk of catheter-related sepsis
- Concurrent monitoring requirements.

Box 1.13 Indications for arterial line insertion

Continuous monitoring
Blood pressure:
- Cardiovascular instability (current or anticipated)
- Non-invasive technique impractical (obesity, burns, etc.) or unreliable (e.g. atrial fibrillation).

Cardiac output:
- Pulse contour analysis (see section 1.7).

Sampling
- Anticipated bleeding (e.g. vascular, cardiac, liver surgery)
- Poor gas exchange
- Anticipated changes in coagulation (e.g. cardiac, liver surgery)
- Repeated sampling required (e.g. diabetic ketoacidosis).

Interpretation of the arterial waveform

Pressure and flow within the proximal aorta reflect the interaction between the heart and the arterial tree. When LV pressure exceeds aortic pressure, blood flows into the ascending aorta. The driving force behind this pressure difference depends on LV contractility, size and shape, and on the heart rate. Assuming no valvular obstruction, opposition to flow is due to *vascular impedance*, which has three components:

- Resistance: related to blood viscosity and vascular geometry.
- Inertia: a function of the mass of blood to be accelerated.
- Compliance: representing the distensibility of the vasculature.

During LV systole, the arterial pressure rises rapidly since blood is being pumped into the arterial tree faster than it can be redistributed. As the ventricle begins to relax, so the pressure falls as aortic blood flow declines. When aortic pressure exceeds LV pressure, the aortic valve closes, generating a small pressure wave—the *incisura* or dicrotic notch, on the arterial waveform (Fig. 1.4). Thereafter, arterial pressure continues to fall towards diastolic pressure before the next systole.

The shape of the aortic pulse wave changes as it is transmitted peripherally: pulse pressure and systolic pressure increase, and the initial upstroke (the anacrotic limb) rises more steeply. The dicrotic notch migrates from a sharp, early position in the waveform to a later, smoother oscillation. A variety of physiological and pathological factors affect the shape of the arterial waveform (see Box 1.14).

Box 1.14 Some factors affecting arterial waveform morphology

Physiological
- *Ageing*: higher systolic pressure and increased pulse wave velocity; loss of diastolic wave.
- *Exercise*: increased pulse pressure (proportional to stroke volume).

Pathological
- *Arteriosclerosis*: increased systolic pressure + pulse pressure.
- *Aortic stenosis*: 'anacrotic' pulse with slow rise, late peak, low pulse pressure.
- *Aortic regurgitation*: 'collapsing' pulse—rapid upstroke, rapid decline, wide pulse pressure.

Central venous cannulation

There are many indications for central venous catheterization:

- Haemodynamic monitoring (CVP, SvO_2, etc.)
- Drug and fluid administration (total parenteral nutrition (TPN), vasopressors, cytotoxic agents, etc.)
- As a route for other procedures (pulmonary artery (PA) catheter, cardiac pacing, liver biopsy, etc.)
- Renal replacement therapy or plasmapheresis
- Poor peripheral venous access.

Interpretation of CVP waveform

The normal CVP waveform is shown in Fig. 1.5.

A wave: atrial contraction

The a wave is pre-systolic. It is caused by right atrial contraction and therefore it is absent in atrial fibrillation. Large a waves occur

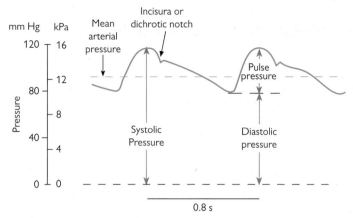

Fig. 1.4 The normal arterial waveform. Reproduced from Pocock and Richards, *Human Physiology: The Basis of Medicine*, third edition, 2006, Figure 15.24, page 285, with permission from Oxford University Press.

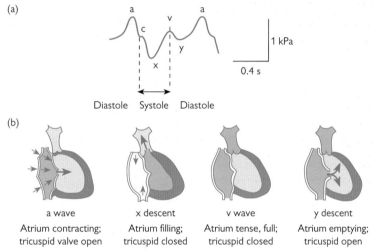

Fig. 1.5 The normal CVP waveform. Reproduced from Pocock and Richards, *Human Physiology: The Basis of Medicine*, third edition, 2006, Figure 15.15, page 275, with permission from Oxford University Press.

when the right atrium is contracting against increased resistance. This happens in three situations:

• Tricuspid stenosis

• Tricuspid valve normal but closed:
  • Regularly: junctional rhythms
  • Irregularly: AV dissociation:
    — Ventricular tachycardia (VT)
    — 3rd-degree heart block

• Increased resistance to right ventricular (RV) filling:
  • Pulmonary hypertension
  • Pulmonary stenosis.

C wave
Unclear origin. Possibly due to:

• Closure of the tricuspid valve

• Bulging of the tricuspid valve into the right atrium during RV isovolumetric contraction

• Transmitted pulsations from the carotid artery.

X descent: atrial relaxation
Occurs during ventricular systole. The CVP decreases because of both atrial relaxation and a downward displacement of the tricuspid valve.

The x descent is larger when the atrium is compressed as in constrictive pericarditis or cardiac tamponade. The x descent is smaller when the right ventricle is dilated, or there is tricuspid regurgitation.

V wave: venous filling of the atria
Occurs in late systole and is due to the increasing volume of blood in the right atrium against a closed tricuspid valve. Tricuspid regurgitation causes the v wave to become more prominent and may obliterate the x descent.

Y descent: yawning open of the tricuspid valve
Occurs when the tricuspid valve opens and the ventricle fills, reducing pressure in the atria. Several variations of the y wave have been characterized:

• Rapid, deep y descent: tricuspid regurgitation

• Rapid, short y descent: constrictive pericarditis, right sided diastolic failure (restrictive RV disease)

• Slow y descent (obstruction to RV filling): tricuspid stenosis, right atrial myxoma.

Complications of central venous cannulation
Many complications have been associated with central line insertion, occurring both at the time of the procedure, and subsequently (Table 1.3).

Table 1.3 Complications of central venous cannulation	
Immediate	Late
Bleeding	Infection
Pneumothorax	Thromboembolism
Arterial puncture	Catheter migration (e.g. right atrial perforation
Dysrhythmia	causing pericardial tamponade)
Air embolism	
Thoracic duct injury	

Particular emphasis has been placed recently on *infectious* complications, since CVCs constitute the largest single source of bloodstream infection in hospitalized patients.

Catheter-related bloodstream infections (CRBSIs) are attributable to four elements: skin colonization, intraluminal or hub contamination, secondary seeding from a current bloodstream infection, and contamination of the infusate (rare). The following reduce the risk of developing a CRBSI:

- Subclavian rather than jugular or femoral approach
- Absence of septic focus elsewhere
- Inserted with maximal barrier precautions
- Totally implantable < tunnelled < non-tunnelled
- Silver-impregnated collagen cuff, or heparin-bonded catheters
- Single-lumen catheters
- Dressings containing sterile gauze, or transparent occlusive dressings
- Catheter site care by specialist teams
- Peripherally inserted central catheters (PICCs).

Interpretation of CVP data

The CVP is often used to assess preload and fluid responsiveness. Volume expansion is considered first-line therapy in haemodynamically unstable patients. However, CVP correlates poorly with circulating blood volume, and the correlation between a change in CVP and a change in stroke volume or cardiac index is poor.

Pulmonary artery catheterization

Flow-directed pulmonary artery catheters (PACs) were developed in the 1970s and initially used to guide fluid therapy following acute MI. They continue to be used for haemodynamic monitoring, but not without controversy (see section 1.7). A variety of data may be obtained from the PAC, either directly or indirectly (see Box 1.15).

Box 1.15 Data obtained from the PAC

Direct
- *Pressure monitoring*: PAC gives direct measurements of central venous, right-sided intracardiac, pulmonary arterial and pulmonary capillary wedge pressures.
- *Mixed venous oxygen saturations*: can be measured directly from the catheter tip either continuously or intermittently.

Indirect
- *Cardiac output*: using thermodilution, PACs can be used to estimated cardiac output using the Stewart–Hamilton equation.
- *Vascular resistance*: pulmonary and systemic vascular resistance can be calculated by combining pressure and flow (cardiac output) data.

Interpretation of the PAC waveform

The pressure trace obtained from a PAC undergoes characteristic changes from chamber to chamber (Fig. 1.6). It is therefore important to have pressure transduction displayed (with an appropriate scale) during insertion and subsequent manipulations.

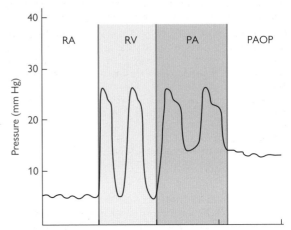

Fig. 1.6 Pressure waveforms recorded during PAC insertion. Reproduced from Catherine Spoors and Kevin Kiff, *Training in Anaesthesia*, 2010, Figure 10.41, Page 285, with permission from Oxford University Press.

Zeroing and referencing

Two separate processes are required when setting up a transduction system for a PAC:

- Zeroing: the process by which the transduction system is exposed ('opened') to air establishing the atmospheric reference pressure (taken as 'zero').
- Referencing: the process by which the air–fluid interface of the transducer is placed at a set level to negate the effects of the weight of the catheter tubing and fluid column. This point (the 'phlebostatic level') is usually taken as the intersection between a coronal plane passing midway between the anterior and posterior surfaces of the chest and a transverse plane lying at the junction of the 4th intercostal space and the sternal margin.

Dynamic response assessment

After placement, the dynamic response of the system to physiological pressure swings should be tested. Response depends on the resonant frequency of the system and damping. Briefly opening and closing the valve in the continuous flush device, producing a square wave followed by a gradual return to baseline, can assess both of these factors. Underdamping exists if there is excessive oscillation before returning to baseline; overdamping exists if there are no oscillations.

- *Underdamping*: caused by short tubing, or resonance within the system due to the natural frequency of the system being too near the oscillatory frequencies of the arterial pressure wave.
- *Overdamping*: most commonly due to air bubbles within the tubing but also from three-way taps, clots, vasospasm, narrow/long/compliant tubing or from kinks in the cannula or tubing.

Interpretation of pressure waveforms

PACs typically only display the *right ventricular trace* during insertion, but some recent devices allow continuous display of RV systolic and diastolic pressures. Normal RV pressures vary from 15–25mmHg systolic and 3–12mmHg diastolic.

- Raised RV systolic pressure: is seen in pulmonary hypertension, pulmonary embolism or left-sided heart failure. In pulmonary stenosis, RV pressure is raised, with a steep fall when the catheter enters the pulmonary artery.
- Raised RV diastolic pressure: is seen in cardiomyopathy, RV ischaemia or infarction, pericardial tamponade or constriction, or in RV failure secondary to pulmonary hypertension.

The *pulmonary artery pressure (PAP) waveform* is similar to the systemic arterial pressure tracing, but at lower pressures. The migration of the PAC into the PA from the RV is evident on the waveform when the diastolic pressure reading increases to 8–15mmHg.

Raised PAP may be seen with normal or high PVR though in practice there is a large degree of overlap between these two groups:

- Raised PAP with high PVR: pulmonary embolism, pulmonary arterial hypertension, hypoxic pulmonary vasoconstriction.
- Raised PAP with normal PVR: mitral valve disease, left-to-right shunts.

The *pulmonary capillary wedge pressure (or pulmonary artery occlusion pressure, PAOP) waveform* is similar to the CVP trace, and described by the same nomenclature (although the c wave, here reflecting *mitral* valve closure, is often not seen). The normal PAOP is between 6mmHg and 15mmHg. Similarities between PAOP and CVP traces extend to the abnormalities seen within them:

- Raised a wave: increased resistance to LV filling, regardless of cause: mitral stenosis, LV systolic or diastolic dysfunction, volume overload, decreased LV compliance (e.g. due to myocardial ischaemia or infarction).
- Raised v wave: occurs when systole results in retrograde flow, e.g. in mitral regurgitation or VSD complicating MI.

Timing of PAC pressure readings

Since spontaneous and positive pressure breathing produce opposite effects on pleural and alveolar pressure, and these pressures influence PAOP, all PAOP readings should be recorded at end-expiration, when intrathoracic pressure is equal to atmospheric pressure.

Potential errors in PAOP interpretation as a surrogate for preload

For pulmonary artery wedge pressure to accurately reflect LV preload, a number of measures must be equivalent. Preload is represented by LV end diastolic volume, measured by assessing LV end diastolic pressure, which in turn is represented by left atrial pressure. Assuming the tip of the PAC lies in West's zone 3 of the lung (where the arterial and venous pressures both exceed the alveolar pressure throughout the cardiac cycle), a continuous column of blood is created between the tip of the catheter and the left atrium.

However if any of these assumptions does not hold, PAOP may not represent LV preload accurately. Readings should be interpreted with caution in a variety of situations: LV diastolic failure, mitral valve disease, raised intrathoracic pressure (e.g. positive end expiratory pressure (PEEP)) or raised pulmonary vascular resistance.

Complications related to PACs

These include all the complications of central venous cannulation together with other procedure-specific risks (see Box 1.16).

Box 1.16 Complications of PA catheterization

- All the complications of central venous cannulation
- Dysrhythmias during insertion (one series reports sustained VT in 3% of cases)
- Knotting of the catheter
- Balloon rupture
- Pulmonary infarction or haemorrhage
- Damage to valves or myocardium
- Mistaken positioning, measurement, or interpretation, and the consequences of decisions thus taken.

1.7 Cardiac output measurement

Cardiac output (CO) monitoring is a routine component of management in respect of critically ill patients in the intensive care unit, and, increasingly, in other areas, including the operating theatre.

Its use rests on the premise that inadequate CO results in organ dysfunction and/or failure, and that maintaining organ perfusion will result in improved patient outcome.

The ideal monitor (see Box 1.17) remains elusive, and there are few high-quality data to support the use of any one existing technique over another.

Box 1.17 Properties of the ideal cardiac output monitor

- Non-invasive or minimally invasive
- Widely applicable in all patient groups (awake/sedated/anaesthetized)
- Real-time beat-to-beat results
- Accurate, precise, and validated
- Short learning curve for implementation and analysis
- Operator independent
- Cost effective
- Safe—with minimal complications.

Bedside measurements and biochemical markers

Assessment of cardiac output using *clinical indicators* (e.g. peripheral skin temperature or neurological status) or *commonly measured parameters* (heart rate, arterial blood pressure, CVP, and urine output) is subject to many confounding factors, including pre-existing cardiovascular disease, intercurrent interventions (e.g. therapeutic cooling), and the effects of intercurrent drug therapy, and correlates poorly with cardiac output.

Biochemical markers such as lactate and acid–base status add to the clinical picture and the trends in these measurements can certainly be used to monitor efficacy of therapy. However, absolute values do not correlate well with CO, and abnormalities tend to be a late feature of inadequate CO.

The pulmonary artery catheter (PAC)

In respect of 'bedside' techniques, the PAC remains the 'gold standard' against which other modalities are validated.

Fick first measured CO in 1870, using the arterio-venous oxygen difference (via mixed venous oxygen saturation sampling) and oxygen consumption (via spirometry). Stewart then adapted the technique to use indicator (indocyanine green) dilution in 1897 followed half a century later by Felger's introduction of thermodilution using boluses of cold fluid.

The PAC was introduced in the 1970s bringing CO measurement to the bedside. To measure CO, the area under the indicator dilution curve (change in concentration of dye as sampled from the PAC or temperature measured by a thermistor at the catheter tip, plotted semi logarithmically against time) is calculated using the Stewart–Hamilton equation. Important assumptions include:

- Complete mixing of blood and indicator (dye or cold fluid) with no loss
- Blood flow remains constant

Errors are thus inevitable in the presence of cardiac shunts, arrhythmias, regurgitant valvular disease, and conditions where there is a marked variation in body temperature (bypass, therapeutic hypothermia) or due to technical difficulties (misplacement or intra/interoperator variation in measurement technique).

By definition, dilutional techniques are intermittent in nature and studies need to be repeated when physiological conditions change. Technological developments have permitted continuous CO monitoring (CCOM) by incorporating specialist thermistors into the PAC to assess either random temperature changes or the amount of energy required to maintain a set temperature. These systems take an average of several readings, and are not, therefore, real time.

The PAC is considered most invasive compared with other CO monitors, as it requires a catheter to be passed via the right atrium and ventricle to reside in a pulmonary artery, and carries a risk of important complications, including arrhythmias and pulmonary haemorrhage. Studies in the 1990s suggesting worse outcomes when using PACs in the critically ill were probably victims of selection bias (PACs were used in the sickest patients). A subsequent multicentre (PAC-Man) study re-evaluated use of the PAC against either no CO monitoring (CVP and clinical evaluation only) or other (non-specified) forms of CO monitoring and found no significant difference in outcome, good or bad, between the three groups.

The PAC remains useful in certain groups (particularly cardiac patients) since, in addition to basic CO parameters, it also provides PA pressures, right- and left-sided filling pressures (PAOP), *and* the potential to measure mixed central venous oxygen saturations.

Transpulmonary dilutional techniques

Invasive monitoring of arterial blood pressure and CVP is a basic standard of care for critically ill patients. New technologies have adapted these to estimate CO using transpulmonary dilutional techniques (TPDTs). The PiCCO® and the LiDCO® are those most widely studied and applied in practice.

TPDT effectively measures the change in concentration of an indicator between the venous and arterial blood—on either side of the pulmonary circulation. Again, it relies on complete mixing, and no loss of indicator, but has been validated in many patient populations when used to monitor physiological trends as a guide to therapy.

Temporal analysis of the transpulmonary dilution curve allows additional variables to be calculated from TPDT:

- *Extravascular lung water (EVLW)*: can be used to differentiate between cardiac and non-cardiac pulmonary oedema, and has been shown to be a predictor of mortality in critically ill patients with acute lung injury
- *Global end-diastolic volume (GEDV)*: represents a *volume-based* assessment of preload that correlates well with stroke volume (SV). When compared to static pressure-based assessments of preload (CVP, PAOP) volume-based measurement has been shown to more reliably predict fluid responsiveness

Pulse contour analysis

Calibrated monitors
Both the PiCCO® and the LiDCO®, in addition to supporting the intermittent transpulmonary thermodilution technique (which is

used to calibrate the system), provide continuous computational analysis of the arterial pulse contour from an indwelling arterial line (see Box 1.18). Since the arterial waveform is dependent on the interaction between SV and systemic vascular resistance, calculated results are affected by changes in resistance, compliance, and impedance at the point of signal detection. For accuracy a good trace is mandatory.

Additional information obtained by pulse wave analysis includes derived 'dynamic' indices such as *stroke volume variation* (SVV), and *pulse pressure variation* (PPV). These indices are not surrogates for preload but can provide an indication that a fluid challenge may be effective in increasing CO. They are only validated in patients who are ventilated, with stable intrathoracic pressures and a constant tidal volume >8mL/kg. They are unreliable in spontaneously breathing patients, or where there is marked ventilator dyssynchrony.

Box 1.18 Comparison of PiCCO® and LiDCO® systems

PiCCO®
- Requires arterial cannula with thermistor tip (brachial or femoral) + central venous catheter.
- Measures area under systolic waveform (from ventricular ejection to dicrotic notch)—averaged over 30sec.
- 8-hourly calibration with cold fluid bolus (TPDT).

LiDCO®
- External sensor attached to conventional arterial line
- Uses harmonic waveform analysis (Fourier transformation).
- Calibrated by TPDT (lithium bolus)—inaccurate in the presence of lithium therapy or muscle relaxants.

Sources of error/limitations (both systems)
- Arrhythmias.
- Poor arterial trace.
- Requires recalibration when changing SVR.
- Use of intra-aortic balloon pump (IABP) or recirculation techniques.

Uncalibrated monitors

Less invasive systems incorporating alternative algorithms for pulse waveform analysis are available. Avoiding the need for intermittent calibration means there is no requirement for central venous access. Lack of calibration would suggest a potential for inaccuracy, but when used to follow trends in response to interventions, studies have shown these systems to be useful, especially in the perioperative setting. As with the calibrated systems, they depend on a high-quality arterial trace and a stable cardiac rhythm.

Examples include the FloTrac® and PRAM® (Pressure Recording Analytical Method) systems.

The oesophageal Doppler

The physical principles behind ultrasound and the Doppler effect are discussed in section 1.8.

Continuous wave Doppler gives a reliable measure of blood flow velocity, which is utilized to calculate stroke volume and hence cardiac output. Inaccurate positioning of the probe may affect results, and certain important assumptions are made during the calculations (see Box 1.19).

The oesophageal Doppler incorporates this technology within a thin semi-rigid tube, inserted either orally or nasally to measure blood flow in the descending thoracic aorta.

The probes are generally only tolerated in anaesthetized or sedated patients, and there is a steep learning curve for optimal use.

Box 1.19 Assumptions for calculations utilizing Doppler measurements

- Constant aortic blood flow: measured as area under velocity: time graph.
- Angle between Doppler beam and blood flow is within 30° of axial flow.
- Aortic radius (r) measurement:
  - Aorta assumed to be a true cylinder (r calculated from estimated cross-sectional area = πr^2).
  - Since r is squared, a small error in measurement will overestimate CO.
  - Derived either from normogram according to height, weight, age, and sex (Cardio Q®) or from direct M-mode measurement (HemoSonic®).
- Fixed ratio of blood supply upper to lower body (assumed 30% cephalic): in reality, this varies with age, pathology, intraoperative manipulations.

In addition to stroke volume and cardiac output, the oesophageal Doppler monitor (ODM) provides additional variables according to the prevailing haemodynamics (see Box 1.20).

Box 1.20 Additional variables from oesophageal Doppler monitoring

FTc (corrected flow time)
- Measured from beginning of upstroke until return to baseline (corrected to HR of 60 beats/min).
- Marker of fluid responsiveness.
- FTc is inversely proportional to SVR—hence FTc low in situations when SVR high (e.g. heart failure, vasopressor therapy) but fluid therapy would be inappropriate.

PV (peak velocity)
- Peak blood flow velocity during systole (cm/sec).
- Marker of contractility.
- Falls linearly with age.
- Affected primarily by LV contractility (low in heart failure/β-blocker therapy; high in inotropic states).

MA (mean acceleration)
- Measured from start of systole to peak velocity.
- Predominantly a marker of contractility.
- Affected by contractility > afterload > preload.

The ODM has been validated in various populations and is now recommended by NICE for perioperative care (see section 4.10).

Echocardiography

There is a wide body of literature supporting the use of TTE and TOE as a monitor of cardiac output, and TOE has good correlation with CO values obtained from PAC data.

The technique is described in more detail in section 1.8.

Thoracic bioimpedance and bioreactance

The techniques of thoracic electrical bioimpedance (TEBI) and bioreactance (TEBR) both rely on the assumption that the thoracic cavity is a cylinder perfused with fluid (blood). The fluid causes a resistance to a current passed between two fixed electrodes on the body wall, which changes according to the amount of fluid within.

Compared to bioimpedance, which measures changes in *amplitude*, bioreactance uses changes in *amplitude* and *frequency* which, analogous to FM versus AM radio waves, is more reliable, has better signal fidelity, better noise filtering capacity and is not affected by the distance between electrodes. Since phase shifts can only occur with *pulsatile* flow bioreactance is not affected by changes in other thoracic cavity fluids (chest wall oedema, effusions, pulmonary oedema, pulmonary and venous circulations). Early studies of bioreactance monitors in clinical practice are encouraging, and further work is ongoing.

Summary

All of the techniques used to measure cardiac output (and derived indices) have specific limitations (see Table 1.4).

Which monitor to use depends upon the patient population, clinical scenario, available equipment, and institutional familiarity. All forms of monitoring are liable to error due to *human* as well as technical factors (see Box 1.21).

Table 1.4 Summary of characteristics of common forms of cardiac output monitoring

	Methods	Examples (indicator)	Invasiveness	Equipment	Continuous or Intermittent	Measured variables	Derived variables	Specific disadvantages	Limitations and errors
Dilution	Thermo dilution	PAFC	++++	CV, PAFC	Int	Temp, CVP, PAOP/PAP/ ScvO$_2$ CO		Invasive line in to RA	Incorrect position, respiratory swing –West's zones
							SV, SVR(I), PVR(I), LVSWI	Complications of centralline insertion	Calculations using non simultaneous data
								Lack of training/ familiarity	Intra/extra-cardiac shunts, arrhythmias
	Transpul-monary indicator dilution	PiCCO (thermal)	+++	CV, thermis-tor tipped FA/BA	Both	Temp, CVP, HR, ABP, CO	GEDV, EVLW, PPV	Specific line	Temperature shifts Rapid changes in vasculomotor tone Arrhythmias
		LiDCO (lithium)	+++	CV or PV, AL			TBV	Muscle relaxants	
								Lithium therapy	
		CO status (ultrasound)	+++	US				Primarily paediatric validation	
		VolumeView (thermal)	+++	CV, specific FA				Specific line	
Pulse analysis	Arterial pulse pressure waveform analysis	PiCCO	+++	CV, specific AL	Cont.	HR, ABP, CO	SVV, SV, SVR(I)	See above	Temperature shifts Rapid changes in vasculomotor tone Arrhythmias
		LiDCO	+++				PPV, SV, SVR(I)	See above	
		Vigileo and FLoTrac sensor	++					Specific kit	
		MostCare	++					Specific kit	
Ultrasound/ Doppler	Doppler-	CardioQ	++	Specific equipment, US machine	Cont.	HR, CO	FT, SV, SVR(I)	Oesophageal pathology	Turbulent flow, skilled operator
	Oesophageal	WAKI						Assumptions re aortic size	
	Doppler-	USCOM	±		Int.			May be difficult with trache/ETT	
	Suprasternal								
	Transoesoph-ageal Echo		++		Int.			Oesophageal pathology	
	Transthoracic Echo		±		Int.			Image quality in critically ill	
	Bioimpedence	Lifegard TEBCO	±	Specific equipment	Cont.		PEP, LVET	Specific kit, validation	Peripheral oedema, pleural effusions
		Hotman							
		BioZ							
	Bioreactance	NICOM	±	Specific equipment	Cont.			Specific kit, validation	Unknown

AL: arterial line (any); BA: brachial arterial access; Cont.: continuous; CV: central venous access; FA: femoral arterial access; Int.: intermittent; PAFC: pulmonary artery flotation catheter; PV: peripheral venous access; US: ultrasound machine.

Box 1.21 Potential human errors in CO monitoring

- Lack of familiarity/training
- Complications during insertion or during use
- Poor positioning
- Poor calibration
- Lack of incorporation of data into entire clinical picture.

Users must be clear about what they are measuring and why, and which values are real and which are derived. This requires a thorough understanding of the physiology of critical illness, and of the techniques used and the physical principles upon which they are based, in order to avoid error. Ultimately, monitoring *per se* cannot improve outcome unless the data obtained are of high quality, *and* used in the correct manner to guide therapeutic interventions that have been shown to improve outcome.

Further reading

Drummond KE & Murphy E (2012). Minimally invasive cardiac output monitors. *CEACCP*, 12(1):5–10. doi:10.1093/bjaceaccp/mkr044.

de Waal EEC, Wappler F, & Buhre WF (2009). Cardiac output monitoring. *Curr Opin Anaesthesiol*, 22(1):71–7. doi:10.1097/ACO.0b013e32831f44d0.

1.8 Echocardiography in anaesthesia and intensive care

Echocardiography is increasingly seen as a safe and accurate method of haemodynamic assessment. In comparison with pressure and flow-based monitoring (see section 1.6), it has the additional advantage of potentially identifying the *cause* of the observed haemodynamics.

Physics of echocardiography

Ultrasound waves are the longitudinal compression of particles that are transmitted via a medium. They reflect off components of the medium according to its echogenicity, and are detected by the same probe. The waves are described in terms of *frequency* (number of oscillations per second, in units of Hertz, Hz) and *wavelength* (λ) in units of metres (m).

Frequency and wavelength are related according to the equation:

$$c = f\lambda$$

c = speed of the wave (m/s); f = frequency (Hz); λ = wavelength (m)

Within a constant medium, doubling the incident frequency will halve the wavelength.

The speed of sound varies according to the medium through which it passes, and is about 1500m/s in most soft tissues. Medical ultrasound typically uses sound wave frequencies of between 1MHz and 20MHz (1MHz = 10^6Hz), which is well above the human auditory spectrum of <20kHz.

The speed (c) of the waves is a function of the compressibility (κ) and density (ρ) of the material, according to the equation:

$$c = \sqrt{1/\kappa\rho}$$

Typical values for various body tissues are given in Table 1.5.

Table 1.5 Physical characteristics of different tissues relevant to ultrasound		
Material	Density ρ (kg/m^3)	Speed c (m/s)
Air	1.2	330
Water	1000	1480
Blood	1060	1570
Fat	920	1450
Bone	1380–1810	4080

When an ultrasound wave passes from one medium to another, the frequency is constant. If the wave speed in the second medium changes, then the wavelength will also change:

$$\text{Frequency}\,(f) = c/\lambda$$

For example, if the speed of the wave in the medium halves, then the wavelength will also halve for the frequency to stay the same.

Generation of ultrasound

A transducer is a device that converts one form of energy to another. In the case of ultrasound this conversion is from electrical to mechanical (sound) energy, and back again when the sound wave returns. The transducer in nearly all medical ultrasound transducers is made of lead zirconate titanate (PZT), a crystalline ceramic, which generates a charge in response to mechanical stress, and vice versa. This quality is known as piezoelectricity.

Returning sound waves are converted to electrical signals via the piezoelectric crystal and converted using software to images. The amplitude of the signal represents the echogenicity of the structure, and is indicated by increasing brightness on the screen.

The Doppler effect

This is the observation that the frequency of an observed wave changes when the source of the wave is moving relative to the observer. In respect of echocardiography, the *source* is the echo-reflective surface (blood or tissue) and the *observer* is the probe.

By measuring the change in frequency, the velocity of the source relative to the medium can be calculated. The Bernoulli equation uses the velocity of flow between the two chambers to calculate the *pressure difference* between them (allowing the technique to provide, for example, a pressure gradient in aortic stenosis). In its simplified form, the Bernoulli equation can be expressed as:

$$\Delta P = 4(V_2^2 - V_1^2)$$

V_1 = proximal velocity (m/s); V_2 = distal velocity (m/s); ΔP = instantaneous pressure gradient (mmHg)

The proximal velocity V_1 can usually be ignored, hence the equation simplifies even further to $\Delta P = 4\,V_2^2$

Colour Doppler

The Doppler effect can be used to indicate simply the direction of blood flow on a 2D image. This is known as colour Doppler. By convention, blood moving away from the probe is coloured blue, and blood moving towards the probe is coloured red (hence the acronym 'BART').

Ultrasound imaging modes

Five modes of echo image representation are recognized, but modern machines use only three (M-mode, 2D, and Doppler).

A (amplitude) mode

Horizontal axis represents *time* or *depth* into the patient. Vertical axis represents *amplitude* of the return echo.

B (brightness) mode

The two dimensions of the display are used to represent a cross section of the patient. The brightness represents the amplitude of the echoes received.

M (motion) mode

The display shows time (horizontal) and brightness (vertical) on the axes. A single plane is chosen by the operator and any echo reflection within this plane is displayed, against time, on the screen.

2D (two-dimensional) mode

Repeated sweeps of M-mode are displayed to reproduce images recognizable as 2D structures. Since multiple M-mode cuts are used to make up each frame, the temporal resolution is inferior to M-mode.

Doppler modes

The Doppler effect can be monitored and colour changes added to a 2D image (colour Doppler). Alternatively, the velocity along a given plane can be tested using either continuous waves (CW Doppler) or pulsed waves (PW Doppler). Collectively these are termed spectral Doppler.

Safety considerations in trans-oesophageal echocardiography (TOE)

In comparison with other imaging and monitoring modalities, TOE has an attractive safety profile: it does not require major vessel cannulation or transfer of a critically ill patient, and does not involve use of ionizing radiation. Significant remaining risks include:

- Physical trauma: to teeth, oropharynx, oesophagus, or stomach. Known oesophageal and/or gastric pathology is a relative contraindication.
- Thermal damage: the probe generates heat, which is normally absorbed by surrounding tissues. There is usually an automatic cut-out if the temperature rises too high.
- Bubble formation: local heat can cause dissolved gases to come out of solution ('cavitation').
- Cardiovascular instability: this is rare, but the procedure may provoke both vagal and sympathetic responses. Tachyarrhythmias and even MI have been reported.

The procedure may be carried out with topical local anaesthesia (LA), light sedation (with/without topical LA), conscious sedation or general anaesthesia (GA). The decision regarding which depends upon the indication for TOE, the clinical status of the patient, resources available, expertise available and patient preference. Of note, pain is often an indicator of significant complications (e.g. oesophageal trauma) and should not simply be relieved by the use of sedative drugs without due consideration as to the cause.

TOE data relevant to anaesthesia and critical care

TOE allows evaluation of several important cardiovascular parameters of immediate relevance to anaesthesia and critical care:

Left ventricular preload
In the presence of mitral regurgitation, LV preload can be estimated using the modified Bernoulli equation by measuring the peak flow velocity of the regurgitant jet to derive the left ventricular-atrial pressure gradient. Subtracting this from the peak systolic blood pressure yields an estimate of left atrial pressure (LAP).

Alternatively, a visual estimation of LV end-systolic and end-diastolic areas (obtained through a transgastric view) readily gives an estimation of volume status.

Global LV systolic function
Doppler TOE can be used to provide continuous measurement of *cardiac output*, classically by the LV outflow tract (LVOT) method: multiplying the LVOT cross-sectional area by the PW Doppler-derived time-velocity integral yields stroke volume.

Alternatively, the fractional change of LV cavity area measured via the transgastric view gives an estimate of *ejection fraction*.

Regional systolic LV function
This is based on a visual (and subjective) assessment of wall motion, graded as normokinesia, hypokinesia, akinesia or dyskinesia. Regional wall motion abnormalities corresponding to the anatomical distribution of the three major coronary arteries are potentially important indicators of ischaemia.

Other TOE observations
TOE will, of course, reveal other potentially important information, including (but not limited to):

- LV diastolic function
- RV function

- Valvular lesions (stenosis or regurgitation)
- Pericardial disease (effusion or constriction).

Intraoperative use of TOE

The use of TOE in *cardiac surgery* is well established: to confirm the diagnosis, refine anaesthetic and surgical management, and to assess the response to the intervention.

There is increasing interest in the use of TOE as a complementary monitoring tool in *non-cardiac surgery*. It is well recognized that perioperative *cardiac* complications constitute a major element of the risk associated with non-cardiac surgery. The factors that make up this risk—the patient's functional status, pre-morbid conditions, and the nature of the proposed surgery—are discussed elsewhere (sections 1.1–1.5).

TOE may be used to guide intraoperative fluid therapy and to identify possible myocardial ischaemia through regional wall motion assessment.

Intraoperative TOE may be especially applicable to certain non-cardiac surgical procedures:

- *Aortic surgery*: aortic occlusion produces an acute rise in afterload that may promote cardiac failure or ischaemia. Reperfusion is frequently associated with myocardial depression.
- *Liver transplantation*: TOE allows rapid identification of possible causes of haemodynamic instability, including hypovolaemia, RV failure, and embolic phenomena.
- *Major orthopaedic surgery*: may be associated with cardiovascular instability due to embolism of fat, air, or bone marrow.
- *Neurosurgery*: procedures in the sitting position carry a particular risk of air embolism. TOE may be used both to screen for a patent foramen ovale and to detect air embolism during surgery.
- *Surgery in the GUCH patient*: in some cases this will pose special challenges (see sections 1.19 and 14.9) and intraoperative TOE may be invaluable.

Use of TOE in critical care

TOE has potentially important applications in the critical care unit, employing the same principles and techniques as described previously. There are several critical care situations in which general consensus and/or evidence supports the use of TOE:

- The haemodynamically unstable patient
- Suspected aortic dissection
- Blunt or penetrating chest trauma
- Suspected pre-existing valvular or myocardial disease in the trauma patient
- Widened mediastinum and suspected aortic injury.

Further reading

American Society of Anesthesiologists and Society of Cardiovascular Anesthesiologists Task Force on Transesophageal Echocardiography. (2010, May). Practice guidelines for perioperative transesophageal echocardiography. *Anesthesiology*, 112(5):1084–96.

Catena, E., & Mele, D. (2008). Role of intraoperative transesophageal echocardiography in patients undergoing noncardiac surgery. *Journal of Cardiovasc Med (Hagerstown, Md.)*, 9(10):993–1003. doi:10.2459/JCM.0b013e32830bf655.

Roscoe, A., & Strang, T. (2008). Echocardiography in intensive care. *CEACCP*, 8(2):46–9.

1.9 Perioperative arrhythmias

The term 'arrhythmia' denotes an abnormality in cardiac rate, rhythm, or conduction. The event may be asymptomatic, or it may cause symptoms such as palpitations, dizziness, or syncope. In some instances, an arrhythmia may result in sudden cardiac death.

Cardiac arrhythmias are an important cause of both morbidity and mortality during the perioperative period, yet there is relatively little guidance in the literature aimed at management in this specific setting.

Mechanisms of arrhythmia generation

Arrhythmias may arise through disorders of impulse *formation* or *conduction*. Essentially, three processes may occur—these are illustrated in Fig. 1.7:

- *Increased automaticity*: either the phase 4 depolarization slope is steeper, or the threshold potential lower.
- *Triggered activity*: 'after'-depolarizations may reach threshold potential—characteristic of the long QT syndrome.
- *Circus movement or re-entry*: non-uniform rates of conduction/refractory periods within a ring of excitable tissue may produce a self-sustaining circus movement: either structural (e.g. Wolff–Parkinson–White syndrome) or, more commonly, functional (e.g. myocardial ischaemia).

A variety of factors may precipitate arrhythmias perioperatively (see Box 1.22).

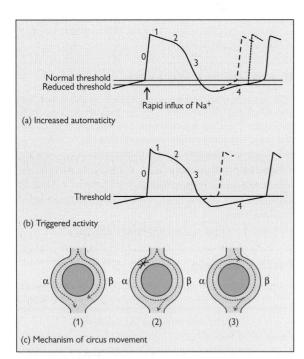

(a) Increased automaticity

(b) Triggered activity

(c) Mechanism of circus movement

Fig. 1.7 Mechanisms of arrhythmogenesis. Image courtesy of Dua et al., 'Management of Perioperative Arrhythmias', *Indian Journal of Anaesthesia*, 2007, Figure 1, 51, 4, pp. 310–323, with permission.

Box 1.22 Common intraoperative factors predisposing to arrhythmias

- Pre-existing cardiac disease:
  - Ischaemic heart disease, cardiomyopathy, etc.
- Fluid and electrolyte imbalance:
  - Hypovolaemia, hypo- or hyperkalaemia, hypocalcaemia or hypomagnesaemia
- Light planes of anaesthesia/excessive stimulation:
  - Especially during endotracheal intubation
- Metabolic upset:
  - Hypo- or hypercarbia, acidosis or alkalosis, hypoxaemia, hypothermia or hyperthermia
- Anaesthetic and other drugs:
  - Volatile agents (e.g. halothane, enflurane), ketamine (blocks catecholamine re-uptake), others (e.g. suxamethonium, atropine, inotropes, β-blockers)
- Mechanical irritation:
  - Central lines, PACs, surgical retraction, etc.
- Vagal stimulation:
  - Peritoneal stretch, oculo-cardiac reflex, etc.
- Intracranial pathology:
  - Subarachnoid haemorrhage, raised intracranial pressure
- Endocrine disorders:
  - Phaeochromocytoma, thyrotoxicosis.

Approach to management

The overriding question is whether the arrhythmia is considered dangerous, or potentially so. If time permits, it is always desirable to record a definitive 12-lead ECG.

If the arrhythmia is causing a haemodynamic disturbance (hypotension, ischaemic ECG changes or signs of cardiac failure), it requires treatment: the degree of disturbance dictates the urgency required. Pseudo-arrhythmias (from diathermy, muscle artefact, or poor ECG electrode contact) should, of course, be ruled out.

Depending on the nature of the arrhythmia, and the clinical status of the patient, there are three categories of treatment:

- Electrical: cardioversion (or defibrillation) or pacing
- Simple clinical intervention: e.g. vagotonic manoeuvre
- Pharmacological.

In all instances, precipitating or aggravating factors should be identified and corrected, and there should be no hesitation in seeking early cardiological advice if needed.

The Resuscitation Council (www.resus.org.uk) provides detailed guidelines on arrhythmia management.

Management of individual rhythm disturbances

Bradycardia

Whilst a bradycardia is defined as HR <60 beats/min, it is perhaps better characterized as a heart rate that is inappropriately slow for the haemodynamic state of the patient. Sinus bradycardia may of course be a normal finding in athletes, but is more usually associated with drug therapy (β-blockers, digoxin, etc.) ± ischaemic heart disease. Other causes include hypothermia and hypothyroidism.

Non-sinus bradycardias may be nodal in origin or occur in the setting of AV block. The presence of adverse signs (HR <40/min, associated hypotension or supercedent ventricular arrhythmias) is an indication for treatment. Anticholinergics (glycopyrronium/atropine) remain first-line (after elimination of obvious precipitants such as peritoneal stretch), but with initial caution in the presence of IHD.

Refractory bradycardias, and those where there is a high risk of deterioration to asystole (e.g. long pauses, Mobitz type II AV block, or 3rd-degree AV block with broad complexes) will require expert assistance and possibly transvenous pacing. Chronotropic infusions (isoprenaline or adrenaline) or transcutaneous pacing may be appropriate interim measures.

Atrial fibrillation

AF is common—it may be seen acutely in theatre, and, perhaps even more commonly, in high-dependency postoperative patients, in whom the incidence may be as high as 15%. It carries a significant mortality and morbidity.

The fundamental consideration remains the haemodynamic status of the patient, whilst the goal of treatment may be to restore sinus rhythm or to control the ventricular rate.

In essence, patients who are severely haemodynamically unstable should undergo prompt synchronized DC cardioversion.

In the case of haemodynamically stable patients with new-onset AF, there is a greater variety of options: DC cardioversion may still be considered, but a pharmacological approach is often employed. Intravenous amiodarone has a conversion rate of up to 80% (and, of course, has efficacy in a wide range of other acute arrhythmias), but there are reports of occasional severe acute pulmonary toxicity. A relatively new class 3 agent, ibutilide, is reported to have high conversion rates, even when amiodarone has been unsuccessful.

Whilst previously, the goal of therapy was to restore sinus rhythm, there is growing interest in *rate control* strategies as a primary endpoint, with similar or even improved mortality and morbidity. A variety of agents may be used, including digoxin, calcium antagonists (diltiazem or verapamil) and β-blockers.

Anticoagulation in AF is discussed in section 1.20.

AV nodal re-entrant tachycardia (AVNRT)

AVNRT is the commonest non-sinus, regular, narrow-QRS complex tachycardia. It is frequently seen in the emergency department and intensive care setting, but may also be encountered in theatre. In many cases, the ventricular rate is extremely high (180–240 beats/min). An awake patient will experience palpitations, light-headedness, and shortness of breath or anxiety. Vagal manoeuvres may slow AV conduction and terminate the arrhythmia. Intravenous adenosine has a rapid onset of action and an extremely short half-life, and is the drug of first choice. Longer-acting agents such as verapamil may be used: it is important *not* to administer verapamil to a patient receiving β-blocker therapy.

Ventricular tachyarrhythmias

Ventricular arrhythmias may be classified according to morphology (monomorphic vs polymorphic) and duration (sustained vs non-sustained). Episodes of non-sustained ventricular tachycardia (NSVT) may be seen in the absence of structural heart disease, but in those with heart disease, NSVT is a predictor of more serious subsequent arrhythmias. Magnesium may reduce the incidence of postoperative NSVT after cardiac surgery.

Sustained VT may be monomorphic (constant QRS amplitude) or polymorphic (continually changing QRS morphology).

Monomorphic VT arises through a re-entry phenomenon: lignocaine was traditionally first-line therapy, but amiodarone is widely used.

In polymorphic VT, the critical deciding factor in choosing therapy is the QT interval during previous sinus rhythm. Polymorphic VT in the setting of a normal QT interval usually occurs in ischaemic heart disease and frequently degenerates into VF. Amiodarone or procainamide may be preferable to lignocaine. By contrast, polymorphic VT with a preceding prolonged QT interval (torsades de pointes) requires a different approach—therapy is focused at reversal of the QT prolongation. Electrolyte imbalance should be corrected, and intravenous magnesium is the first-line treatment. Both class I and III anti-arrhythmics may themselves prolong the QT interval (procainamide, for example, is contraindicated in torsades)—the incidence of torsades is lowest with amiodarone (see Box 1.23), which may, therefore, be a rational therapy for refractory polymorphic VT of unknown aetiology.

In all cases, it must be stressed that DC cardioversion remains first-line treatment in the unstable patient.

Box 1.23 Some causes of prolonged QT syndrome

Congenital
- Jervell–Lange–Nielsen and Romano–Ward syndromes.

Acquired
- Metabolic:
  - Hypokalaemia, hypocalcaemia, hypomagnesaemia
- Bradyarrhythmias:
  - Sinus node dysfunction
  - 2nd- or 3rd-degree AV block
- Antiarrhythmic drugs:
  - Quinidine, procainamide, disopyramide, amiodarone, sotalol
- Antimicrobial drugs:
  - Erythromycin, clarithromycin, some azole antifungals
- Antihistamines:
  - Terfenadine, astemizole
- Psychotropic drugs:
  - Thioridazine, phenothiazines, SSRIs, risperidone
- Other:
  - Droperidol, myocardial ischaemia, hypothermia.

Pulseless cardiac arrest

The four most common lethal rhythms are ventricular fibrillation (VF), pulseless VT, pulseless electrical activity (PEA), and asystole. The most critical intervention is immediate CPR, and in the case of a shockable rhythm (VF or VT), defibrillation should be performed as early as possible.

The exact mechanism of successful defibrillation remains unknown, but it may act to prolong the refractory period of the cardiac action potential. Most defibrillators now employ a biphasic shock waveform that possibly increases the termination rate of VF.

In the case of asystole or PEA, survival is poor unless a reversible cause (e.g. hyperkalaemia or hypovolaemia) is identified and treated.

Further reading

Dua N & Kumra V (2007). Management of perioperative arrhythmias. *Indian J Anaesth*, 51(4):310–23.

Thompson A (2004). Perioperative cardiac arrhythmias. *Br J Anaesth*, 93(1):86–94.

Trappe H-J, Brandts B, & Weismueller P (2003). Arrhythmias in the intensive care patient. *Curr Opin Crit Care*, 9(5):345–55.

1.10 Pacemakers and defibrillators

There are important considerations in respect of patients with permanent pacemakers and/or implantable defibrillators who present for surgery. It is essential to have a basic understanding of the function of these so-called cardiac rhythm management devices (CRMDs) and a strategy for safe management during the perioperative period.

Overview of pacemakers

Pacemaker systems consist of an *impulse generator* (usually implanted in the subpectoral region) and *leads* (usually attached to the endocardium via a transvenous approach).

Pacemakers may be single chamber (RV), dual chamber (RA + RV), or even tri-chamber (RA+RV+LV)—the latter are used in resynchronization therapy for heart failure (see section 1.13, in which the LV lead is usually placed via the coronary sinus).

Single-chamber devices sense intrinsic activity within that chamber, which will either inhibit or trigger pacing activity. Dual-chamber systems seek to maintain atrioventricular synchrony to optimize cardiac output. Some systems incorporate a rate-modulating mode that enables patients without intact sinus node function to increase their heart rate in response to exercise—commonly used sensors detect motion/vibration or minute ventilation (via changes in thoracic impedance). It is crucial to be aware of such configurations preoperatively, since certain functions may need to be altered or disabled.

An internationally recognized 5-position code is used to describe pacemaker location and function (Table 1.6). The 5-position code is often shortened to the first 3, and the most commonly used mode is a dual chamber (DDD) mode. Multisite pacing (position V) refers either to the presence of more than one lead in a single chamber, or more commonly, biventricular pacing to promote resynchronization.

Implantable cardioverter defibrillators

Implantable cardioverter defibrillators (ICDs) have all the capabilities of a pacemaker, together with the potential for defibrillation (± overdrive pacing) of tachyarrhythmias (usually ventricular). ICDs measure each cardiac R–R interval, and categorize the rate as normal, too fast (short R–R) or too slow (long R–R). When enough short R–R intervals are detected, an antitachycardia event (pacing or shock) is begun. Most ICDs will also start pacing when the R–R interval is too long. Like pacemakers, ICDs are described by an international generic code (Table 1.7).

Preoperative assessment of patients with CRMDs

Preoperative evaluation should focus on three main questions (see Fig. 1.8):
1. What type of device is present?
2. How dependent is the patient on the device's pacing function, and what is the underlying escape rhythm (Box 1.24)?
3. What are the device settings and is it functioning correctly?

A detailed history and examination should determine the indication for the CRMD, any coexisting pathology, and the location of the impulse generator. Many patients with CRMDs will have

> **Box 1.24 Major indications for pacemaker implantation**
>
> - 3rd-degree and advanced 2nd-degree AV block at any level.
> - Higher level AV block of any type with associated bundle branch block.
> - Sinus node dysfunction with documented symptomatic bradycardia.
> - Bradycardia–tachycardia syndrome.
> - Recurrent carotid sinus syncope.

important coexisting disease, including IHD, cardiomyopathy, valvular heart disease, or congenital heart disease.

Patients will ideally carry a card showing the make, model, and serial number of the device. Pacemaker dependency will be suggested by a preceding history of symptomatic bradycardia or AV node ablation. A chest X-ray (CXR), whilst not routinely required, will confirm whether the device is single- or dual-chamber and whether an ICD is *in situ* (visible shock coil on the ventricular lead).

A 12-lead ECG will demonstrate whether or not the pacing function is being used, and which chamber(s) are sensed and/or paced.

The only reliable assessment of a CRMD is direct interrogation by a cardiac electrophysiologist—this will reveal battery status, settings, pacemaker dependency, and event log (e.g. shock history); additionally, whether or not a magnet will convert the device to an asynchronous mode (Box 1.25).

> **Box 1.25 Key points in preoperative evaluation of CRMDs**
>
> - Has the device been interrogated by an electrophysiologist?
> - Consider replacement if device nearing end of battery life.
> - What is the patient's underlying rate and rhythm?
> - Identify the magnet rate and rhythm.
> - Ensure that rate-responsiveness functions (e.g. via minute ventilation) are turned off.
> - Consider increasing the pacing rate to optimize oxygen delivery during major surgery.
> - Disable antitachycardia therapy if ICD *in situ*.

Sources of electromagnetic interference (EMI) in theatre and use of magnets

EMI may cause pacemaker output to be inhibited, or it may produce inappropriate triggering. Additionally, the pacemaker may revert to an asynchronous mode that may provoke arrhythmias if there is a competing underlying rhythm.

The operating theatre environment may generate numerous sources of EMI (Box 1.26).

> **Box 1.26 Sources of EMI in theatre**
>
> - Surgical diathermy (esp. 'coag' or 'blend'); MRI
> - External cardioversion or defibrillation; lithotripsy
> - Radio-frequency ablation; electroconvulsive therapy (ECT).

Table 1.6 Generic pacemaker codes

Position 1	Position II	Position III	Position IV	Position V
Chamber(s) paced	Chamber(s) sensed	Response to sensing	Rate modulation	Multi-site pacing
O = None	O = None	O = None	O = None	O = None
A = Atrium	A = Atrium	T = Triggered	R = Rate modulation	A = Atrium
V = Ventricle	V = Ventricle	I = Inhibited		V = Ventricle
D = Dual (A + V)	D = Dual (A + V)	D = Dual (T + I)		D = Dual (A + V)

Table 1.7 Generic defibrillator codes

Position 1	Position II	Position III	Position IV (or use pacemaker code)
Shock chambers	Antitachycardia pacing chambers	Tachycardia detection	Antibradycardia pacing chambers
O = None	O = None	E = Electrogram	O = None
A = Atrium	A = Atrium	H = Haemodynamic	A = Atrium
V = Ventricle	V = Ventricle		V = Ventricle
D = Dual (A + V)	D = Dual (A + V)		D = Dual (A + V)

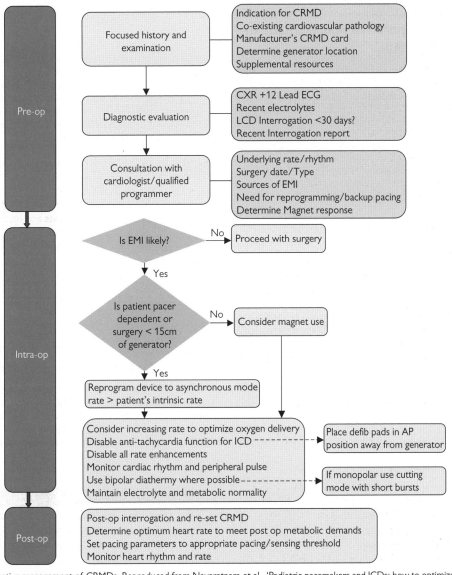

Fig. 1.8 Perioperative management of CRMDs. Reproduced from Navaratnam et al., 'Pediatric pacemakers and ICDs: how to optimize perioperative care', *Pediatric Anesthesia*, 21, 5, pp. 512–521, with permission, © 2011, Blackwell Publishing Ltd.

Modern devices are less susceptible, but the risk remains. Patients who are pacemaker dependent *and* in whom there is deemed a significant risk of EMI should be reprogrammed to an asynchronous mode at a rate higher than the patient's intrinsic rate. Rate-responsive functions, as discussed previously, should be disabled, as should the antitachycardia function of an ICD.

Reprogramming should take place under appropriate monitoring, and external defibrillator pads applied if an ICD has been disabled—these should be placed as far away from the pulse generator as possible.

It is usually advised that a magnet be made available for emergency use in theatre if EMI occurs. It is important to remember, however, that different devices respond in different ways. The device's individual magnet response settings can be revealed by interrogation as part of the preoperative work-up. In most cases, placing a magnet over the pulse generator will cause the pacemaker to revert to an asynchronous pacing mode (AOO, VOO, or DOO). ICDs will usually suspend antitachycardia therapy in the presence of a magnet.

The availability of a magnet does, not, however, replace the need for preoperative evaluation of a CRMD and for re-programming by a cardiac electrophysiologist if the risk of EMI is deemed significant.

Intra- and postoperative management of patients with CRMDs

ECG monitoring is essential, and the monitor settings should be altered to detect pacemaker activity. Pulse oximetry is, of course, routine, and the waveform should be displayed. For patients with significant cardiac disease or those undergoing major surgery, invasive arterial monitoring is invaluable. Major electrolyte disturbances, acid–base imbalance or hypoxaemia may affect pacemaker function and should be corrected.

If a device was altered preoperatively, it will of necessity require reprogramming postoperatively, and in the case of ICDs, full monitoring should continue until the anti-tachycardia function has been re-enabled.

Further reading

Allen M (2006). Pacemakers and implantable cardioverter defibrillators. *Anaesthesia*, 61(9):883–90. doi:10.1111/j.1365-2044.2006.04722.x.

Navaratnam M & Dubin A (2011). Pediatric pacemakers and ICDs: how to optimize perioperative care. *Paediatr Anaesth*, 21(5):512–21. doi:10.1111/j.1460-9592.2011.03562.x.

Rozner MA (2007). The patient with a cardiac pacemaker or implanted defibrillator and management during anaesthesia. *Curr Opin Anaesthesiol*, 20(3):261–8. doi:10.1097/ACO.0b013e32814f1c4a.

Salukhe TV, Dob D, & Sutton R (2004). Pacemakers and defibrillators: anaesthetic implications. *Br J Anaesth*, 93(1):95–104. doi:10.1093/bja/aeh170.

1.11 Cardiomyopathy

Cardiomyopathy is defined as a myocardial disorder in which the heart muscle is structurally and functionally abnormal, in the absence of coronary artery disease, hypertension, valvular or congenital heart disease.

Classification

The phenotypes described are:
- Dilated cardiomyopathy (DCM)
- Hypertrophic (obstructive) cardiomyopathy (HCM)
- Restrictive cardiomyopathy (RCM)
- Arrhythmogenic right ventricular dysplasia (ARVD)
- Unclassified (encompassing Tako-tsubo cardiomyopathy and left ventricular non-compaction).

Each may be subclassified into familial/non-familial, genetic/non-genetic, and idiopathic/acquired forms (for a summary, see Table 1.8).

General investigations and perioperative management

The management of heart failure is discussed in section 1.13.

Brain natriuretic peptide (BNP) levels are useful in diagnosing and assessing the severity of both acute and chronic heart failure.

Echocardiography (see section 1.8) is crucial for objective assessment of both structural and functional cardiac abnormalities. Determining the LV ejection fraction (LVEF) allows for a broad classification of heart failure syndromes into two types:
- HFREF (heart failure with reduced ejection fraction): LVEF <50%
- HFPEF (heart failure with preserved ejection fraction): LVEF >50% with diastolic dysfunction.

Cardiac MRI may be useful in assessing possible aetiologies, since it may reveal cardiac inflammation, infiltration or fibrosis. Myocardial biopsy may be useful in cases of myocarditis and infiltrative diseases such as amyloidosis.

Certain categories of drug are disease modifying in HFREF (see Box 1.27).

Box 1.27 Drug therapy in HFREF

Disease modifying
- Angiotensin-converting enzyme inhibitors (ACEIs).
- β-blockers.
- Mineralocorticoid receptor antagonists (e.g. spironolactone).
- Angiotensin receptor antagonists (ARAs) if ACEI intolerant.

Drugs of less certain benefit
- Ivabradine—if HR >70/min (in addition to β-blocker, or as an alternative if β-blocker intolerant).
- Digoxin (even in sinus rhythm).
- Nitrates and hydralazine (alternative to ACEI or ARA).
- Diuretics (loop or thiazide) for fluid retention.

For HFPEF, there are no convincing data to suggest a survival benefit with ACEI or ARA therapy. Diuretics are useful for treating fluid retention. Comorbidities such as hypertension and myocardial ischaemia should be treated.

There are certain fundamental principles of perioperative management of patients with cardiomyopathies or heart failure (see Box 1.28).

Box 1.28 Perioperative management of heart failure syndromes

- Undertake risk scoring prior to anaesthesia (see sections 1.1–1.5).
- Optimize heart failure medication.
- Consider invasive monitoring, including TOE.
- Avoid tachycardia, and aim to maintain sinus rhythm (low threshold for DC cardioversion if arrhythmia develops).
- Avoid large-volume infusions.
- Consider inotropic support *only* if measured CO and patient's clinical state suggest indicated (patient's normal BP may be significantly lower than in normal population).
- If longstanding heart failure on maintenance diuretics, IV diuretics or even ultrafiltration may be required in the early postoperative period.

Dilated cardiomyopathy

DCM is the most common of the cardiomyopathies, defined by the presence of LV dilatation and systolic dysfunction (with or without RV dysfunction), in the absence of abnormal loading conditions or coronary artery disease.

In addition to familial and genetic causes, alcohol, viruses, tachycardia, nutritional deficiencies, pregnancy, and drugs (including chemotherapeutic agents) are known causes.

Many patients are asymptomatic, but may present acutely with decompensated heart failure. There is an important risk of life-threatening arrhythmias and sudden death, and symptomatic patients with LVEF <30% should be considered for an ICD. There is growing use of cardiac resynchronization therapy (see section 1.13).

In terms of surgical treatment, severely impaired patients may be candidates for cardiac transplantation. Other therapies have been tried, including LV volume reduction surgery (the Batista procedure), attempting to improve the mechanics of LV function.

Peripartum cardiomyopathy (PPCM)

PPCM is a form of DCM that occurs during the last month of pregnancy or within 5 months of delivery, in the absence of another cause for heart failure or structural and functional abnormality of the heart. The LV systolic function is reduced (LVEF <45%). Risk factors include: age >30 years, multiparity, African origin, multiple fetuses, history of pre-eclampsia, eclampsia, or hypertension, cocaine use, or oral tocolytic therapy.

Management goals are similar to those in all heart failure syndromes, but some important aspects are specific to PPCM (see Box 1.29).

- ACEIs, ARAs, and aldosterone antagonists are contraindicated in pregnancy (consider hydralazine).
- β-blockers (especially selective β1-receptor blockers such as bisoprolol) can safely be used during pregnancy.
- IV GTN can be given during pregnancy.
- Anticoagulation is recommended: pregnancy and the postpartum period are hypercoagulable states and in the context of LV systolic dysfunction there is a high risk of embolic events.
- Breastfeeding is not recommended, as the aim is to reduce prolactin levels, which is thought to play an important role in the pathophysiology of the condition, and bromocriptine may be considered.
- In cardiogenic shock, urgent mechanical circulatory support should be considered.
- Expedite delivery of patients with advanced or unstable heart failure.

Hypertrophic cardiomyopathy

Hypertrophic (obstructive) cardiomyopathy (HCM) is characterized by the presence of myocardial hypertrophy in the absence of an obvious precipitant such as hypertension or valvular heart disease. Several different subtypes exist, any of which may be associated with diastolic dysfunction, myocardial ischaemia or dynamic or fixed LV outflow tract (LVOT) obstruction. The dynamic LVOT obstruction is secondary to systolic anterior motion of the mitral valve apparatus (SAM), which may or may not result in mitral regurgitation. HCM is additionally a phenotypic presentation for several conditions e.g. Anderson–Fabry's disease or Friedreich's ataxia, and an association exists with bicuspid aortic valve, and Wolff–Parkinson–White syndrome.

Patients with HCM are at particular risk of *sudden cardiac death* (SCD). Risk factors include:

- Family history of SCD
- Severe LV hypertrophy (>30mm)
- Abnormal BP or HR response to exercise
- Sustained or multiple non-sustained VT on Holter monitoring.

β-blockers, verapamil, or disopyramide are treatments of choice in HCM, especially in the context of LVOT obstruction. Control of AF through pharmacotherapy or ablation (with anticoagulation as appropriate) is important, as AF is poorly tolerated. Patients with reduced ejection fraction should be on standard heart failure medication for HFREF.

Surgical management includes septal myomectomy for obstructive HCM and severe symptoms unresponsive to pharmacotherapy. An alcohol septal ablation procedure in the cardiac catheter laboratory may be a preferred strategy in selected patients. Dual chamber pacing can be considered although the benefits of this strategy are questionable. Patients with end-stage heart failure should be considered for cardiac transplantation.

Restrictive cardiomyopathy

RCM is defined as restrictive ventricular physiology in the presence of normal or reduced diastolic volumes (of one or both ventricles), normal or reduced systolic volumes, and normal ventricular wall thickness. However a degree of increased LV wall thickness is seen in some cases such as infiltrative disease (e.g. amyloidosis) or storage disease (Pompe's disease or Fabry's disease). RCM is rare in the developed world, where it is most commonly associated with cardiac amyloidosis.

Other potential causes include haemochromatosis, sarcoidosis, carcinoid syndrome, endomyocardial fibrosis (subtropical Africa, Asia, and central America) and radiation. The most important differential diagnosis is constrictive pericarditis, where surgical pericardectomy can be considered.

Table 1.8 Summary of essential features of the cardiomyopathies

	Dilated	Peri-partum	Hypertrophic	Restrictive	Arrhythmogenic
Sex	M > F	F	M = F	M = F	M = F
Prevalence	36:100 000	1:100–1:4000	1:500	1:1000–1:5000	1:5000
Aetiology	Multiple: 25% genetic (predominantly autosomal dominant, but X-linked with muscular dystrophies); drugs, alcohol, viral, nutritional	? pregnancy-related inflammation/altered prolactin processing	Predominantly autosomal dominant inheritance	Multiple–including deposition disorders and genetic	Predominantly autosomal dominant inheritance
Histology	Myocyte hypertrophy, fibrosis, lymphocyte infiltration	Lymphocytic infiltrate, myocyte oedema, variable fibrosis	Myocyte disarray and fibrosis	Myocyte hypertrophy, fibrosis, lymphocyte infiltration ± evidence of storage disease	Replacement of RV myocardium with adipose tissue and fibrosis
Examination	Features of LV ± RV failure. May be functional mitral ± tricuspid regurgitation	Features of LV ± RV failure. May be functional mitral ± tricuspid regurgitation	Double LV impulse, sharp rising pulse, ejection systolic murmur ± mitral regurgitation	Features of LV ± RV failure. May be functional mitral ± tricuspid regurgitation	Features of RV ± LV failure
ECG	Normal or bundle branch block, tachyarrhythmias, abnormalities of ST segment, T wave, QT interval	Normal or bundle branch block, tachyarrhythmias, abnormalities of ST segment, T wave, QT interval	Usually abnormal, with features of LVH, various ST segment and T wave abnormalities	AF, sick sinus syndrome, VT, inferior Q waves, low QRS voltages	ECG normal at presentation in 40-50%. May show RBBB, T wave inversion, epsilon waves, LBBB or VT
Outlook	Depends on aetiology	Ranges from full recovery to progressive fibrosis and DCM	Mortality 1% per year	Depends on aetiology	Depends on risk factors for sudden cardiac death

LBBB/RBBB: left/right bundle branch block

In RCM, the stroke volume is limited and small. Further, infiltrative disease involving the sino-atrial or atrio-ventricular node may lead to bradyarrhythmias in the perioperative situation. Maintenance of an adequate SVR and heart rate are key to maintain CO.

Arrhythmogenic right ventricular dysplasia

ARVD is an inherited disorder in which there is progressive replacement of RV myocardium by adipose and fibrous tissue. The principal complication is arrhythmia, and certain factors increase the risk of SCD in ARVD:

- Young age.
- Competitive sport activity.
- Family history of SCD.
- Significant RV involvement with impaired systolic function.
- Involvement of the LV.
- History of syncope or previous ventricular arrhythmia.

Such patients should undergo ICD placement and refrain from competitive athletics. Sotalol is often a highly effective antiarrhythmic agent in ARVD. Patients with intractable arrhythmias and progressive heart failure should be assessed for cardiac transplantation.

Further reading

Elliott P, Andersson B, Arbustini E, *et al.* (2008). Classification of the cardiomyopathies: a position statement from the European Society Of Cardiology Working Group on Myocardial and Pericardial Diseases. *Eur Heart J*, 29(2), 270–276. doi:10.1093/eurheartj/ehm342.

1.12 Inotropes and vasodilators

The development of a low cardiac output state necessitates urgent intervention to restore adequate perfusion before multiorgan failure develops. Current consensus recommends that inotropes and vasodilators be used *early* in selected patients whose shocked state persists despite volume resuscitation. Appropriate monitoring should be instituted to guide therapy (see sections 1.6 and 1.7). Inotrope therapy should be weaned as soon as adequate organ perfusion is restored and can be maintained.

Inotropes and inodilators

Adrenaline (epinephrine)

Adrenaline is an endogenous catecholamine formed by the methylation of noradrenaline (norepinephrine). It acts predominantly on cardiac β_1 and peripheral α_1 receptors, resulting in positive inotropic, chronotropic, and vasoconstrictor effects. The net effects on systemic vascular resistance (SVR) are less predictable than with noradrenaline, since adrenaline also causes concomitant peripheral β_2 receptor activation with vasodilatation.

Adrenaline also exhibits positive *dromotropic* (increased AV node conduction) and *bathmotropic* (increased myocyte excitability) effects.

There are a number of important potential adverse effects associated with adrenaline therapy:

- Significantly increased myocardial work and O_2 consumption (positive chronotropy and inotropy).
- Potential myocardial ischaemia from coronary vasoconstriction.
- Pro-arrhythmogenic effects.
- Regional vasoconstriction, e.g. of splanchnic circulation.
- Increased lactic acid production: via stimulation of Emden–Meyerhof pathway via pyruvate: makes interpretation of lactate levels potentially challenging.

Adrenaline is not recommended for the routine treatment of acute heart failure, but is frequently used at low doses in patients with severe refractory haemodynamic instability. It remains widely used in anaphylaxis and as part of current Advanced Life Support (ALS) guidelines in the management of cardiac arrest.

Dopamine

Dopamine is a naturally occurring precursor of noradrenaline with varying receptor effects depending on dosage. At low doses (0.5–3mcg/kg/min) its predominant activity is on dopaminergic (DA_1 and DA_2) receptors, whilst at higher doses (3–10mcg/kg/min), β_1 effects predominate, with some β_2 mediated peripheral vasodilatation. Doses higher than these should be used with caution, as they are associated with an increasing risk of tachycardia, dysrhythmias, and α_1 stimulation resulting in increased SVR.

The routine use of dopamine remains contentious. It was thought that low-dose 'renal' dopamine to increase renal blood flow could be used to prevent renal failure, before a randomized clinical trial, comparing dopamine to placebo, demonstrated no difference in primary or secondary outcome. Nonetheless, in diuretic-resistant hypotensive chronic heart failure, dopamine (2.5mcg/kg/min) in conjunction with a furosemide infusion may optimize haemodynamics and renal perfusion sufficient to facilitate diuresis.

Adverse systemic effects of dopaminergic stimulation include confusion, nausea and vomiting, and altered immune regulation, which may also be associated with adverse outcomes.

Isoprenaline

Isoprenaline is a synthetic derivative of dopamine, with potent β_1 and β_2 effects. Chronotropic effects predominate, and it is rarely used as an inotrope. More frequently, it is used to provide a temporary increase in heart rate pending institution of definitive pacing. Isoprenaline may be useful in the presence of significant pulmonary hypertension where it acts both as an inotrope and a pulmonary vasodilator.

Dobutamine

Dobutamine is a synthetic derivative of isoprenaline, and an agonist at β_1 and β_2 receptors. It therefore increases cardiac output whilst also decreasing SVR. Current guidelines recommend using dobutamine in low-output states provided there is adequate blood pressure. Dobutamine may exacerbate tachycardia and tachyarrhythmias, and in the presence of hypovolaemia may result in profound hypotension. It is often used in combination with vasopressor agents, especially in refractory septic shock, where cardiogenic and vasodilatory shock may coexist.

Milrinone and enoximone

These agents are phosphodiesterase (III) inhibitors (PDEIs), and act as *inodilators* to cause:

- Increased stroke volume and cardiac output.
- Reduced PA pressure, PAOP, SVR, and PVR.

The haemodynamic effects of the PDEIs are similar to dobutamine, with some important differences:

- More potent peripheral and pulmonary vasodilatation.
- Less tachycardia and myocardial O_2 consumption.

Levosimendan

Levosimendan is a calcium sensitizer that exerts its inotropic effects through several important mechanisms:

- Binds to calcium saturated troponin-C in cardiac myocytes to cause a positive inotropic effect.
- Acts on ATP-sensitive potassium channels (KATP) on vascular smooth muscle causing vasodilatation.
- Exerts a cardioprotective effect via mitochondrial KATP channels.
- At high doses, has a mild PDEI action.

Overall these manifest as an increased cardiac output and stroke volume along with reduced pulmonary capillary wedge pressure and reduced SVR and PVR.

Initial studies produced conflicting results, with no improvement in overall survival, but these were performed in the context of chronic heart failure rather than haemodynamically compromised critically ill patients. More recent studies have supported its safety and efficacy in various patient populations.

Levosimendan would appear to be an ideal inotrope in the critically ill patient, increasing cardiac output without increasing oxygen requirements, and whilst exerting cardioprotective effects. Further studies are currently evaluating its potential applications.

Vasodilators

Vasodilator therapy is recommended early in the treatment of acute heart failure in the absence of hypotension (SBP <90mmHg) or severe obstructive valvular disease. The aim is to reduce both right- and left-sided filling pressures, and SVR, resulting in improved symptoms and haemodynamics.

Pulmonary vasodilators are indicated in right heart failure secondary to pulmonary hypertension (mean PAP >25mmHg).

There are numerous triggers for pulmonary hypertension during anaesthesia, surgery, and critical care. Hypoxia, hypercarbia, hypothermia, high airway pressures, acidosis, PEEP, hypovolaemia, and ischaemia can all contribute to acute increases in PAP or PVR, which if not recognized and corrected promptly, can result in a downward spiral of worsening pulmonary hypertension and decompensated heart failure. The failing right ventricle has little ability to compensate for acute changes in afterload. RV dilatation can in turn compromise *left* heart function and coronary perfusion.

Nitric oxide (NO) is an endogenous vasodilator produced by the vascular endothelium. NO donors form the mainstay of vasodilator therapies. These agents undergo biotransformation in smooth muscle cells to form NO, which produces venous and arterial vasodilatation via cyclic GMP. cGMP is broken down by phosphodiesterase (PDE) (in particular isoenzyme PDE-V). NO rapidly diffuses into the bloodstream and reacts with haemoglobin forming metabolites that are excreted in the urine. In heart failure, the resultant reduced systemic and pulmonary vascular venous tone, increased vascular compliance, and reduced afterload have the net effect of increasing cardiac output and reversing myocardial ischaemia.

Organic nitrates

The organic nitrates are systemic vasodilators that can be administered by a variety of routes (enteral, sublingual, subcutaneous, or intravenous). In the acute setting, nitrate therapy is usually titrated intravenously to the maximum tolerated dose without haemodynamic compromise. Limitations include the development of tolerance, with a marked attenuation of initial effects in up to 50% of patients.

Nitroprusside

Sodium (or potassium) nitroprusside is perhaps the gold standard against which other vasodilators are evaluated. It has a complex structure, containing a ferrous iron molecule bound to five cyanide molecules and nitric acid. Nitroprusside mediates its effects by decomposition to produce nitrosothiol on contact with red blood cells. Clearance is via hepatic metabolism to thiocyanate, which is then renally excreted with a half-life of 3–4 days. The main limitation of the drug relates to the toxicity of its metabolites. Suspected thiocyanate toxicity (lactic acidosis, confusion, and seizures) may require haemofiltration.

Inhaled nitric oxide

When administered by inhalation, NO diffuses rapidly across the alveolar capillary membrane into the smooth muscle cell causing local pulmonary vasodilatation. Other actions include bronchodilatation, anti-inflammatory, and antiproliferative effects. Compared to other agents, it also enhances ventilation-perfusion matching, since it increases blood flow only in well-ventilated lung areas.

It has a variety of clinical applications (Box 1.30).

> **Box 1.30 Clinical applications of inhaled nitric oxide**
>
> - Pulmonary hypertension of the newborn.
> - Pulmonary vasoreactivity testing in cardiac catheterization.
> - Preventing RV failure due to pulmonary hypertension after cardiac transplantation.
> - Supporting RV function in the critically ill or after left ventricular assist device (LVAD) insertion.
> - Treatment of ischaemia-reperfusion injury after lung transplantation.
> - Improving oxygenation in severe acute respiratory distress syndrome (ARDS) or in chronic obstructive pulmonary disease (COPD).

Potential complications include toxicity due to the formation of nitrogen dioxide (causing pulmonary oedema) or methaemoglobinaemia (causing tissue hypoxia), although this is less likely at inhaled concentrations <80ppm.

Prostacyclin

Prostacyclin (prostaglandin I_2) is a naturally occurring vasodilator produced within endothelial cells from arachidonic acid. It also inhibits platelet aggregation and smooth muscle proliferation, and has anti-inflammatory effects. Synthetic analogues are epoprostenol (Flolan®), and iloprost, which are currently licensed for the treatment of New York Heart Association (NYHA) class III/IV pulmonary hypertension via specialized intravenous or aerosol devices. In the context of pulmonary hypertension and right heart failure in critically ill mechanically ventilated patients these agents have been found to be effective in decreasing pulmonary pressures without reducing systemic perfusion, and with minimal adverse effects. However, an effect on outcome has yet to be determined in clinical trials.

Phosphodiesterase inhibitors

Sildenafil is one of several phosphodiesterase V inhibitors used as a pulmonary vasodilator in the treatment of pulmonary hypertension. It can be administered orally, intravenously, or via inhalation. Only oral sildenafil is commercially available. It has been used effectively to treat RV dysfunction in transplant recipients and in weaning patients from NO therapy.

Other vasodilator agents

Neseritide is a recombinant DNA preparation of human ventricular brain natriuretic peptide (BNP). It binds to the guanylate cyclase receptor and converts GTP to cGMP, resulting in smooth muscle relaxation. Systemic hypotension limits its use.

L-Citrulline is metabolized to L-arginine in the pulmonary vascular endothelium. As a NO precursor, supplementation of citrulline is under evaluation in the prevention and treatment of pulmonary hypertension in children with congenital heart disease.

Bosentan is an antagonist at endothelin A and B receptors to inhibit endothelin-1 induced vasoconstriction. It produces pulmonary vasodilatation and improved haemodynamics in patients with chronic thromboembolic pulmonary hypertension.

Conivaptan is a vasopressin receptor antagonist. The vasoconstrictor effects of arginine vasopressin have led to development of antagonists proposed for the use in acute heart failure. Conivaptan reduces pulmonary capillary wedge pressure and right atrial pressure, with no significant change in other haemodynamic parameters.

Further reading

Hollenberg SM (2011). Vasoactive drugs in circulatory shock. *Am J Respir Crit Care Med*, 183(7):847–55. doi:10.1164/rccm.201006-0972CI.

1.13 Heart failure

Heart failure is a complex clinical syndrome in which the heart's ability to fill or eject is impaired. It is becoming more frequent in an ageing population. A new classification by the ACC and AHA emphasizes that heart failure is an *evolving* entity: if screening and treatment are instituted *early*, its course and outcome can be improved.

Causes of heart failure

Heart failure may be caused by a primary defect in the heart muscle, or be secondary to a circulatory disorder (Box 1.31). Ischaemic heart disease and hypertension are the commonest causes in the Western world.

> **Box 1.31 Causes of heart failure**
>
> *Primary myocardial disease*
> - Ischaemic heart disease; toxic (e.g. alcohol/cytotoxic drugs)
> - Infective (e.g. viral myocarditis)
> - Idiopathic or pregnancy-related cardiomyopathy.
>
> *Circulatory disease*
> - Hypertension; valvular heart disease; pericardial constriction
> - High output (e.g. anaemia or AV fistula).

Pathophysiology

This reflects the normal physiological response to cardiac injury. Raised end-diastolic volume (EDV) initially causes stretch of myocytes and hence increased contractility, but stroke volume eventually declines with continuing volume overload due to ventricular dilatation (Fig. 1.9).

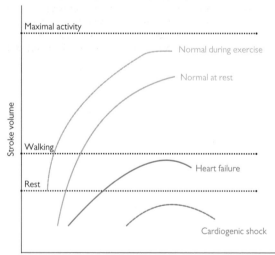

Fig. 1.9 Frank–Starling relationship.

Central sympathetic outflow and vasopressin release both increase, causing increased HR, peripheral vasoconstriction, and water reabsorption.

Sympathetic stimulation and renal hypoperfusion promote renin release from the juxtaglomerular apparatus: increased angiotensin II and aldosterone causes further vasoconstriction together with salt and water retention. These defences may be useful in the short-term response to injury, but *cause* harm as a long-term response to disease.

The result is a sustained haemodynamic burden on an already failing heart. The myocardium becomes thickened and hypertrophied with eventual fibrosis. This impairs both contractility and filling and may provoke arrhythmias.

The term *remodelling* describes how mechanical and neurohumoral factors act to alter ventricular size, shape and function. Therapies such as ACEI/β-blockers/resynchronization aim to induce so-called 'inverse remodelling' and a return to a more normal ventricular size and shape.

Diagnosis and staging of heart failure

The diagnosis requires typical symptoms and signs (shortness of breath/fatigue/oedema/gallop rhythm) *plus* objective evidence of ventricular dysfunction. Appropriate investigations include:

- Serum BNP: an important biomarker in patients with heart failure, secreted by ventricular myocytes in response to stress. It inhibits the renin–angiotensin–aldosterone system (RAAS), reducing renal Na^+ reabsorption and increasing glomerular filtration rate (GFR). Levels of BNP reflect the severity of heart failure and are useful in screening, diagnosis, and in assessing prognosis.
- ECG: usually abnormal—may show AF/hypertrophy or strain/conduction disease/signs of ischaemia or previous infarction.
- ECHO: may indicate severity ± cause, e.g. valvular heart disease.
- MRI/radionuclide scanning/cardiac catheterization: may add further information (see also section 1.3).

The ACC/AHA propose a four-stage classification for chronic heart failure. During stage A only risk factors for heart failure are present. At Stage B, structural heart disease, e.g. LVH, is present but the patient remains asymptomatic. At Stage C heart failure symptoms of dyspnoea or fatigue are present. Finally, Stage D represents refractory heart failure requiring specialist intervention.

Medical management of chronic heart failure

Treatment is aimed towards breaking the vicious cycle of neurohumoral activation and remodelling. The aims are both to reduce symptoms *and* to slow disease progression:

In *Stage A* disease, the goal is to prevent remodelling by aggressive control of risk factors: treat hypertension (aiming for diastolic BP <80mmHg); control diabetes/hyperlipidaemia; stop smoking; consider ACEI or ARA in some patients.

In *Stage B* disease, risk factor control continues: all patients should receive ACEI or ARA. NSAIDs should be avoided (fluid retention/renal impairment), and some patients should also receive β-blockers.

In *Stage C and D* disease (symptomatic heart failure), *all* patients should receive both ACEI/ARA *and* β blockers unless contraindications. Diuretics (spironolactone or loop diuretics) may improve symptoms, and digoxin may help in some cases. Consider hydralazine + nitrate combination in patients intolerant of ACEI/ARA.

Angiotensin-converting enzyme inhibitors

These are first-line treatment for LV dysfunction, *with or without symptoms*. Reduced angiotensin II and aldosterone causes less vasoconstriction/salt and water retention. Bradykinin breakdown is also reduced (promotes vasodilatation and natriuresis, but may produce chronic cough).

In surgical patients taking ACEIs, there is often concern about hypotension during or after induction: however, this is usually readily treated with vasopressors/sympathomimetics/judicious volume challenges. *Stopping* ACEIs may be even more harmful: the RAAS recovers rapidly, and the resultant adverse effects are less easily treatable.

The other concern is the possibility of renal impairment in the presence of hypovolaemia, when renal flood flow and GFR become dependent upon afferent arteriolar vasoconstriction via angiotensin II. A combination of hypovolaemia and ACEI may set up a vicious cycle of hypotension → reduced GFR → reduced clearance of ACEI. Regular monitoring of renal function is required: stop ACEI if there are significant intraoperative losses and/or renal dysfunction develops postoperatively.

Angiotensin receptor antagonists

These are an alternative to ACEIs in patients who develop cough or angioedema. They may also be used in combination when ACEIs and β-blockers fail to relieve symptoms. Similar concerns apply as with ACEI re: low BP and renal dysfunction. Hypotension may be relatively resistant to first-line sympathomimetics and sometimes associated with bradycardia: prophylactic glycopyrrolate has been recommended. ARAs are relatively long acting: if they are to be stopped perioperatively, this should be done at least 24h before surgery.

β-blockers

These promote inverse remodelling by counteracting the harmful effects of sympathetic stimulation. All patients with stable, chronic heart failure should be considered for β-blocker therapy (metoprolol, bisoprolol, or carvedilol). Caution is required, however, in patients with bradyarrhythmias (without a pacemaker), in reactive airways disease, and in patients with diabetes complicated by frequent hypoglycaemia (see section 1.5).

Diuretics

Evidence supports the use of spironolactone in advanced heart failure. By antagonizing the effects of aldosterone it reduces sodium retention, but interestingly, it may also act directly to reduce collagen synthesis and myocardial fibrosis. Loop diuretics (e.g. furosemide) are often used to control symptoms, but often at the expense of electrolyte imbalance, hypovolaemia and arrhythmias, especially in the elderly.

Cardiac resynchronization therapy in heart failure

Some 25% of patients with moderate-to-severe heart failure have LBBB. LV contraction becomes asynchronous, and ejection fraction and cardiac output are reduced. Simultaneous pacing of left and right ventricles (biventricular pacing) aims to resynchronize ventricular contraction (see section 5.7). Current guidelines for CRT include:

- Dilated cardiomyopathy with ejection fraction <35%.
- QRS duration >120ms.
- Poor functional status despite maximal medical therapy.

Diastolic heart failure

Between 30% and 50% of patients with chronic heart failure have a preserved ejection fraction. This proportion is at its highest in older patients and reflects age-related changes in the cardiovascular system (CVS; including systemic hypertension and changes in cardiac muscle structure) that cause impaired *relaxation*. Abnormal ventricular filling causes pulmonary congestion manifesting as shortness of breath and oedema. The ventricular pressure–volume relationship is characteristically altered (Fig. 1.10): the diastolic compliance curve is shifted upwards and to the left, i.e. increased LVEDP for a given LVEDV, resulting in pulmonary congestion. ACEIs and β-blockers remain first-line treatments.

Anaesthetic management of the patient with heart failure

No firm evidence exists to support any one technique (GA or regional anaesthesia) over another. The aim is to maintain preload, and to avoid myocardial depression, tachycardia, or increases in afterload. Invasive monitoring may allow anticipation or earlier detection of changes in haemodynamics. Neuraxial blockade may cause hypotension, but afterload reduction and good postoperative analgesia may be beneficial (see also section 1.5).

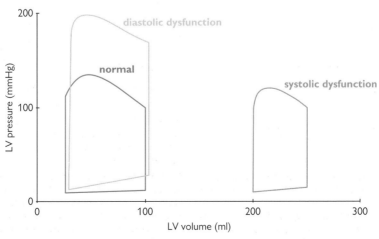

Fig. 1.10 Pressure–volume loops in heart failure.

Management of acute heart failure

Many patients presenting with acute heart failure and pulmonary oedema are hypertensive with relatively well-preserved LV function (as already discussed).

Vasodilators—typically nitrates—form the mainstay of therapy. Nesiritide, is a recombinant form of human BNP and acts as both a venous and arterial dilator (given by IV bolus then infusion). Diuretics are frequently used inappropriately as first-line agents in acute heart failure. Most patients are normo- or even hypovolaemic and are in pulmonary oedema because of a hypertrophied, stiff LV, not primarily because of fluid overload.

Patients who present with hypotension (i.e. in cardiogenic shock) may need early inotropic support (e.g. dobutamine, milrinone) ± vasopressors (e.g. noradrenaline) to maintain systolic BP. Levosimendan is a novel agent with an interesting dual action: it binds to troponin C in cardiac muscle to exert a positive inotropic effect, but also opens ATP-sensitive K^+ channels to cause peripheral arterial and venous dilatation.

Non-invasive ventilation should be considered *early* in *all* forms of acute heart failure. Both CPAP and BiPAP offer multiple benefits, reducing afterload, work of breathing, and the need for intubation in patients with acute pulmonary oedema.

Further reading

Groban L & Butterworth J (2006). Perioperative management of chronic heart failure. *Anesth Analg*, 103(3):557–75.

Hunt SA, Abraham WT, Chin MH, *et al*. (2005) ACC/AHA 2005 Guideline Update for the Diagnosis and Management of Chronic Heart Failure in the Adult: A Report of the American College of Cardiology/American Heart Association Task Force on Practice Guidelines (Writing Committee to Update the 2001 Guidelines for the Evaluation and Management of Heart Failure): Developed in Collaboration With the American College of Chest Physicians and the International Society for Heart and Lung Transplantation: Endorsed by the Heart Rhythm Society, *Circulation*, 112(12):154–235.

Jessup M & Brozena S (2003). Heart failure. *NEJM*, 348(20):2007–18. doi:10.1056/NEJMra021498.

Pirracchio R, Cholley B, De Hert S, *et al*. (2007). Diastolic heart failure in anaesthesia and critical care. *Br J Anaesth*, 98(6):707–21. doi:10.1093/bja/aem098.

Shock is a physiological state where there is a decrease in perfusion such that the oxygen delivery to tissues is inadequate to meet demand. Shock is a life-threatening condition, which if not treated promptly can lead to irreversible organ dysfunction and death.

The signs and symptoms of shock will differ according to the aetiology. However, signs of poor tissue perfusion would usually be expected, including oliguria, tachycardia, hypotension, tachypnoea, and altered conscious level.

Neurohumoral response to shock

The neural and humoral responses to shock happen concurrently although at different speeds. They are in fact seamlessly integrated, but can be considered separately to aid comprehension. Understanding the response can perhaps be best explained by considering the events that accompany an acute severe haemorrhage.

Neural response

The immediate response to acute blood loss is a decrease in venous return to the heart. This directly results in a decrease in stroke volume according to Frank–Starling's law. The decreased stroke volume manifests physiologically as a decrease in mean arterial pressure.

Baroreceptors in the arch of the aorta and carotid sinus are stretch sensitive mechanoreceptors. The baroreceptors detect hypotension and respond by decreasing afferent outflow to the nucleus tractus solitarius (NTS). In turn the NTS will decrease inhibitory outflow to the rostral ventrolateral medulla (the major pressor centre). This will result in an increased sympathetic outflow to the CVS, leading to tachycardia, increased inotropy and vasoconstriction, and thus an increase in blood pressure.

The sympathetic outflow will, via the splanchnic nerves directly stimulate the adrenal medulla leading to the release of adrenaline and noradrenaline into the bloodstream. This 'neural response' happens within seconds of hypotension.

Humoral response

The humoral response takes place concurrently with the neural response although is slower in both onset and effect (minutes rather than the seconds of the sympathetic response).

The endocrine responses are intrinsically interlinked to one another although can be usefully categorized by organ system.

Renal

Hypotension directly results in hypoperfusion of the kidneys. This gives rise to a decrease in afferent arteriolar pressure and a fall in GFR. The decreased flow of filtrate and crucially sodium delivery is detected by the cells of the macula densa, located in the wall of the distal convoluted tubule. In response to this, the cells release prostaglandins, which stimulate juxtaglomerular cells to release renin (cAMP mediated). Renin hydrolyses angiotensinogen to angiotensin I, which is in turn converted to angiotensin II.

Angiotensin II has a number of important acute functions:

- Direct arteriolar vasoconstriction via AT II receptors.
- Stimulation of aldosterone release from the adrenal cortex.
- Stimulates vasopressin release from the posterior pituitary.
- Stimulatory effect on sympathetic nervous system.

These functions serve to increase mean arterial pressure, divert blood flow away from non-vital organ systems and increase sodium and water retention in an attempt to restore normal circulating volume.

Adrenal

The adrenal response to volume loss has already been alluded to. Sympathetic outflow leads to direct adrenal medullary stimulation and catecholamine release.

The cortex responds to angiotensin II by stimulating aldosterone synthesis. Aldosterone is a steroid hormone, which has the overall effect of increasing sodium and water reabsorption at the distal tubule and collecting duct of the nephron.

Hypothalamo-pituitary axis

The shock state leads to adrenocorticotrophic hormone (ACTH) release from the anterior pituitary, which leads to increased cortisol levels. Cortisol augments vascular reactivity to catecholamines. Relative or absolute cortisol deficiency states may worsen outcome.

The hypothalamus receives direct input from the ventrolateral medulla following decreased baroreceptor firing in response to hypotension. This stimulates a release of arginine vasopressin (antidiuretic hormone, ADH) into the plasma. Plasma hyperosmolarity directly leads to a release of ADH. Plasma tonicity will be minimally affected in acute hypovolaemia but this mechanism may play a more significant role in other shock states—for example, sepsis where the onset of shock is more gradual.

ADH is an octapeptide with two significant roles in shock:

- Vasoconstriction: acts directly on V1 receptors in the peripheral vasculature. These same receptors lead to platelet aggregation when stimulated.
- Water retention: activates the V2 receptor in the renal collecting duct generating an increase in water permeability and reabsorption.

Cardiac

Not traditionally considered an endocrine organ, the heart has an important humoral role in shock states. Atrial natriuretic peptide (ANP) is produced and stored in cardiac myocytes. ANPs physiological role is to promote sodium and water loss via the kidneys and peripheral vasodilatation via specific receptors. The fall in venous return during shock decreases the amount of ANP release thus promoting vasoconstriction and water conservation in keeping with the other humoral responses.

Degrees of shock

The physiological responses explain the progressive clinical features that accompany shock states. As the condition worsens, the adverse effects of these protective measures become apparent with dysfunction of different organ systems. Haemorrhagic shock (as adapted from Advanced Trauma Life Support, ATLS) is usefully classified into four categories of severity (see Table 1.9).

Not all patients will present within these discrete groups, but despite this, the classification provides a useful reference for degrees of volume loss.

Table 1.9 Stages of shock				
Stage	I	II	III	IV
Blood loss	<15%	15–30%	30–40%	>40%
Blood pressure	Normal	Normal	Decreased	Decreased
Heart rate (beats/min)	<100	100–120	120–140	>140
Respiratory rate (breaths/min)	14–20	20–30	30–40	>35
Urine output	>30mL/h	20–30 mL/h	5–15mL/h	Negligible
Mental state	Slightly anxious	Mildly anxious	Anxious, confused	Confused, lethargic

Reproduced from *ATLS Student Course Manual*, 8th edition, Table 3.1, p. 61, with permission from the ATLS and the American College of Surgeons.

Types of shock

The aetiology of shock falls into the following groups:
- Hypovolaemic
- Anaphylactic (distributive)
- Septic
- Neurogenic
- Cardiogenic
- Obstructive (often combined with cardiogenic).

Although some of the physiological responses are similar between groups there are key differences between them.

Hypovolaemic shock

The physiological response is essentially as already described whether the cause is blood loss or dehydration although the humoral aspects may be more established in dehydration that is by its nature of a slower onset.

Shock following trauma has a number of key differences. Rapid correction of shock states in patients with ongoing haemorrhage may promote further bleeding and worsen outcome and indeed hypotension is often tolerated with minimal resuscitation until haemorrhage control is achieved.

The combination of shock and tissue injury in these patients promotes an early coagulopathy and fibrinolysis. Volume replacement, when undertaken, should involve packed red cells with aggressive use of plasma and platelets.

Anaphylactic shock

Uncontrolled and widespread mast cell granulation leads to massive histamine and cytokine release. This inflammatory response overcomes the ability to vasoconstrict in response to hypotension. Gross vasodilatation and systemic capillary leak follow rapidly, possibly accompanied by a degree of direct cardiac impairment. The clinical picture may differ with generalized flushing rather than impaired peripheral perfusion. Often accompanied by bronchoconstriction and angio-oedema, emergent treatment is required with adrenaline the priority rather than volume replacement.

Sepsis

A commonly encountered condition which mandates prompt therapy. Patients may exhibit the typical vasoconstricted picture but may also be vasodilated and apparently well perfused (previously termed warm shock). Without management this picture will change to the more typical picture as perfusion becomes more inadequate. Septic shock is similar to anaphylactic shock with vasodilatation and capillary leak due to a significant inflammatory cascade component. There may be specific impairments in cortisol and vasopressin function, which further contribute to the shock. Volume replacement requirements are often large and may require concurrent vasopressor therapy. Early broad-spectrum antibiotics are crucial, with possible roles for steroid and vasopressin therapy in certain cases (see section 20.3).

Neurogenic

Spinal cord injury results in an immediate vasoplegia below the level of injury secondary to sympathetic injury. The severity of the shock state depends on the level of the injury with higher lesions yielding more severe signs. Lack of sympathetic innervation peripherally explains the clinical picture of warm dry peripheries. Injuries above T4 may interrupt sympathetic supply to the heart leading to a paradoxical bradycardia. It is crucial to exclude concomitant hypovolaemia, but in a likely injury early vasopressor therapy may be indicated (see section 6.6).

Cardiogenic

A very typical picture of sympathetic overactivity (clamminess and tachycardia) accompanies hypotension and impaired perfusion. Acute myocardial insufficiency carries a high morbidity and mortality. It is important to distinguish this aetiological category, as therapeutic options may be quite different. Fluid offloading rather than resuscitation may be necessary and inotropes may be helpful whereas vasopressor therapy may worsen the failing myocardium. Treatment of the cause, if possible (e.g. coronary artery occlusion) is important to facilitate resolution.

Obstructive

Massive pulmonary embolus, tension pneumothorax, and pericardial tamponade cause a mechanical obstruction to cardiac output. The pathophysiology variously encompasses changes in preload and afterload depending on underlying cause. The clinical picture is one of sympathetic hyper-activity in keeping with cardiogenic or hypovolaemic shock states. Distended veins although often described in texts are unreliable indicators, whether positive or negative. History, clinical examination, timely investigation, and a high index of suspicion are key to identification. Treatment of the underlying cause will often give rise to a rapid and significant resolution of the impaired perfusion.

Further reading

Sethi AK, Sharma P, Mohta M, *et al.* (2003). Shock – a short review. *Indian J Anaesth*, 47(5):345–59.

1.15 Ischaemic heart disease

Ischaemic heart disease (IHD) remains extremely prevalent in the Western world and its incidence is now increasing in developing countries. In the UK, it remains the commonest cause of death (88 000 deaths in 2008), and also of *premature* death (28 000 deaths in 2008). Notwithstanding its obvious significance in respect of health and healthcare in general, IHD also has important implications for the safe delivery of anaesthesia. 60% per cent of patients who die within 30 days of surgery have evidence of IHD.

Aetiology

The usual cause of IHD is coronary artery disease (CAD). Atheromatous plaques, composed principally of lipid and smooth muscle proliferation, are deposited within coronary arteries, causing luminal narrowing sufficient to restrict myocardial blood flow. Subsequently, when myocardial oxygen demands exceed supply in times of stress, ischaemia occurs. Plaque rupture may precipitate thrombosis, leading to total occlusion of the vessel and MI.

Risk factors for IHD

- Age: incidence increases with age.
- Gender: more prevalent in males (5× at age 50 years).
- Serum cholesterol: IHD risk increases dramatically when LDL:HDL ratio >4:1.
- Smoking: increases incidence by 60%.
- Hypertension: increases risk whether systolic or diastolic.
- Diabetes mellitus.
- Positive family history.

Pathophysiology of myocardial ischaemia

Ischaemia manifests when there is an imbalance between oxygen *supply* and *demand* within the myocardium (see Table 1.10).

Table 1.10 Myocardial ischaemia: supply and demand	
Supply	**Demand**
Heart rate: Max diastolic coronary flow with low/normal heart rate	*Heart rate:* Tachycardia increases myocardial VO_2 *and* reduces diastolic filling time
Coronary perfusion pressure: Aortic diastolic BP − LVEDP	*Contractility:* Increases during stress due to sympathohumoral activation
Coronary artery diameter: Narrowed with atheroma	*Ventricular wall tension:* According to preload and afterload
Arterial oxygen content: Dependent on Hb and arterial PO_2	

Management of chronic stable IHD

Patients with chronic stable angina have an average annual mortality of 2–3%. Treatment can be broadly divided into medical and mechanical interventions.

Drug therapy

Pharmacological treatments involve:

- Antianginal agents: β-blockers, nitrates and calcium channel blockers (CCBs). β-blockers reduce myocardial oxygen demand. Nitrates reduce myocardial oxygen demand and improve perfusion with effects augmented by co-administration with CCBs and β-blockers. CCBs improve coronary blood flow by reducing coronary vascular resistance and reduce myocardial oxygen demand by reducing peripheral SVR.
- Antiplatelet agents (aspirin, clopidogrel): aspirin inhibits formation of thromboxane A2, reducing platelet activation but having no effect on adhesion. It remains the mainstay of treatment for chronic IHD and may reduce risk of death in unstable angina by up to 50%. Clopidogrel inhibits ADP-mediated platelet aggregation and can act in synergy with aspirin.
- Antithrombotic agents: low-molecular-weight heparin (LMWH) reduces fibrinogen levels and does not require monitoring of activated partial thromboplastin time (APTT).
- Lipid-lowering agents: HMG CoA reductase inhibitors (statins) have been shown to reduce fatal and non-fatal MI.
- ACEIs: shown by HOPE trial (Heart Outcomes Prevention Evaluation) to reduce risk of MI and stroke in patients with vascular disease but no heart failure. Recommended by trial to be of use in routine secondary prevention for patients with CAD.

Revascularization

Non-pharmacological treatments involve re-vascularization techniques. A cardiological opinion should be sought if it is felt that the patient may benefit from coronary angioplasty or CABG.

Acute coronary syndromes

The term 'acute coronary syndrome' (ACS) comprises three conditions: unstable angina (UA), non-ST elevation MI (NSTEMI), and ST-elevation MI (STEMI). UA and NSTEMI occur when non-occluding thrombus develops over plaque rupture. Myonecrosis in this scenario may develop as a result of distal vasospasm or embolization.

Treatment of STEMI is focused on rapid restoration of coronary blood flow by pharmacological and catheter-based means. Suppression of recurrent ischaemic events is achieved through subsequent antithrombotic therapy. Re-perfusion in STEMI is achieved by fibrinolysis or catheter-based means. Bolus dose fibrin-specific agents (tPA) have replaced non-fibrin-specific agents (streptokinase), achieving greater vessel patency with similar mortality benefits.

Catheter-based reperfusion is resource intensive and harder to implement but appears to offer improved clinical outcomes. Meta-analysis of over 20 trials reveals that percutaneous coronary intervention (PCI) reduces rates of early death, reinfarction and haemorrhagic stroke when compared to fibrinolysis.

Treatment of UA and NSTEMI is aimed at reducing ischaemia and achieving plaque stabilization:

- Reducing platelet aggregation (aspirin, glycoprotein 2b/3a inhibitors, clopidogrel).
- Preventing thrombus propagation (unfractionated or LMWH). Unfractionated and LMWH have been shown to be beneficial when given with aspirin in patients presenting with UA. LMWH has the benefits of a longer half-life and the lack of need to monitor the APTT, but absence of an antidote and the long half-life make the risk of bleeding potentially higher.
- Anti-ischaemic agents: β-blockade remains the treatment of choice with more cardio-selective agents (e.g. bisoprolol) preferred.

- Symptomatic relief of chest pain achieved with nitrates (oral or buccal) and opiates.
- Statins: given at high dose at time of presentation may reduce further ischaemic events.
- Thrombolytics: not shown to have any benefit in NSTEMI/UA and are associated with increased morbidity and mortality in these patients.
- Intervention with PCI or CABG soon after presentation with UA has been shown to reduce recurrent chest pain and MI (in those with troponin rises), but there is little evidence that mortality is altered, with one British study showing higher mortality in this group as compared to a conservative treatment group. PCI for NSTEMI/UA should only be considered for high-risk patients.

Anaesthesia in patients with IHD

The perioperative period may provoke myocardial ischaemia for a number of reasons:
- As part of the stress response to surgery, increased circulating catecholamines promote tachycardia, increased afterload, and coronary vasoconstriction.
- Most anaesthetic agents cause a reduced aortic diastolic pressure which reduces coronary perfusion pressure.
- Blood loss reduces oxygen supply.
- Hypercoagulability increases susceptibility to thrombosis.

Preoperative evaluation
A careful history should elicit:
- The patient's functional capacity and frequency of anginal symptoms.
- Previous MI (high risk of reinfarction if surgery undertaken within 3 months).
- Previous coronary revascularization procedures (including presence and types of stents).
- Current medications (including antiplatelet therapy).

In general, non-cardiac surgery is considered safe in patients with good functional capacity and stable angina. However, the nature of surgery is also an independent risk factor for perioperative ischaemia with major vascular surgical patients three times more likely to suffer a perioperative ischaemic event than non-vascular patients.

Cardiological advice and support should be sought for perioperative care of high-risk patients (those with a history of MI, PCI, or CABG within the past 6 weeks, patients with unstable angina, or those with recurrent ischaemia post-MI) and only emergency surgery should be considered in this group. Advice may be required regarding pre-optimization of medication (e.g. β-blockers or antiplatelet therapy). For many years, β-blocker therapy was suggested to reduce perioperative ischaemia: recent studies suggest reduced mortality in high-risk (but not low-risk) patients. If the history is suggestive of unstable angina, a cardiology opinion should be sought since PCI or coronary bypass surgery may be required prior to elective surgery. See sections 1.1–1.5 for further details.

Anaesthetic technique
The essential tenet for safe anaesthesia in IHD is to keep myocardial oxygen delivery greater than demand. Choosing drugs and techniques that avoid tachycardia whilst maintaining normotension assists this fundamental requirement.

Premedication
- Anxiety-related tachycardia should be avoided (preoperative benzodiazepines may be indicated).
- Continue antianginal medications (in the knowledge that these may augment the hypotensive effects of anaesthetic agents).

Induction
- Consider arterial line insertion (under LA ± sedation) prior to induction for close BP monitoring.
- Nearly all IV agents cause direct myocardial depression and may reduce SVR: the resulting tachycardia and hypotension can usually be minimized by slow and careful agent administration. Vasopressors should be immediately available.
- The pressor response to intubation should be attenuated with fast-acting opioid prior to laryngoscopy (having also ensured complete neuromuscular relaxation).

Monitoring
- Requirements depend on the surgical procedure and the severity of the underlying cardiac disease.
- Arterial and central venous lines are required if vasoactive infusions are likely to be needed.
- Intraoperative TOE can be used to monitor ventricular function and regional wall motion abnormalities during cardiac or high-risk general surgery.

Analgesia/regional techniques
- Opioids attenuate the surgical stress response.
- Regional techniques may avoid the depressant effects of GA.
- Epidural analgesia reduces preload and afterload, and thoracic sympathetic blockade attenuates the cardiac response to stress: associated hypotension should be treated promptly and aggressively to reduce ischaemia.

Postoperative care
- Ensure oxygen delivery exceeds demand throughout postoperative period.
- Avoid early postoperative ischaemic precipitants (hypoxia, pain, tachycardia, hypotension, shivering, anaemia).
- Monitoring on HDU/ITU post-op if indicated.

Further reading

Lindenauer PK, Pekow P, Wang K, et al.(2005). Perioperative beta-blocker therapy and mortality after major noncardiac surgery. *NEJM*, 353(4):349–61.

Sheppard LP & Channer KS (2004). Acute coronary syndromes. *CEACCP*, 4:175–80. doi:10.1093/bjaceaccp/mkh048.

White HD & Chew DP (2008). Acute myocardial infarction. *Lancet*, 372(9638):570–84. doi:10.1016/S0140-6736(08)61237-4.

1.16 Valvular heart disease

Aortic stenosis

Epidemiology
Aortic stenosis (AS) is the commonest major valve lesion, present in 3% of people aged >75 years, rising to 4% in those >85 years of age.

Aetiology
- Age-related progressive calcification of normal tri-leaflet valve (50% of cases)
- Calcification of a congenital bicuspid valve
- Rheumatic heart disease

Pathophysiology
LV outflow obstruction occurs due to narrowing of the aortic orifice. This leads over time to concentric LV hypertrophy and a reduction in LV compliance. The eventual result is a fixed low cardiac output state and—importantly—an inability to compensate for systemic vasodilatation. This process typically occurs as the valve area decreases over time from a normal 2.5–3.5cm² to about 1cm² (Table 1.11). The hypertrophied, non-compliant LV requires high filling pressures (normal LVEDP may reflect hypovolaemia), making AS patients sensitive to both preload and rhythms other than sinus (Fig. 1.11). The contribution of atrial contraction to LV filling in sinus rhythm may be up to 20% in a normal heart but may rise to 40% in AS. Patients with AS have a higher risk of myocardial ischaemia due to increased oxygen demands and wall tension within the hypertrophied LV. Up to 30% of patients with AS get angina even in the context of normal coronary arteries.

Clinical progression of AS
As the valve area narrows to around 1cm², symptoms develop as cardiac output becomes compromised. Angina may develop due to increased work of the heart and reduced compliance. With disease progression the LV begins to dilate, the atria may develop fibrillation, and the patient may experience exertional syncope or pulmonary congestion. The onset of angina is associated with an average survival of 5 years, syncope 3 years, and congestive heart failure 2 years. Valve replacement is recommended with a valve area of 0.8cm² or evidence of ventricular dysfunction.

Table 1.11 Severity grading of aortic stenosis		
Degree of AS	Mean ΔP (mmHg)	Valve area (cm²)
Mild	<25	<1.5
Moderate	25–40	1–1.5
Severe	>40	<1.0
Critical	>70	<0.6

Reproduced from Bonow RO, et al., '2008 Focused Update Incorporated Into the ACC/AHA 2006 Guidelines for the Management of Patients With Valvular Heart Disease: A Report of the American College of Cardiology/American Heart Association Task Force on Practice Guidelines (Writing Committee to Revise the 1998 Guidelines for the Management of Patients With Valvular Heart Disease): Endorsed by the Society of Cardiovascular Anesthesiologists, Society for Cardiovascular Angiography and Interventions, and Society of Thoracic Surgeons', *Circulation*, 118, 15, pp. 523–661, copyright 2008 American Heart Association, published by Wolters Kluwer, with permission. Adapted from *Journal of the American Society of Echocardiography*, 16, 7, Zoghbi WA et al., 'Recommendations for evaluation of the severity of native valvular regurgitation with two-dimensional and doppler echocardiography', pp.777–802, copyright 2003, with permission from American Society of Echocardiography.

Clinical management

Investigations
ECG (LVH/strain pattern), ECHO, cardiac catheterization (assessment of pressure gradient either side of valve, and coronary patency).

Preoperative care
Symptomatic patients for elective non-cardiac surgery should have their valve replaced beforehand (if sufficiently fit). Transcatheter aortic valve replacement (TAVI) may be considered in elderly patients.

Asymptomatic patients for major elective surgery associated with major fluid shifts (major abdominal, orthopaedic, vascular) and with a valve gradient >50mmHg should have valve replacement beforehand.

Monitoring
Arterial line (pre-induction) ± CVC, TOE and/or PAC.

Anaesthetic goals
- Maintain normal (low) HR.
- Maintain sinus rhythm (have defibrillator attached).
- Maintain adequate volume loading (preload).
- Maintain high (normal) SVR.

Anaesthetic techniques should aim to maintain afterload and avoid tachycardia. To facilitate this, regional techniques are relatively contraindicated, and all anaesthetic agents must be administered in such a way as to cause minimal haemodynamic disturbance. Patients with AS have a fixed low cardiac output and can't compensate for falls in SVR which may cause severe hypotension, myocardial ischaemia, reduced contractility, and further falls in BP and coronary perfusion. Consequently, hypotension must be recognized and treated promptly.

Postoperative care
Patients should be monitored in a HDU or ITU setting so that close attention may be paid to fluid filling status, BP maintenance, and cardiac rhythm. Blood loss, tachycardia, and hypotension should all be recognized early and treated aggressively.

Aortic regurgitation

Aetiology
- Commonest adult causes are post-rheumatic fever, bacterial endocarditis, and aortic dissection (trauma)
- Connective tissue disorders (ankylosing spondylitis, Marfan's syndrome and tertiary syphilis) dilate the aortic root, causing secondary aortic regurgitation (AR)

Pathophysiology
There is volume overload of the LV causing dilation and eccentric hypertrophy (Fig. 1.11). Afterload and heart rate determine the regurgitant load. A lower aortic pressure lowers LV afterload, thus increasing forward flow. HR is usually elevated so reducing the time spent in diastole and reducing AR.

Clinical progression of AR

Acute AR
Usually secondary to bacterial endocarditis or aortic dissection. Presents with acute LV failure/pulmonary oedema and requires emergency surgical correction.

Chronic AR

Regurgitation occurs over many years giving the LV time to adapt to an increased volume load. Symptoms of LV failure arise following a rise in LVEDP and herald progressive LV dysfunction. The onset of dyspnoea usually signifies mortality within 2–4 years.

Investigations

ECG (voltage criteria for LVH), CXR (cardiomegaly/LVF), ECHO.

Clinical management

Preoperative care

Patients with functional capacity <4 METs (a flight of stairs) should be considered for valve surgery prior to elective surgery.

Monitoring

Invasive BP monitoring ± CVC ± TOE.

Anaesthetic aims

- High (normal) HR (approximately 90bpm)
- Adequate preload
- Low/normal SVR
- Maintain contractility.

Unlike in AS, regional anaesthetic techniques may be well tolerated in AR. Invasive monitoring may facilitate rapid appropriate responses to haemodynamic change and drugs that have negative inotropic or positive chronotropic effects should be used with extreme caution.

Mitral stenosis

Aetiology

Rheumatic fever remains the commonest cause. Mixed mitral valve disease (mitral stenosis (MS) and regurgitation (MR)) is more common than isolated MS.

Pathophysiology

The LV is chronically under-filled causing both volume and pressure increases proximal to mitral valve (Fig. 1.11). The LV functions normally despite poor filling. LV filling is aided when the HR is low (increased diastolic filling time). As valve area reduces, so the pressure gradient across valve must increase to maintain stroke volume. The LA dilates to maintain normal PA pressures but as the disease worsens, the PA pressure rises, causing chronic pulmonary hypertension. The RV hypertrophies in response and then eventually fails.

Clinical progression of MS

The normal valve area is 4–6cm². Exertional dyspnoea, fatigue, palpitations may develop when valve area <1.5cm².

Investigations

ECG, CXR (valve calcification, splaying of carina, pulmonary congestion), ECHO.

Clinical management

Preoperative care

Corrective valvular surgery is required prior to elective non-cardiac surgery if functional capacity <4 METs.

Monitoring

Invasive BP monitoring ± CVC and/or TOE.

Anaesthetic aims

- Maintain adequate diastolic filling time (low/normal rate sinus rhythm) and control ventricular rate if in AF (β-blockers, CCBs).
- Maintain adequate pre-load.
- Avoid factors causing raised pulmonary artery pressures (hypercarbia, acidosis, hypoxia).
- Maintain contractility and high/normal SVR.
- Maintenance of haemodynamic stability necessitates careful management of fluid /volume status, and therefore epidural/spinal anaesthesia is particularly hazardous. In the context of primary cardiac surgery, the chronically underfilled LV may fail to cope with the sudden increase in pre-load associated with mitral valve repair. In such cases, inotropic support may be necessary.

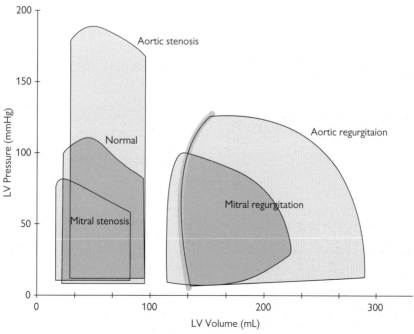

Fig. 1.11 Pressure–volume loops in valvular heart disease.

Mitral regurgitation

Aetiology
This occurs either as a primary valvular dysfunction or secondary to LV dysfunction. Leaflet MR may occur after endocarditis, rheumatic fever, or MV prolapse. Chordal MR occurs when chordae rupture during endocarditis or after MI. Papillary muscle MR arises due to ischaemic papillary muscle dysfunction. LV failure may cause varying amounts of MR due to annular dilatation.

Pathophysiology
The regurgitant fraction is determined by afterload, the size of the regurgitant orifice, and the HR. Like AR, there is compensatory peripheral vasodilatation to reduce regurgitation. Regurgitation occurs during systole (diastole in AR) from the LV to the LA. MR fractions >60% of SV compromise cardiac output. Dilatation of the LA occurs over decades in chronic MR thus keeping LA pressure low until late in the disease (pulmonary congestion may present late) (Fig. 1.11).

Clinical history
Acute MR (endocarditis, MI) presents with sudden volume overload of the LV and LA and warrants urgent surgical correction. Chronic MR may present with symptoms of fatigue, weakness dyspnoea and palpitations (AF).

Investigations
ECG, CXR, ECHO.

Clinical management

Preoperative care
Patients with reduced functional capacity (<4 METS) should be considered for corrective surgery prior to elective surgery.

Anaesthetic aims
- Avoid bradycardia (may cause acute ventricular dilation thus increasing MR), and maintain normal/high HR.
- Adequate pre-load.
- Maintain low/normal SVR (to reduce regurgitant fraction).
- Avoid precipitants of raised PAPs (hypercarbia, hypoxia, acidosis).
- As in AR, epidural analgesia may be relatively well tolerated (reducing afterload/SVR thus maintaining forward flow whilst reducing the regurgitant fraction).
- Acute LV failure may occur after valve repair as the low-resistance MR pathway is lost. A requirement for inotropic support should be anticipated, and high-dependency aftercare sought.

Further reading

Frogel J & Galusca D (2010). Anesthetic considerations for patients with advanced valvular heart disease undergoing non-cardiac surgery. *Anesthesiol Clin*, 28:67–85.

1.17 Systemic hypertension

Hypertension is present in some 30% of the UK adult population. It is an important risk factor for IHD, heart failure, renal failure, and stroke, and is one of the commonest intercurrent diseases in patients presenting for anaesthesia.

Aetiology of hypertension

Some 95% of cases fall into the category of 'essential hypertension', implying that there is no identifiable underlying cause. In the remaining 5%, the hypertension occurs secondary to an underlying medical condition (see Box 1.32).

Box 1.32 Aetiology of hypertension

Essential (primary) hypertension
- Elevated BP without obvious secondary cause.

Secondary hypertension
- Vascular: coarctation of the aorta, renal artery stenosis
- Endocrine: phaeochromocytoma, Conn's syndrome, Cushing's syndrome, acromegaly, thyroid dysfunction
- Renal disease
- Pregnancy-induced hypertension
- Drug induced: clinical or recreational (e.g. corticosteroids, sympathomimetics).

Classification of hypertension

Hypertension is generally classified into various stages, according to well-defined and widely accepted bands (see Table 1.12).

Table 1.12 Stages of hypertension

Category	Systolic pressure (mmHg)		Diastolic pressure (mmHg)
Optimal	<120	and	<80
Normal	<130	and	<85
High normal	130–139	or	85–89
Hypertension			
Stage 1: mild	140–159	or	90–99
Stage 2: moderate	160–179	or	100–109
Stage 3: severe	180–209	or	110–119
Stage 4: very severe	>210	or	>120
Isolated systolic hypertension	>140	and	<90

Reproduced from Mancia G, De Backer G, Dominiczak A, *et al.*, '2007 ESH-ESC Practice Guidelines for the Management of Arterial Hypertension: ESH-ESC Task Force on the Management of Arterial Hypertension', *Journal of Hypertension*, 25, 9, pp. 1751–1762, copyright 2007, with permission from Wolters Kluwer.

Pathogenesis of hypertension

Systolic BP rises continuously with age, whilst diastolic BP reaches a plateau in late middle age and may then decrease. Pulse pressure therefore rises. It was previously thought that *diastolic* BP was the most important determinant of outcome, but more recent work suggests that *systolic* hypertension is the crucial issue and that this should be the target for blood pressure control.

The concept of *pulse pressure hypertension* has gained prominence as a recognized important risk factor for stroke and MI.

A raised pulse pressure induces stress forces on the vascular tree, causing endothelial dysfunction and an increased risk of plaque rupture.

The autonomic nervous system and RAAS are key in maintaining normotension. Dysfunction in these systems is thought to play a role in pathological hypertension.

Sympathetic overactivation has been implicated in causing a rise in BP through baroreceptor activation. Once hypertension is established, the baroreceptors 'reset' to the new level and the condition persists. Some patients are noted to have exaggerated sympathetic responses to stressors and exogenous vasopressors.

RAAS disorders will be contributory in some groups of patients, and in fact renin activity is normal or increased in 75% of hypertensive patients (where it might be expected to fall through negative feedback). Many patients have an impaired natriuretic reaction to volume excess.

Once hypertension is established it becomes self-propagating without treatment. Baroreceptor resetting, vascular remodelling (with consequent luminal narrowing and increased vascular resistance), and LV hypertrophy will predispose to further rises in BP.

Chronic arterial hypertension produces end-organ damage, predominantly of the heart, kidney. and brain.

Effects on heart and vascular tree

Chronic hypertension increases arterial and arteriolar wall stress. The high pressure induces endothelial dysfunction, altering physiological NO function. This dysfunction promotes atherosclerotic plaque formation.

Similarly, the elevated pressure and resulting increased wall tension accelerate the pathological process by which arterial aneurysms form.

Increased myocardial wall tension results in concentric LV hypertrophy. This hypertrophied muscle exhibits poorer diastolic relaxation and as such the coronary arterial transmural pressures are higher. Thus, diastolic blood flow to the heart is impaired. This is further impaired by accelerated coronary atherosclerosis. This leads to cardiac ischaemia and potentially infarction.

Long-term 'pressure overload' can lead to LV failure.

Renal manifestations

The renal vasculature is affected by atherosclerotic plaque formation. The resultant ischaemia can lead to tubular atrophy and glomerular injury. Nephropathy can lead to proteinuria, haematuria, and ultimately renal failure.

With established hypertension, renovascular autoregulation becomes defective with a shift to higher pressure. This increases the likelihood of renal injury in the presence of hypotensive insults.

Cerebral

Cerebral pathology occurs following a similar pattern. Atherosclerotic change in the carotid arteries and subsequent stenosis can lead to both embolic events and global ischaemia secondary to relative hypotension.

A 'right shift' occurs in the cerebral autoregulation curve (see section 22.5). Patients are thus predisposed to both ischaemic and haemorrhagic strokes.

Management of hypertension

Numerous guidelines and consensus statements exist for the management of hypertension. In the UK, these are produced by the National Institute for Health and Clinical Excellence (NICE) in partnership with the British Hypertension Society (BHS).

Outpatient BP readings >140/90mmHg should be investigated further with ambulatory blood pressure monitoring (ABPM). Patients with average ABPM >135/85 should be considered for treatment, depending on cardiovascular risk factors and coexisting disease.

Patients with stage 2 or above hypertension should be offered treatment independently of coexisting disease, and those <40 years old should be referred for specialist review.

The type of pharmacological intervention varies according to the patient group. Six major classes of drug are available for treatment of essential hypertension (see Box 1.33).

> **Box 1.33 Drug therapies for essential hypertension**
>
> - Calcium channel blockers (CCBs)
> - Angiotensin-converting enzyme inhibitors (ACEIs)
> - Angiotensin-2 receptor antagonists (ARAs)
> - Thiazide diuretics
> - β-blockers
> - α-blockers.

Calcium channel blockers

CCBs have a proven efficacy, especially in stroke prevention, and are first-line therapy in the over 55s and in black patients. They have few major side effects, and can safely be continued perioperatively if the patient has a normal mean arterial pressure. Metabolism is via CYP3A4, in common with many other drugs and therefore affected by enzyme induction or inhibition.

ACEIs and ARAs

These are usually withheld on the day of surgery to avoid post-induction hypotension. The arguments for continuing these or stopping them in patients with coexistent heart failure are more complex, and are discussed in section 1.13.

They can be associated with renal failure postoperatively especially if patients are hypovolaemic or in combination with NSAIDs or diuretics.

Electrolyte disturbances include hyperkalaemia secondary to decreased aldosterone levels.

Thiazide diuretics

These are commonly used, typically as second-line therapy. The antihypertensive effect appears to be beyond the simple volume reduction effect of the drugs. They present a number of potential problems including hypovolaemia, hyponatraemia, hypo/hyperkalaemia, and hypercalcaemia.

β-blockers

β-blockers were previously the mainstay of treatment, but within the last decade, studies such as the ASCOT and VALUE trials have drawn attention to their potential adverse effects (all β-blockers have a pre-diabetic potential) and to the greater efficacy of CCBs, especially in terms of stroke protection.

β-blocker therapy should be continued throughout the perioperative period. An important perioperative consideration is bradycardia especially in procedures likely to increase vagal tone or in combination with high-dose opioids. Non-dihydropyridine calcium channel antagonists (e.g. verapamil) are contraindicated in patients with established β-blockade.

α-blockers

Selective α₁ adrenergic blockers are used as second- or third-line therapy. Their important adverse effect is hypotension, especially orthostatic hypotension. The 'first-dose' phenomenon of a significant drop in BP should be borne in mind when reinstituting therapy after a prolonged omission perioperatively.

Perioperative approach to the hypertensive patient

Preoperative assessment

The emphasis should be on detecting end-organ dysfunction (cardiovascular, cerebral, and renal), the presence of which is a better predictor of adverse outcome than hypertension alone. As a minimum, this should include ECG, urea and electrolytes, GFR, blood glucose, and a urine dipstick.

Patients with mild-to-moderate hypertension, and no additional risk factors nor evidence of end-organ dysfunction, can safely proceed to anaesthesia and surgery.

Patients with poorly controlled (stage 3) hypertension should as a minimum be screened for end-organ damage. Patients with stage 4 disease pose a significant perioperative risk, and should be deferred for treatment if at all possible.

A suggested algorithm for a patient with previously undiagnosed hypertension who requires surgery is presented in Fig. 1.12.

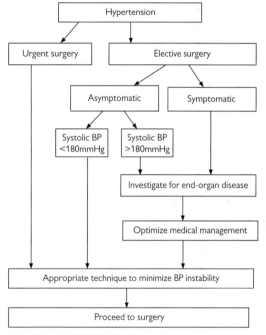

Fig. 1.12 Suggested algorithm for the hypertensive surgical patient. Adapted from Figure 1 in *South African Journal of Anaesthesia and Analgesia*, 17, 2, 'A modern look at hypertension and anaesthesia', MFM James, RA Dyer, and BL Rayner, Copyright 2011, with permission from South African Society of Anaesthesiologists

Anaesthetic technique

Hypertensive patients show greater cardiovascular lability under anaesthesia. Prolonged hypotension (<40% normal) is independently associated with cardiac events. One should have a low threshold for invasive arterial BP monitoring, aiming to maintain BP within 20% of baseline throughout the procedure. Controlling the response to intubation (or avoiding intubation altogether) is important. Consideration should be made for continuing management in a HDU postoperatively, and ensuring good analgesia.

Further reading

James MFM, Dyer RA, & Rayner BL (2011). A modern look at hypertension and anaesthesia. *S Afr J Anaesth Analg*, 17(2):168–73.

Sear JW (2008). Perioperative control of hypertension: when will it adversely affect perioperative outcome? *Curr Hypertens Rep*, 10(6):480–7.

1.18 Pulmonary hypertension

Pulmonary hypertension is a disease state characterized by abnormally high blood pressure within the pulmonary vessels, which leads to strain on the usually low pressure bearing right ventricle. Whilst there are numerous aetiologies and associated disease processes, the eventual outcome is right ventricular failure.

Patients with pulmonary hypertension who require surgery are at high risk of perioperative morbidity and mortality (up to 7% mortality after non-cardiac surgery).

Normal pulmonary system physiology

The pulmonary circulation is a low pressure, low resistance system with mean arterial pressures of around 8–20mmHg at rest. The pulmonary vessels are thin-walled and highly distensible with enormous capacitance and have the unique property of vasoconstriction with hypoxia and relaxation with hyperoxia. Because of the extreme compliance within the pulmonary circulation, changes in CO and gravity may affect the pulmonary vessels more than the systemic circulation.

Classification

Pulmonary hypertension is defined as a mean pulmonary artery pressure (MPAP) ≥25mmHg at rest or 30mmHg on exercise.

There are multiple aetiologies of pulmonary hypertension and identification of the underlying cause is crucial in order to manage the disease. Five major groups have been classified (Box 1.34).

Box 1.34 Classification of pulmonary hypertension

- Pulmonary arterial hypertension (PAH).
- Pulmonary hypertension with left heart disease.
- Pulmonary hypertension associated with lung diseases and/ or hypoxaemia.
- Pulmonary hypertension due to thrombotic and/or embolic disease.
- Miscellaneous, e.g. metabolic or haematological disorders.

PAH that is *not* associated with a precipitating disease (formerly known as primary pulmonary hypertension) is the rarest of these groups (1–2 cases per million) with the majority of pulmonary hypertension being secondary to cardiac, pulmonary, or respiratory disease.

Pathogenesis

The pathological process central to development of pulmonary hypertension is increased PVR, which places an increased workload on the right side of the heart.

In non-PAH pulmonary hypertension, the precise cellular changes occurring within the vessels vary according to underlying disease. For example, in pulmonary hypertension associated with thromboembolic disease, the cross section of the pulmonary vascular bed is reduced by obstruction due to organized thrombus.

In PAH there are numerous pathogenic pathways, which result in medial smooth muscle hypertrophy and thickening or fibrosis of the vessel intima, some of which may be targeted for therapeutic intervention:

- There is a reduction in the expression and activity of endothelial nitric oxide synthase (NOS), leading to a reduction in production of endothelial NO. This leads to a reduction in pulmonary artery smooth muscle cell relaxation and an increase in cell proliferation via a reduction in cyclic guanylate monophosphate (cGMP).
- There is increased production and decreased clearance of the potent vasoconstrictor and stimulator of cell proliferation endothelin-1 (ET-1). This leads to vasoconstriction and increased proliferation of pulmonary artery smooth muscle cells.
- There is a reduction in the production of prostacyclin (due to reduction in prostacyclin synthase), which is a powerful vasodilator and platelet antagonist and inhibitor of smooth muscle cell proliferation.

However, these cellular changes may also be seen in non-PAH pulmonary hypertension, due to chronic hypoxia, resulting in similar pulmonary vascular remodelling.

Clinical features

In many cases, there is a considerable delay from the onset of disease until display of symptoms. In addition, the cardinal symptom of pulmonary hypertension is breathlessness, which may be present with any of the associated causes. As such, patients with non-PAH pulmonary hypertension may be found to have pulmonary hypertension incidentally during investigations for their underlying condition.

Late symptoms include severe dyspnoea, chest pain, and syncope on exercise, which reflect a low CO due to a failing right ventricle. Accompanying late signs are those of right ventricular failure with tachycardia, elevated jugular venous pressure, right ventricular heave, tricuspid regurgitation, and a loud pulmonary component of the 2nd heart sound.

Investigations

Patients with suspected pulmonary hypertension require specific investigations to confirm and quantify the severity of the disease as well as a myriad of general tests to identify any associated underlying cause.

Echocardiography and Doppler studies

The TTE and TOE are the commonest and least invasive methods of demonstrating pulmonary hypertension and assessing the right ventricular function. The systolic PAP can be estimated from the velocity of the tricuspid regurgitation jet on Doppler and an estimation of the right atrial pressure (RAP) using the modified Bernoulli equation (see section 1.8). In addition, any cardiac cause of pulmonary hypertension can be diagnosed (valvular heart disease, congenital heart disease, LV dysfunction).

Right heart catheterization

The definitive diagnosis is obtained by right heart catheterization, which enables direct measurement of the PAP, RAP, CO and pulmonary artery occlusion pressure (PAOP). PVR can therefore be calculated. In addition it allows assessment of a patient's response to pharmacological therapy by administering a short-acting vasodilator, e.g. adenosine, whilst monitoring the haemodynamics.

Exercise capacity

Tests of functionality provide important prognostic information as well as enabling monitoring of treatment response and clinical deterioration. The 6-minute walk test (6MWT) has traditionally been used, as the distance walked correlates with CO and peak oxygen consumption (VO_2). Studies have shown that the mean survival in PAH patients who can walk further than 332m on 6MWT is significantly greater than those who could not.

Although CPET can be useful to assess the maximal aerobic capacity of the patient, this may be difficult in patients with advanced disease.

General tests

ECG

The ECG may be normal and lacks the sensitivity and specificity to be used for diagnosis of pulmonary hypertension. However this should be considered in unexplained breathless patients presenting for theatre with sinus tachycardia or right ventricular strain on their ECG.

Chest X-ray

The CXR may reveal any underlying cause of pulmonary hypertension, e.g. LV failure or chronic respiratory disease. Specific signs of PAH are cardiomegaly, with prominent pulmonary arteries and pruning of vessels.

Pulmonary function tests

Pulmonary function tests may be performed to identify those patients who have pulmonary hypertension secondary to intra-pulmonary disease. Patients with PAH often have a degree of breathlessness that is out of proportion to their results, which may be normal.

General treatments

Perioperative optimization of the patient and aggressive treatment of any underlying conditions is essential. This can be supported by general measures to reduce PVR and increase pulmonary blood flow:

- Oxygen therapy to keep oxygen saturations >90% and avoid hypoxic pulmonary vasoconstriction.
- Diuretics to prevent RV volume overload.
- Anticoagulation for patients with severe disease who are at increased risk of thromboembolism.

Specific treatments

Drug therapies are used both to reduce the PVR as well as to suppress the pathogenic pathways, which may lead to pulmonary vascular remodelling. Patients will be established on optimal dose regimens in specialist clinics after careful assessment and should be continued on these in the perioperative period.

Calcium channel blockers may be useful in the small population of patients (around 10%) who demonstrate a significant vasodilator response at cardiac catheterization. They have no role in patients who are non-responders and may be hazardous in patients with impaired RV function.

Prostacyclin analogues are used to counteract the reduction in production of prostacyclin seen in PAH. These drugs have powerful pulmonary vasodilatory effects as well as being potent inhibitors of platelet aggregation. Administration may be by continuous infusion (epoprostenol, treprostinil) or nebulized solution (iloprost).

Endothelin receptor analogues, bosentan and ambrisentan are newer drugs that act by blocking endothelin receptors to reduce the vasoconstrictive effects of ET-1 on the pulmonary vasculature. Currently their use is limited by their adverse side effect profiles.

PDE5 inhibitors, e.g. sildenafil, act by reducing the breakdown of cGMP, which leads to pulmonary arterial vasodilatation.

NO is a highly specific pulmonary vasodilator (acting via stimulation of guanylate cyclase to increase cGMP), which is unsuitable for outpatient use due to its obligatory inhalational route of delivery. It may be used in an acute pulmonary hypertensive crisis, where it is administered via a ventilator circuit at a dose of 20–40ppm (see section 2.9).

Anaesthetic technique

The key aim is to prevent RV decompensation:

Prevent rise in PVR

- Aggressive treatment of triggers of pulmonary vasoconstriction e.g. pain, cold, stress, hypoxia, hypercarbia, acidosis.
- Use of selective pulmonary vasodilator, e.g. NO.
- Avoidance of lung hyperinflation: low tidal volume/low PEEP ventilation.

Maintain adequate RV filling

- Sinus rhythm (to allow atrial emptying to contribute maximally to RV preload).
- Adequate preload and contractility using target directed fluid therapy.

Maintain systemic perfusion pressures

- Vasoconstrictors to counteract vasodilator effects of anaesthetic agents.
- Slow titration epidural (instead of spinal) technique if neuraxial blockade is technique is required.
- Inotropic support with inodilators (to reduce PVR), e.g. dobutamine or milrinone.

Monitoring

All patients will require ECG, invasive BP measurements, and regular arterial blood gas sampling. Central venous catheters provide limited additional information, but a PAC permits constant monitoring of changes in pulmonary PAP, CO, PCWP, PVR, and SVR, which may be required in some patients.

Minimally invasive CO monitors (oesophageal Doppler and pulse contour analysis devices) have the advantage of avoiding the complications associated with pulmonary artery catheterization (such as arrhythmias and pulmonary haemorrhage) and are useful for early detection of low CO states. However, they are unable to measure haemodynamic changes of the right heart and pulmonary vasculature. Intra-operative echocardiography (TOE, TEE) can be used to visualize the RV filling and contractility as well as monitoring the left side for signs of poor cardiac output.

Further reading

Ramakrishna G, Sprung J, Ravi BS, et al. (2005). Impact of pulmonary hypertension on the outcomes of non-cardiac surgery: predictors of perioperative morbidity and mortality. *J Am Coll Cardiol*, 45:1691–9.

Simonneau G, Robbins IM, Beghetti M, et al. (2009). Updated clinical classification of pulmonary hypertension. *J Am Coll Cardiol*, 54(1 Suppl):S43–S54.

Congenital heart disease (CHD) is common, occurring in 8 per 1000 live births. Approximately 90% of children born with cardiac abnormalities now survive to adulthood.

Grown-up patients with CHD (so-called 'GUCH' patients) pose a particular challenge for the non-specialist. The most common acute presentations are with arrhythmia, heart failure, or endocarditis.

This section is concerned predominantly with the underlying *pathophysiology* of the more common forms of CHD: further clinical aspects are discussed elsewhere (see section 14.9).

Classification

The underlying pathophysiology forms the basis of the most useful classification of CHD from a clinical perspective. In essence, there are two types of defect: *shunts* and *obstructive lesions* (see Box 1.35).

Box 1.35 Classification of the more common congenital heart lesions

Shunts
- Left to right:
  - Atrial level: atrial septal defect (ASD), patent foramen ovale (PFO)
  - Ventricular level: ventricular septal defect (VSD)
  - Great artery level: patent ductus arteriosus (PDA)
- Right to left:
  - Tetralogy of Fallot.

Obstructive lesions
- Left heart:
  - Coarctation of the aorta
- Right heart:
  - Pulmonary stenosis.

Left-to-right shunts

A left-to-right shunt is the commonest pathophysiology seen in patients with CHD. The shunt causes volume overload of the heart, and increased pulmonary blood flow.

The prevailing systemic and pulmonary vascular resistances (SVR and PVR) will affect the magnitude of the shunt and its haemodynamic consequences. The high PVR *in utero* limits pulmonary blood flow. At birth, PVR falls and SVR rises, and a left-to-right shunt may become manifest with cardiac failure during the first weeks of life.

Factors reducing PVR result in increased left-to-right shunt and reduced systemic CO: these include administration of oxygen or NO, reduced arterial CO_2 tension, and systemic alkalosis.

Persistent left-to-right shunting ultimately damages the pulmonary vasculature, resulting in pulmonary hypertension and potential shunt reversal (Eisenmenger's syndrome).

Atrial septal defect

In normal fetal life the formation of the atrial septum occurs due to the growth and partial reabsorption of two tissue membranes, the *septum primum* and *septum secundum*. The *foramen ovale* is the opening between the upper and lower limbs of the septum secundum.

Several types of ASD are described:
- An *ostium primum* defect (deficiency of endocardial cushion tissue).
- An *ostium secundum* defect (excessive reabsorption of septum primum).
- *Sinus venosus* defect (an error in the incorporation of the sinus venosus chamber into the right atrium).

Flow across the defect occurs in both systole and diastole, with a predominant left-to-right shunt in adults. Thus, patients with an ASD exhibit signs and symptoms of bi-atrial volume overload and right ventricle overload.

Patent foramen ovale

A PFO is a communication across the atrial septum, and a remnant of the normal fetal circulation. The foramen ovale comprises overlapping portions of the septum primum and septum secundum, acting as a one-way valve. Postpartum there is an acute increase in pulmonary blood flow, with a corresponding increase in LA pressure. When the LA pressure exceeds the RA pressure, the septum primum becomes approximated to the septum secundum, closing the flap of the PFO. Subsequent intermittent rises in RA pressure (from a Valsalva manoeuvre, for example, or other isometric strain) may cause the foramen ovale to re-open, permitting flow from RA to LA.

In 20–25% of people, there is incomplete fusion leading to the persistence of an inter-atrial connection. The magnitude of shunt is not usually haemodynamically significant, but a PFO may result in paradoxical embolism. In the critically ill ventilated patient, persistent left–right shunting through a PFO may be the cause of disproportionate hypoxaemia.

Ventricular septal defect

VSD is the most common form of congenital heart defect in children (approximately 20% of human cardiac malformations), resulting from an abnormal connection between the two ventricles.

The hemodynamic effects of VSD differ from those of ASD. Blood flow during systole in the presence of a VSD can take two possible pathways: through the usual outflow tract of that ventricle, or through the VSD to the outflow tract of the other ventricle. Thus, the direction and volume of systolic flow across a VSD is principally determined by:
- *The size of the VSD*: the smaller the VSD, the higher the resistance of the defect itself, limiting the left-to-right shunt even with low pulmonary resistance. Conversely in a large, non-restrictive VSD with normal pulmonary vascular resistance, the sum of resistors from the LV to pulmonary artery is very low compared with resistance of flow from across the defect, resulting in large left-to-right systolic flow across the VSD.
- *The PVR*: if PVR is high in the presence of a large VSD, the sum of the resistors may approximate the aortic resistance and net shunting will be minimal. If pulmonary resistance is higher than systemic resistance, the shunt will be right-to-left regardless of the size of the VSD.

A left-to-right shunt at ventricular level reduces the LV output by the amount of the shunt. Compensatory mechanisms act to increase intravascular volume until LVEDV is sufficient to achieve both a normal CO and the proportionate left-to-right shunt resulting in a significant LV volume overload. High LV volume elevates LA filling pressures and may cause pulmonary congestion at rest and/or during exertion.

A secondary effect of a larger VSD is the transmission of LV pressure to the pulmonary vascular bed. Here, the ventricles become functionally a common chamber. In the absence of RV outflow/pulmonary obstruction, the pulmonary artery systolic pressure equals that in the aorta. Elevation of pulmonary artery pressure may help to differentiate a shunt at ventricular level from one at atrial level. The combination of volume and pressure overload contributes to the development of pulmonary vascular disease or Eisenmenger's syndrome.

Patent ductus arteriosus

The ductus arteriosus is an arterial structure connecting the aorta and main PA, which *in utero* allows blood flow from the PA to bypass the non-functioning lungs to return to the placenta via the descending aorta. Usually it closes within 72h of birth. Incomplete obliteration of the ductus results in a persistent arterial connection remaining between the systemic and pulmonary circulations.

Shunt direction and volume depend on the relative resistances to flow in each direction. In most patients, SVR is higher than PVR, resulting in left-to-right flow.

The *size* of the PDA is the principal determinant of the volume of flow. With large PDAs the LVEDV (preload) must increase to allow the stroke volume to supply both the normal CO and the left-to-right shunt. LA pressures rise and pulmonary venous congestion may limit exertion. There is flow during both diastole and systole and the diastolic flow may result in impaired coronary and splanchnic perfusion.

Right-to-left shunts

Tetralogy of Fallot

As its name suggests, the tetralogy of Fallot comprises four cardiac malformations (see Box 1.36).

Box 1.36 Tetralogy of Fallot

- *Pulmonary stenosis:* either at the pulmonary valve, or proximal to it, within the infundibulum.
- *Overriding aorta:* an aortic valve with a biventricular connection—situated above the VSD, and connected to both ventricles.
- *Ventricular septal defect:* usually a single large hole within the ventricular septum.
- *Right ventricular hypertrophy:* as a consequence of RV outflow tract obstruction.

Right-to-left shunting occurs across the VSD, and the patient is cyanosed due to lack of pulmonary blood flow. In 'Fallot's spells', pulmonary infundibular spasm causes all RV blood to shunt across the VSD, and there is no pulmonary venous return to the left heart.

Manoeuvres that increase SVR—e.g. squatting, or administration of 100% oxygen—will decrease right-to-left shunting and increase blood flow across the pulmonary valve.

Obstructive lesions

Under normal conditions the ventricular outflow tracts, semilunar valves and great vessels present no significant obstruction to flow. Congenital narrowing of any of these pathways increases ventricular afterload, reducing downstream flow. The effective increase in afterload may result in ventricular hypertrophy,

reduced compliance, and higher filling pressures. When severe, venous congestion occurs on exertion, limiting cardiac output and exercise tolerance. Symptoms in general are related to the severity of the obstruction and the side of the heart involved.

Coarctation of the aorta

Coarctation is a congenital narrowing of the aorta accounting for 5–8% of all cases of CHD. The obstruction classically occurs just distal to the origin of the left subclavian artery where the fetal ductus arteriosus had previously inserted into the aorta. Coarctation of the aorta is associated with a bicuspid valve in 50% to 85% of patients. With fixed obstruction at the coarctation and maintenance of flow (cardiac output), the result is a significant blood pressure elevation proximal to the lesion. Over time, the body develops alternate pathways from the ascending to descending aorta in the form of collateral arterial vessels. This results in the rib notching seen on chest radiographs in patients with coarctation. Significant collaterals may 'mask' the extent of the severity of obstruction.

Pulmonary stenosis

The normal response of the RV to increased afterload is to develop hypertrophy and increase systolic pressures. In CHD, right-sided stenotic lesions are generally relatively well tolerated until or unless they become severe. Pulmonary stenosis may be subvalvar, valvular, or supravalvar.

Most often, isolated *subvalvar pulmonary obstruction* in adults is a residuum of earlier surgical intervention (usually for tetralogy of Fallot), but it can be seen in adult patients with CHD who have not undergone surgery. Severe subvalvar obstruction may rarely present *de novo* in adults with a double-chambered RV.

Isolated *valvular pulmonary stenosis* is present in 8–10% of patients with CHD. In mild degrees of obstruction (<30mmHg), the natural history is similar whether or not patients undergo surgery. Moderate gradients, whilst well tolerated in children, become more important in adults. This may be due to the decreased ventricular compliance associated with ageing. More severe obstructive gradients increase RV afterload resulting in chamber hypertrophy. Symptomatic patients tend to present with serious dysrhythmic events and exercise intolerance.

Supravalvular pulmonary stenosis can occur as an isolated abnormality or be associated with complex cardiac malformations. These include tetralogy of Fallot, exposure to fetal teratogens (e.g. rubella or toxoplasmosis), or genetic syndromes such as Noonan's or Williams' syndrome.

Alternatively, it may the result of surgical scarring from previous surgery, including PA banding or after an arterial switch operation (for transposition of the great arteries).

The haemodynamic effects are identical to those of valvular pulmonary stenosis.

Further reading

Baumgartner H, Bonhoeffer P, De Groot NM, *et al*. (2010). ESC Guidelines for the management of grown-up congenital heart disease (new version 2010). *Eur Heart J*, 31(23):2915–57.

Chowdhury D (2007). Pathophysiology of congenital heart diseases. *Ann Cardiac Anaesth*, 10(1):19–26.

Warnes CA, Williams RG, Bashore TM, *et al*. (2008). ACC/AHA 2008 Guidelines for the Management of Adults with Congenital Heart Disease: a report of the American College of Cardiology/American Heart Association Task Force on Practice Guidelines (writing committee to develop guidelines on the management of adults with congenital heart disease). *Circulation*, 118(23):e714–833.

1.20 Thromboprophylaxis and anticoagulant therapy

Prevention and treatment of thrombosis—both venous *and* arterial—is an important and, in some respects, rapidly changing field, and will be discussed in the context of a number of key clinical situations:

- Perioperative prophylaxis against venous thromboembolism (VTE).
- Prevention of *arterial* thrombosis.
- Antithrombotic therapy in patients with atrial fibrillation.
- Perioperative management of anticoagulant and antiplatelet therapy.

Prophylaxis against VTE

This remains a core priority. One widely quoted estimate in 2005 put the number of preventable deaths in the UK from VTE as high as 25 000 per year, prompting an intervention from a House of Commons Select Committee.

Pathophysiology of venous thrombosis

Venous thrombi result from an accumulation predominantly of red cells and fibrin, with a lesser contribution from white cells and platelets. The risk factors for VTE are immortalized in Virchow's triad (1856):

- Alterations in blood flow (stasis or turbulence).
- Injury to the vascular endothelium.
- Alterations in the components of the blood (increased coagulability).

This remains an accurate and convenient classification, although an extended version may provide a more complete mechanistic view of the risk factors (see Box 1.37).

Box 1.37 Mechanisms of VTE

Venous stasis causing local hypoxia and endothelial activation
Prolonged stasis lowers oxygen tension within the vein. This induces a pro-inflammatory state within the endothelium. There is local recruitment of white cells, platelets and micro-particles, and activation of coagulation pathways, e.g. surgery, trauma, indwelling venous catheters, bedrest and immobilization, pregnancy, and obesity.

Activation of innate and acquired immunity
An increased risk of VTE is present in acute infections and also in chronic inflammatory disease (e.g. inflammatory bowel disease and rheumatoid arthritis).

Activation of platelets
Compared to arterial thrombi, the number of platelets in venous clots is relatively low. Nonetheless, successive layers of thrombus do contain platelets. In addition, platelets are important catalysts of thrombin generation and fibrin production.

Microparticles (MPs)
These are submicron particles shed from endothelial cells, platelets, and white cells that have emerged as potential key players in thromboembolic events. They provide a membrane surface for assembly of clotting cascade components. Tissue factor (TF)-bearing MPs are found in high numbers in patients with malignant disease, and are believed to have an important role in cancer-associated thrombosis.

Altered coagulation factor concentrations
These have been widely studied, and are well recognized to affect VTE risk. Alterations may be:

- *Congenital*: deficiencies of protein S, protein C, and antithrombin III.
- *Acquired*: pregnancy and use of oral contraceptives or HRT causes a hypercoagulable state marked by decreased anticoagulant activity, increased procoagulant activity, and decreased fibrinolysis.

Specific aspects of risk reduction

Graduated compression stockings remain the first-line NICE recommendation, but their efficacy has been challenged, particularly in medical patients and certainly if used as sole therapy in high-risk cases. Care should be taken in peripheral vascular disease and in cases of significant sensory impairment (including epidural analgesia, when careful inspection of the skin should be undertaken daily).

Medical patients should be offered pharmacological VTE prophylaxis (LMWH, UFH, or fondaparinux). If pharmacotherapy is contraindicated, then mechanical method(s) should be employed (stockings and/or intermittent pneumatic compression devices).

Extended thromboprophylaxis (up to 4 weeks postoperatively) may be indicated after surgery for cancer, and after major joint replacement surgery.

Novel oral anticoagulants in VTE thromboprophylaxis

Dabigatran is a direct thrombin (IIa) inhibitor, first developed for orthopaedic surgery. It is administered once or twice daily and excreted unchanged in the urine. Dose reduction is required in moderate renal impairment (creatinine clearance <50mL/min). Dabigatran binds competitively and reversibly to the catalytic site of thrombin. Because it is a thrombin inhibitor, administration of coagulation factors (FFP or prothrombin complex concentrates) may not wholly reverse its effects. Activated factor VII may be required in cases of uncontrolled bleeding.

Dabigatran was found to be comparable to enoxaparin for thromboprophylaxis after major joint replacement surgery, and has recently been licensed for use in AF as discussed later.

Rivaroxaban is a highly selective, reversible direct factor Xa inhibitor and has been found superior to enoxaparin for extended thromboprophylaxis after major joint replacement surgery. Since it is an 'upstream' inhibitor of coagulation, administration of coagulation factors may be expected to reverse its effects in cases of bleeding or overdose.

Fondaparinux acts via antithrombin as an indirect factor Xa inhibitor. It is delivered as a daily subcutaneous injection and may be superior to LMWH in thromboprophylaxis, and a useful alternative in cases of heparin-induced thrombocytopenia (HIT).

Prevention of arterial thrombosis

Arterial thrombosis is the result of a sequence of events that includes platelet adhesion, activation, and aggregation, the endpoint of which is vascular occlusion. It is the primary pathological complication of atherosclerotic disease, with potentially devastating consequences when it occurs in the coronary or cerebral circulations.

In terms of pharmacological strategies to prevent arterial thrombosis, three categories of drug have emerged.

- Aspirin
- Thienopyridines
- GP IIb–IIIa antagonists.

Anticoagulants (UFH or LMWH) may be used in conjunction with antiplatelet agents in the acute setting, and also as bridging therapy when antiplatelet therapy is interrupted.

Aspirin

Aspirin has a remarkable history and remains the most widely used of current antithrombotic agents. It causes acetylation of the cyclo-oxygenase (COX)-1 enzyme that persists for the lifetime of an affected platelet. Data showing a 25% risk reduction in fatal vascular events (MI or stroke) across multiple trials led to the widespread use of aspirin in both primary and secondary prevention.

Thienopyridines

Clopidogrel, and its predecessor ticlopidine, causes irreversible inhibition of the platelet $P2Y_{12}$ receptor. Studies have demonstrated greater efficacy than aspirin, particularly in high-risk situations (e.g. diabetes or previous revascularization), see Box 1.38.

GP IIb–IIIa antagonists

Drugs such as tirofiban and abciximab act on the final common pathway mediating platelet aggregation. They are administered intravenously in the acute setting of an ischaemic event (acute MI and/or PCI).

Box 1.38 Current recommendations for antithrombotic therapy in practice (Vandvik et al, 2012)

- Low-dose aspirin (75mg once a day) for primary prevention of cardiovascular disease in patients >50 years.
- Long-term low-dose aspirin or clopidogrel 75mg once a day in patients with established coronary artery disease.
- Dual antiplatelet therapy for 1 year in patients who undergo PCI with stent placement, and single antiplatelet therapy thereafter.

Data from Vandvik, P. O., Lincoff, A. M., Gore, J. M., Gutterman, D. D., Sonnenberg, F. A., Alonso-Coello, P., et al. (2012). Primary and secondary prevention of cardiovascular disease. *Chest*, 141(2 suppl), e637S–e668S.

Antithrombotic therapy in AF

Aside from the haemodynamic consequences of the arrhythmia itself (see section 1.9), an important consideration in AF is anticoagulation to reduce the risk of thromboembolic complications.

The stroke risk in AF is most simply stratified according to the $CHADS_2$ (**c**ongestive heart failure, **h**ypertension, **a**ge, **d**iabetes, **s**troke) score (see Table 1.13). $CHADS_2$ scores of 1 and 6 equate to an estimated annual stroke risk of 1 and 18% respectively.

Table 1.13 $CHADS_2$ score to predict stroke risk in AF

Risk factor	Score
LV dysfunction/heart failure	1
Hypertension	1
Age ≥75 years	1
Diabetes	1
Previous stroke or TIA	2

Reproduced from Gage BF, et al., 'Selecting patients with atrial fibrillation for anticoagulation: stroke risk stratification in patients taking aspirin', *Circulation*, 110, pp. 2287–2292, copyright 2004 American Heart Association, published by Wolters Kluwer.

In terms of anticoagulation, numerous trials support the use of warfarin or other vitamin K antagonists (VKAs) in all patients with AF in whom ≥1 risk factor is present, provided there are no absolute contraindications and after a careful assessment of the risk:benefit ratio. VKA therapy is clearly superior to antiplatelet therapy in terms of stroke risk reduction in AF.

VKAs obviously have a narrow therapeutic index and exhibit complex interactions with other drugs and foodstuffs, necessitating careful monitoring of the INR.

More recently, newer anticoagulant drugs have been studied, of which dabigatran has been recommended by NICE as a possible alternative to warfarin to prevent stroke and systemic embolism in patients with AF.

Perioperative management of anticoagulant and antiplatelet therapy

The perioperative management of patients receiving warfarin or antiplatelet therapy requires an assessment of the balance of risks between bleeding and thromboembolic complications.

Patients receiving warfarin therapy

Stratify risk according to the underlying indication for anticoagulation (mechanical heart valve, AF, previous VTE, etc.). For example:

- High risk: mechanical mitral valve/AF with $CHADS_2$ score 5–6/recent VTE.
- Moderate risk: bileaflet aortic valve/AF with $CHADS_2$ score 3–4.
- Low risk: AF with $CHADS_2$ score 1–2/single previous VTE.

This risk stratification is used to inform the decision for bridging therapy:

- High risk: bridging with therapeutic dose UFH or LMWH.
- Moderate risk: bridging with therapeutic or low-dose heparin.
- Low risk: either no bridging or low-dose heparin.

There is a widely held view that LMWH is unsafe as bridging therapy in patients with mechanical heart valves, but recent studies do not support this view. It is, however, important to carefully consider both the timing *and* dose of LMWH when restarting bridging therapy postoperatively.

Perioperative management of antiplatelet therapy in patients with coronary stents

Preoperative evaluation should include the following:

- Type of stent: bare metal or drug eluting.
- When was each stent implanted and were there any complications?
- Is there a past history of stent thrombosis?
- What is the current antiplatelet regimen?
- What other comorbidities might contribute to the overall cardiac risk? (Diabetes, renal insufficiency, poor LV, etc.)
- Discuss with patient's cardiologist re: optimal management strategy.

The appropriate strategy in respect of non-cardiac surgery in the presence of coronary stents has been widely discussed, and a number of guidelines exist, from the ACC/AHA and others. Delaying non-urgent surgery for the recommended periods is the most sensible approach (see also section 1.5):

- After a bare metal stent, delay elective or non-urgent surgery by a minimum of 6 weeks (preferably at least 3 months).
- If urgent surgery is required in a patient with bare metal stent *in situ* <6 weeks, continue dual antiplatelet therapy perioperatively.
- After a drug-eluting stent, delay non-urgent procedures preferably for 12 months.
- For essential surgery in the presence of a recently-inserted drug-eluting stent, continue *at least* single antiplatelet therapy.

Further reading

Vandvik PO, Lincoff AM, Gore JM, *et al.* (2012). Primary and secondary prevention of cardiovascular disease. *Chest*, 141(2 suppl): e637S–e668S.

1.21 Pulmonary embolism

Pulmonary embolism (PE) is a cardiovascular emergency. The clinical presentation is highly variable, often with non-specific features, and therefore easily missed. Symptoms range from none at all, or mild breathlessness, through to cardiopulmonary collapse. If the diagnosis is made early, treatment is usually highly effective, both in respect of managing a major occlusion *and* in preventing more major recurrences when the initial presentation is less severe.

Despite advances in the prophylaxis (see section 1.19), diagnosis, *and* treatment of VTE, PE remains an important cause of in-hospital morbidity and mortality, not least amongst perioperative patients and those in critical care.

In most cases, PE occurs as a consequence of deep venous thrombosis (DVT). Lower limb DVT can be detected in about 70% of patients with PE. Similarly, amongst patients with proximal DVT, some 50% will be found to have PE, which is usually asymptomatic. It is worth remembering that most patients with *symptomatic* DVT will, in fact, have proximal thrombi.

The factors predisposing to VTE are discussed in section 1.19.

Pathophysiology

The clinical consequences of acute PE largely reflect the *haemodynamic* insult—symptoms and signs of respiratory insufficiency occur secondary to the haemodynamic disturbance.

The key insult is an increase in PVR and RV afterload that occurs when >30% of the pulmonary arterial tree is occluded by a large embolus or by multiple smaller emboli.

Massive PE produces an insurmountable RV afterload and causes circulatory arrest, usually as pulseless electrical activity.

Patients who survive the initial episode may develop secondary haemodynamic deterioration, typically within the first 24–48h, reflecting either recurrent embolism, and/or a failure of compensation of the right ventricle.

The hypoxaemia observed in acute PE has several causes, including reduced CO and V:Q mismatch.

Classification of severity

It is immediately obvious that PE varies in severity, and previous classifications have used the terms 'massive', 'submassive', and 'non-massive' to reflect this.

The latest guidelines suggest that a more relevant classification should be according to the estimated early (in-hospital or 30-day) mortality. On this basis, three categories of severity are recognized (see Box 1.39), according to the presence or absence of three categories of risk factors:

1. Clinical signs: shock or hypotension
2. Evidence of RV dysfunction (e.g. on ECHO)
3. Signs of myocardial injury (raised troponins or BNP)

> ### Box 1.39 Risk stratification of PE according to early mortality
>
> - *High risk* (>15% early mortality): presence of shock or hypotension, even without confirmation of RV dysfunction or myocardial injury, i.e. the presence of shock or hypotension is the single most important predictor of prognosis.
> - *Intermediate risk* (3–15% early mortality): no features of shock, but demonstrable RV dysfunction and/or myocardial injury.
> - *Low risk* (<1% early mortality): no adverse risk factors present.
>
> Data from Torbicki A, et al., (2008) 'Guidelines on the diagnosis and management of acute pulmonary embolism: the Task Force for the Diagnosis and Management of Acute Pulmonary Embolism of the European Society of Cardiology (ESC)', *European Heart Journal*, 29, 18, pp. 2276–2315. doi:10.1093/eurheartj/ehn310.

Diagnostic tools in suspected pulmonary embolism

For the reasons already stated, the diagnosis of a PE is a crucial one to make. It is important, therefore, to be aware of the accuracy and limitations of the various diagnostic modalities available.

Clinical features

The 'typical' symptoms of PE are sudden onset breathlessness, pleuritic chest pain, and cough, sometimes with haemoptysis, but these are neither sensitive nor specific for PE.

Untreated or massive PE may present with cardiovascular collapse and sudden death.

In the theatre or critical care environment, where patients are typically sedated and ventilated, a high index of suspicion is required in patients who develop unexplained hypoxaemia or arterial hypotension.

A CXR may show atelectasis, effusion, or peripheral oligaemia.

New ECG changes suggestive of right heart strain (anterior T-wave inversion, right bundle branch block, or the classic S1Q3T3 pattern) may be helpful.

Arterial blood gas analysis usually demonstrates hypoxaemia, but may be normal in 20% of patients.

In summary, the results of clinical assessment and simple investigations may increase suspicion, but are insufficient to confirm or refute the diagnosis of PE.

Clinical prediction tools (Wells and revised Geneva scores)

Whilst *individual* symptoms, signs and common test results may be non-specific, particular combinations may be more discriminating. The most commonly used (and similar) scores are the Wells and the revised Geneva scores, each of which can be used to suggest low, moderate, and high probabilities of PE, corresponding to actual prevalences of 10%, 30%, and 60% respectively (see Box 1.40). The revised Geneva score of PE probability combines scores for predisposing factors, symptoms and signs. Scores indicate clinical probability of PE: 0–3 low, 4–10 intermediate, ≥11 high probability.

> ### Box 1.40 Scoring systems for estimation of clinical probability of PE
>
> Current recommendations support the use of validated clinical prediction scores to estimate pre-test probability of PE. The two algorithms in common use are the Wells score and the revised Geneva score. These grade the clinical probability of PE as low, intermediate, or high, depending on the presence or absence of:
> - Risk factors (e.g. malignancy or recent surgery)
> - Symptoms (e.g. haemoptysis)
> - Clinical signs (e.g. tachycardia or signs of DVT).
>
> Scoring systems are not intended to replace clinical judgement, but may assist in prioritizing salient features in the history or clinical examination.

Plasma D-dimer levels

D-dimer is a fibrin degradation product, and levels are elevated in the presence of an acute clot because of simultaneous coagulation and fibrinolysis. A normal D-dimer has a high negative predictive value (DVT or PE unlikely), but a low positive predictive value since fibrin is produced in a wide variety of other conditions, including malignancy, infection, and inflammation.

Using a highly sensitive assay, a negative D-dimer result usefully excludes PE in patients with a low or moderate clinical probability.

Ventilation–perfusion scintigraphy (V/Q scan)

V/Q scan is a widely used diagnostic test in suspected PE. The perfusion scan is based on an intravenous injection of technetium (Tc)-99m-labelled albumin particles. The ventilation component typically uses xenon (Xe)-133 gas.

The interpretation of V/Q scan findings has been a process of revision and debate. By consensus, *a normal perfusion scan safely excludes PE*. Similarly, a high probability scan result confirms the diagnosis when the clinical probability is also high. Many scans are, however, non-diagnostic or of intermediate probability, or the scan results do match the clinical probability, and in these situations, further tests are indicated.

Computed tomography pulmonary angiography (CTPA)

With the advent of high-resolution techniques, CTPA has become the imaging technique of choice for suspected PE. Sensitivities and specificities are high. A positive scan is diagnostic, and a negative scan safely excludes PE in cases of low to intermediate clinical probability. In the rare situation of a negative scan in a patient with high clinical probability, there may be a case for further testing.

Pulmonary angiography

Pulmonary angiography was traditionally the gold standard test for diagnosis or exclusion of PE, but has largely been superseded by non-invasive CTPA. Pulmonary angiography is invasive and carries a mortality risk of 0.2%. In patients who undergo thrombolysis, there is a markedly increased risk of local bleeding complications after pulmonary angiography, which is now only performed if non-invasive tests yield equivocal results.

Echocardiography

The finding of RV dilatation is useful in risk stratification of patients with suspected PE. Bedside ECHO is particularly advantageous in critically ill patients who may be too unstable to be transferred for CTPA.

In a patient with shock or hypotension, the absence of RV strain on ECHO practically excludes PE as the cause.

Diagnostic strategy in suspected PE

The strategy differs according to whether the suspected PE is high risk (i.e. with shock or hypotension) or low-to-intermediate risk (Boxes 1.41 and 1.42).

Box 1.41 Diagnostic strategy in suspected high-risk PE

Transfer for CTPA if immediately available and the patient is fit for transfer:
- A +ve result justifies treatment: consider thrombolysis or embolectomy.
- A −ve result should prompt a search for other causes.

If CT not available or patient unfit for transfer, perform ECHO:
- If ECHO shows RV overload, confirm diagnosis of PE with CT if possible, but otherwise treatment justified as for fit-for-transfer patient.
- A negative ECHO should prompt a search for other causes.

Box 1.42 Diagnostic strategy in suspected non-high-risk PE

Assess clinical probability i.e. 'high' or 'low-intermediate' risk:
- In high-risk probabilities, proceed to CTPA: decision to treat based on CT result.
- In lower probability cases, a sensitive D-dimer assay can be used:
  - If negative, treatment may safely be withheld.
  - If positive D-dimer, proceed to CT (V/Q scanning is a viable option for patients with a raised D-dimer and a contraindication to CT).

Therapeutic strategies in pulmonary embolism

Thrombolytic therapy

Thrombolytic therapy is the first-line treatment for patients presenting with shock or hypotension. There is little to choose between different agents, and no advantage of local thrombolysis over systemic intravenous therapy. A typical regimen is streptokinase 250 000IU over 30min, followed by an infusion of 100 000 IU/h over 12–24h.

Surgical embolectomy

Surgical embolectomy remains a valuable therapeutic option in high-risk patients in whom thrombolysis is absolutely contraindicated or has failed, and should be considered early—the surgical procedure is relatively straightforward in an appropriate centre.

Anticoagulant therapy

Anticoagulant therapy should be initiated in all patients with *confirmed* PE, using UFH, LMWH, or fondaparinux. Additionally, patients with suspected high-risk PE should receive anticoagulation whilst the diagnostic process is continuing. LMWH (e.g. enoxaparin 1.5mg/kg/24h) is a typical starting regimen.

Venous filters

Venous filters may be used if there is an absolute contraindication to anticoagulation and/or a high risk of recurrence, typically in the immediate postoperative period after major surgery when thrombolysis or anticoagulation would be hazardous.

Long-term anticoagulation

Treatment with VKAs or LMWH is indicated for a minimum of 3 months following a PE when there has been a transient, identifiable cause. In cases of recurrent PE, or where the risk is persistent (e.g. in malignant disease), treatment should be continued in the longer term.

Further reading

Bahloul M, Chaari A, Ben Algia, N, *et al.* (2012). Pulmonary embolism in intensive care unit 'literature review.' *Trends Anaesth Crit Care*, 2:25–9.

Le Gal G, Righini M, Roy PM, *et al.* (2006). Prediction of pulmonary embolism in the emergency department: the revised Geneva score. *Ann Intern Med* 144(3):165–71.

Takach Lapner S & Kearon C (2013). Diagnosis and management of pulmonary embolism. *BMJ*, 346:f757.

Torbicki A, Perrier A, Konstantinides S, et al. (2008). Guidelines on the diagnosis and management of acute pulmonary embolism: the Task Force for the Diagnosis and Management of Acute Pulmonary Embolism of the European Society of Cardiology (ESC). *Eur Heart J*, 29:2276–315.

Chapter 2

Respiratory system

2.1 Assessment of respiratory function

As with many clinical assessments, the majority of essential information about a patient is gained from a thorough history and examination. Due attention should be paid to known pathology, previous hospital and critical care admissions, and medications taken (including home oxygen). Specific tests can be sought to confirm and quantify respiratory dysfunction.

Respiratory function tests (RFTs) objectively assess distinct components of the respiratory system, but no single test can evaluate either the whole system or its limitations during periods of increased demand. Appropriate tests must therefore be ordered to answer specific questions and values obtained should be considered in the context of the proposed perioperative period. Comparison of individual results to tables of predicted values provide a measure of normality.

Limitations of RFTs include their dependence on patient co-operation and motivation, and the 'snap-shot' single resting view of respiratory function.

Spirometry

Spirometry is a test that measures the capacity to inhale and exhale air. The spirometer either measures *volume* or *flow* in order to allow the calculation of useful respiratory values. It is the most commonly used RFT and provides information that can be used to stratify risk in the perioperative period. The test is straightforward but requires a skilled technician and the full cooperation and motivation of the patient. Failure of the latter can result in falsely low readings. All spirometry values should be reported as body temperature and pressure saturated, i.e. fully saturated with water at body temperature and ambient barometric pressure. Guidelines exist that describe the conduct, validity, and interpretation of spirometry.

Wet spirometers consisted of a chamber containing water and a second chamber inverted over it connected to an indicator gauge or marker pen. Breathing via a tube connected to the water chamber led to a corresponding movement of the chamber above and the indicator displayed the change in volume. These have been surpassed by a variety of dry devices that measure volume displacement by bellows, or airflow by pneumotachometer or ultrasound. If flow is measured then volume is calculated automatically by microprocessors contained within the spirometer. Peak expiratory flow rate can be measured using a simple hand-held device but no other data can be obtained using this method.

The spirometer is able to generate a spirogram (Fig. 2.1), a graphical plot of either volume-time or a flow–volume loop, along with the selected numerical data listed:

- *Forced vital capacity* (FVC): the volume during a forceful and maximal expiration after starting from full inspiration (litres). FVC is not a reliable indicator of total lung capacity: reduced FVC can occur despite a normal or increased total lung volume particularly in the setting of airflow obstruction in COPD. FVC is markedly affected by restrictive lung pathology such as pulmonary fibrosis.
- *Forced expiratory volume in 1 second* (FEV_1): the volume delivered in the first second of an FVC manoeuvre (litres). The majority of the FVC should occur in the first second of a forced expiration and it is a measure of the mechanical properties of the large and medium-sized airways. It is reduced in both restrictive and obstructive disorders.

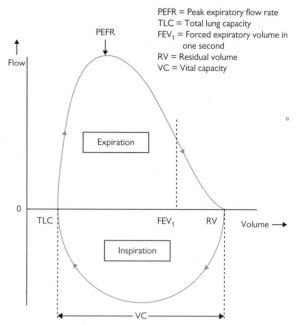

PEFR = Peak expiratory flow rate
TLC = Total lung capacity
FEV_1 = Forced expiratory volume in one second
RV = Residual volume
VC = Vital capacity

Fig. 2.1 Normal spirometry trace.

- *FEV_1/FVC ratio*: in health this is >75%. Obstructive pathology, such as asthma and COPD, leads to a disproportionate decrease in FEV_1 causing a decline in the FEV_1/FVC ratio. In restrictive lung disease FEV_1 and FVC decrease equally so the ratio remains unchanged.
- *Peak expiratory flow rate*: the maximal flow rate generated during forced exhalation, starting from full lung inflation.

The spirogram itself can provide useful information in its shape: certain respiratory pathologies lead to typical changes in the outline of the plot. Obstructive pathology, such as asthma and COPD, tends to affect the expiratory limb of the spirogram, causing concavity of the curve (Fig. 2.2).

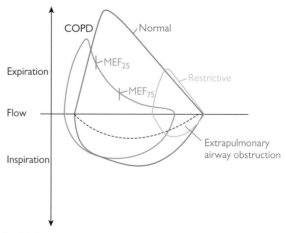

Fig. 2.2 Spirometry patterns in health and disease. Reproduced from Catherine Spoors and Kevin Kiff, *Training in Anaesthesia*, 2010, Figure 13.28, page 353, with permission from Oxford University Press.

Reversibility testing

This tends to be performed in patients with demonstrable air-flow limitation to assess the effectiveness of potential therapies. These are usually short-acting inhaled drugs such as salbutamol and ipratropium bromide, although long-acting drugs such as salmeterol and aminophylline can also be assessed. Spirometry is performed before and after a dose of the selected medication is administered, and the data compared.

Lung volume testing

Body plethysmography

Functional residual capacity (FRC) and total lung volume (TLV) can be measured by body plethysmography. The patient sits within a small air-sealed container and breathes quietly through a mouthpiece attached to an open shutter. When the shutter is closed, the patient pants against the shutter whilst pressure and volume changes are measured within the container and used to calculate lung volumes by the application of Boyle's law.

Gas dilution techniques

TLV can also be measured by gas dilution techniques. However, these techniques are less accurate than the body plethysmograph since they do not include in their measurements any non-communicating bullae that are present within the lungs. The two methods commonly used are the closed-circuit *helium dilution* or open-circuit *nitrogen washout* tests.

In the helium dilution test, the patient breathes a known concentration of helium in a closed circuit system for a period of approximately 7min. An analyser continuously monitors the helium concentration within the circuit, and, being an inert gas, the final reduction in concentration will be proportional to its dilution within the lungs. Since the test is usually commenced at the end of normal tidal expiration, the dilution represents the FRC.

The nitrogen washout test requires the patient to breathe 100% oxygen for approximately 7min through a one-way valve to wash all of the nitrogen out of the lungs. During that time the concentration of nitrogen is analysed and breath volume measured until the nitrogen concentration drops below 1.5%. Lung volumes can be calculated along with closing volume (the volume of air remaining in the lungs when the flow from the lower sections of the lungs ceased).

Diffusion capacity

The capacity for gas to diffuse across the alveolar membrane can be assessed by measuring the diffusing capacity for carbon monoxide (DLCO) in the lungs.

During the test, a low concentration of carbon monoxide is inhaled in a single breath and held in the lungs for a short period of time. Some of the inhaled CO is taken up by haemoglobin in the pulmonary circulation and exhaled gas is analysed for its CO concentration.

DLCO is calculated by comparing inhaled and exhaled CO concentrations. DLCO can be affected by:

- Alveolar-capillary surface area
- Pulmonary capillary blood volume
- Thickness of the alveolar-capillary membrane
- V/Q mismatching
- Haemoglobin concentration.

Diseases affecting the alveolar membrane and pulmonary capillary tend to reduce DLCO.

Arterial oxygenation

Benefit can be gained by knowing the arterial oxygenation of a patient preoperatively and this can be achieved by pulse oximetry and blood gas analysis. Whilst these provide little diagnostic or prognostic information, they can serve as a useful baseline measurement during the perioperative and recovery period.

Further reading

Miller MR, Hankinson J, Brusasco V, *et al.* (2005). ATS/ERS Task force: Standardisation of lung function testing. *Eur Respir J*, 26:319–38.

2.2 Capnography

Capnography is a graphical display of the change in CO_2 concentration during breathing, and is arguably the most informative monitoring modality available to the anaesthetist. It is therefore a popular (and perhaps the correct!) answer to the classic viva question of 'If you could monitor only one parameter during anaesthesia, which would it be?'. The measurement of CO_2 in expired gas can provide information relating to metabolism, perfusion, and ventilation.

End-tidal CO_2 monitoring should be a standard of care during anaesthesia, ventilation of the critically ill patient, and transportation of mechanically ventilated patients.

The measurement of CO_2 in gas mixtures

Infrared CO_2 analyser

This is the commonest method of CO_2 detection utilized in anaesthetic equipment. The underlying principle is that diatomic gases (those containing two or more different atoms) such as CO_2 absorb infrared light.

As other diatomic gases may also be present in the breathing system (nitrous oxide and volatile anaesthetic agents), thus causing inaccuracy, a wavelength that corresponds to the peak absorbance by CO_2 (4.25μm) is used.

Due to collision broadening, a phenomenon where the infrared absorption spectrum of CO_2 is broadened by the presence of other gases (such as oxygen and nitrous oxide), modern anaesthetic analysers also measure the concentration of these other gases to correct this source of error.

The basic design of the capnograph consists of a source of infrared light emitted across a sapphire windowed gas analysis chamber, and a detector on the opposite side of the chamber.

Sample gas passes through the chamber either as a result of it being placed in the direct path of the gas to be measured (main-stream) or via a sampling line that is connected between the two (side-stream). Side-stream detection requires an additional pump that actively draws gas away from the respiratory gas to the capnograph (usually at 150mL/min).

Detection works on the Beer–Lambert law such that the amount of absorption of infrared light is directly proportional to the concentration CO_2 in the sample. Continuous analysis permits the generation of a graphical representation of the change in CO_2 concentration during breathing, the capnogram.

Water can lead to erroneous capnograph readings by condensing within tubing: this can be reduced by the addition of a water trap into the transit tube of a side-stream analyser.

Mass spectrometry

CO_2 concentrations can also be measured by mass spectrometry, a rapid and highly accurate analysis technique. Due to the expense of the equipment it is rarely used in clinical practice.

The capnogram

The cyclical rise and fall that occurs during expiration and inspiration respectively leads to a square-wave capnogram (Fig. 2.3). For infrared detectors the measurements will usually be in partial pressure (rather than fractional concentration), and this is plotted against time on the horizontal axis of the trace. The trace is commonly described in four phases (see Box 2.1).

> **Box 2.1 Phases of the capnogram**
>
> 0: Inspiration
> I: CO_2 'free' gas from the apparatus and anatomical dead space
> II: Rapidly rising limb resulting from a mixture of dead space and alveolar gas
> III: Plateau of alveolar gas, the final peak of which is the end-tidal CO_2.

Two angles are also described (α and β) that provide quantification of abnormalities on the capnogram.

The response time of the capnograph also needs to be considered. Two phenomena, the *transit time* and the *rise time*, describe why capnography does not respond to a change in CO_2 concentration immediately. When combined, they describe the response time.

Transit time refers to the time taken for the gas sample to move from the respiratory gas flow into the capnograph, and only really applies to side-stream analysers. From the time there is a rise in CO_2 concentration to detection will therefore be represented on the capnogram by an extended baseline trace.

Rise time is the speed at which the analyser responds to a true change in CO_2 concentration and is measured as the time between 10% and 90% of a step-change in concentration. Rise time can be improved by reducing the size of the analysis chamber in a main-stream capnograph. Table 2.1 shows the advantages and disadvantages of main-stream and side-stream capnography.

Table 2.1 Advantages and disadvantages of main-stream and side-stream capnography

Main-stream capnography	
Advantages	**Disadvantages**
Faster response time than side-stream	Does not allow analyses of anaesthetic gases
Will work during active humidification systems	Expensive, fragile probe on breathing circuit
	Additional weight on the ventilator circuit
	Increased circuit dead space
Side-stream capnography	
Advantages	**Disadvantages**
Cheaper and more robust than main-stream capnography	May not work with active humidification due to moisture accumulation in transit tubing
Will also measure anaesthetic gases	Slower response time than main-stream
	Waveform may be prone to damping
	Multiple sites for disconnection away from the circuit

Common capnogram patterns

Pattern recognition of common changes in the capnogram can be useful in coming to a rapid diagnosis during mechanical ventilation (see patterns in Fig. 2.3):
1. Normal
2. Flat line:
   - Disconnection
   - Apnoea/respiratory arrest
   - Cardiac arrest.

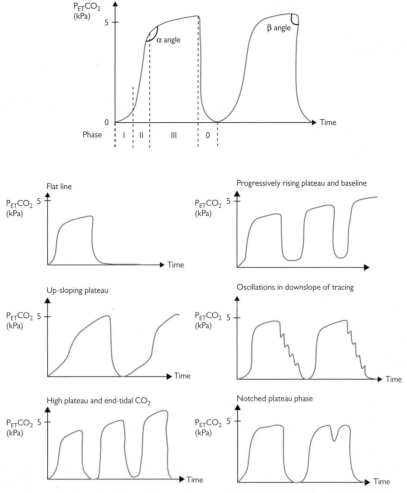

Fig. 2.3 Common capnograph patterns. Reproduced from Catherine Spoors and Kevin Kiff, *Training in Anaesthesia*, 2010, Figure 4.15, Page 77, with permission from Oxford University Press.

3. Up-sloping plateau phase (increased alpha-angle):
   - Ventilation-perfusion mismatch
   - Lower airway obstruction (bronchospasm/asthma/COPD)
   - Partial airway obstruction (pathological/secretions/tube kinking).
3. High plateau and end-tidal CO_2:
   - Hypoventilation
   - Increased CO_2 production (metabolic), e.g. malignant hyperpyrexia.
4. Low plateau and end-tidal CO_2:
   - Hyperventilation.
5. Progressively rising plateau and baseline:
   - Re-breathing within an anaesthetic breathing system.
6. Oscillations in down slope of tracing:
   - Cardiac oscillations.
7. Notched plateau phase:
   - Spontaneous inspiration within the expiratory phase during mechanical ventilation
   - External pressure on the chest wall.

Relationship between end-tidal and arterial CO₂

$EtCO_2$ reflects $PaCO_2$ but is usually lower than $PaCO_2$ by 0.3–0.6kPa in health. An increase in the difference between $EtCO_2$

and $PaCO_2$ develops in the presence of ventilation-perfusion mismatch, due to an increase in physiological dead space. Arterial − end-tidal PCO_2 (a-ET PCO_2) difference is therefore a good measure of dead space ventilation, except when the phase III plateau is steeply up-sloping, which can result in a zero or negative a-ET PCO_2 difference. Reduced cardiac output, poor pulmonary perfusion, and pulmonary embolism are common situations that result in an increased a-ET PCO_2. These conditions will cause an underestimation of $PaCO_2$ from $EtCO_2$.

Colorimetric CO₂ detectors

Colorimetric detectors are small disposable devices that can be attached directly to an endotracheal tube to confirm the presence of CO_2 in respiratory gas. They comprise a pH sensitive chemical that changes colour as gas containing CO_2 in the range of 2–5% CO_2 passes over it but will remain unchanged if lower than this. It is therefore a useful aid to help confirm correct placement of an endotracheal tube when formal capnography is unavailable.

Further reading

Bhavani-Shankar K, Moseley H, Kumar AY, *et al*. (1992). Capnometry and anaesthesia. *Can J Anaesth*. 39(6):617–32.

Intensive Care Society: *Standards for Capnography in Critical Care*. <http://www.ics.ac.uk>

2.3 Pulse oximetry

Although a relatively modern invention, it would now be highly unusual to administer anaesthesia or sedation without using a pulse oximeter.

Oximetry reveals the presence of *hypoxaemia* and thereby may allow its potentially harmful effects to be avoided. Cyanosis, the presence of 5g/dL of deoxygenated haemoglobin, is a clinical sign of hypoxaemia but is notorious for being poorly detected by clinicians. Pulse oximetry facilitates the objective, non-invasive measurement of peripheral arterial haemoglobin oxygen saturation (SpO_2).

The pulse oximeter

The device combines oximetry, plethysmography, and a microprocessor in order to provide continuous SpO_2 monitoring. Measurement of SpO_2 (an estimation of true arterial oxygen saturation (SaO_2) measured on a co-oximeter) by the pulse oximeter occurs by calculating the absorbance of transmitted light through tissue in which there is an arterial pulsation.

Light transmission and absorption

Oxygenated (HbO_2) and deoxygenated haemoglobin (Hb) possess different light absorptive capacities, a phenomenon observed clinically when bright red arterial blood changes to a deep blue colour in veins.

The ratio of light absorbance by each haemoglobin species can, therefore, be used to determine their relative quantities. The amount of light energy absorbed by haemoglobin is governed by the Beer–Lambert law. This states that absorbance is dependent upon the concentration of the haemoglobin within the blood, the path length of the light beam and the molar extinction coefficient (a wavelength-dependent constant of absorptivity).

Light emitting diodes (LEDs) on one arm of the pulse oximeter illuminate the tissue, whilst a photodetector on the other side measures how much light has been absorbed. The digits are commonly used for pulse oximetry since they present a reasonably short path length for the transmitted light. Pulse oximeters use two wavelengths of light: visible red (660nm) and infrared (940nm), at which HbO_2 and Hb display markedly different absorbing characteristics (Fig. 2.4). SpO_2 is calculated using the ratio of light absorbance between the two wavelengths with reference to electronic tables within the device's algorithm. Also, haemoglobin exhibits isobestic points at wavelengths of 590nm and 805nm, at which light absorbance is the same for both HbO_2 and Hb, allowing an approximation of total haemoglobin concentration.

Interference from ambient light

Ambient light can distort pulse oximetry readings, and systems are built in to try to minimize this. In rapid succession, every 5–10 microseconds, the visible red LED switches on and off, followed by the infrared LED and a subsequent period of no light. The two independent signals received by the photodetector during LED illumination are successively amplified and equalized, and the signal received whilst the LEDs are off is subtracted to allow for ambient light.

Signal interpretation

The light absorbed by the photodetector is composed of a pulsatile and non-pulsatile component (Fig. 2.4). Whilst the pulsatile

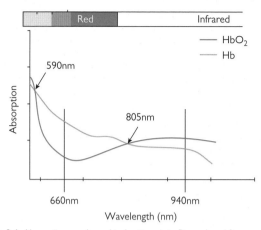

Fig. 2.4 Absorption graphs and isobestic points. Reproduced from Catherine Spoors and Kevin Kiff, *Training in Anaesthesia*, 2010, Figure 4.20, page 79, with permission from Oxford University Press.

fraction represents the arterial signal, the remainder is derived from tissues and other parts of the circulation (venous blood, bone, fingernail.) The algorithm within the oximeter separates the pulsatile and non-pulsatile components and assumes that the pulsatile signal is arterial blood, therefore discarding the remaining information. Three seconds of data are averaged to display on a screen: a longer averaging time can lead to delayed detection of hypoxaemia.

Different haemoglobin types

In order to detect other types of haemoglobin, the pulse oximeter would need to use several wavelengths of light in a similar manner to a co-oximeter. This is not the case, and therefore pulse oximeters unfortunately mistake carboxyhaemoglobin for oxyhaemoglobin and over-read the true SaO_2 in its presence. Similarly, methaemoglobin reduces the SpO_2 value to 85% regardless of the patient's actual oxygenation status. Neither fetal haemoglobin nor anaemia affects the signal quality to any significant degree.

Pulse oximetry in the clinical context

As with all medical devices, the value obtained from a pulse oximeter is valid only if the device is used correctly *and* if consideration is given to the clinical scenario in which it is being used.

Accuracy

The accuracy of a pulse oximeter depends upon several factors:

- The specific design of the device
- The algorithm by which it has been programmed (derived from volunteer studies)
- Various patient and environmental factors.

Most commercially available oximeters are accurate only above an SpO_2 of 70% since ethical considerations prevent human volunteer studies below this threshold. Pulse oximeters cannot be calibrated after manufacture, so accuracy is variable and differs between manufacturers. Most devices offer an accuracy approximately ±2% of the actual SaO_2.

Signal quality

The pulse oximeter reading can be affected by a number of patient specific factors that may be suspected by observing the graphical plethysmograph trace. Hypothermia, hypotension, and peripheral vasoconstriction will all lead to a poor plethysmograph trace and unreliable SpO_2 values.

The presence of other compounds can also significantly alter the pulse oximeter readings. Intravenous dyes used perioperatively and in intensive care such as methylene blue and indocyanine green may cause transient falsely low readings. Hyperbilirubinaemia, even if severe, should not affect the accuracy of pulse oximetry. Coloured nail varnish and pigmented skin may detrimentally affect readings.

Safety considerations

It is important that unnecessarily high levels of energy are not inflicted on the tissues, as this could cause heat damage, particularly in those with poor peripheral perfusion.

Clinical relevance

Pulse oximetry is an almost ubiquitous monitoring device in modern hospitals yet its usefulness has been brought in to question. A 2009 Cochrane Database review taking data from 22 992 patients concluded that whilst pulse oximetry reduced the incidence of hypoxaemia in the operating and recovery room its use did not reduce rates of transfer to intensive care or overall mortality.

Other manifestations of oximetry

In contrast to *transmission* pulse oximetry as described, *reflectance* oximetry relies on the reflection of light back to a photodetector that lies next to the source of transmission.

This allows a simple sticker-type probe to be applied to a flat surface of tissue, since light need not be transmitted through a tissue.

Hand-held devices now exist that utilize pulse oximeter technology to acquire other useful non-invasive data from patients. Using extra wavelengths of light, carboxyhaemoglobin detection can be incorporated. Further integration of the processed signal can generate an estimate of total haemoglobin concentration (Masimo®, CA, USA).

Further reading

Jubran A (1999). Pulse oximetry. *Crit Care*, 3(2):R11–7.

Moyle, JTB (2002). *Pulse Oximetry* (2nd edn). London: BMJ Books.

Pedersen T, Møller AM, Hovhannisyan K (2009). Pulse oximetry for perioperative monitoring. *Cochrane Database Syst Rev*, 4:CD002013.

2.4 Arterial blood gas analysis

Arterial blood gas (ABG) measurements provide information about acid–base balance and respiratory function that cannot be achieved from simple non-invasive measurements such as pulse oximetry. ABGs are particularly useful in patients with respiratory and circulatory failure in order to assess both the severity of the condition, and the effectiveness of innate compensatory mechanisms and implemented therapies. Modern blood gas analysers can provide additional measurements that include the concentration of haemoglobin, glucose, lactate, and common electrolytes.

Arterial blood gas measurement

Acquiring arterial blood from patients is not without risk: it can lead to haematoma, thrombosis, arterial dissection, aneurysm formation, or infection. The incidence of these depends upon the skill of the operator, the method used (puncture or cannula insertion), the site, and a number of patient-related factors.

Pain from the procedure causes patient distress and hyperventilation. It should, therefore, be performed following the administration of local anaesthesia. The syringes used must contain heparin (to avoid blood clotting within the blood gas machine) and pre-filled syringes are preferred. Care must be taken to remove excess air from the syringe before a cap is placed on it and if analysis will not be immediate, the sample should be stored on ice.

The blood gas analysis machine will have electrodes for each of the primary measurements it takes and as a minimum these will be pH, $PaCO_2$, and PaO_2 (see Box 2.2).

SaO_2, bicarbonate concentration, and base excess are then calculated according to standardized formulae.

> **Box 2.2 Measurement of pH, $PaCO_2$, and PaO_2**
>
> - pH is measured by the potential across a pH sensitive glass membrane that separates a sample of known pH and the sample being tested.
> - $PaCO_2$ is measured with a Severinghaus electrode, in which CO_2 is able to pass through a membrane and alter the pH of a bicarbonate electrolyte solution.
> - PaO_2 is measured by passing a voltage across the sample, between a platinum cathode and silver anode in a Clark electrode.

Oxygen

The oxygen electrode measures the PaO_2, and from this SaO_2 is calculated by the analyser using a standard algorithm. Samples may have a falsely high PaO_2 if left exposed to air for a prolonged period as the higher partial pressure of oxygen in the air will lead to its diffusion into the sample.

Hypoxaemia

The definition of hypoxaemia is a level of arterial oxygenation that falls below 'normal'. Guidelines suggest the normal range of PaO_2 in a healthy population is 10.7–13.3 kPa. PaO_2 must always be interpreted in the knowledge of FiO_2 and can be expressed as the PaO_2: FiO_2 (P/F) ratio. P/F ratio is used as part of the diagnostic criteria for acute lung injury (ALI) and acute respiratory distress syndrome (ARDS) where diagnostic thresholds of <40kPa and <26.7kPa respectively exist. In addition, the alveolar–arterial (A–a) oxygen partial pressure difference can be estimated in order to assist in elucidating the cause of hypoxaemia. However, the alveolar gas equation (Box 2.3) must be used to estimate PaO_2 as it cannot be easily measured.

> **Box 2.3 The alveolar gas equation**
>
> $PaO_2 = PiO_2 - PaCO_2 \times (FiO_2/RQ)$
> $PiO_2 = FiO_2 (PB - PH_2O)$
> RQ = respiratory quotient (0.8 in healthy resting individuals)
> PB = barometric pressure
> PH_2O = saturated vapour pressure of air at 37°C (6.3kPa).

In health the A–a difference is approximately 1kPa at rest, but increases with age due to a decline in PaO_2. V/Q mismatch and high FiO_2 levels also increase the A–a difference.

The causes of hypoxaemia broadly fit into five categories (see Box 2.4). These should all be considered when low arterial oxygenation is detected.

> **Box 2.4 Causes of hypoxaemia**
>
> - Hypoventilation
> - Low inspired oxygen tension
> - Right-to-left shunt
> - Ventilation–perfusion mismatch
> - Impaired diffusion.

Hypoventilation

$PaCO_2$ is raised, causing a respiratory acidosis, but the A–a oxygen difference remains normal. This may be due to respiratory depressant drugs, neurological disease (central and peripheral), pathology of the respiratory muscles, chest wall abnormalities, defects of the neuromuscular junction, and abdominal pathology causing pain and diaphragmatic splinting. Increasing the FiO_2 will raise PaO_2 but invasive or non-invasive ventilation may be required to resolve hypoventilation.

Low inspired oxygen tension

$PaCO_2$ is decreased and if extreme, the A–a oxygen difference may also be reduced. $PaCO_2$ decreases due to the compensatory hyperventilation caused by hypoxaemia and will lead to a respiratory alkalosis. This is observed at high altitude (hypobaric hypoxia) and is corrected by increasing the FiO_2.

Right-to-left shunt

In this scenario the A–a oxygen difference is increased and $PaCO_2$ normal. Blood passes from the venous to arterial circulation without being oxygenated in the lungs. Examples would include tetralogy of Fallot (see section 1.19) and pulmonary AV malformations. The hypoxaemia cannot be corrected by administering a higher FiO_2: the shunted blood will never be exposed to this additional oxygen at the alveolar membrane and therefore remains desaturated.

Ventilation–perfusion (V/Q) mismatch

A–a oxygen difference is increased and $PaCO_2$ remains normal. This is a very common cause of hypoxaemia and can result from alterations in ventilation and/or the pulmonary circulation.

At the two extreme ends of the spectrum, a V/Q ratio of 0 would indicate no ventilation but normal blood flow (shunt), whilst a V/Q ratio of >>1 indicates ventilation but no blood flow (dead space). In reality the situation is rarely so distinct. Because of the sigmoid shape of the oxygen–haemoglobin dissociation curve, a lung unit with a high V/Q ratio will have a minimal effect on PaO_2, whilst blood from a lung unit with a low V/Q ratio tends to cause significant hypoxaemia. Low V/Q shunting is seen in pulmonary consolidation caused by pneumonia and the hypoxaemia does not respond well to increasing the FiO_2.

Diffusion impairment

Both $PaCO_2$ and the A–a oxygen difference remain normal. Pathologically this can be due to thickening of the alveolar membrane such as is observed in interstitial lung disease. Pulmonary diffusion limitation can also occur in elite athletes at maximum exercise due to the reduced transit time of pulmonary capillary blood at the alveolar membrane when cardiac output is so high. It is also seen in healthy individuals exercising at high altitude because the diffusion gradient of oxygen across the alveolar membrane is so low.

Carbon dioxide

The normal partial pressure of dissolved carbon dioxide in the blood is 4.7–6.0kPa. Alterations in $PaCO_2$ will give information about ventilatory effort, with hypoventilation resulting in hypercarbia and hyperventilation in hypocarbia. In turn, changes in $PaCO_2$ will alter pH according to the carbonic acid equation. $PACO_2$ is usually equal to $PaCO_2$ as CO_2 dissolves so readily in blood, although with substantial V/Q mismatch or shunt $PaCO_2$ can be lower than $PACO_2$.

Dead space

Dead space is the volume of the respiratory tract that does not participate in gas exchange. This is approximately 2.2mL per kg, equating to 150mL in an average adult.

Anatomical dead space consists of the conducting part of the respiratory tract and can be measured using a nitrogen washout technique (Fowler's method).

Alveolar dead space is that caused by high V/Q mismatch in areas of lung with good ventilation but poor pulmonary blood flow. It can be calculated by use of the Bohr equation, which requires knowledge of a patient's $PaCO_2$ and $PetCO_2$.

Respiratory acidosis

When ventilation is insufficient to remove the carbon dioxide produced in tissues, $PaCO_2$ will rise, leading to increased H^+ and HCO_3^- concentrations from carbonic acid. The strong ion difference (SID) will remain constant, so there is no change in the base excess.

Respiratory failure can be caused by neurological, musculo-skeletal, parenchymal, and pharmacological factors as well as air flow obstruction and V/Q mismatch.

Compensation for acute respiratory acidosis is via a limited buffering capacity provided by the extrarenal (primarily intracellular) HCO_3^- buffering systems. A rise in serum HCO_3^- may be noted. With time, renal retention of HCO_3^- enhances this buffering effect and there is normalization of the pH. The renal response is said to take effect after 6–12h of respiratory acidosis and have a maximal effect in 3–4 days. Those with renal impairment will find it more difficult to adapt to respiratory acidosis. The administration of sodium bicarbonate solution in an attempt to treat acute respiratory acidosis can lead to worsening of the clinical situation because of the increased carbon dioxide load. Mechanical ventilation may then be needed to resolve this.

Respiratory alkalosis

Respiratory alkalosis is observed in hyperventilation and causes include pregnancy, salicylate poisoning and hepatic failure, head injury, psychiatric disorder, and ascent to high altitude. Initial HCO_3^- buffering by haemoglobin and tissues is followed by a more lasting compensatory mechanism whereby increased renal excretion of HCO_3^- occurs.

Metabolic acid–base disturbances

These are discussed in section 3.3.

Haemoglobin

Some blood gas machines may estimate haemoglobin concentration via a photometric system. A more accurate way to measure the various species of haemoglobin, however, is to use a co-oximeter. It uses a number of optodes that emit light at specific frequencies that can differentiate between total, fetal, carboxy-, met-, and sulpha-haemoglobin. This is particularly useful in smoke inhalation injury when carboxyhaemoglobin will be detected as oxyhaemoglobin by a pulse oximeter.

Further reading

Lumb AB (2010). *Nunn's Applied Respiratory Physiology* (7th edn). London: Churchill Livingstone.

O'Driscoll BR, Howard LS, Davison AG (2008). BTS guideline for emergency oxygen use in adult patients. *Thorax*, 63(Suppl 6): 1–68.

Scheer BV, Perel A, Pfeiffer U (2002). Clinical review: Complications and risk factors of peripheral arterial catheters used for haemodynamic monitoring in anaesthesia and intensive care medicine. *Crit Care*, 6(3):198–204.

2.5 Respiratory mechanics

Ventilation involves the mechanical process of expanding and diminishing the volume of the thorax. It is an active muscular process that is affected by alterations in tissue compliance and gas flow.

Control of ventilation

The respiratory centre is situated on the floor of the 4th ventricle in the medulla. A dorsal inspiratory group and ventral expiratory group use reciprocal innervation to maintain rhythmical ventilation.

Afferents from the cortex, hypothalamus, and pons, alongside those from the apneustic and pneumotaxic centres sanction control and differentiation from this automated pattern.

Fluctuations in PaO_2 and $PaCO_2$ are detected both centrally and peripherally by chemoreceptors, and alter ventilation accordingly.

Central chemoreceptors, located on the anterolateral surface of the medulla, respond to the hydrogen ion concentration in the surrounding CSF. CO_2 must therefore diffuse out of the blood and across the blood–brain barrier for this to occur.

Peripheral chemoreceptors, comprising the carotid bodies, (glossopharyngeal nerve), and aortic bodies (vagus nerve), respond primarily to a fall in PaO_2, and less so to a rise in CO_2. Their resultant actions on the respiratory centre are rapidly effected.

Ventilatory effectors: the muscles of respiration

In order to generate flow into or out of the lungs, a pressure gradient ($\pm 5cmH_2O$) is required. This is created by expanding or decreasing the thoracic volume. On inspiration, the diaphragm moves downwards, and the thoracic cage outwards (external intercostals, sternocleidomastoid, anterior serrate, and scalenes), to create a subatmospheric pressure within the alveoli. Expiration is a mainly passive process, using the elastic recoil of the lungs and chest wall to increase alveolar pressure. During exercise, coughing, or forced exhalation, the abdominal and internal intercostal muscles are used to aid the process.

These thoracic movements only allow expansion of the lung due to the presence of a negative intrapleural pressure (−0.5 kPa) between the lung and chest wall (parietal and visceral) pleura. If this is compromised, as seen in a pneumothorax, the lung will collapse.

Compliance

At rest, the lung will naturally lie at the point of functional residual capacity (FRC). In this instance, the inwards collapse of the lung is balanced by the chest wall recoil. On inspiration, in order for the lungs to expand, both airway resistance and compliance must be overcome. Compliance is defined as the change in lung volume per unit change in pressure.

$$\text{Compliance} = \Delta \text{ volume} / \Delta \text{ pressure}$$

Overall compliance is comprised of two components: lung compliance and chest wall compliance. These may both be measured, using dynamic or static measurements depending on whether pressure–volume changes of the lung are measured continuously or given time to equilibrate respectively. Since lung and chest wall function is a single entity, moving in parallel, total compliance is taken as the sum of each reciprocal value (C_T = 100mL/cmH$_2$O, C_L = 200mL/cmH$_2$O, C_W = 200mL/cmH$_2$O).

The relationship between lung compliance (C_L), chest wall compliance (C_W) and total compliance (C_T) can be seen in Fig. 2.5.

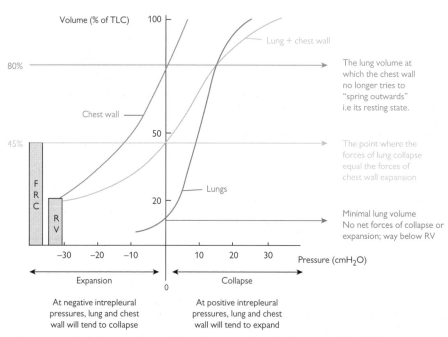

Fig. 2.5 Pressure–volume relationships for lung and chest wall. Reproduced from Catherine Spoors and Kevin Kiff, *Training in Anaesthesia*, 2010, Figure 13.17, Page 345, with permission from Oxford University Press.

Note that total compliance is not linear, but instead varies with volume. At low volumes, the alveoli are collapsed and initially hard to inflate (as in blowing up a balloon) whilst at high volumes further expansion is limited due to attainment of maximal alveolar volumes (see Box 2.5).

Box 2.5 Factors affecting compliance

- Increased compliance:
  - Emphysema
  - Ageing.
- Reduced compliance:
  - ARDS
  - Pulmonary oedema
  - Ankylosing spondylitis.

In healthy lungs, compliance would be markedly decreased if it were not for the presence of surfactant. Containing dipalmitoyl phosphatidylcholine (DPPC), this amphiphilic phospholipid substance produced by type II alveolar cells, reduces surface tension throughout the lung air–water interface. It furthermore stabilizes the alveoli to prevent atelectasis, and prevents transudation of fluid.

Airway resistance and gas flow

The flow of air through the bronchial trees is dependent upon a pressure difference between each end, and thus affected by airway resistance. It may be considered analogous to the electrical equation: current = voltage/resistance. Flow within the airways may be laminar or turbulent.

Laminar flow describes a smooth flowing gas stream with a uniform direction of flow. Gas flow in the middle of the column is two times faster than the average velocity, and this can be described by the velocity profile. The Hagen–Poiseuille equation describes the pressure-flow characteristics of laminar flow (Box 2.6).

Box 2.6 Poiseuille equation for laminar flow

$$Q = \frac{P\pi r^4}{8\eta l}$$

(Q flow rate, P is the driving pressure, r radius, η viscosity, l length)

An essential point to note from this equation is that if tube length is doubled, flow rate will halve. Halving the radius, however, decreases flow rate by 16-fold.

Turbulent flow describes disorderly flow, with eddies disrupting flow dynamics. Flow in this instance is proportional to the square root of pressure.

Whether flow in an airway is turbulent or laminar may be predicted by calculation of Reynolds number (Box 2.7).

Box 2.7 Reynolds number to predict laminar or turbulent flow

$$R_e = \frac{\rho v d}{\eta}$$

(ρ density, v velocity, d diameter, η viscosity)

This dimensionless number provides a measure of the ratio of inertial forces to viscous forces, and if >2000 is associated with turbulent flow, and <1000 with laminar flow.

The former is likely in scenarios when the flow velocity is high, and the diameter large (i.e. an upper airway), and the latter in small airways and bronchioles. The major site of resistance for the lung as a whole is not the bronchioles as would be expected, but rather the medium-sized airways and bronchi. The sheer magnitude of number of small airways makes this the case. See Box 2.8 for factors that increase or decrease airways resistance.

Box 2.8 Factors affecting airways resistance

- Increased airways resistance:
  - Vagal stimulation
  - Cigarette smoke
  - Histamine, acetylcholine
  - Cold air
  - Reduced CO_2.
- Decreased airways resistance:
  - Adrenergic stimulation
  - β2 agonists, anticholinergics
  - Increased CO_2.

Work of breathing

Pressure volume curves can used to demonstrate the inspiratory and expiratory cycles of a lung (Fig. 2.6).

As evident from Fig. 2.6, the two curves do not match and this is known as hysteresis. The loop produced describes the total work of breathing, and thus demonstrates energy lost (as heat) in overcoming viscous elastic tissues of the lung and chest, and airway resistance frictional forces. The larger the loop, the greater the work required. In an ideal elastic lung, no energy would be dissipated as heat, and a straight line would be evident with no respective energy loss. Evidently this is not the case, and efficiency of breathing is believed to be in the region of 5–10%.

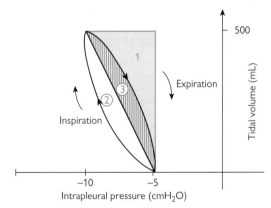

Fig. 2.6 Work of breathing. Reproduced from Catherine Spoors and Kevin Kiff, *Training in Anaesthesia*, 2010, Figure 13.23, page 347, with permission from Oxford University Press

Further reading

Lumb AB (2010). *Nunn's Applied Respiratory Physiology* (7th edn). London: Churchill Livingstone.

West JB (2011). *Respiratory Physiology: The Essentials* (9th edn). Philadelphia, PA: Lippincott Williams and Wilkins.

2.6 Pulmonary circulation

The pulmonary circulation delivers deoxygenated blood to the pulmonary capillaries so oxygen can be replenished, and carbon dioxide removed. Blood leaves the right ventricle via the thin-walled pulmonary artery, which sequentially branches alongside the airways, and ends up as a dense capillary network encompassing the 300 million alveoli. Within this circulation, which contains 10% of circulating blood volume (500mL) at any one time, deoxygenated blood traverses the capillaries in 0.5–1.0sec. Whilst both the systemic and pulmonary circulations working in series must accept essentially the same cardiac output (the bronchial circulation arising from the thoracic artery is approximately 2% of the cardiac output), the latter represents a low-pressure, low-resistance system. In fact a sixfold difference is seen between the two mean arterial pressures (MAPs) (Table 2.2).

Table 2.2 Pressures within the pulmonary and systemic circulations (mmHg)		
	Right	**Left**
Atrium	2	5
Ventricle	25/0	120/0
Artery	25/8 (pulmonary artery)	120/80 (aorta)
MAP	15	100

A PAC is traditionally used to assess right heart, pulmonary circulation, and left atrial ('wedge') pressures; however, the pressure in the pulmonary capillaries remains uncertain. Normal mean pulmonary artery pressures are 12–16mmHg with pulmonary hypertension defined as >25mmHg as rest, and >30mmHg on exercise. Pulmonary blood flow may also be calculated using the Fick principle or indicator dilution techniques.

Regulation of pulmonary circulation and pulmonary vascular resistance

Both passive and active factors are responsible for the regulation of pulmonary blood flow. At rest, two passive factors predominate: recruitment and distension. Recruitment describes the process of increased blood flow opening up previously closed capillaries, and thus increasing blood flow and lowering resistance. Distension involves increasing the thin-walled vessel dimensions, again enhancing flow. Both of these processes usually occur in unison, as does the alteration of blood flow in relation to lung volumes. At large lung volumes, extra-alveolar vessels are pulled open and capillaries stretched, whilst at low volumes, vessels are compressed and tortuous. In both cases, PVR increases (Fig. 2.7).

Whilst the pulmonary circulation is minimally affected by neural regulation, (innervation is via the sympathetic nervous system with alpha and beta adrenergic fibres responsible for vasoconstriction and vasodilatation respectively), numerous humoral and pharmacological factors may affect it (Table 2.3; see also section 1.18).

Table 2.3 Factors affecting pulmonary vascular resistance	
Increased PVR	Decreased PVR
Hypoxia	Hyperoxia
Hypercapnia	Hypocapnia
Histamine, serotonin, prostaglandin, angiotensin, thromboxane A2	Bradykinin, acetylcholine, prostacyclin, nitric oxide
Drugs: COX inhibitors, β-blockers	Drugs: calcium channel blockers, volatiles, phosphodiesterase inhibitors

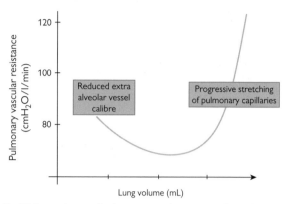

Fig. 2.7 Lung volume and pulmonary vascular resistance. Reproduced from Catherine Spoors and Kevin Kiff, *Training in Anaesthesia*, 2010, Figure 13.39, page 359, with permission from Oxford University Press.

Hypoxic pulmonary vasoconstriction

In an attempt to minimize V/Q mismatch, vasoconstriction occurs in poorly ventilated, and thus hypoxic areas of the lung. This diverts blood to better-ventilated areas of the lung. The mechanism behind this response is yet to be determined; however it is the alveolar PO_2, and *not* the oxygen content of the pulmonary circulation that governs it. Though beneficial at sea level (and *in utero*), at altitude it may exacerbate the problems of hypobaric hypoxia leading to high-altitude pulmonary oedema (HAPE).

Distribution of pulmonary blood flow

Blood flow throughout the lung is not evenly distributed and two models have been used to describe its distribution.

The gravitational model for pulmonary blood flow uses the notion that within the lung, a hydrostatic pressure difference exists. As pressure is directly related to the height of the fluid column, (as well as the density of fluid, and acceleration due to gravity (P=phg)), in the upright position between the main pulmonary artery and lung base (30cm), this is approximately 25mmHg. Increased pressure towards the lung bases consequently increases blood flow.

The structural model for the distribution of blood flow maintains the concept that alterations in vessel resistance have the main impact on blood flow—which is minimized when the lung is over- or underexpanded. PVR is least, and therefore, blood flow greatest, at FRC.

Lung zones

The importance of PVR and blood flow may be illustrated when considering functional lung zones (Fig. 2.8). These are defined by the pressure difference between the alveoli and surrounding pulmonary vessels, the transmural pressure, and describe the interaction between gravity and extravascular pressures in the alveoli. As blood pressure, and thus arterial and venous flow, increases descending down the lung, and alveolar pressure remains constant, the relative values in each lung zone effectively determines the blood flow.

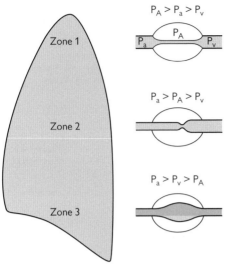

Fig. 2.8 Zones of blood flow within the lung. Reproduced from Catherine Spoors and Kevin Kiff, *Training in Anaesthesia*, 2010, Figure 13.40, page 359, with permission from Oxford University Press.

Zone 1: PA > Pa > Pv

At the apices of the lung, alveolar pressure is greater than the hydrostatic pressure within the pulmonary vasculature, hence vessels collapse with no blood flow. In health, this does not occur, as pulmonary artery pressure is sufficiently greater than alveolar pressure. However, if arterial pressure decreases (e.g. haemorrhage) or alveolar pressure increases (e.g. PEEP) this may occur and alveolar dead space will be present.

Zone 2: Pa > PA > Pv

In this zone, pulmonary arterial pressure is greater than alveolar pressure, but venous pressure remains lowest. Flow is thus determined by the arterial and alveolar pressure difference, and partial obstruction may occur due to vessel collapse.

Zone 3: Pa > Pv > PA

In zone 3 (10cm above heart to base of lungs) blood flow is normally uninterrupted. As alveolar pressure is less than both arterial and venous pressure, the arterial and venous pressure difference determines flow.

Ventilation–perfusion mismatch

In an ideal scenario, the blood supply to an area of lung would perfectly match the ventilation. The V/Q ratio in this instance would be 1 and no shunting or dead space would be present. In reality, both perfusion and ventilation vary throughout the lung in both good and poor health.

Ventilation across the lung is dependent on lung compliance. With a normal inspiratory effort starting from FRC, the lung bases lie on a more favourable part of the compliance curve and experience a greater change of volume for pressure applied. Ventilation is therefore greater. During IPPV, the FRC moves to the left of the compliance curve, and thus the apex now resides at the most favourable part of the curve (Fig. 2.9).

Shunt and dead space

Two extremes of V/Q mismatch may be used to illustrate the associated issues of shunt and dead space. Shunt describes an area of lung that is perfused but not ventilated. In this instance the V/Q ratio will approach 0, depending on the severity of the shunt, and blood will leave the lung deoxygenated. The severity of shunt, and consequent hypoxaemia, may be calculated using the shunt equations as outlined here:[1]

$$\frac{Qs}{Qt} = \frac{CcO_2 - CaO_2}{CcO_2 - CvO_2}$$

As perfused blood does not come into contact with the ventilated areas of lung, increasing the inspired fraction of oxygen (FiO_2) will have no effect on the hypoxaemia. Ventilated areas elsewhere in the lung will not compensate as haemoglobin is already fully saturated by oxygen. Potentially CPAP, PEEP, and physiotherapy may help in this setting to re expand collapsed areas of lung.

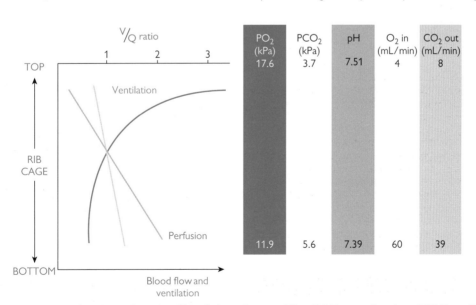

Fig. 2.9 Blood flow, ventilation, and V/Q ratio. Reproduced from Catherine Spoors and Kevin Kiff, *Training in Anaesthesia*, 2010, Figure 13.42, page 361, with permission from Oxford University Press.

1 Qs = shunted blood flow; Qt = cardiac output; CcO_2 = oxygen content of end pulmonary capillary blood; CaO_2 = oxygen content of arterial blood; CvO_2 = oxygen content of mixed venous blood.

At the other end of the scale, dead space describes an area of lung that is ventilated but not perfused. This alveolar dead space, in addition to anatomical dead space results in physiological dead space. An example of this may be a PE, and in this instance the V/Q ratio will approach infinity.

Other functions of the lung

See Box 2.9 for other functions of the lung.

Box 2.9 Other functions of the lung
• Blood reservoir
• Blood filter
• Angiotensin I activation
• Metabolism of vasoactive substances and drugs.
• Immunoglobulin (IgA) production
• Phospholipid and protein synthesis.

Further reading

Peacock A, Naeije R, & Rubin L (2011). *Pulmonary Circulation* (3rd rev. edn). London: Hodder Arnold.

West JB (2011). *Respiratory Physiology: The Essentials* (9th edn). Philadelphia, PA: Lippincott Williams and Wilkins.

2.7 Respiratory failure

Respiratory failure is defined as a *failure of gas exchange*. It can be divided into two distinct types (Box 2.10).

Box 2.10 Classification of respiratory failure

- *Type 1:* hypoxaemia with normal or low $PaCO_2$
- *Type 2:* hypoxaemia with high $PaCO_2$.

Whilst there are numerous underlying causes, the symptoms and signs are generally similar regardless of type or pathology. The commonest symptom is breathlessness whilst signs include tachypnoea, tachycardia, cyanosis, and confusion or reduced level of consciousness.

Causes of respiratory failure

A number of pathologies can result in hypoxaemia (see section 2.4). Calculation of the alveolar–arterial oxygen partial pressure $(P(A–a)O_2)$ gradient may assist in diagnosing the cause of hypoxaemia. The normal $P(A–a)O_2$ is approximately 1kPa but increases with age due to worsening ventilation–perfusion (V/Q) mismatching (see Table 2.4).

Reduced FiO_2/PiO_2
This can be experienced during ascent to high altitude where the barometric pressure declines with ascent (reduced PiO_2) and is resolved via administration of supplemental oxygen. $PaCO_2$ is often reduced due to hypoxic ventilatory drive.

Hypoventilation
This is caused either by a reduction in minute ventilation or an increase in the proportion of dead space ventilation (anatomical or physical). It can be caused pharmacologically (typically by opiates), by neurological abnormalities (central or peripheral), and by muscular weakness. It is characterized by a raised $PaCO_2$ and is usually alleviated by the administration of supplemental oxygen unless severe, when ventilatory assistance will be required.

Ventilation–perfusion mismatch
This is the most common cause of respiratory failure clinically. Diseased lungs will have increasing levels of mismatch causing systemic hypoxaemia. $PaCO_2$ tends to be normal in V/Q mismatch and the hypoxaemia is alleviated to a limited extent by the administration of supplemental oxygen.

Shunt
This occurs when blood in the right side of the circulation bypasses the lungs (extrapulmonary shunt) or passes through poorly ventilated areas of lung (intrapulmonary shunt), thus failing to become oxygenated. Intrapulmonary shunting represents an extreme form of V/Q mismatching and may be seen in a collapsed or severely consolidated area of lung. Extrapulmonary

shunts usually occur due to congenital heart disease where right-to-left shunt may occur. Shunts cannot be fully corrected by the administration of supplemental oxygen. The response to increasing PaO_2 depends on the shunt fraction (Fig. 2.10). $PaCO_2$ tends to be normal even in severe shunting.

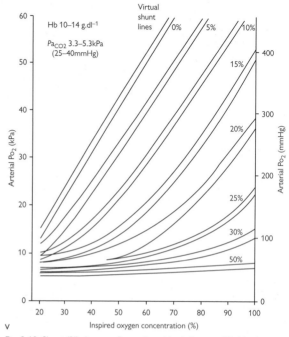

Fig. 2.10 Shunt (%) diagram. Reproduced from Benator SR, Hewlett AM, and Nunn JF, 'The use of iso-shunt lines for control of oxygen therapy', *British Journal of Anaesthesia*, 1973, 45, pp. 711–718, by permission of The Board of Management and Trustees of the British Journal of Anaesthesia and Oxford University Press.

Diffusion limitation
This relatively uncommon cause of respiratory failure reflects damage to the alveolar membrane, which prevents effective gas transfer between the alveolus and circulation – for example, in pulmonary fibrosis. The hypoxaemia due to diffusion limitation tends to be exacerbated by exercise, leading to a rise in $P(A–a)O_2$.

Treatment of respiratory failure

Respiratory failure can be diagnosed clinically and confirmed by the measurement of arterial oxygen saturation (with pulse oximetry) or by analysis of an ABG. Only the latter will enable differentiation between type 1 and type 2 respiratory failure. Neither will necessarily highlight the underlying cause.

Treatment of respiratory failure requires improvement of abnormal blood gases with oxygen administration or ventilation *in combination* with treatment of the underlying cause.

Oxygen administration
Management of the acutely hypoxaemic patient requires administration of oxygen to restore arterial oxygenation towards normal. Whilst high flow oxygen is unlikely to cause adverse effects in the acutely unwell, FiO_2 should then be titrated downwards to maintain the desired SpO_2 in order to administer the minimum FiO_2 necessary.

Table 2.4 Causes of hypoxaemia	
Cause of hypoxemia	$P(A–a)O_2$
Reduced FiO_2 (or PiO_2)	Normal
Hypoventilation	Normal
Ventilation–perfusion mismatch	Elevated
Right-to-left shunt	Elevated
Diffusion limitation	Normal

There are a small number of patients in whom hypoxic respiratory drive is an important component of the balance of their lung disease (typically, patients with severe COPD who have compensated type 2 respiratory failure with a high serum bicarbonate concentration and a high $PaCO_2$). In these patients, FiO_2 should be carefully titrated upwards and the response observed with repeated ABGs. Excessive administration of oxygen may result in hypoventilation and a dangerous rise in $PaCO_2$.

Oxygen may be administered via a number of different methods (Fig. 2.11).

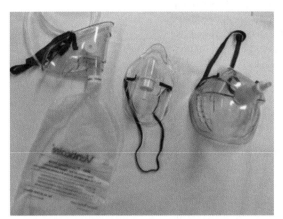

Fig. 2.11 Modes of oxygen delivery. High concentration reservoir mask, simple facemask and Venturi mask.

High concentration reservoir mask
Also known as the non-rebreathing mask, this mask has a reservoir bag and delivers oxygen at concentrations between 60% and 90% when used at flow rates of 10–15L/min. This type of mask is commonly used in the emergency situation. The precise FiO_2 provided will depend on the oxygen flow rate and on the patient's breathing pattern.

Simple facemask
Previously referred to as a 'Hudson' mask, this can deliver between 40% and 60% oxygen, depending upon oxygen flow rate and the patient's breathing pattern. Flow rates of <5L/min can lead to rebreathing and the possibility of a rise in $PaCO_2$. This mask should be avoided in those patients with type 2 respiratory failure.

Venturi mask
These provide a very accurate FiO_2 by using the Venturi effect of entraining air through a fixed constriction incorporated into the design of the mask. Different masks can be used to provide a range of different FiO_2s but the correct oxygen flow rate must be selected to achieve this. Commonly available Venturi masks administer oxygen concentrations of 24%, 28%, 35%, 40%, and 60%. They are ideal for patients who require an accurately titrated FiO_2.

Nasal cannulae
These are used to administer low additional quantities of oxygen in which the actual FiO_2 is not particularly important. Nasal cannulae set at 1–4L/min can deliver approximately 24–40% oxygen, depending on the patient's breathing pattern.

Non-invasive ventilation

Gas exchange may be improved by application of a tight fitting mask that enables positive pressure to be applied during ventilation. There are essentially two forms of non-invasive ventilation (NIV):

Continuous positive airway pressure (CPAP)
Oxygenation may be improved by the maintenance of a continuous amount of pressure throughout the respiratory cycle, analogous to the PEEP that can be provided during invasive ventilation. It can improve oxygenation, but will not improve a high $PaCO_2$ in type 2 respiratory failure. CPAP is commonly provided at a level of 5–15cmH$_2$O.

Bi-level positive airway pressure (BiPAP)
With a similar mask to that commonly used for CPAP, alternative devices can provide a cyclical changing pressure that is timed to inspiration and expiration so as to provide true inspiratory assistance and PEEP. A typical setting might be 20/5cmH$_2$O (inspiratory pressure of 20cmH$_2$O and PEEP of 5cmH$_2$O). The benefit of BiPAP over CPAP is that the increase in minute ventilation that it produces can reduce hypercapnia in type 2 respiratory failure.

Invasive ventilation
Severe respiratory failure may require the use of mechanical ventilation to provide adequate oxygenation and removal of CO_2. The point at which to commence mechanical ventilation will involve consideration of the risks (anaesthesia and insertion of an endotracheal tube) and benefits (potential for improved gas exchange and a secured airway). Particular thought should also be given to those patients with end-stage chronic lung disease, as mechanical ventilation may be inappropriate or perhaps unwanted. There is no evidence that one particular mode of mechanical ventilation is superior to another in the management of respiratory failure.

Further reading

O'Driscoll R (2008). BTS guideline for emergency oxygen use in adult patients. *Thorax*; 63: suppl VI68.

2.8 Asthma

Asthma is a common respiratory condition affecting 5–10% of the population. Acute life-threatening asthma may be encountered throughout the hospital and in the perioperative setting. Over 1000 people die annually in the UK from asthma. The recognition and treatment of asthma is essential knowledge for all clinicians.

Pathophysiology

Asthma is a chronic inflammatory disorder that affects the airways. Whilst the fundamental lesion is reversible airways obstruction, its pathophysiology is multifactorial. Under the influence of the parasympathetic nervous system (vagal nerve and muscarinic cholinergic receptors), altered bronchial smooth muscle tone leads to bronchoconstriction and hypersecretion of mucus. Mast cell and basophil degranulation cause mucosal inflammation, oedema, and subsequent worsening of the airway narrowing. Airway hyper-responsiveness is a prominent feature of asthma: triggers that provoke airway obstruction include cold air, exercise, viral upper respiratory infections, cigarette smoke and respiratory allergens. Asthma undoubtedly has an inherited component, but the genetics involved are complex and highly interactive with environmental factors.

Signs and symptoms

Asthma is characterized by recurrent episodes of dyspnoea, cough, and wheeze, often worse in the morning due to diurnal variation. Patients may be able to identify a specific trigger factor. During an exacerbation of asthma, tachypnoea, tachycardia, and a widespread polyphonic wheeze may be present. The signs may, however, vary according to the severity of the attack. Immediate assessment of disease severity should be made according to the British Thoracic Society (BTS) guidelines (Box 2.11). Normal or raised $PaCO_2$ demonstrates exhaustion and an inability to maintain adequate ventilation. This would place the patient in the 'life-threatening' asthma category.

In children, assessment may be difficult as wheezing attacks are often viral in nature and unresponsive to asthma treatment. However, children unable to talk or feed, with heart and respiratory rate parameters outside the 'normal for age' should warrant serious concern.

Treatment

Treatment in the community usually follows the BTS stepwise guidelines (see Box 2.12).

Pharmacological treatment in the emergency setting again follows a stepwise approach (see Box 2.13).

Aminophylline, which is metabolized to theophylline, demonstrates a narrow therapeutic range, and thus must be administered with great caution to avoid toxicity that could lead to seizures and arrhythmias.

Referral to intensive care may be required in the event of:

- Acute or life-threatening asthma failing to respond to therapy
- Worsening gas exchange
- Exhaustion or imminent respiratory arrest.

Currently no studies demonstrate a benefit of NIV in asthma, however it is still frequently used. Intubation and ventilation may

---

Box 2.11 British Thoracic Society guidelines re: asthma severity

Moderate asthma
- Worsening symptoms
- PEFR >50–75% of best or predicted
- No features of acute severe asthma.

Acute severe asthma
- PEFR 33–50% of best or predicted
- Respiratory rate >25/min
- Heart rate >110/min
- Inability to complete sentences in one breath.

Life threatening asthma
- PEFR <33% of best or predicted
- SpO_2 <92%
- PaO_2 <8kPa
- Normal $PaCO_2$
- Silent chest
- Cyanosis
- Poor respiratory effort
- Arrhythmia
- Exhaustion
- Confusion.

Data from BTS/SIGN Asthma Guideline: 2011. http://www.brit-thoracic.org.uk.

---

be required. Whilst this secures the upper airway and allows control of ventilation, it will *not* treat the underlying pathology. Moreover, it is an extremely hazardous procedure in this setting, and may precipitate arrhythmias, cardiovascular collapse, and worsening bronchospasm. The decision to intubate should be taken at the most senior level available.

Appropriate IV bronchodilator therapy may be effective even in severe hypercarbia, and prevent the need for intubation. Therapy should take place in a controlled environment with the equipment and expertise for emergency intubation immediately available.

Adequate fluid resuscitation is an essential component of management to avoid dehydration.

Asthma during the perioperative period

Most asthmatics who are well controlled have an uneventful course during the perioperative period. Whilst the asthmatic population is more liable to sputum retention, atelectasis, and chest infection, the incidence of intraoperative bronchospasm is under 2%.

Box 2.12 Community management of asthma

1. Inhaled short acting β-2-agonist (salbutamol, terbutaline)
2. Inhaled steroid (beclomethasone)
3. Inhaled long acting β-2-agonist (salmeterol, formoterol)
4. Leukotriene receptor antagonist (montelukast) or theophylline
5. Daily oral steroids.

Data from BTS/SIGN Asthma Guideline: 2011. http://www.brit-thoracic.org.uk.<

Box 2.13 Management of acute severe asthma

1. Oxygen
2. Nebulized salbutamol (5mg) and nebulized ipratropium bromide (0.5mg)
3. Hydrocortisone (100mg IV) and/or prednisolone (40mg PO)
4. Magnesium sulphate (1.2–2g IV infusion). If not improving then consider:
5. Aminophylline (5mg/kg IV loading dose)
6. Salbutamol (3–20mcg/min IV infusion)
7. Nebulized adrenaline (5mL 1:1000)
8. Other agents: Volatile agents, ketamine, Heliox (see section 2.9).

Data from BTS/SIGN Asthma Guideline: 2011. http://www.brit-thoracic.org.uk.

Box 2.14 Management of intraoperative bronchospasm

1. Switch to 100% oxygen and call for help
2. Identify a precipitant where possible
3. Use sevoflurane to maintain general anaesthesia
4. Administer salbutamol nebulizer via breathing circuit
5. Consider IV magnesium
6. Consider IV salbutamol.

Laryngoscopy and intubation are common culprits for inducing an exacerbation of asthma: deep intubation with local anaesthetic administration may abate this if intubation is truly required.

In the event that intraoperative bronchospasm does occur, an appropriate management plan should be followed (see Box 2.14).

Alternative diagnoses should always be considered: for example, breathing circuit obstruction or anaphylaxis.

Postoperative management

In the immediate hours following surgery, patients should be monitored both in recovery and on the ward. Regular asthma medication should be instigated as soon as possible, steroid cover prescribed if necessary, and adequate analgesia provided as pain may provoke an exacerbation.

Anaesthetic considerations in the management of acute life-threatening asthma

In the event that anaesthesia is required during an acute asthmatic episode, overzealous administration of induction agent may precipitate cardiovascular instability, as patients are often severely dehydrated and reliant on their sympathetic nervous system. Maintenance of anaesthesia may be provided by sevoflurane and muscle relaxation continued to improve chest wall compliance.

Bronchospasm may necessitate the use of high inflation pressures to achieve adequate ventilatory volumes and this increases the risk of developing pneumothoraces. Pressure-limited ventilation and permissive hypercapnia may be employed as strategies in acute asthma. Gas trapping occurs due to the long time constants of alveoli associated with constricted small airways. This leads to 'autopeep', which can greatly increase intrathoracic pressure and cause cardiovascular instability in severe cases. This can be managed with prolongation of the ventilator expiratory phase. In severe cases, manual deflation by chest compression during ventilator disconnection may be required to reduce gas trapping.

Further reading

BTS/SIGN (2011). *Asthma Guideline*. <http://www.brit-thoracic.org.uk>

Browne GJ & Wilkins BH (2003). Use of intravenous salbutamol in acute severe asthma. *Anaesthesia*, 58(8):729–32.

Currie G (2008). *Asthma* (Oxford Respiratory Medicine Library). Oxford: Oxford University Press.

Preoperative considerations

Prior to surgery, during the preoperative assessment, a full history and examination should be undertaken. Attention should be paid to asthma-inducing precipitants, exercise tolerance, medications, and frequency of inhaler use. Recent oral steroid use or long-term inhaled steroid use may induce adrenocortical suppression. In this instance supplementary steroids may be required. Tolerance of NSAIDs should also be elicited as their administration may precipitate an exacerbation of asthma in up to 5% of children and 20% of adults.

Investigations may include serial measurements of peak expiratory flow rate (PEFR) and comparison to predicted peak flow or, more usefully, individual best flow rates. In the elective setting, should signs and symptoms suggest a worsening disease state, surgery should be postponed.

Bronchodilator therapy should be continued preoperatively, and many anaesthetists advocate the use of a salbutamol inhaler immediately preoperatively. Anxiolytics may also be used if anxiety is a precipitant.

Conduct of anaesthesia

Whilst most volatile agents are bronchodilators, desflurane may precipitate bronchospasm in high concentrations. Halothane is a particularly powerful bronchodilator (Table 2.5) and many ICUs maintain an anaesthetic machine with a halothane vaporizer for treating life-threatening asthma. Histamine-releasing drugs (e.g. atracurium and mivacurium) should be avoided. Opiate use, though considered low risk, may be minimized in brittle asthmatics by using regional anaesthesia.

Table 2.5 Drugs safe to use in asthma	
Induction agents	Propofol, ketamine, etomidate, midazolam
Muscle relaxants	Suxamethonium, rocuronium, vecuronium
Opioids	Fentanyl, alfentanil, pethidine
Volatiles	Isoflurane, sevoflurane, enflurane, halothane

2.9 Helium and nitric oxide

Properties of helium

Helium is a colourless, odourless, tasteless gas with a boiling point of −269°C. With a valence of zero, helium is chemically inert under normal conditions. It is the second lightest and second most abundant element in the universe, hydrogen being first in both categories. Helium is extremely scarce within the Earth's atmosphere, only 0.00052% by volume (5.2 parts per million), but is present in higher proportions within natural gas (up to 7%), providing a useful commercial source of the gas. The manufacturing process involves liquefaction of air or natural gas to remove easily condensable fractions followed by adsorption of contaminant gases. A report by the US National Research Council in 2010 predicted that because of diminishing natural gas supplies and issues surrounding underground reserves, the world supply of helium may be exhausted within 30 years.

Properties of helium–oxygen mixtures

For clinical purposes helium is commonly available as Heliox (21% oxygen and 79% helium) and supplied in cylinders (Fig. 2.12) that have a brown body with brown and white quadrants on the shoulder. Cylinder pressure is 137 bar when full. As an inert gas with a similar viscosity to air but a density that is approximately three times lower, helium can replace nitrogen in gas mixtures breathed by patients in order to reduce the work of breathing.

Air flow within the respiratory tract can be laminar or turbulent and the tendency for turbulence is described by the calculated Reynolds number. A higher Reynolds number predicts more turbulent air flow (see section 2.5).

A reduction in gas density lowers the Reynolds number and therefore increases the propensity for laminar flow. Work of breathing is directly proportional to gas flow during laminar flow but is proportional to the square of the gas flow under turbulent conditions. Consequently, the lower density of Heliox, as compared to air, reduces both turbulence and work of breathing. Whilst this is particularly effective in the large upper airways, it should be noted that in the smaller distal airways of the respiratory tract where flow tends to be predominantly laminar, resistance is proportional to gas viscosity (rather than density) so Heliox is relatively ineffective at improving gas flow properties.

Clinical use of helium–oxygen mixtures

Since 1935, helium–oxygen mixtures have been used to reduce the work of breathing and it was the mainstay of treatment in acute asthma prior to the advent of bronchodilators. Today, Heliox is most commonly used in emergency situations involving acute obstruction of the upper airway. Whilst this is ineffective in treating the cause of an airway obstruction, it can provide a window in which definitive treatment may be initiated. Situations where this has been shown to be effective include epiglottitis, laryngitis, tracheal stenosis, post-extubation stridor, foreign bodies, and tumours.

Despite the theoretical limitations of using Heliox in the treatment of asthma, and noting that maximum inspired fractional concentration of oxygen is limited with its use, evidence supports its effectiveness in reducing work of breathing and improving symptoms during acute exacerbations. Recently, the use of Heliox for nebulizing drugs for asthma has been investigated, as molecules diffuse up to four times faster through a helium–oxygen mixture than through an equivalent nitrogen–oxygen mixture. Heliox has also been used during the weaning of patients off mechanical ventilation in the critical care setting and special ventilators are available to deliver accurate mixtures of helium–oxygen.

Other uses of helium

MRI
The superconducting magnet within an MRI scanner has almost no electrical resistance when cooled to a temperature close to absolute zero (−273°C). This can be achieved by immersing the magnet in liquid helium.

Diving
Divers use helium as part of as gas mixture that also includes oxygen and nitrogen called 'Trimix.' Its purpose is to reduce the fractions of nitrogen and oxygen in the mixture to below that of air, in order to minimize the effects of nitrogen narcosis and oxygen toxicity when high-pressure gas is breathed at great depth.

Other
Helium is used in preference to hydrogen when filling airships and balloons because it is non-flammable. Helium is also used to clean out rocket engines, to condense hydrogen and oxygen to make rocket fuel, and to pressurize the interior of liquid fuel rockets.

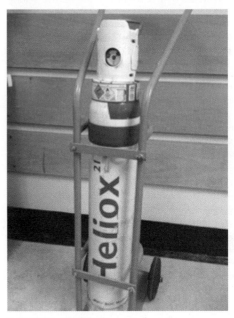

Fig. 2.12 The Heliox cylinder.

Properties of nitric oxide

Gaseous nitric oxide

Nitric oxide (NO) is a colourless, highly reactive, gas with a boiling point of −152°C: it reacts rapidly with oxygen to form toxic nitrogen dioxide (NO_2). NO is highly lipid soluble and therefore diffuses rapidly across biological membranes. In the UK, NO is available as INOmax (Ikaria), 800 parts per million (ppm) in nitrogen; these are white aluminium cylinders with a turquoise coloured shoulder, at 137 bar.

Endogenous nitric oxide

NO is also an important biological signalling molecule that was previously known as endothelium-derived relaxing factor (EDRF) until its true identity was discovered in the 1980s. NO is generated *in vivo* from L-arginine and oxygen via one of the isoforms of the enzyme nitric oxide synthase. Under certain conditions NO can also be produced by the reduction of nitrate (NO_3^-) via nitrite (NO_2^-), utilizing the enzyme xanthine oxidase. In whole blood NO is rapidly metabolized to nitrite and nitrate, by interaction with the haem group of haemoglobin. The half-life of NO is only a few seconds: rapid oxidation close to the site of release, ensure its actions are highly localized.

Endogenously, NO is primarily released from endothelial cells where its principal role is to regulate vascular tone. Most of the effects of NO are mediated through activation of the soluble haem-containing enzyme guanylate cyclase which produces guanosine 3′,5′-cyclic monophosphate (cGMP). Its most well-known effect is relaxation of vascular smooth muscle leading to vasodilatation but it also plays a key role in neurotransmission, platelet aggregation, leucocyte adhesion, the inflammatory and immune responses, and mitochondrial function.

Inhaled nitric oxide therapy

Acute respiratory distress syndrome (ARDS)

The major use of NO gas in medicine has been to reverse the hypoxic pulmonary vasoconstriction that results from ARDS in mechanically ventilated neonates and adults on critical care units (see section 20.4). ARDS is characterized by a heterogeneous pattern of altered V/Q mismatch leading to profound hypoxaemia.

Administered within the gas flow of a standard ventilator, NO can be delivered to lung units with good ventilation, causing selective pulmonary vasodilatation and improving V/Q mismatch and arterial oxygenation. The inhalational route and short half-life of NO tends to avoid systemic vasodilatation and consequent hypotension. Conversely, administration of alternative systemic agents that also bring about pulmonary vasodilatation (e.g. nitroglycerin and sodium nitroprusside) will result in pulmonary vasodilatation throughout the lung and will invariably exacerbate V/Q mismatching and hypoxaemia along with sometimes profound hypotension.

Administration of inhaled nitric oxide

The INOvent (Ikaria) delivery system can be used to deliver a closely monitored dose of NO into the inspiratory limb of a patient breathing circuit. It uses an injector system and can be incorporated into most ventilator configurations, including high-frequency oscillatory (HFO) ventilators. When used at concentrations of <20ppm, environmental contamination with NO_2 is extremely low. Maximum recommended exposure levels in the environment are 25ppm of NO and 3ppm of NO_2 over an 8h period. Environmental monitors are available and the use of scavenging systems should therefore be considered in areas where NO administration is to be performed.

Reported effective doses of inhaled NO range from 10–80ppm, whilst a dose of >100ppm is likely to be detrimental. Some authors advocate doses in the range of only 1–10ppm, claiming this to be equally as effective in improving oxygenation. The individual response to inhaled NO therapy is highly variable and a slow dose-response approach to administration is advised, titrating the dose to optimum oxygenation. Some patients may exhibit no response to inhaled NO and a small proportion may exhibit early adverse effects such as worsening oxygenation and systemic hypotension. Treatment should be stopped in the latter cohort.

Benefits of inhaled nitric oxide therapy

Whilst NO is reasonably effective at improving arterial oxygenation in the majority of hypoxaemic patients with acute lung injury (ALI) and ARDS, meta-analyses have failed to demonstrate an improvement in survival, and consequently NO therapy is not recommend for routine use in severely hypoxaemic adult patients. However, some clinicians still advocate its use as a bridging therapy. Cost must also be taken into consideration when administering NO: in 2010 the price of administering inhaled NO was approximately £85 per hour.

Adverse effects of inhaled nitric oxide

The binding of NO to haemoglobin results in the production of methaemoglobin. Whilst methaemoglobin is not toxic per se, it is unable to transport oxygen and thus reduces the oxygen-carrying capacity of the blood. This dose-dependent effect is particularly noticeable in neonates, but levels of methaemoglobin should be monitored in all patients. Administration of NO donor compounds, such as prilocaine, sodium nitroprusside, and nitroglycerine, may have an additive effect on the risk of developing methaemoglobinaemia.

Rapid withdrawal of NO can lead to rebound pulmonary vasoconstriction and profound hypoxaemia leading to circulatory collapse. NO must therefore be weaned slowly with careful observation of oxygenation and haemodynamic parameters.

Further reading

Adhikari NK, Burns KE, Friedrich JO, *et al.* (2007). Effect of nitric oxide on oxygenation and mortality in acute lung injury: systematic review and meta-analysis. *BMJ*, 334(7597):779.

Barrington KJ & and Finer N (2010). Inhaled nitric oxide for respiratory failure in preterm infants. *Cochrane Database Syst Rev*, 12:CD000509.

Branson RD (2010). Respiratory care controversies II. *Respir Care*, 55(2):217–24.

Chevrolet JC (2001). Helium oxygen mixtures in the intensive care unit. *Crit Care Med*, 5:179–81.

Manthous CA, Morgan S, Pohlman A, *et al.* (1997). Heliox in the treatment of airflow obstruction. *Respir Care*, 42:1034–42.

Chapter 3

Kidney and body fluids

83

3.1 Fluid balance

Physiological fluid balance refers to the movement of fluids into and out of the body, and between the different compartments that exist within it. Homeostatic mechanisms attempt to maintain euvolaemia in the face of the natural variation in water intake, but this process may fail during illness or iatrogenic intervention.

Fluid compartments

The human body is made up of approximately 60% water; in an 'ideal' 70kg man this is 42L but this value is slightly lower in women due to their greater proportion of adipose tissue. Neonates have a higher percentage of body water than adults (75–80%), and total body water declines progressively with age.

The total water volume is divided roughly between the intracellular (28L) and extracellular (14L) compartments (Fig. 3.1). The extracellular compartment is further divided ⅔:⅓ between the interstitial (11L) and intravascular (3L) compartments. A small component of the extracellular compartment is termed *transcellular fluid*, which refers to fluid contained within epithelial-lined spaces, for example, pleural, pericardial, and synovial fluid. Interstitial fluid is that which lies between cells, bathing them in oxygen and nutrients. The intravascular space also contains red blood cells (in addition to water) to make up the total intravascular volume to approximately 5L in a 70kg male (blood volume in adults is 75mL/kg in males and 65mL/kg in females). The ratio between red blood cell volume and plasma volume is the haematocrit value:

$$\text{Blood volume} = \text{plasma volume} \times (100 / 100 - \text{haematocrit})$$

An additional fluid compartment that is frequently referred to, but for which there is no evidence for its existence, is the so-called 'third space'. This was a theory popularized in the 1960s which has led to the overadministration of intravenous fluid in order to replace losses 'into it'.

Internal fluid balance

This describes the movement of water through compartments within the body. The intracellular and extracellular compartments are separated by the cell membrane but movement of water occurs easily between them. Water crosses membranes by osmosis, the process whereby a solvent moves through a semi-permeable membrane from an area of low solute concentration (hypotonic) to a high solute concentration (hypertonic). Water will move in this way until the osmotic gradient across the semi-permeable membrane is zero. As water is able to move between the intracellular and extracellular compartments freely, their overall tonicity is equal, even though the composition is different. The osmolarity of extracellular fluid (ECF) is primarily governed by its sodium concentration and this in turn determines the intracellular fluid (ICF) volume through osmosis.

Movement of water between the interstitial and intravascular compartments is determined by Starling's forces (Fig. 3.2), which are the net effect of hydrostatic and oncotic (osmotic pressure generated by the presence of proteins) pressures in these two compartments.

In general, high hydrostatic pressure in the arteriolar end of capillaries leads to a net outflow of fluid into the interstitial space,

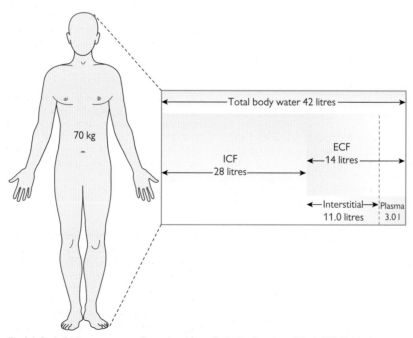

Fig. 3.1 Body fluid compartments. Reproduced from Catherine Spoors and Kevin Kiff, *Training in Anaesthesia*, 2010, Figure 11.1, page 291, with permission from Oxford University Press.

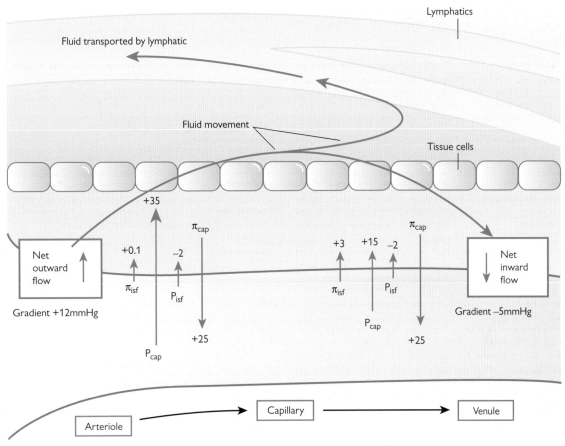

Fig. 3.2 Starling's forces. Reproduced from Catherine Spoors and Kevin Kiff, *Training in Anaesthesia*, 2010, Figure 11.8, page 299, with permission from Oxford University Press.

whilst high oncotic pressure in the venous end of the capillaries draws fluid back in. In this way fluid is circulated past cells to bathe them in oxygen and nutrients and remove waste products. As net filtration into the interstitial space (20mL/min) tends to exceed net reabsorption back into the intravascular space (18mL/min), excess fluid in the interstitial space is collected into the lymphatic system and returned to the circulation.

External fluid balance

Most adults require somewhere in the region of 1.5–2.5L of water per day (i.e. 25–35mL/kg/24h) to maintain adequate hydration. The volume of water entering the body must equal that leaving (see Box 3.1) otherwise there will be either a net gain or loss, leading to hyper- or hypovolaemia. Compensatory mechanisms exist to address these states but are limited in their effectiveness.

Box 3.1 Average daily water losses in the resting adult
• Urine: 1000–1500mL
• Respiratory tract: 400mL
• Evaporation from skin: 500mL
• Stool: 100mL.
Total = 2000–2500mL per 24h.

'Insensible' loss is a term used to describe the combined loss from evaporation and the respiratory tract, as it is very difficult to measure. These figures will alter according to activity and the availability of water but will need to be matched by an equal input. This will include water in fluids, pre-formed foods and that produced during oxidation in cells (approximately 5mL/kg/24h).

Clinical assessment of fluid balance

Determining volume status in patients is notoriously difficult as there is no specific measure of 'volaemia'. A combination of symptoms, signs, and readings must be used to gauge a decision as to whether a patient is hypo-, hyper-, or euvolaemic. None of the methods is infallible, but used in combination they may provide a reasonable indication (Table 3.1).

Management of fluid imbalance

Hypovolaemia
This can be managed by the administration of oral or intravenous fluids. It is important to consider from which compartment depletion has occurred in order to rectify the deficit correctly. ICF loss requires pure water replacement whilst ECF loss requires salt and water replacement. Oral fluids are usually the preferable route of replacement, but if this is not possible then appropriate intravenous fluids must be selected. Consideration must be given to the type, quantity, and duration of fluid given intravenously in order to avoid harm. Excessive intravenous fluid administration can be as detrimental as hypovolaemia and

Table 3.1 Clinical assessment of intravascular volume status	
Indicator	Clinical significance and reliability of indicator
Patient history	May highlight possible underlying abnormalities e.g. hypovolaemia following prolonged vomiting/diarrhoea or hypervolaemia due to excessive IV fluid administration.
Fluid balance charts	Should indicate net loss or gain of fluid over time but do not include evaporative losses and may be inaccurately completed.
Weight change	Can be useful over time if weighing is possible and other factors are constant.
Tissue oedema	May indicate excessive body water accumulation but not intravascular volume status. It may also be due to hypoalbuminaemia or cardiac failure.
Skin turgor	Reasonable indicator of water depletion but can be affected by factors such as age and temperature.
Dry mucus membranes	Can indicate water depletion but also produced by a number of other factors.
Capillary refill time	An increased time (>3 sec) can be caused by hypovolaemia, but cold and peripheral vascular disease can mimic this.
Blood pressure	Hypotension is a late marker of hypovolaemia. Postural hypotension (lying/standing BP difference) and narrowing of the pulse pressure tend to occur before a reduction in systolic BP.
Central venous pressure	Progressive decline in CVP (and hence clinically observed JVP) can indicate hypovolaemia but is influenced by many other factors too. Trends in change are more useful than absolute values.
Urine output	Commonly 1 mL/kg/hr is desirable but frequently a lower volume is normal perioperatively (0.3-0.5 mL/kg/hr).
Stroke volume	Only obtainable with cardiac output monitoring. Low absolute value (< 1mL/kg) may indicate hypovolaemia. Lack of response to a fluid bolus may indicate normo- or hypervolaemia.
Serum biochemistry	Hyponatraemia is most commonly caused by water excess whilst hypernatraemia may (or may not) be caused by dehydration. This must be interpreted considering changes in sodium and fluid levels. A raised urea (without a rise in creatinine) may indicate dehydration, but could also be due to renal failure. High plasma osmolality (> 500 mOsm/kg) suggests possible fluid deficit.
Urine biochemistry	Urine sodium concentration reflects renal perfusion and a low value (<20mmol/L) indicates renal hypoperfusion
Autonomic responses	Pallor, sweating, tachycardia and cold peripheries may suggest intravascular volume deficit but are not specific.

should be avoided. In the perioperative period this may be guided by technologies that measure blood flow (oesophageal Doppler monitor) or those that calculate it from an arterial waveform (see section 4.7). Blood pressure and urine output are poor indicators of volume status perioperatively. Care must also be given to the management of electrolytes, particularly sodium, when administering fluid both orally and intravenously (see section 3.2).

Hypervolaemia

Water overload may be managed by restricting fluid intake although in many instances this is insufficient. Diuretics are used to increase the efflux of salt and water from the body but should be used with care as they may cause deterioration in renal function, particularly if the intravascular space is depleted. In an acutely unwell patient, haemofiltration can be used to remove intravascular water but this is an invasive procedure associated with significant risks.

Further reading

Powell-Tuck J, Gosling P, Lobo D, et al. (2011). British Consensus Guidelines on Intravenous Fluid Therapy for Adult Surgical Patients (GIFTASUP). <http://www.bapen.org.uk/pdfs/bapen_pubs/giftasup.pdf> accessed 31 October 2012.

3.2 Electrolyte disturbances

Electrolyte homeostasis is essential: at a cellular level it is important for maintaining membrane potentials and stability. This affects all organs but is particularly important for cardiovascular, renal, and neurological function. Many cellular processes depend upon specific electrolyte concentrations as cofactors in chemical reactions. On a broader scale, electrolyte disturbances can cause significant fluid imbalance between different compartments.

Sodium

Sodium is the main extracellular cation and so the major determinant of osmolarity and ECF volume. The normal plasma value is 135–145mmol/L. Sodium is actively pumped out of the cells against its concentration gradient by the Na-K ATPase to help maintain the resting membrane potential of cells.

Sodium is absorbed from the intestine, and is filtered and actively reabsorbed by the kidney. Levels of sodium are regulated by the hypothalamus (via osmoreceptors) and the renin–angiotensin system. Atrial natriuretic peptide also has a role via fluid volume changes.

Abnormalities of sodium balance are the result of excessive or insufficient sodium intake and/or changes in extracellular water volume. Imbalance will affect ICF volume, hypernatraemia reducing it and hyponatraemia increasing it, through osmosis.

Hyponatraemia (serum Na <135mmol/L)

This is a common condition, seen in 15–30% of hospitalized patients and is caused by either increased sodium loss or excessive water intake. Symptoms of hyponatraemia range from lethargy, irritability, nausea, and vomiting to confusion, drowsiness, seizures, and coma. Rapid correction of hyponatraemia should be avoided as this can lead to central pontine myelinolysis. Sodium levels should generally be corrected at <0.5mmol/L/h. Causes of hyponatraemia are given in Table 3.2 according to the volaemic status of the patient. Treatment should primarily be directed at the cause of the hyponatraemia.

Table 3.2 Causes of hyponatraemia

Hypovolaemic	Normovolaemic	Hypervolaemic
Cerebral salt wasting syndrome (CSWS)	Syndrome of inappropriate antidiuretic hormone (SIADH)	SIADH
Diuretic therapy	Thiazide diuretics	Congestive cardiac failure
Diarrhoea/vomiting	Adrenal insufficiency	Nephrotic syndrome
Sweating	Hypothyroidism	Cirrhosis
Adrenal insufficiency	Iatrogenic	Renal failure
Blood loss		Iatrogenic (excessive fluid administration)
		'TUR' syndrome

Causes of SIADH include CNS pathology (traumatic brain injury, subarachnoid haemorrhage) and pulmonary pathology (typically carcinoma of the bronchus). It may also be drug-induced (seen, e.g. as part of MDMA toxicity—see section 7.3). SIADH can be treated with fluid restriction, hypertonic saline, demeclocycline (an antibacterial which reduces the renal response to ADH) and lithium. Newer drugs are available, such as conivaptan and tolvaptan, which bind to the ADH receptor.

Hypernatraemia (serum Na >145mmol/L)

Hypernatraemia is less common than hyponatraemia and can be caused by decreased water intake, excess water loss, or excess salt intake. Neurological symptoms such as weakness, lethargy, and seizures can occur when it is severe. The most common cause is fluid loss or 'dehydration'.

Diabetes insipidus (DI) is relatively common following brain injury, particularly in patients selected for organ donation in whom brain stem death has been diagnosed. DI results from decreased secretion of ADH leading to decreased water reabsorption by the kidney and a diuresis. Nephrogenic DI exists where the kidney does not respond to ADH. In DI plasma osmolarity is high (>305mosm/L) and the patient produces large volumes of dilute urine (osmolarity <350mosm/L). A simple test is to use a urine dipstick to measure specific gravity: dilute urine will be <1.005.

Treatment of hypernatraemia should be directed at the cause but may also involve the administration of water either enterally or intravenously as 5% dextrose. Excessively rapid correction of hypernatraemia can lead to cerebral oedema.

Potassium

Potassium is the main intracellular cation. The normal plasma concentration is 3.5–5.0mmol/L. Potassium's most important action is in the maintenance of the cell membrane potential and action potentials. Potassium is absorbed from the intestine and excreted via the kidney. Abnormalities of potassium homeostasis are generally due to excessive or insufficient intake or excretion, or movement into or out of cells.

Hypokalaemia (serum K <3.5mmol/L)

This common electrolyte abnormality is frequently asymptomatic but can lead to weakness and malaise. Common causes are listed in Table 3.3.

Table 3.3 Causes of hypokalaemia

Reduced intake	Increased loss	Shift into cells
IV fluids without K	Renal: • Diuretics • Hyperaldosteronism	Metabolic alkalosis
Low potassium diet (rare)	Gastrointestinal: • Vomiting • Diarrhoea • Fistulae	Insulin
		Catecholamines (β agonists)

Severe adverse effects are unlikely until the level is <2.5mmol/L when muscle weakness and cardiac arrhythmias can occur. ECG changes include prolongation of the PR interval, ST depression, prolonged QT interval, T wave inversion and prominent U waves. Treatment is by potassium replacement, but high concentrations of potassium given quickly IV can cause cardiac arrest: maximum recommended infusion rates are 10–20mmol/h.

Hyperkalaemia (serum K >5.0mmol/L)

Severe hyperkalaemia is a life-threatening condition and requires immediate treatment. ECG changes are progressive: tall tented T waves, diminished P waves, ultimately leading to a sinusoidal trace and asystole. Causes of hyperkalaemia are given in Table 3.4. Muscle weakness is reported when hyperkalaemia is severe.

Table 3.4 Causes of hyperkalaemia

Increased intake	Shift from inside cells	Decreased excretion
Potassium replacement	Drugs: • Suxamethonium	Renal failure
Blood transfusion	Metabolic acidosis	Drugs: • ACE inhibitors • A2 blockers • NSAIDs • Potassium-sparing diuretics
Potassium-containing drugs	Tissue necrosis	Hypoaldosteronism

Management is initially directed at driving potassium into the cells with insulin and dextrose (e.g. 15 units fast-acting insulin and 50mL 50% glucose) and β-agonists (nebulized salbutamol). Calcium gluconate should also be given to protect from cardiac arrhythmias (10mL of 10% calcium gluconate). However, these are only temporizing measures and ultimately the excess potassium needs to be removed from the body. This may require renal replacement therapy, although potassium exchange resins (e.g. calcium resonium) can be used if renal replacement is not possible, or delayed.

Calcium

The majority of the body's calcium is stored within bone. The normal plasma level is 2.12–2.65mmol/L, a significant proportion of which is bound to proteins, mostly albumin. It is therefore important that the reported value is corrected for the albumin level. Free ionized calcium is approximately 1.2mmol/L. Free calcium is important for cardiac and skeletal muscle contraction: it acts as a second messenger and neurotransmitter, and it is an important cofactor for some enzymatic reactions, notably in coagulation.

Calcium homeostasis is regulated by the actions of vitamin D, parathyroid hormone, and calcitonin.

Parathyroid hormone is secreted from the parathyroid gland in response to hypocalcaemia and hypomagnesaemia and it acts to increase absorption from the intestine, kidney, and bone, and increases conversion of vitamin D to the active form.

Vitamin D is formed in the skin or absorbed in the gut. The active metabolite 1,25-dihydroxycholecalciferol is formed in two stages by the liver and then the kidney. It also acts to increase reabsorption of calcium.

Calcitonin is secreted by the parafollicular cells of the thyroid gland in response to hypercalcaemia. It acts to inhibit calcium resorption from bone and increases renal excretion of calcium and phosphate.

Hypocalcaemia (serum Ca <2.12mmol/L)

Hypocalcaemia is associated with reduced parathyroid hormone or vitamin D activity, renal failure, pancreatitis, and alkalosis. It is particularly important to check for hypocalcaemia following thyroidectomy.

Features include:

- Neuromuscular excitability: paraesthesia (or convulsions in severe cases), +ve Chvostek's and Trousseau's signs
- Cardiac manifestations: low cardiac output state + ECG changes (prolonged QT interval)

Treatment is directed at the predisposing cause together with calcium replacement (10mL 10% calcium chloride or gluconate administered slowly intravenously).

Hypercalcaemia (serum Ca >2.65mmol/L)

Common causes of hypercalcaemia are hyperparathyroidism and malignancy (both primary and bony metastases). The clinical features are classically memorized as *bones* (bone pain), *stones* (renal stones), *groans* (abdominal pain), and *moans* (psychiatric disorders). Treatment is to administer normal saline by IV infusion to dilute the plasma level, sometimes combined with diuretics to promote excretion of calcium. Bisphosphonates also have a role some cases.

Magnesium

Magnesium is mostly found in the ICF. The normal plasma level is 0.7–1.05mmol/L. Whilst an oversimplification, magnesium can be thought of as an antagonist to calcium in its actions. It is a cofactor in many reactions including ATP and nucleic acid production.

In anaesthesia it is used for the treatment of bronchospasm in asthma, as an anticonvulsant in pre-eclampsia and eclampsia, and as an antiarrhythmic. It has also been used as an adjuvant to postoperative analgesia. Magnesium decreases acetylcholine release at the neuromuscular junction and can increase the action of non-depolarizing muscle relaxants.

Hypomagnesaemia (serum Mg <0.7mmol/L)

Hypomagnesaemia is reasonably common amongst hospitalized patients. Causes include poor dietary intake, GI losses (diarrhoea, vomiting), renal losses, and drug therapy (e.g. diuretics). Magnesium losses often coexist with other electrolyte deficiencies, particularly hypokalaemia. Features include arrhythmias, tremors, cramps, and neurological symptoms. Hypomagnesaemia can be treated with an IV infusion (10–20mmol) of magnesium sulphate (note that 1g is equivalent to 4mmol of $MgSO_4$). It is common in critical care to aim for plasma levels of >1.0mmol/L.

Hypermagnesaemia

Hypermagnesaemia is rare. It is caused most commonly by excessive magnesium supplementation, especially in renal failure. Features include hypotension, vasodilatation, confusion, and muscle weakness (including respiratory muscles), together with loss of deep tendon reflexes. It is treated by stopping magnesium supplementation and inducing a diuresis. In severe cases IV calcium should be given.

Further reading

Arora SK. (2013). Hypernatremic disorders in the intensive care unit. *J Intensive Care Med*, 28(1):37–45.

Elliott MJ, Ronksley PE, Clase CM, et al. (2010). Management of patients with acute hyperkalemia. *CMAJ*, 182(15):1631–5.

Parikh M, Webb ST (2012). Cations: potassium, calcium, and magnesium. *CEACCP*, 12(4):195–8.

Rassam SS (2005). Perioperative electrolyte and fluid balance. *CEACCP*, 5(5):157–60.

3.3 Acid–base abnormalities

Definitions

Hydrogen ions

The pH is the negative logarithm of the H+ion concentration and the normal range is 7.35–7.45. It is important to remember that pH is a logarithmic scale therefore small changes in pH reflect dramatic changes in the concentration of H+. Abnormalities of acid–base balance detrimentally affect enzymatic processes and membrane potentials leading to metabolic failure. The majority of H+ ions come from CO_2:

$$CO_2 + H_2O \leftrightharpoons H_2CO_3 \leftrightharpoons HCO_3^- + H^+$$

Acid–base abnormalities have traditionally been considered using the Henderson–Hasselbach (HH) equation:

$$pH = pK + \frac{Log\left[HCO_3^-\right]}{Dissolved\ CO_2}$$

Acid–base abnormalities can originate from respiratory or metabolic causes. The abnormality can then be 'compensated' by respiratory or metabolic measures, for example, a respiratory acidosis with metabolic compensation, or a metabolic acidosis with respiratory compensation.

Respiratory abnormalities are caused by an increase or decrease in the partial pressure of CO_2 (low pCO_2 causing a respiratory alkalosis and high pCO_2 causing a respiratory acidosis). Excessive CO_2 causing a respiratory acidosis can be buffered with HCO_3- through a leftwards shift of the HH equation. Respiratory abnormalities are discussed in section 2.4.

Base excess (BE)

BE is a calculated value (reported in mEq/L) representing the amount of strong acid that would be needed to bring the pH to 7.4 when pCO_2 is 5.3 kPa. A positive BE indicates a metabolic alkalosis whereas negative BE is a metabolic acidosis.

Standard bicarbonate

In a similar manner to BE, standard bicarbonate is defined as the calculated blood bicarbonate concentration corrected to a PCO_2 of 5.3kPa. Abnormal values for the standard bicarbonate reflect the metabolic component of an acid–base abnormality.

Metabolic acidosis

In metabolic acidosis the pH is <7.35 with a decreased bicarbonate and a negative BE. It may be due to excessive acid or a lowered buffering capacity as a result of a reduced bicarbonate concentration. Respiratory compensation occurs by generating tachypnoea to decrease pCO_2 thereby reducing the acid load. When a metabolic acidosis is present the *anion gap* should be calculated to determine the cause.

Anion gap (AG)

The AG is used to help distinguish the cause of a metabolic acidosis: it is calculated using the following formula:

$$Anion\ gap = ([Na^+] + [K^+]) - ([Cl^-] + [HCO_3^-])$$

The normal range for anion gap is 8–14mmol/L. The 'gap' represents unmeasured negatively charged ions (anions) in the blood (usually negatively charged proteins). A raised anion gap indicates the presence of extra 'unmeasured' ions. These may be exogenous acids (e.g. ethylene glycol, salicylate and methanol) or endogenous (e.g. lactic acid and ketones). Determining the cause of a metabolic acidosis has become easier since blood gas machines now commonly measure lactate concentration. If the cause is purely due to hyperlactataemia the anion gap should be of similar magnitude to the rise in lactate concentration, otherwise another causative anion should be sought.

Causes of 'normal' anion gap acidosis include:

- Renal tubular acidosis
- GI causes (pancreatic/small bowel drainage and fistulae)
- Iatrogenic causes (parenteral nutrition and other infusions).

Albumin is a significant contributor to the anion gap. The anion gap can be falsely elevated in hypoalbuminaemia, which is very common in the critically ill. It can be corrected for hypoalbuminaemia using the following formula:

$$AG(albumin\ corrected)$$
$$= AG + 0.25 \times \left(40 - measured\ albumin(g/l)\right)$$

The Stewart approach

Peter Stewart developed an alternative approach to acid–base balance. His 'physicochemical' approach is based on fundamental principles:

- Electroneutrality—there must be equal numbers of positively and negatively charged ions.
- Conservation of mass—the amount of a substance cannot change unless it is added or removed.
- Mass action—dissociation is a dynamic equilibrium.

As all biological solutions are aqueous, water can always dissociate to provide H+ or OH−

$$H_2O \leftrightharpoons H^+ + OH^-$$

pH is determined by the amount of hydrogen ions. The balance of this equilibrium equation is determined by Stewart's three independent variables:

1. Strong ions (Na^+, K^+, Mg^{2+}, Cl^-)
2. CO_2
3. Weak acids (mostly phosphate and proteins e.g. albumin)

Strong ions dissociate completely in solution. Significantly, bicarbonate is not a strong ion.

The strong ion difference (SID) can be calculated:

$$SID = \left(Na^+ + K^+ + Mg^{2+} + Ca^{2+}\right) - \left(Cl^- + Lactate\right)$$

Normal SID is 40–44mmol/L. The SID is balanced by CO_2 and the weak acids (A^-) such that:

$$SID - \left(A^- + CO_2\right) = 0$$

Where the SID is low this represents a metabolic acidosis; conversely in a metabolic alkalosis the SID is high. It is easy to understand why hyperchloraemia causes a metabolic acidosis using this approach.

Stewart described six simultaneous equations for all of his variables. This is too complex to calculate by hand in clinical practice. It is, however, an easy process using a computer: there are web- or even smartphone-based apps that will do the calculations.

Metabolic alkalosis

Metabolic alkalosis is far less common than metabolic acidosis. It may be due to excessive H^+ loss or a gain in bicarbonate or alkali. It occurs when there is an increase in the SID. Metabolic alkalosis can be classified somewhat artificially according to 'response' to chloride in urine; some causes are listed in Table 3.5.

Table 3.5 Causes of metabolic alkalosis	
Chloride responsive (urine Cl <10mmol/L)	Chloride unresponsive (Urine Cl >20mmol/L)
Gastrointestinal: • Vomiting • Gastric drainage	Mineralocorticoid excess: • Cushing's syndrome • Conn's syndrome • Iatrogenic
Correction of a compensated respiratory acidosis	Alkalotic medication: • Antacids • Bicarbonate
Contraction alkalosis	Hypokalaemia
Diuretics	

Loss of hydrochloric acid from the stomach causes a low chloride metabolic alkalosis. Patients with chronic retention of CO_2 who are ventilated with inappropriately high minute volumes will have a metabolic alkalosis. This is common perioperatively and in ICU. A 'contraction alkalosis' occurs when free water is lost from the kidney but bicarbonate is retained.

The administration of sodium bicarbonate causes a decrease in the SID by adding sodium without chloride. Severe hypokalaemia causes intracellular shift of hydrogen ions thus causing a metabolic alkalosis.

As with all abnormalities, treatment should be directed at the cause. Chloride responsive alkalosis is easy to treat with saline; chloride unresponsive states are often more difficult.

Further reading

Badr A & Nightingale P (2007). An alternative approach to acid-base abnormalities in critically ill patients. *CEACCP*, 7(4):107–11.

Chawla G & Drummond G (2008). Water, strong ions, and weak ions. *CEACCP*, 8(3):108–12.

Kitching AJ & Edge CJ (2002). Acid base balance: a review of normal physiology. *CEACCP*, 2(1):3–6.

Sirker AA, Rhodes A, Grounds RM, *et al.* (2002). Acid-base physiology: the 'traditional' and the "modern" approaches. *Anaesthesia*, 57(4):348–56.

3.4 Renal tubular acidosis

Definition of renal tubular acidosis

Renal tubular acidosis (RTA) is a rare disorder of the secretion of acid (H^+) or re-absorption of bicarbonate (HCO_3^-) in the kidney. It is primarily a defect of tubular function, with maintenance of overall glomerular function. Unlike in renal failure where there can be a failure to excrete acid, in RTA the GFR is approximately normal. RTA tends to result in a hyperchloraemic metabolic acidosis, with a normal anion gap (raised H^+ concentration). By contrast, renal failure tends to cause a high anion gap due to accumulation of fixed acids.

There are three types of RTA, traditionally called I, II, and IV (type III is now thought to be a subset of types I and II). Alternatively they can be classified by the defect site: proximal, distal, and aldosterone deficiency (Table 3.6).

RTA should be suspected whenever there is a normal anion gap metabolic acidosis. Urinary pH should be measured and a value of >5.3 is supportive of the diagnosis, although it can be less than in proximal RTA.

Table 3.6 Types of renal tubular acidosis		
Proximal (type II)	Distal (type I)	Aldosterone deficiency (type IV)
Urine pH <5.5	Urine pH >5.5	Urine pH <5.5
Often hypokalaemia	Variable serum K^+	Hyperkalaemia

Normal tubular physiology

The acidification of urine takes place as a result of two processes: secretion of H^+ and re-absorption of HCO_3^-. These mostly take place in the proximal tubule of the nephron where H^+ ions are excreted in exchange for Na^+ ions by an 'antiport' carrier (Fig. 3.3). H^+ ions then combine with HCO_3^- ions in the tubular lumen to form carbonic acid (H_2CO_3). This dissociates under the influence of carbonic anhydrase to form CO_2 and H_2O. The CO_2 is able to diffuse back into the tubular cell where it is combined with water to form carbonic acid. The carbonic acid can again dissociate, producing another H^+ ion that can be secreted into the tubule and HCO_3^-, which is pumped into the capillary lumen. Thus HCO_3^- filtered at the glomerulus is absorbed.

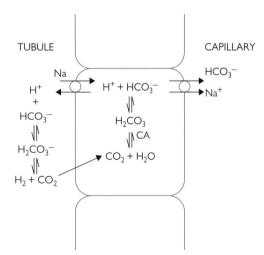

Fig. 3.3 Acid balance in the proximal convoluted tubule.

This process also takes place in the distal tubule but to a lesser extent than in the proximal. As almost all of the filtered bicarbonate is reabsorbed and H^+ is excreted, normal urine contains little bicarbonate and is slightly acidic (normal pH range of 5–7).

The second part of urinary acidification is the secretion of acid at the distal tubule. Again H^+ ions are formed by the generation of carbonic acid by carbonic anhydrase (Fig. 3.4). $H^+ATPase$ secretes the H^+ ions into the lumen where it is buffered by ammonium or phosphate ions. The bicarbonate is exchanged for chloride at the basolateral membrane.

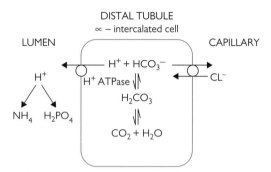

Fig. 3.4 Urinary acidification in the distal convoluted tubule.

Proximal RTA (type II)

In proximal RTA there is failure of bicarbonate reabsorption in the proximal tubule. This can be inherited as either an autosomal recessive or dominant trait. Type II RTA can also occur as part of other abnormalities of tubular function (e.g. Fanconi's syndrome). Other acquired causes include drugs (carbonic anhydrase inhibitors and heavy metals), hyperparathyroidism, amyloid, renal transplant, and nephritic syndrome.

Although distal acidification mechanisms are intact, as the plasma bicarbonate level falls the urine will become acidic (pH <5.5). There is often an associated hypokalaemia.

Proximal bicarbonate reabsorption can be tested by measurement of bicarbonate excretion following an infusion of bicarbonate.

Treatment of RTA type II is enteral alkali supplementation either with bicarbonate or potassium citrate (the latter tastes nicer and also provides potassium). In severe acute cases with hypokalaemia, the potassium should be monitored closely because as the bicarbonate is replaced the potassium will fall further.

Distal RTA (type I)

In distal RTA there is impairment of acidification of urine by the distal tubule, caused by a failure of H^+ secretion. Urinary pH is usually high (>5.5) even when the patient is challenged with an acid load or given furosemide or fludrocortisone. The diagnosis of RTA type I is suggested by the presence of hyperchloraemic acidosis with an alkaline urine, particularly if there is evidence of renal stone formation.

Causes of RTA type I include inherited cases, drugs (amphotericin B, lithium, toluene, amiloride, trimethoprim, pentamidine), autoimmune disorders (Sjögren's syndrome, systemic lupus erythematosus (SLE), primary biliary cirrhosis) and disorders of calcium (primary hyperparathyroidism, hypercalciuria). Treatment is with alkali supplementation (bicarbonate or citrate).

Aldosterone deficiency (type IV RTA)

Aldosterone deficiency or aldosterone resistance characterizes RTA type IV. The renal response to aldosterone is normally to excrete potassium and hydrogen in exchange for sodium. Type IV RTA is also known as 'hyperkalaemic RTA' since excretion of potassium is also affected, leading to increased plasma levels. The underlying defect is impairment of cation exchange in the distal tubule with reduced secretion of H^+ and K^+. There will also be a hyperchloraemic metabolic acidosis, as in types I and II, and urine pH will be low.

A number of different conditions have been associated with RTA type IV but most patients have renal failure associated with disorders affecting the renal interstitium and tubules. Causes include inherited defects, mineralocorticoid deficiency (e.g. Addison's disease), chronic interstitial nephropathy and drugs (ciclosporin, NSAIDs, ACEIs).

Potassium restriction should be initiated in these patients, and non-potassium-sparing diuretics may have a use. In severe cases, fludrocortisone can help to reduce serum potassium levels.

Further reading

Laing CM & Unwin RJ (2006). Renal tubular acidosis. *J Nephrol*, 19(Suppl 9):S46–52.

Rodriguez Soriano J (2002). Renal tubular acidosis: the clinical entity. *J Am Soc Nephrol*, 13(8):2160–70.

3.5 Acute kidney injury

Acute kidney injury

The term 'acute kidney injury' (AKI) has replaced 'acute renal failure' to emphasize its potential reversibility in the early stages. Early identification and appropriate management are essential. AKI should be viewed as a spectrum of injury and is characterized by a reduction in kidney function that results in a failure to maintain fluid, electrolyte, and acid–base balance.

AKI occurs in up to 7% of all patients admitted to hospital, whilst 5–20% of all critically ill patients have an episode of AKI during the course of their illness. Approximately 5% of all critically ill patients will at some point require renal replacement therapy (RRT) during their admission. Patients with AKI are also vulnerable to additional harm perioperatively, and care must be taken to reduce long-term risk in this cohort.

The international definition of AKI is the presence of one of the following criteria:

– Serum creatinine rising by ≥26μmol/L within 48 hours.
– Serum creatinine rising ≥1.5-fold from the reference value, which is known or presumed to have occurred within 1 week.
– Urine output is <0.5mL/kg/h for >6 consecutive hours.

The reference serum creatinine should be the lowest creatinine value recorded within 3 months of the event.

RIFLE Classification

In 2004, the Acute Dialysis Quality Initiative (ADQI) group developed the RIFLE system to standardize the classification of AKI. AKI is classified according to the acronym RIFLE, which includes three classes of severity (risk/injury/failure) and two outcome classes (loss and end-stage).

The three severity classes are based on changes in either serum creatinine or urine output. The two outcome criteria are defined by the duration of loss of kidney function at 4 weeks and 3 months, respectively. The RIFLE criteria are summarized in Table 3.7.

Table 3.7	The RIFLE criteria	
	GFR criteria	Urine output criteria
Risk	Creatinine ↑ 1.5× GFR ↓ >25%	<0.5mL/kg/h for 6h
Injury	Creatinine ↑ 2× GFR ↓ >50%	<0.5mL/kg/h for 12h
Failure	Creatinine ↑ 3× GFR ↓ >75%	<0.3mL/kg/h for 24h Or anuria for 16h
Loss	Persistent renal failure for >4 weeks	
ESRF	Persistent renal failure for >3 months	

Copyright 2004, Acute Kidney Injury Network, with permission.

Causes of AKI

Traditionally the causes of AKI have been classified as pre-renal, intrinsic renal, and post-renal.

Pre-renal

This represents a functional response to renal hypoperfusion, without any structural damage to the kidneys. It is characterized by the fact that restoration of normal renal perfusion should result in a prompt recovery of renal function. However, prerenal injury is a potent risk factor for intrinsic renal injury, which can result in permanent kidney dysfunction.

Renal hypoperfusion activates the sympathetic nervous system and the renin–angiotensin system, causing postglomerular vasoconstriction and increased proximal tubular sodium and water reabsorption. Aldosterone and vasopressin (antidiuretic hormone) secretion are stimulated, resulting in increased sodium, urea, and water reabsorption in distal nephron segments. Thus the overall response leads to maintenance of the glomerular filtration rate (GFR) by concentration of urine and reduction in sodium excretion. However, if renal hypoperfusion is persistent these compensatory mechanisms fail and GFR begins to decline.

The usual urinary features of prerenal injury are:

– Low urine sodium concentration (<20mmol/L)
– Low fractional excretion of sodium (<1%)
– Low fractional excretion of urea (<35%)
– High urine osmolality.

Examples of scenarios that could lead to pre-renal injury are: haemorrhage, burns, vomiting, diarrhoea, excessive drain fluid loss, osmotic diuretics, cirrhosis, and hepatorenal syndrome.

Intrinsic

This category describes parenchymal failure of the kidneys in which there is intrinsic damage to parts of the glomerulus or nephron. The commonest type is acute tubular necrosis (ATN) as a result of ischaemic or nephrotoxic processes, although it is frequently due to a combination of causes. Causes of intrinsic AKI include hypotension, cardiogenic shock, radiocontrast media, rhabdomyolysis, sepsis, acute glomerulonephritis, acute interstitial nephritis, and systemic diseases such as sarcoidosis and SLE.

Post-renal

This occurs as a result of obstruction anywhere within the urinary tract, e.g. urethra, bladder, or ureters. Unilateral obstruction may simply present with renal colic and hydronephrosis with preserved renal function if the contralateral kidney function is normal. The presence of an obstructive cause should be sought in all patients with AKI as it may be easily reversible. This can be performed by ultrasound or CT imaging.

In reality the cause of AKI in many patients tends to be multifactorial with various aetiologies contributing to the injury, e.g. sepsis, IV contrast, antibiotics, and hypoperfusion. The pathophysiology is complex but is thought to involve haemodynamic changes, inflammation, and endothelial and epithelial cell injury.

Prevention of AKI

AKI is asymptomatic, and it is therefore important to identify individuals at risk and maintain a high level of vigilance. Identified risk factors include advanced age, pre-existing renal disease, cardiac and liver disease, diabetes and vascular disease, and nephrotoxic medication. In addition, there are acute insults known to precipitate AKI. The mnemonic 'STOP' has been proposed to describe these:

● Sepsis and hypoperfusion
● Toxicity (nephrotoxic drugs and IV contrast)
● Obstruction
● Parenchymal disease.

The key to prevention is to treat the underlying cause whilst maintaining renal perfusion and avoiding renal insults. For perioperative patients this necessitates careful preoperative assessment, optimization of haemodynamic status, avoidance of nephrotoxins, and vigilant postoperative care. Careful consideration must be given to the withholding and reintroduction of diuretic medications in the perioperative period.

Nephrotoxins

Nephrotoxic drugs include:
- Aminoglycosides
- Amphotericin
- Immunosuppressive agents
- NSAIDs
- ACEIs
- IV radiocontrast media.

IV contrast media are given during radiological investigations and angiographic procedures (e.g. cardiac and vascular). The use of low osmolarity media has been shown to reduce the risk of AKI when compared to high osmolarity agents. Anaesthetists should encourage the use of low osmolarity media whenever a patient is at risk of AKI. Hypovolaemia is a potent risk factor for developing contrast nephropathy and should be avoided in any patient having contrast. There is some evidence (low quality) that sodium bicarbonate is beneficial compared to saline when given prior to and after the administration of contrast. N-acetylcysteine has also been used to prevent contrast nephropathy, although there is no robust evidence of benefit to date. The most effective way to reduce the risk of AKI when contrast media must be administered is IV volume expansion with isotonic crystalloid, the use of low osmolar contrast media, and minimizing overall contrast dose.

Management

Once a patient has developed AKI the therapeutic options are limited, with the mainstay of treatment being RRT. Haemodynamic status should be optimized to prevent further renal hypoperfusion. This may include fluid resuscitation, followed by vasopressor or inotropic drugs. Cardiac output monitoring is useful to guide therapy and prevent fluid overadministration. Renal autoregulation can fail in AKI and the patient may need a higher mean arterial pressure for adequate renal perfusion.

Post-renal causes of AKI (i.e. obstruction) should be excluded early in any patient suspected of having AKI (either with ultrasound or other imaging). Any nephrotoxic agents should be stopped immediately.

Unless the cause of AKI is obvious (e.g. sepsis, multiorgan failure) consideration should be given to other parenchymal causes in the history or examination. Urine dipstick and microscopy should be performed: this may show haematuria, proteinuria or casts. None of these are diagnostic, but they should prompt review by a nephrologist.

The optimal timing of RRT is unknown.

Specific treatments

No specific treatment for AKI has yet been shown to be beneficial. However, the following treatments have been shown not to be of benefit and are possibly harmful:
- Low-dose dopamine
- Loop diuretic at high dose
- Natriuretic peptides.

Biomarkers

Various biomarkers are being developed to aid in the early prediction of AKI. It is hoped that these will allow the prediction of AKI before there is a change in the serum creatinine. N-GAL (neutrophil gelatinase-associated lipocalin) is one of several that are under investigation and there is a significant body of literature to support its use clinically.

Prognosis

Mortality from AKI is high—in critically ill patients, it is in the order of 40–50%. Some studies have linked the development of AKI to later chronic renal failure and other morbidity and mortality. Whether AKI is a marker of other risk factors or the AKI itself affects long-term health is unknown.

Further reading

Bellomo PR, Kellum JA, & Ronco C (2012). Acute kidney injury. *Lancet.* 380(9843):756–66.

Lewington A & Kanagasundaram S (2011). *Clinical Practice Guidelines Acute Kidney Injury.* (5th edn), London: UK Renal Association. <http://www.renal.org/guidelines>

London Acute Kidney Injury Network: <http://www.londonaki.net/>

Webb ST & Allen JSD (2008). Perioperative renal protection. *CEACCP*, 8(5):176–80.

3.6 Renal replacement therapy

Approximately a third of critically ill patients will develop an AKI and 5% will require RRT as a result. The in-hospital mortality of patients with an AKI requiring RRT is approaching 60%. Whilst the underlying cause of renal injury should always be sought, support of renal function may be required, either temporarily or permanently. The aim of RRT is to mimic the main functions of the kidney in terms of fluid balance and clearance of waste products. This section focuses on provision of RRT for AKI.

Continuous versus intermittent RRT

RRT can be performed continuously or intermittently. The principal difference is the speed at which water and wastes are removed.

With intermittent techniques (e.g. intermittent haemodialysis (IntHD)), patients are connected to a renal replacement circuit for 3–5h per session. Typically patients require two to three sessions per week but this can vary. Large volumes of fluid and solute can be removed in a short period of time using IntHD.

With continuous techniques (e.g. continuous renal replacement therapy (CRRT)) patients are connected to the circuit for several days at a time. There is no overwhelming evidence for the benefit of continuous over intermittent techniques, but most ICUs use continuous RRT since it tends to be advantageous with regards to haemodynamic stability. Intermittent techniques require the removal of a day or several days' worth of fluid in only a few hours, which can lead to large fluid and electrolyte shifts.

There are a number of hybrid techniques, e.g. sustained low efficiency (daily) dialysis (SLEDD), where standard IntHD equipment can be used with reduced dialysate and blood flow rates.

Haemodialysis versus haemofiltration

Both haemodialysis and haemofiltration involve blood being removed from the body and pumped in an extracorporeal circuit through a filter (artificial kidney) that is composed of small hollow fibres to maximize the surface area in contact with the blood flowing within them. Haemofiltration uses hydrostatic pressure in the circuit to drive fluid across the semi-permeable membrane of the fibres, and into bags that are then removed. This is termed ultrafiltration and is similar to what happens at the glomerulus (Fig. 3.5).

The physical process in ultrafiltration is *convection*. Large molecules (approximately >50KDa) cannot pass through the membrane, but smaller solutes are pulled through with the fluid (termed solvent drag). Exogenous fluid is then added to the circuit after the filter to achieve the required fluid balance. Thus a haemofiltration rate of 1L/h means that 1L of fluid is filtered from the patient's blood and eliminated in the drainage fluid and 1L of replacement fluid is returned to the circuit before it reaches the patient to achieve neutral fluid balance. The filtration fraction (fraction of 'water' removed from blood) is optimal at about 20–25%. If the filtration fraction is too high the filter will clot due to haemoconcentration. The additional fluid can also be added prior to the filter (pre-dilution) in order to prolong filter life but leads to a reduction in solute clearance. Post-dilution concentrates the blood in the filter, enhancing clearance.

Haemodialysis also involves a semipermeable membrane but uses a dialysis fluid (dialysate) on the other side from the blood. Solutes move across the membrane according to their concentration gradient (Fick's law of *diffusion*). The dialysate is a crystalloid solution in which the concentrations of the various solutes have been carefully chosen. The dialysis fluid usually flows in the opposite direction to the blood (countercurrent) in order to maximize the concentration gradient along the length of the filter.

Both principles can be utilized at the same time in haemodiafiltration, and this is particularly useful for the clearance of small solutes.

Indications for RRT

The classical indications for RRT are:
- Hyperkalaemia (>6.5mmol/L)
- Acidosis (pH<7.2)
- Fluid overload
- Symptomatic uraemia (encephalopathy, pericarditis, etc.)
- Anuria (for >6h) or oliguria (for >12h).

In addition RRT can also be used for the removal of unwanted drugs and other toxins (see section 7.2). Drugs that are removed by RRT include lithium, metformin, ethylene glycol, salicylates, and many antibiotics. Digoxin, tricyclics, phenytoin, warfarin, and macrolide and quinolone antibiotics are not removed. There has been some interest in the use of RRT in the management of severe sepsis (even without AKI) in order to remove inflammatory mediators.

Venous access

Most ICUs use continuous veno-venous haemofiltration (CVVHF) or haemodiafiltration (CVVHDF). A dual lumen catheter is inserted into a large central vein. Blood can then be drawn

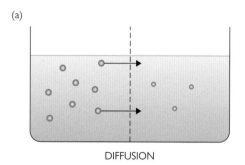
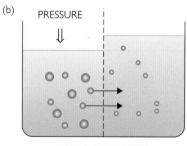

Fig. 3.5 Diffusion and ultrafiltration.

from the vein in one lumen, passed through the filter and then returned to the circulation via the other lumen.

Historically arterio-venous haemofiltration (CAVF) was employed. This is no longer used due to arterial complications. Chronic intermittent haemodialysis is commonly performed via an arterio-venous fistula that has been surgically created in the upper limb.

Anticoagulation

The extracorporeal circuit of a haemofilter (see Fig. 3.6) usually requires anticoagulation to prevent clotting. However, anticoagulation is unnecessary and contraindicated if the patient has a coagulopathy (INR >2.0, APTT >60sec, platelet count <60) or there is a high risk of haemorrhage.

Anticoagulation can be achieved in a number of ways:

Heparin infusion
Heparin is commonly added to the circuit immediately pre-filter. This inevitably leads to anticoagulation of the patient and APTT should be monitored. LMWHs are used rarely as they are difficult to monitor and reverse should haemorrhage occur.

Prostacyclin
Prostacyclin can also be administered by infusion into the circuit. This acts to prevent platelet aggregation but can cause some vasodilatation. Prostacyclin is useful when heparin is contraindicated or when heparin-induced thrombocytopaenia is a complication.

Regional citrate anticoagulation
This involves adding citrate pre-filter. Citrate binds to calcium and thus prevents clotting within the filter. The filter then removes the calcium–citrate complex and calcium needs to be added post filter. Anticoagulant effects are limited to within the filter. This technique is common in the US, but less common in Europe and the UK.

Pre-dilution is not strictly an anticoagulant but it is a method of preventing clotting within the filter. Some of the replacement fluid that is normally given back after the filter is added pre-filter. This causes a reduction in the haematocrit and reduces clot formation. This is, however, at the cost of a reduction in the filtration fraction.

Replacement fluids

These are all balanced crystalloid solutions. They use either bicarbonate or lactate as a buffer. Bicarbonate is unstable in storage so lactate is cheaper and easier although can cause problems especially if there is impaired liver function, as lactate is normally converted to bicarbonate within the liver. Lactate-free solutions should also be used in severe hyperlactataemia.

Dose of RRT

The 'dose' of RRT is the volume of solute that is filtered (and therefore replaced) per hour. Current evidence suggests that the optimum prescribed dose is approximately 20mL/kg/h, i.e. 1400mL/h in a 70kg adult.

Complications of RRT

Complications of RRT relate to venous access, the extra-corporeal circuit, and the replacement therapy itself (see Box 3.2).

Box 3.2 Complications of RRT
• Haemorrhage
• Infection (catheter-related bloodstream infection)
• Air emboli
• Platelet consumption and coagulation abnormalities
• Electrolyte abnormalities
• Haemodynamic instability
• Hypothermia.

Further reading

Hall NA (2006). Renal replacement therapies in critical care. *CEACCP*, 6(5):197–202.

Ronco C & Ricci Z (2008). Renal replacement therapies: physiological review. *Intensive Care Med*, 34(12):2139–46.

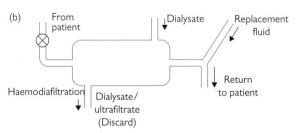

Fig. 3.6 Typical circuits for haemofiltration and haemodiafiltration.

Chapter 4

Gastrointestinal tract and liver

99

4.1 Perioperative nausea and vomiting

Incidence and impact of PONV

Perioperative nausea and vomiting (PONV) is a common problem with an incidence of 30–80%. It impacts in many ways on the postoperative course:

- Delayed day surgery discharge
- Unplanned admission from day surgery
- Raised intraocular pressure
- Raised intracerebral pressure
- Secondary haemorrhage from raised venous pressure
- Increased wound dehiscence
- Reduced patient satisfaction.

Risk factors for PONV

Three categories of risk factor impact upon the risk of PONV:

Patient factors

- History of PONV
- Female
- Children, young adults
- Anxiety
- History of motion sickness
- Non-smokers
- Dehydration
- Delayed gastric emptying.

Type of surgery

- ENT surgery
- Gynaecological procedures
- Squint surgery
- Abdominal procedures
- Prolonged surgery.

Anaesthetic factors

- Opioid analgesia
- Nitrous oxide
- Gastric insufflation
- Volatile anaesthetic agents
- Neostigmine
- Hypotension.

Physiology of vomiting

The vomiting centre

The vomiting centre is contained within the reticular formation of the medulla (Fig. 4.1) and is closely related to the nucleus tractus solitarius, which contains the nuclei of the vagus, glossopharyngeal, and accessory nerves.

Afferents are received from the GI tract, peritoneum, vagal afferents from the heart, vestibular apparatus and the chemoreceptor trigger zone (CTZ). The vomiting centre also has afferents from higher centres related to thought, smell, and emotion (Fig. 4.2).

Vomiting centre receptors include:

- Muscarinic M_3 receptors (cholinergic input from the vestibular apparatus and vagal innervation)
- Histamine H_1 receptors from the nucleus tractus solitarius.

The chemoreceptor trigger zone

The CTZ is in the area postrema of the medulla and lies outside the blood–brain barrier allowing stimulation by chemicals carried within the blood.

The receptors involved are:

- Dopamine D_2 receptors
- Serotonin 5-HT_3 receptors
- Chemical receptors, e.g. opioids.

Efferent pathway from the vomiting centre

Efferent nerves from the vomiting centre are the vagus, phrenic, glossopharyngeal, and accessory nerves (Fig. 4.2). The motor nucleus of the vagus is within the nucleus tractus solitarius and is closely related to the dorsal motor nucleus of the vagus, which controls parasympathetic output to the GI tract.

The vomiting reflex starts with swallowing and increased respiratory rate. Following closure of the pylorus, which prevents retropulsion of duodenal contents, the oesophageal sphincters relax. A high intra-abdominal pressure is created by contraction of the abdominal muscles and diaphragm, and then the stomach contracts to expel the contents. The laryngeal inlet is protected by the glottis closing and epiglottis moving down.

Prophylaxis of PONV

Modification of anaesthetic technique

Regional anaesthesia or neuraxial anaesthesia may be used as the sole anaesthetic technique or as an opioid-sparing technique. Total intravenous anaesthesia may decrease the incidence of PONV by 25%. Known triggers for PONV such as nitrous oxide and hypotension can be avoided.

Pharmacological

For patients at risk of PONV, evidence would support the use of dexamethasone 8mg given shortly after induction, in combination with a 5-HT_3 antagonist at the end of the procedure.

Acupressure/acupuncture

Many studies show comparable results to those with antiemetic medication by using Chinese P6 pressure point stimulation *prior* to anaesthesia.

Management of PONV

The large number of receptors involved in the control of vomiting makes PONV difficult to treat. Many of the drugs used commonly act on multiple receptors and often need to be used in combination. If pharmacological prophylaxis has failed, drugs from another class should be used.

Dopamine antagonists (D_2)

Metoclopramide: may also have an effect via peripheral 5-HT3 receptors and increases gastric emptying. It is often ineffective in the treatment of PONV and may be associated with extrapyramidal side effects.

Phenothiazines: Prochlorperazine is available as an intramuscular preparation. It also has antimuscarinic effects and is associated with extrapyramidal side effects and sedation.

Butyrophenones: e.g. droperidol which has been recently relicensed. Droperidol can be associated with a distressing dissociative state and with arrhythmias.

Histamine antagonists (H₁)

Cyclizine: also has antimuscarinic effects and causes sedation. Cyclizine may have higher efficacy for motion sickness or PONV due to middle ear surgery.

Serotonin receptor antagonists (5-HT₃)

Studies have indicated a number-needed-to-treat (NNT) of 4–7 with better results at higher doses. There are very few associated side effects although rarely dystonia may occur.

Corticosteroids

Dexamethasone is an effective prophylactic antiemetic with a NNT of 4. The mechanism of effect is unknown. Steroid side effects are unlikely with single use but need to be considered with repeat anaesthesia in a short time frame.

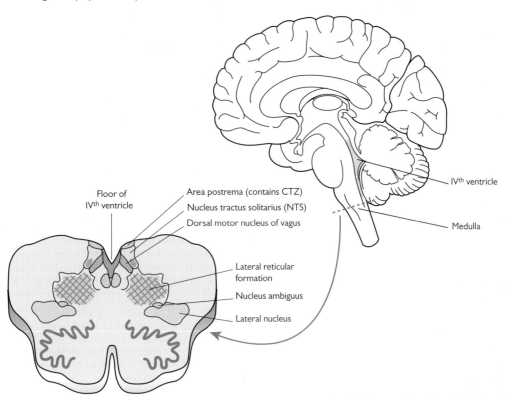

Fig. 4.1 Anatomical location of the vomiting centre. Reproduced from Catherine Spoors and Kevin Kiff, *Training in Anaesthesia*, 2010, Figure 17.12, page 431, with permission from Oxford University Press.

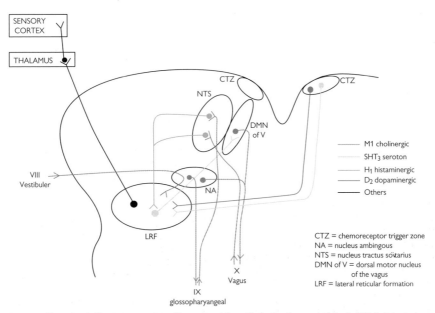

Fig. 4.2 The vomiting centre: afferent and efferent connections. Reproduced from Catherine Spoors and Kevin Kiff, *Training in Anaesthesia*, 2010, Figure 17.13, page 431, with permission from Oxford University Press.

4.2 Oesophageal reflux and acid aspiration prophylaxis

Oesophageal reflux

The overriding concern in respect of gastro-oesophageal reflux disease (GORD) is the aspiration of acidic contents into the tracheobronchial tree during anaesthesia with resultant aspiration pneumonitis. Chemical injury is caused by acidic gastric contents, and any solid/semi-solid components may lead to airway obstruction and atelectasis.

Oesophageal reflux is due to four main factors:

1. Increased gastric volume
2. Decreased gastric emptying
3. Gastro-oesophageal junction incompetence
4. Reduced gastro-oesophageal barrier pressure.

Increased gastric volume

The gastric volume is routinely reduced preoperatively by fasting. The normal production of about 2L/day of gastric secretion is also reduced by fasting. In an emergency situation, the stomach may be full or gastric emptying delayed.

Delayed gastric emptying

Factors that delay gastric emptying

- Pain, anxiety, stress
- Sympathetic stimulation
- Autonomic neuropathy, e.g. diabetes, vagotomy
- Anticholinergics
- Opioids
- Alcohol
- Pyloric stenosis, ileus, obstruction.

Factors that increase gastric emptying

- Metoclopramide
- Domperidone
- Erythromycin.

Metoclopramide is a dopamine receptor (D_2) antagonist, which increases gastric emptying and small bowel transit by improving cholinergic function as well as oesophageal sphincter tone.

Domperidone has a similar action but has less central nervous system side effects.

Erythromycin is a macrolide antibiotic which acts as a motilin agonist causing antral contraction.

Gastro-oesophageal junction incompetence

This is related to the lower oesophageal sphincter (LOS) tone as well as the acute angle that the oesophagus communicates with the stomach and the muscle fibres surrounding this at the diaphragmatic hiatus. These anatomical factors are lost with the formation of a hiatus hernia. The LOS can be disrupted by the presence of a nasogastric tube or replaced by fibrous tissue in scleroderma.

The LOS is an area of circular smooth muscle in the distal 3–5cm of the oesophagus, which is in a state of tonic contraction to separate the two lumens. This generates a LOS pressure of 15–25mmHg.

Factors that reduce lower oesophageal sphincter tone

- Swallowing
- Anticholinergics—atropine, glycopyrrolate
- Dopamine
- Oestrogen and progesterone
- Opioids
- Alcohol
- Anaesthetic agents.

Factors that increase lower oesophageal sphincter tone

- Cholinergic stimulation—anticholinesterases, cyclizine
- Dopamine antagonist—metoclopramide, domperidone, prochlorperazine
- Suxamethonium.

Some patients have transient relaxation of the LOS that is unprovoked and results in oesophageal reflux even in the presence of a competent LOS and normal LOS pressures.

Reduced gastro-oesophageal barrier pressure

The gastro-oesophageal barrier pressure is the difference between the LOS pressure and the intragastric (or intra-abdominal) pressure.

A raised intragastric or intra-abdominal pressure due to obesity, pregnancy, bowel obstruction, laparoscopic surgery or Trendelenburg position reduces the barrier pressure and may cause reflux.

Acid secretion and antacid prophylaxis

About 2L of gastric juice containing hydrochloric acid, potassium, pepsinogens, and mucus is produced per day. The pH is 1–1.5. Gastric secretion is increased by the presence of food in the mouth or stomach. Raising the pH of gastric secretions and reducing the volume reduces the risks of aspiration pneumonitis (Box 4.1).

Antacids

Sodium citrate is a clear, non-particulate alkali which is effective at raising intragastric pH for 45min after 30mL 0.3M solution. It does, however, increase gastric volume. Magnesium trisilicate is particulate and may be harmful if aspirated.

Ranitidine

Ranitidine is a histamine (H_2) receptor antagonist which reduces gastric secretion and hydrogen ion secretion from parietal cells (Fig. 4.3). 150mg is given orally 2h prior to anaesthesia. IM/IV doses are effective within 4min.

Proton pump inhibitors

These are irreversible, non-competitive inhibitors of the $H^+K^+ATPase$, which is the final pathway of acid secretion by the parietal cell. They cause dramatic reductions in acid secretion for up to 48h.

Box 4.1 Methods of reducing acid aspiration

Physiological

- Fasting (2h clear fluid, 6h solids).
- Siting and aspirating nasogastric tube if gastric outlet obstruction.
- Positioning head-up for induction of anaesthesia.
- Cricoid pressure and avoidance of gastric insufflation as in rapid sequence induction techniques.

Pharmacological

- Sodium citrate to raise pH.
- Ranitidine 150mg orally 2h prior to anaesthesia (or IV 1h prior if not absorbing).
- Dose may also be given the night before, especially obstetrics.
- Proton pump inhibitor, e.g. omeprazole.
- Metoclopramide to increase gastric emptying. 10mg orally 2h prior to anaesthesia.

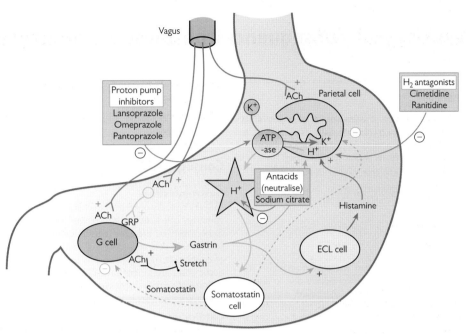

Fig. 4.3 Gastric acid regulation and the effects of drugs. Reproduced from Catherine Spoors and Kevin Kiff, *Training in Anaesthesia*, 2010, Figure 17.3, page 417, with permission from Oxford University Press.

4.3 Physiological consequences of bowel obstruction

Pathogenesis

Bowel obstruction is a *physical* impairment of gastrointestinal transit, as opposed to ileus which is a physiological impairment. It is a common cause of surgical admission and may affect the small or large intestine. There are many aetiologies including:

- Postoperative adhesions—the commonest cause
- Stricture from tumour, inflammatory bowel disease, or diverticulitis
- Volvulus or intussusception
- Incarceration in hernial orifice
- Occlusion by foreign body.

Bowel proximal to the obstruction increases peristalsis to oppose the blockage. Gaseous distension occurs due to bacterial overgrowth and digestive enzymes. The bowel dilates and peristalsis decreases, which reduces blood flow requirements as a protective measure. The bowel wall becomes oedematous and eventually leaks fluid into the peritoneum causing contamination and peritonitis. Intramural blood supply becomes compromised from a combination of bowel distension and hypovolaemia and eventually ischaemic bowel wall will perforate. Bacterial translocation causes local then systemic sepsis.

X-ray findings in small bowel obstruction (see Figure 4.4):

- Small bowel dilatation (>30mm)
- Multiple air or fluid levels
- 'Slit sign' (slit of air in the valvulae conniventes)
- 'String of pearls sign' (small gas bubbles in the valvulae conniventes)
- 'Coiled spring sign' (stretched perpendicular valvulae)
- Collapsed large intestine if small bowel pathology
- Large intestine x-ray findings if pathology there

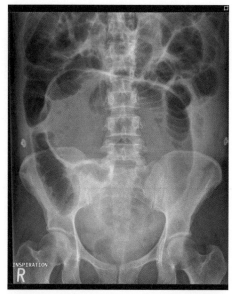

Fig. 4.4 X-ray appearance of small bowel obstruction.

Large bowel obstruction:

- Caecum >9cm
- Other colon >6cm
- Gas-fluid levels

Consequences of obstruction

Gastrointestinal

Patients typically present with colicky abdominal pain, distension, vomiting, and constipation. Bowel sounds may be hyperactive. Generalized or localized peritonitis may be present indicating perforation. Poor absorption of medication may cause instability of concurrent medical problems and if chronic, malnutrition may occur. Intra-abdominal pressure is increased and may result in abdominal compartment syndrome. Perforation will precipitate a systemic inflammatory response.

Cardiovascular

Dehydration and hypovolaemia are common. This results from GI losses, such as vomiting, and also from fluid sequestration in the gut. Fluid loss is frequently underestimated and is difficult to measure.

Respiratory

Abdominal distension causes splinting of the diaphragm with basal atelectasis, reduced functional residual capacity, and ventilation:perfusion mismatch.

Metabolic

Metabolic derangements occur due to loss of sodium and water as well as the particular losses from GI secretions. The electrolyte derangements may reflect the level of obstruction:

- Proximal bowel obstruction may present with hypokalaemic, hypochloraemic alkalosis as in gastric outlet obstruction.
- More distal obstruction is associated with acidosis due to bicarbonate loss.

Anaesthetic management

Preoperative

The urgency of the surgery must be assessed. Where possible, NCEPOD guidelines suggest operating within routine hours, as there is significant morbidity and mortality associated with the procedure. Bowel obstruction with a high risk of ischaemia (e.g. incarcerated hernias or closed-loop obstruction) requires urgent surgery.

Preoptimization may have an important impact. Preoperative fluid resuscitation should aim to restore intravascular volume and replace interstitial fluid and electrolyte losses. This may require preoperative central venous pressure measurement as well as monitoring end-organ function. In severe hypovolaemia, preoperative inotropic support may be required. Oxygen therapy should be commenced and analgesia provided to improve respiratory function. A NGT should be inserted to decompress the proximal bowel, allow measurement of GI losses and empty the stomach prior to anaesthesia. Postoperative high-dependency or intensive care should be arranged.

Perioperative

A rapid sequence induction technique will be required, following aspiration of the NGT, due to the high risk of aspiration. The importance of an NGT *prior* to induction cannot be over-stated. Invasive monitoring is often required and non-invasive cardiac output monitoring should be instituted to guide perioperative fluid resuscitation. Goal-directed fluid therapy, i.e. fluid management targeted to stroke volume (see section 13.10), improves tissue perfusion and has been shown in some studies to improve both patient and surgical outcome with:

• Reduced length of stay
• Reduced requirement for critical care
• Reduced length of time until restoration of normal diet
• Reduced GI morbidity
• Reduced overall morbidity.

Epidural analgesia may improve postoperative respiratory function but is contraindicated in the septic patient when a combination of transversus abdominis plane (TAP) blocks and opiate analgesia may be more appropriate. Nitrous oxide should be avoided as it increases bowel distension and is associated with raised intra-abdominal pressure.

Postoperative

Postoperatively, high-dependency care is optimal. There may be an ongoing need for cardiovascular monitoring as well as attention to fluid and electrolyte balance. Optimization of respiratory function is possible with good analgesia and respiratory physiotherapy. CPAP may be required to reduce basal atelectasis or treat hypoxia. Enteral nutrition should be commenced as soon as possible and parenteral nutrition instituted if this fails.

Further reading

Gemmel LW & Rincon C (2001). Anaesthetic management of intestinal obstruction. *CEPD Rev*, 1(5):138–41.

4.4 Management of massive gastrointestinal haemorrhage

Incidence/causes

Upper GI haemorrhage causes about 5000 deaths per year in the UK. It presents with haematemesis or melaena and is most commonly due to peptic ulcer disease or oesophagitis/gastric erosions. Massive upper GI haemorrhage is more likely to be due to varices, vascular malformations, malignancy, or, rarely, aorto-enteric fistula. Lower GI haemorrhage is less likely to cause haemodynamic compromise and mortality.

Initial assessment

Airway and breathing

Failure to protect the airway is an important cause of delayed mortality with massive upper GI haemorrhage. Aspiration is common in severe bleeding and protective reflexes are lost due to impaired conscious levels secondary to haemorrhagic shock or encephalopathy. Intubation is also indicated for impaired ventilation. A difficult intubation should be anticipated and adequate suction is essential.

Circulation

An early assessment of volaemic status and end-organ function is essential. Early targeted management of haemorrhagic shock (see section 1.14) improves outcome. Large bore IV access and fluid therapy should be commenced. All IV fluid infusions should be warmed. Resuscitation should be guided by frequent haematological investigation:

- Transfusion is indicated for massive haemorrhage or Hb <7g/dL. Higher transfusion thresholds may be associated with greater mortality and rebleeding rates.
- Coagulopathy (INR >1.5) should be reversed with FFP or prothrombin complex concentrate (e.g. Beriplex®).
- Platelet transfusion is indicated if platelet count is <50 × 10⁹/L.
- Hypofibrinogenaemia is managed with cryoprecipitate (fibrinolysis can also be inhibited with tranexamic acid which may also confer a benefit in overall mortality).

The response to resuscitation should be monitored clinically including central venous pressure and urine output measurement, as well as biochemical and haematological investigation. Vasopressor support may be necessary.

Adequate resuscitation should precede endoscopic or surgical intervention where possible, but in some situations these will need to be concurrent to gain control of the circulation. In variceal bleeding, a Sengstaken–Blakemore tube may be used to prevent ongoing haemorrhage.

Disability/exposure

Defining any comorbidity of the patient allows some prediction of expected mortality as well as the cause of GI bleeding (Table 4.1). Increasing age (>65 years) and renal or hepatic disease are particularly associated with increased mortality. Stigmata of chronic liver disease may well suggest variceal bleeding which has implications for management. Broad-spectrum antibiotics reduce hospital mortality by 20%. Gram-negative bacteria are a common cause of infection.

Table 4.1 Predicting mortality from GI bleeding—the Rockall score

Variable	Score			
	0	1	2	3
Age	<60 years	60–79 years	>80 years	
Shock	SBP >100 HR <100	SBP >100 HR >100	SBP <100 HR >100	
Comorbidity	None		Heart failure	Renal failure Malignancy

High-risk endoscopy findings (active arterial bleed, adherent clot, visible vessel, large ulcer and varices) also add points post endoscopy.
Rockall score >5 = 10% mortality
Rockall score >8 = 40% mortality

Reproduced from *Gut*, TF Rockall et al., 'Risk assessment after acute upper gastrointestinal haemorrhage', 38, 3, pp. 316–321, copyright 1996, with permission from BMJ Publishing Group Ltd.

Management of variceal bleeding

In the presence of chronic liver disease and portal hypertension, oesophageal and gastric varices may occur as portosystemic vessels dilate. These carry a 30% lifetime risk of GI bleeding which has a mortality of 50%.

A Sengstaken–Blakemore tube (a double-cuffed gastric tube) may be used to compress varices. It is inserted into the stomach and the gastric cuff inflated with 150–250mL of air. With gentle traction, this compresses gastro-oesophageal varices in most cases. If bleeding continues, the oesophageal cuff is inflated to pressures of 30–40mmHg. This can be left *in situ* for 24h and is effective in controlling haemorrhage in about 90% of cases. Due to a high rebleeding rate on deflation, balloon tamponade is often used as a bridging procedure to other forms of intervention. The use of Sengstaken tubes carries certain important risks (Box 4.2).

Box 4.2 Complications of Sengstaken–Blakemore tubes

- Airway obstruction
- Pulmonary aspiration
- Necrosis of gastric mucosa
- Oesophageal ulceration (deflate oesophageal balloon every 12h to prevent necrosis)
- Oesophageal rupture.

Management of variceal bleeding also includes pharmacological manipulation of portal pressures and splanchnic blood flow. Terlipressin, a vasopressin analogue (2mg IV then 1–2mg 4–6h for 72h) and octreotide (50mcg then 50mcg/h) are used. Terlipressin increases SVR, reduces CO, and reduces coronary blood flow, which may precipitate myocardial ischaemia. Octreotide may be more effective and has fewer side effects.

Endoscopy/surgical intervention

Endoscopy

- Injection of adrenaline
- Thermocoagulation

- Mechanical clips
- Banding of varices
- Sclerotherapy of varices.

Endoscopy may not identify the source of bleeding in 20% of cases. Visceral angiography may be required. Endoscopic intervention should take place in the theatre environment in massive haemorrhage.

Surgical
- Oversewing of ulcer
- Partial gastrectomy
- Portosystemic shunt procedures.

Surgical intervention is reserved for rebleeding following endoscopic intervention and is associated with high morbidity and mortality rates.

Prevention of recurrence

Proton pump inhibitors
Proton pump inhibitors may reduce the risk of rebleeding, surgical intervention and death, although a Cochrane review found no significant difference. Suppressing gastric mucosal acid secretion prevents mucosal fibrinolytic activity and allows clot formation. Proton pump inhibitors are the only reliable way of raising gastric pH >6 to prevent clot lysis after upper GI bleeding.

Propranolol
Propranolol is used to reduce portal hypertension and reduce further risk of variceal bleeding. Low doses are commenced initially as these patients have reduced first-pass metabolism. Propranolol is contraindicated during acute bleeding. Propranolol reduces rebleeding risk by about 40%.

Endoscopy
Endoscopic band ligation of varices is effective, particularly in conjunction with β-blockade.

Transjugular intrahepatic portosystemic shunt (TIPS)
TIPS may be used in variceal bleeding after failed endoscopy or to prevent recurrent bleeding by reducing portal pressures. The hepatic vein is cannulated via an internal jugular vein approach under X-ray guidance. A tract is created through liver parenchyma to the portal vein and an expandable stent is deployed into this tract connecting the portal and systemic circulations. This reduces portal pressures but at the expense of encephalopathy in 25% cases. The procedure is associated with a 1% mortality although this compares favourably to the surgical shunt techniques, which may have a mortality of 20%. The shunts may become occluded by thrombosis or stenosis.

Further reading

Jairath V, Hearnshaw S, Brunskill SJ, et al. (2010). Red cell transfusion for the management of upper GI haemorrhage. *Cochrane Database Syst Rev*, 7:CD006613.

McKay R & Webster NR (2007). Variceal bleeding. *CEACCP*, 7(6):191–98.

Sreedharan A, Martin J, Leontiadis GI, et al. (2010). PPI treatment prior to endoscopic diagnosis in upper GI bleeding. *Cochrane Database Syst Rev*, 7:CD005415.

4.5 Severe acute pancreatitis

Incidence/pathogenesis

The incidence of acute pancreatitis is 10–30 per 100 000 of the population. There is interstitial inflammation and oedema but acinar cells are initially spared. Most cases are self-limiting with simple, supportive treatment. In about 20% of cases, however, the disease process progresses to a severe acute pancreatitis in which necrosis involves the functional acinar cells and where there is associated organ dysfunction and/or local complications.

Pancreatitis is triggered by the release and activation of proteases secondary to hyperstimulation (e.g. alcohol, fat) and pancreatic duct obstruction (e.g. gallstones). See Box 4.3. Proteases autodigest pancreatic tissue as well as the surrounding tissues as there is a poor capsular barrier. The proteases also trigger a systemic inflammatory response as they enter the bloodstream.

Box 4.3 Causes of pancreatitis

Common
- Gallstones (>90% cases)
- Alcohol
- Iatrogenic

Less common
- Post ERCP/surgery
- Trauma
- Drugs, e.g. diuretics, steroids, azathioprine, TPN
- Hypercalcaemia, hyperlipidaemia
- Hypothermia
- Infection, e.g. mumps, CMV, EBV

Symptoms and signs

- Severe constant abdominal pain which typically radiates to the back.
- Nausea and vomiting.
- Epigastric tenderness (peritonism may be absent as the pancreas is largely retroperitoneal).
- Haemorrhagic pancreatitis may lead to Grey Turner's or Cullen's signs (flank or periumbilical discolouration) due to retroperitoneal bleeding.
- Evidence of associated systemic response with signs of shock, respiratory failure, and renal failure.

Investigations

Serum amylase >1000 IU/L

Amylase may be elevated within the first 24h but is then rapidly excreted by the kidneys. More prolonged elevation may suggest pseudocyst formation. Urinary amylase levels remain elevated.

Serum lipase >600 IU/L

May be more specific and remains elevated for 14 days.

CT imaging

Defines the extent of necrosis, allows severity scoring, and demonstrates associated complications.

Ultrasound imaging

Demonstrates the presence of gallstones.

Complications

Within the first 2 weeks, most complications are the result of pancreatic necrosis and the systemic inflammatory response (Boxes 4.4 and 4.5). Beyond this period there is potential for infection of the necrotic tissue, which may cause local complications as well as sepsis, and multiorgan failure, which is associated with a high mortality.

Box 4.4 Local complications of acute pancreatitis

- Pancreatic pseudocyst: pseudocysts are extra-pancreatic collections of pancreatic secretions from disrupted pancreatic ducts. The surrounding capsule becomes fibrinous, and large pseudocysts may cause ongoing symptoms and require surgery.
- Pancreatic abscess: this is infected pancreatic necrosis, which requires radiological or surgical drainage.
- Ascites/effusions: pancreatic duct secretions leak into peritoneal cavity.
- Ileus: from intra-abdominal inflammation/peritoneal irritation.
- Abdominal compartment syndrome: see section 4.6
- Portal vein thrombosis: due to surrounding inflammation and microthrombi. Portal vein thrombosis may lead to portal hypertension.
- Massive haemorrhage: this is a rare complication but can occur late due to rupture of splenic artery pseudoaneurysms.

Box 4.5 Systemic complications of acute pancreatitis

- Shock: circulatory kinins increase vascular permeability causing relative hypovolaemia.
- Respiratory failure: diaphragmatic splinting, pleural effusions, ARDS and microthrombi in the pulmonary circulation may all contribute.
- Renal failure: prerenal failure is common due to hypovolaemia and low perfusion pressure.
- Hyperglycaemia: the Islets of Langerhans and insulin secretion are affected.
- Hypocalaemia: calcium sequestration in fat necrosis lowers corrected plasma calcium.
- Hypoalbuminaemia: occurs due to vascular permeability.

Management of severe pancreatitis

Trials of antiproteolytic drugs (e.g. aprotinin), antisecretory drugs (e.g. somatostatin or glucagon), antioxidants, e.g. N-acetylcysteine and drugs that target the inflammatory response have all failed to demonstrate any improvement in outcome. Management is therefore supportive with appropriate radiological or surgical intervention.

Patients have high fluid requirements and these should be guided by central venous pressure, urine output, and cardiac output monitoring. Vasopressors may be required to maintain adequate perfusion pressures. Early management of cardiovascular disturbance may prevent renal failure although some units practice early haemofiltration to reduce cytokine load and inflammatory response. Ventilatory support is usually required and pleural effusions may require draining. Hyperglycaemia is managed with insulin infusions and hypocalcaemia corrected. Early nutrition is required and TPN should be considered promptly if nasogastric/jejunal feeding fails due to ileus.

Although prophylactic antibiotics are not recommended, close surveillance for evidence of infection is necessary with early, targeted treatment. Management of sterile necrosis is conservative but infected necrosis requires a more interventional approach. Evidence of infection may require CT diagnosis, FNA culture or an increase in procalcitonin levels (CRP is chronically elevated). Gram-negative bacteria are commonly implicated but fungal infection may also occur.

Surgical intervention is generally reserved for infected necrosis. Open necrosectomy may be required and this is generally followed with frequent laparotomies with washout and packing to reduce debris. Laparostomy may be necessary and surgery is associated with high mortality, especially if required in the initial 3 weeks before demarcation of necrotic tissue has occurred. Less invasive hydroscopic debridements may be possible in some patients.

Mortality is increased in infected necrosis, with older age and with higher BMI, and is usually due to multiorgan failure. Ranson's criteria (Box 4.6) and the Glasgow score (Box 4.7) help to predict the need for ITU care and expected mortality.

Box 4.6 Ranson's criteria in severe acute pancreatitis
At presentation
• Age >55 years
• WCC >16 × 10^9/L
• Glucose >11mmol/L
• LDH >350IU/L
• AST >60IU/L
During first 24h
• Hct fall >10%
• Urea >10mmol/L
• Calcium <2mmol/L
• Base excess >−4
• PaO$_2$ <8kPa
• Fluid sequestration >6L
Predicted mortality
• 0–2 points – 2%
• 3–4 points – 15%
• 5–6 points – 40%
• 7–8 points – 100%

Reprinted with permission from the *Journal of the American College of Surgeons*, formerly *Surgery Gynaecology & Obstetrics*. 'Prognostic signs and the role of operative management in acute pancreatitis'. Ranson JHC, Rifkind KM, Roses DF, et al., *Surg Gynecol Obstet* 1974; 139:69–81.

Box 4.7 Glasgow score for pancreatitis severity	
PO$_2$ <8kPa	Glucose >11mmol/L
WCC > 15 × 10^9/L	Urea >16mmol/L
Albumin <30g/L	LDH > 600IU/L
Calcium < 2mmol/L	Age >55 years

A score ≥3 indicates severe acute pancreatitis.
Patients should be referred for critical care evaluation early.

Reprinted from *The Lancet*, 326, 8452, Corfield AP et al., 'Prediction of severity in acute pancreatitis prospective comparison of three prognostic indices', pp. 403–407, Copyright 1985, with permission from Elsevier.

A reminder of pancreatic physiology is summarized in Box 4.8.

Box 4.8 Reminder of pancreatic physiology
• Acinar cells are the main functional unit and comprise the parenchyma of the pancreas.
• Centroacinar cells secrete bicarbonate.
• Basophilic cells secrete digestive enzymes.
• Exocrine products produced are secreted into a tubular system that forms the main pancreatic duct. This then joins the common bile duct to form the ampulla of Vater, which opens into the duodenum surrounded by the Sphincter of Oddi.
• 1500mL/day of alkaline pancreatic secretion is formed containing trypsin, lipases, amylase, and elastase.
The endocrine function of the pancreas is performed by the islets of Langerhans. These are embedded within the exocrine pancreas:
• Beta cells secrete insulin
• Alpha cells secrete glucagon
• Delta cells secrete somatostatin.

Further reading

Swaroop VS, Chari ST, & Clain JE (2004). Severe acute pancreatitis. *JAMA* 291(23):2865–2868. doi:10.1001/jama.291.23.2865.

Young SP & Thompson JP (2008). Severe acute pancreatitis. CEACCP, 8(4):125–8.

4.6 Abdominal compartment syndrome

Incidence/pathogenesis

The normal intra-abdominal pressure (IAP), the intrinsic pressure in the abdominal cavity, is around 5–7mmHg and slight increases can be seen with morbid obesity, during positive pressure ventilation, and post-surgery (see Box 4.9). Intra-abdominal pressure depends on intra-abdominal *volume* and abdominal wall *compliance*. A rapid increase in volume will result in abdominal hypertension.

> **Box 4.9 Factors affecting intra-abdominal pressure**
>
> *Factors that increase intra-abdominal volume*
> - Haemorrhage, e.g. trauma, AAA, peptic ulcer
> - Capillary leak/oedema, e.g. pancreatitis, sepsis, large volume fluid resuscitation
> - Bowel obstruction, ileus
> - Ascites
> - Surgical packs.
>
> *Factors that reduce abdominal wall compliance*
> - Pain
> - Burns
> - Dressings.

Intra-abdominal hypertension is defined as a sustained IAP >12mmHg (Table 4.2). Abdominal compartment syndrome occurs when IAP >20mmHg with at least one organ dysfunction. Abdominal compartment syndrome occurs in about 10% of trauma ICU admissions and is associated with a mortality in excess of 60%.

Table 4.2 Grades of intra-abdominal hypertension

Grade	IAP	Management
1	10–15mmHg	Monitor IAP, medical management
2	16–25mmHg	As above, and consider early decompression to prevent end-organ damage
3	26–35mmHg	Organ dysfunction will occur >25mmHg. Surgical decompression is required
4	>35mmHg	Repeat decompressions required

Reprinted from *Surgical Clinics*, 76, 4, Jon M Burch et al., 'The Abdominal Compartment Syndrome', pp. 833–842, Copyright 1996, with permission from Elsevier.

Multiorgan effects of abdominal compartment syndrome

Gastrointestinal effects
Reduced oxygen delivery resulting from compression and congestion of mesenteric veins and capillaries causes mucosal ischaemia. Histamine and serotonin release from ischaemic tissue results in oedema, which causes a further increase in IAP, and which also allows bacterial translocation. Surgical anastomoses may break down. Hepatic blood flow is also reduced, decreasing the capacity for lactate clearance.

Cardiovascular effects
Inferior vena cava obstruction reduces venous return and a compensatory rise in SVR occurs. This effect is compounded by hypovolaemia and raised intrathoracic pressure. Reduced venous return from the lower limbs may increase the incidence of DVT.

Diaphragmatic elevation raises PVR and also reduces ventricular compliance. Myocardial contractility is further reduced by the developing metabolic acidosis.

Blood pressure is often maintained, or may increase, due to increased SVR. CVP appears elevated as the IAP is transmitted to the central venous pressure recording. The true CVP should be calculated by subtracting IAP from the measurement. Fluid resuscitation should be guided by cardiac output measurement.

Respiratory effects
Diaphragmatic elevation increases intrathoracic pressure and causes atelectasis, which increases A-a gradient, reduces dead space and increases V/Q mismatch. Both pulmonary and chest wall compliance decrease. High inspiratory pressures, high levels of PEEP and high respiratory rates to maintain normocapnia may be required.

Renal effects
Both renal blood flow and glomerular filtration rate decrease, causing oliguria. Renin, aldosterone, and antidiuretic hormone secretion is increased.

Central nervous system
Acute rises in IAP cause a reciprocal rise in ICP. In traumatic head injury this compromises cerebral perfusion pressure and is associated with higher mortality.

Diagnosis: IAP measurement

In order to diagnose abdominal compartment syndrome, elevated IAP must be demonstrated in the presence of organ dysfunction. Abdominal pressures may be measured indirectly by monitoring intravesical pressures. Following the introduction of 25mL sterile saline via a urinary catheter, the drainage tube is clamped beyond the aspiration port. An 18G needle attached to a pressure transducer can then be introduced into the sample aspiration port and zeroed at the level of the symphysis pubis in the supine patient. Urinary catheters with pressure monitoring devices are also available commercially. Direct measurement is only possible surgically.

A CT scan may show a collection of signs to support the diagnosis. These include:
- Compression of the IVC
- Tense infiltration of the retroperitoneum
- Bowel wall thickening
- Bilateral inguinal herniation
- The 'round belly sign' where the anteroposterior diameter is increased (>0.8 in ratio) in comparison to the transverse abdominal diameter.

Management of abdominal compartment syndrome

Medical management
- *Improve abdominal wall compliance:* good analgesia, neuromuscular blockade, position (stretch out, avoid prone), removal of dressings.
- *Evacuate intraluminal contents:* nasogastric drainage, rectal tube, use of prokinetics and enemas

- *Evacuate intraperitoneal collections:* drain collections/abscesses percutaneously.
- *Optimize fluids:* cardiac output guided fluid management may improve intra-abdominal blood flow and oxygen delivery at lower IAP. Over-resuscitation will compound the problem. The aim should be for neutral balance and colloid should be used. If over-resuscitation has occurred, haemofiltration may remove fluid and reduce bowel and mesenteric oedema.
- *Optimize systemic and local perfusion:* as well as goal directed fluid therapy, vasoactive support may be required to optimize systemic circulation, aiming for abdominal perfusion pressures >60mmHg.

Surgical decompression

Surgical decompression has been shown to improve morbidity and mortality. Studies have shown that early decompression is an independent predictor of survival and also facilitates early primary closure. Mortality is reduced to about 20% if decompression is performed before organ dysfunction develops. If IAP >25mmHg and/or abdominal perfusion pressure <50mmHg with new organ dysfunction refractory to medical management, surgical decompression is warranted urgently. See Box 4.10.

Prevention

IAP should be monitored in high-risk cases. Supra-normal fluid resuscitation should be avoided in trauma and burns patients, with adherence to transfusion protocols.

Consideration should be given to leaving the abdomen open following trauma or ruptured aneurysm cases where large volume fluid resuscitation or periods of prolonged shock have occurred. In organ transplantation, organs should be matched for size. Massive hernia reduction may require careful planning to prevent raised IAP. Good analgesia techniques should be used to improve abdominal wall compliance.

Further reading

Cheatham ML (2009). Abdominal compartment syndrome. *Curr Opin Crit Care*, 15(2):154–62. doi:10.1097/MCC.0b013e3283297934.

The World Society of Abdominal Compartment Syndrome. Lectures and guidelines: <http://www.wsaca.org>.

Box 4.10 Anaesthesia for surgical decompression of abdominal compartment syndrome

Decompression may need to be performed on ICU in the critically unstable patient. Potential consequences include:
- CVS:
  - Sudden reduction in SVR as IAP released.
  - Fluid preload/vasopressor may be required to maintain cardiovascular stability.
- RS: sudden reduction in intrathoracic pressures may cause volutrauma during mechanical ventilation.
- Reperfusion syndrome: products of anaerobic metabolism, free radicals, and lactate are suddenly released into the circulation as blood flow is restored. Sudden myocardial depression, arrhythmia, and vasodilatation may lead to cardiac arrest. Inotropic support may be necessary as well as correction of acidosis with bicarbonate, and treatment of hyperkalaemia.
- Postoperative considerations: patients with open abdomens have increased fluid requirements and are prone to hypothermia. Invasive monitoring and goal-directed fluid therapy should be continued. Enteral feeding may be commenced. IAP monitoring must be continued as raised intra-abdominal pressures can still recur.

4.7 Jaundice

Definition

Jaundice is the yellow appearance of skin, sclera, and mucous membranes resulting from increased bilirubin concentration within the body fluids (Box 4.11). Jaundice becomes clinically detectable when plasma bilirubin exceeds 50μmol/L and is usually first evident in the sclerae. Table 4.3 compares the features of haemolytic, hepatocellular and cholestatic jaundice.

> **Box 4.11 Classification of jaundice**
>
> - *Pre-hepatic:* increased bilirubin production (haemolysis)
> - *Hepatic:* hepatocellular disease
> - *Post-hepatic:* cholestasis.

Bilirubin metabolism

Bilirubin is a product of the catabolism of haem. This unconjugated form of bilirubin is protein bound and not water- soluble. About 400–550mmol a day is produced but this increases with excess breakdown of haemoglobin or other haem containing proteins, or ineffective erythropoesis.

Unconjugated bilirubin is conjugated by glucuronyl transferase in the endoplasmic reticulum of the liver hepatocytes to form bilirubin monoglucuronide and diglucuronide. Carriers on the hepatocyte membrane transport the conjugated bilirubin to the bile canaliculi. Conjugated bilirubin is water-soluble.

Conjugated bilirubin is carried in bile to the bowel where it is metabolized by bacteria to form stercobilinogen. Further oxidization forms stercobilin, which colours the stool. A small amount of stercobilinogen is absorbed from the bowel and excreted as urobilinogen in the urine.

Haemolytic jaundice

Increased red blood cell and haemoglobin breakdown increases levels of unconjugated bilirubin. The liver has the capacity to increase the metabolism of bilirubin up to about 6 times the normal amount, thus levels of conjugated bilirubin and urobilinogen also increase. For this reason haemolytic jaundice is usually mild. Stools remain a normal colour and urine contains no bilirubin as unconjugated bilirubin is not water soluble.

An increased reticulocyte count suggests haemolysis, as red blood cells regenerate. Haptoglobin levels may decrease as free haemoglobin is bound.

Causes of haemolysis include:
- Haemoglobinopathies, e.g. sickle cell
- Glucose-6-phosphate dehydrogenase (G6PD) deficiency (Box 4.12)
- Immune
- Mechanical, e.g. prosthetic heart valves, burns
- Infections, e.g. malaria
- Drug-induced
- Pre-eclampsia
- Disseminated intravascular coagulation.

> **Box 4.12 Drugs causing haemolysis in G6PD-deficient patients**
>
> - Quinolones, e.g. ciprofloxacin
> - Sulphonamides
> - Nitrofurantoin
> - Dapsone
>
> *Drugs with possible risk*
> - Aspirin (usually acceptable up to 1g/day)
> - Quinine
> - Chloroquine

Hepatocellular jaundice

Liver parenchymal disease disrupts both the conjugation of bilirubin and its transport into the bile canaliculi. Hepatocellular jaundice implies severe liver disease which may be acute or chronic. Transaminases will be elevated, prothrombin time increased, and stigmata of chronic liver disease such as ascites may be present.

Cholestatic jaundice

Conjugated bilirubin is unable to drain via intrahepatic bile canaliculi or extrahepatic ducts and accumulates in the plasma. Cholestasis may be intra- or extrahepatic:

Intrahepatic cholestasis
Causes include:
- Primary biliary cirrhosis
- Primary sclerosing cholangitis
- Alcohol
- Drugs—erythromycin, chlorpromazine
- Viral
- Autoimmune
- Obstetric cholestasis.

Extrahepatic cholestasis
This represents obstruction in the portal tracts or extrahepatic bile ducts due to:
- Gallstones
- Carcinoma of the pancreas
- Cholangiocarcinoma
- Cystic fibrosis.

Cholestatic jaundice is often severe. Urine is dark as it contains conjugated bilirubin and stools are pale as reduced stercobilin is formed. Liver function tests will demonstrate raised alkaline phosphatase levels with a lesser degree of transaminase disturbance.

Anaesthetic considerations in jaundice

Perioperative renal failure is a real risk in jaundiced patients, especially in those with the very high bilirubin levels that often accompany cholestatic jaundice. Volaemic status should be optimized preoperatively and a urine output of >1mL/kg/h maintained with fluid resuscitation and possibly the use of mannitol or frusemide where necessary.

Other considerations relate to the underlying cause of the jaundice such as chronic liver disease (see section 4.8). Haemolytic jaundice may have implications for care such as avoiding tourniquet use in sickle cell disease or avoiding drugs that may trigger haemolysis in glucose-6-phophate dehydrogenase deficiency (see Box 4.12).

Postoperative jaundice

There are a variety of causes of postoperative jaundice, including:
- Underlying chronic disease (e.g. viral hepatitis).
- Acute liver dysfunction from hypotension or hypoxia.
- Following liver surgery or surgical damage to the liver or extrahepatic structures.
- Gilbert's syndrome (congenital non-haemolytic hyperbilirubinaemia): jaundice is triggered by fasting or intercurrent illness.
- Drugs e.g. halothane (see section 7.1).
- Haemolysis, e.g. transfusion reaction, breakdown of haematoma.
- Sepsis.

Table 4.3 Differentiating features of jaundice			
	Haemolytic	Hepatocellular	Cholestatic
Jaundice	Mild	Moderate	Severe
Symptoms	None	Variable	Dark urine, pale stools, itching
Bilirubin	↑ unconjugated	Mixed	↑ conjugated
Urobilinogen	High	Mixed	Low
Urine	Bilirubin −ve	Bilirubin +ve	Bilirubin ++ve
Transaminases	↑	↑↑↑	↑↑
Alkaline phosphatase	Normal	↑	↑↑
Other investigations	↑ reticulocytes	↑ INR	Ultrasound

4.8 Liver failure

Acute liver failure

Acute liver failure presents within 8 weeks of the onset of a precipitating illness and is characterized by progressive hepatic encephalopathy and jaundice. The most common cause in the UK is paracetamol overdose (Box 4.13; also see section 7.3). Complications include cerebral oedema, respiratory failure, hypotension, bleeding, hypoglycaemia, renal failure, acid–base disturbance with lactic acidosis, electrolyte disturbance, and infection. Management is supportive and ideally on a specialist liver ITU as urgent transplantation is often necessary. N-acetylcysteine infusion has been associated with minor improvement in mortality regardless of the aetiology of acute hepatic failure (Box 4.14).

Box 4.13 Causes of acute hepatic failure

- Paracetamol overdose
- Viral hepatitis
- Circulatory shock
- Drugs, e.g. aspirin, rifampicin
- Acute fatty liver of pregnancy.

Box 4.14 Predictors of mortality in acute hepatic failure

A mortality in excess of 90% is predicted if:
- PT >100s

or three of the following factors are present:
- PT >50s
- Age <10 or >40 years
- Jaundice to encephalopathy time >7 days
- Bilirubin >300µmol/L
- Cryptogenic aetiology.

Chronic liver disease

Chronic liver disease is much more common than acute liver failure. It is associated with high morbidity and mortality in the perioperative period. The Child–Pugh classification, originally designed for portocaval shunt surgery, may be used to stratify risk (Table 4.4). For causes, see Box 4.15.

Table 4.4 Child–Pugh classification and perioperative mortality

	Points		
	1	2	3
Serum bilirubin	<40	40–50	>50
Serum albumin	>35	28–35	<28
Ascites	None	Mild	Moderate–severe
Encephalopathy	Absent	Grade 1-2	Grade 3-4
INR	1–4	4–6	>6

Score 5–6 (Child A) = low mortality <5%
Score 7–9 (Child B) = moderate risk 25%
Score 10–15 (Child C) = high risk >50%

Reproduced from R.N.H. Pugh et al., 'Transection of the oesophagus for bleeding oesophageal varices', *British Journal of Surgery*, 60, 8, pp. 646–649, 1973, Wiley, with permission.

Box 4.15 Causes of chronic liver disease

- Alcoholic liver disease
- Viral hepatitis (B, C)
- Autoimmune
- Cryptogenic
- Cholestatic:
  - Primary biliary cirrhosis
  - Sclerosing cholangitis
- Venous outflow obstruction, e.g. Budd–Chiari syndrome
- Metabolic—Wilson's disease, haemochromatosis

Portal hypertension

Portal hypertension (>10mmHg) occurs due to increased intrahepatic vascular resistance and increased portal blood flow. Reduction in systemic and splanchnic vascular resistance further increases portal blood flow. As the portosystemic gradient increases, collaterals form varices at the gastro-oesophageal junction and rectum. Portal hypertension causes splenomegaly and, combined with water retention, produces ascites. Ascites may impair respiratory and renal function and is usually managed with salt/water restriction or diuretics, but paracentesis may be required. Propranolol starting at 40mg twice daily is used to reduce portal pressures. TIPS may be performed.

Respiratory system

Patients with chronic liver disease commonly have respiratory compromise due to ascites, which reduces functional residual capacity and may cause pleural effusions. Many patients may have associated COPD from smoking.

Hepatopulmonary syndrome (see section 13.5) may occur in chronic liver disease and causes hypoxia, increased A–a gradient and is associated with evidence of intrapulmonary shunting. Basal intrapulmonary vessels become dilated causing physiological shunt demonstrable by contrast echocardiography or perfusion scan. This produces *orthodeoxia*, worsening oxygenation in the upright position, when V/Q mismatch is increased. Oxygen therapy and transplantation may be required.

Portopulmonary syndrome is pulmonary hypertension associated with portal hypertension. It is a diagnosis of exclusion and is confirmed by right heart catheter studies demonstrating increased pulmonary vascular resistance. Management is as for primary pulmonary hypertension but the condition has a high mortality.

Cardiovascular system

Patients with chronic liver disease have a hyperdynamic circulation with high cardiac output, low systemic vascular resistance, and a low–normal blood pressure. There is an increased intravascular volume due to sodium and water retention. There may be associated ischaemic heart disease although this may not be revealed as the left ventricle work is low in the hyperdynamic circulation. Some aetiologies of chronic liver disease may be associated with cardiomyopathy, e.g. alcohol and haemochromatosis.

Renal system

Increased antidiuretic hormone, secondary hyperaldosteronism, and reduced glomerular filtration rate all cause sodium and water retention, which manifests as ascites and oedema. Hyponatraemia occurs due to relative excess water retention. Other electrolyte disorders are common. Treatment with spironolactone or loop diuretics may reduce oedema but possibly at the expense of relative hypovolaemia. Hepatorenal syndrome is functional renal failure in liver disease with histologically normal kidneys. It can be precipitated by any factor that further alters renal blood flow such as volume depletion, sepsis and high intra-abdominal pressures. Dialysis has little impact on outcome.

Central nervous system

Hepatic encephalopathy (Box 4.16) is a neuropsychiatric disorder that occurs with disease progression or may be precipitated by infection, GI bleeding, metabolic disturbance, drugs, surgery, portosystemic shunt formation, or uraemia. It is associated with increased plasma ammonia. Management centres on correcting the underlying cause, airway protection, and dietary protein restriction. Lactulose is used to acidify the gut converting ammonia to ammonium, which is non-absorbable.

Box 4.16 Grades of encephalopathy	
1: drowsy, orientated	tremor, apraxia
2: drowsy, disorientated	asterixis, ataxia
3: agitated, aggressive	asterixis, hyper-reflexia
4: unresponsive to pain	decerebration

Data from Conn H, Lieberthal M. The hepatic coma syndromes and lactulose. Baltimore: Williams & Wilkins; 1979. p. 7.

Haematological system

Anaemia in chronic liver disease may be due to malnutrition, chronic disease, or GI bleeding.

Thrombocytopenia occurs with splenic sequestration due to portal hypertension.

Disordered coagulation reflects a combination of reduced synthesis of clotting factors and increased fibrinolysis. The vitamin K dependent clotting factors (II, VII, IX, and X) are particularly affected. Coagulopathy is particularly a feature when liver disease is due to a hepatocellular aetiology as opposed to obstructive.

Metabolic effects

Unlike acute hepatic failure, hypoglycaemia is not usually a feature of chronic disease. A mild respiratory alkalosis due to tachypnoea, and metabolic alkalosis due to hypokalaemia or vomiting may be seen. Metabolic acidosis is an ominous sign, usually reflecting associated complications. In an acutely failing liver, lactate accumulates (since its metabolism to bicarbonate is dependent upon hepatic function).

Malnutrition is common in chronic liver disease and is associated with poor wound healing, increased rates of infection and muscle weakness.

Anaesthesia in patients with chronic liver disease

Preoperative investigation/optimization

- GI: ascites should be optimally managed and portal hypertension treated with propranolol.
- RS: pulmonary function tests and CXR should be performed if dyspnoea is present. Restrictive defects are common due to ascites. Pleural effusions may need to be drained.
- CVS: echocardiography is necessary in the presence of poor exercise tolerance or possible associated cardiomyopathy. Stress testing is performed if ischaemic symptoms are present.
- Renal: GFR should be measured as urea and electrolytes are unreliable. Volaemic status and electrolyte levels should be optimized.
- Haematological: most surgery will require platelet count >50, INR <1.5, and fibrinogen >1g/dL.

Perioperative aims

The main aim is to optimize hepatic blood flow and oxygen delivery. Hepatic blood flow is maintained by optimizing volaemic status, which requires CVP and urine output monitoring, using vasopressors if required to maintain MAP and maintaining normocarbia. All major surgery requires full invasive monitoring and consideration of cardiac output monitoring.

The pharmacokinetics of drugs are altered by decreased protein binding and high volume of distribution, e.g. reduced thiopentone dose and sensitivity to non-depolarizing muscle relaxants. Reduced pseudocholinesterase levels may prolong the duration of suxamethonium. Many drugs have prolonged elimination due to lack of liver metabolism or excretion, e.g. vecuronium and morphine.

Postoperative care

Following major surgery fluid balance is challenging and patients require high dependency or intensive care. Acute on chronic liver failure may occur.

Further reading

Wildlund R (2004). Pre-optimisation of patients with liver disease. *Crit Care Med*, 32:4 Suppl.

4.9 Porphyria

Definition

The porphyrias are a group of disorders caused by an inherited or acquired abnormality in the enzymes relating to haem synthesis. This leads to an excess accumulation of porphyrins and their precursors, particularly aminolaevulinic acid (ALA) and porphobilinogen (PBG), which precede the enzyme in the biochemical pathway. ALA synthetase is an important, early, rate-limiting enzyme in the pathway with positive feedback from decreasing haem levels. Porphyrias are rare with an incidence of 1/20 000 but are of relevance to anaesthetic practice as acute attacks may be precipitated by anaesthetic drugs and acute crises may require high dependency or intensive care.

The acute porphyrias

The acute porphyrias consist of acute intermittent porphyria which presents with acute attacks, and variegate and hereditary coproporphyria which are similar and present with acute attacks and skin photosensitivity. Within this group of porphyrias, an acute attack may be precipitated by alcohol, fasting, dehydration, stress, infection, menstruation, pregnancy, and enzyme-inducing drugs. All these factors reduce haem levels, increase activity of ALA synthetase, and hence production of porphyrins.

An acute attack may present with a variety of symptoms (Box 4.17). Abdominal pain is often severe and accompanied by vomiting so may present surgically as an acute abdomen, although signs of peritonitis will be absent. Autonomic instability with tachycardia and hypertension occur, and in the long term this may cause renal dysfunction. Neurological presentations include peripheral nerve palsies, cranial nerve palsies which may lead to aspiration pneumonitis, seizures, and neuromuscular weakness, which may lead to respiratory failure and necessitate ventilation. Psychiatric disturbance is also common. An attack may last 1–2 weeks. Diagnosis is confirmed by detecting high levels of urinary ALA and porphobilinogen. These urinary porphyrins may be visible as a red-brown discolouration when urine is left to stand.

Box 4.17 Symptom presentation during acute porphyria	
• Abdominal pain	95%
• Tachycardia	80%
• Peripheral neuropathy	60%
• Altered mental status	55%
• Hypertension	40%
• Postural hypotension	21%
• Bulbar involvement	30%
• Seizures	10%

Reproduced from Jensen et al., 'Anaesthetic considerations in porphyrias', *Anaesthesia and Analgesia*, 80, 3, pp. 591–599, copyright 1995 International Anaesthesia Research Society and Wolters Kluwer, with permission.

Management of acute porphyria

Supportive measures
Management of acute porphyria is supportive. Hydration and carbohydrate intake must be well maintained. Electrolyte imbalances, commonly hyponatraemia, hypokalaemia, and hypomagnesaemia, should be corrected. Autonomic overactivity is managed with β- or α-blockade. Pain is controlled with opiates. Bulbar symptoms may herald the onset of respiratory failure and neuromuscular weakness should be monitored with forced vital capacity bedside measurement to allow early detection of ventilatory failure.

Specific treatment
In a severe attack, a haematin infusion may be required to halt the haem biosynthetic pathway temporarily and prevent further build-up of porphyrins via negative feedback on ALA synthetase. Haematin may cause dramatic clinical improvement, reducing intensity and duration of symptoms, but is associated with serious side effects, including renal failure and dose-related coagulopathy. Haem arginate is used in the UK. Cimetidine may also be used to inhibit haem oxidase activity, reducing haem consumption and providing some negative feedback on ALA synthetase activity.

Mortality of an acute attack is 10% with most deaths occurring due to concurrent infection, respiratory failure, or cardiac dysrhythmia.

Anaesthetic pre-assessment

A patient with quiescent porphyria may be asymptomatic. If anaesthesia is required during an acute attack, a careful assessment of mental status, cardiovascular stability, bulbar symptoms and ventilatory function is required. If regional anaesthesia is considered, neurological examination should be performed and peripheral neuropathy recorded.

If a patient has a family history of porphyria, screening is possible. As urinary porphyrin levels may be normal in quiescent disease, this may require referral to a specialist porphyria centre for genetic testing. In urgent cases, such patients should be managed as if they have porphyria.

Anaesthesia in acute porphyria

Premedication and preparation
Fasting should be minimized and dextrose infusion (or dextrose-saline) commenced to maintain carbohydrate load. Anxiolytic premedication is advisable since stress may precipitate an acute attack.

Induction
Propofol is the safest induction agent and can be combined with opiates. If neuromuscular blockade is required, suxamethonium and rocuronium are non-porphyrinogenic. Other muscle relaxants are probably safe.

Maintenance
Volatile maintenance with isoflurane, sevoflurane and desflurane has been reported without complication. Nitrous oxide is also safe. Propofol infusions should be avoided.

Analgesia
Opiates are safe to use, although partial agonists should be avoided and there is little evidence currently to support the use of tramadol. Diclofenac and ketorolac should be avoided.

Regional anaesthesia
Bupivacaine appears to be the local anaesthetic of choice. Some reports of lidocaine-related problems exist and ester drugs should be avoided.

In general, using multiple potential inducers should be avoided. There seems to be a trend for more porphyrinogenic activity with repeat or prolonged exposure to drugs (e.g. propofol induction vs propofol maintenance). Short-acting drugs are potentially safer for this reason. In an acute attack, the drugs that are known to be safest should be used. See Table 4.5.

There are many reports of patients with acute porphyria having major surgery without complication under general anaesthesia. The biggest risk is for patients with undiagnosed disease.

Post anaesthesia, if 'unsafe' drugs have inadvertently been given, it is good practice to monitor urinary porphyrins for 5 days.

Further reading

Jensen NF, Fiddler DS, & Striepe V (1995). Anesthetic considerations in porphyrias. *Anesth Analg*, 80:591–9.

The Drug Database for Acute Porphyria website: <http://www.drugs-porphyria.org>.

UK National Centre for Porphyria: <http://www.cardiff-porphyria.org>.

Table 4.5 Drugs used during anaesthesia and porphyria		
	Safe	Unsafe
Premedication		Diazepam Metoclopramide
Induction agents	Propofol	Thiopentone Etomidate Ketamine
Maintenance	Most volatiles, nitrous oxide	Propofol infusion Halothane
Analgesia	Paracetamol Aspirin Fentanyl, alfentanil Morphine, pethidine Codeine	Diclofenac Ketorolac Oxycodone
Local anaesthetics	Bupivacaine Prilocaine	Lidocaine Cocaine
CVS stabilisers	α-agonists β-agonists β-blockers Atropine, glycopyrrolate	Amiodarone Hydralazine Clonidine Phenoxybenzamine Calcium channel blockers
Reversal	Neostigmine Naloxone	
Antibiotics		Metronidazole, macrolides, trimethoprim
Uterotonics	Oxytocin	Ergometrine

Chapter 5

Endocrinology, metabolism, and body temperature

119

5.1 Anaesthesia and the adrenal cortex

Adrenal cortex

The adrenal cortex secretes steroid hormones of three main types;

- Mineralocorticoids from the outer *zona glomerulosa*
- Glucocorticoids from the middle *zona fasciculata*
- Androgens from the inner *zona reticularis*.

All the steroid hormones are synthesized from cholesterol, which is converted to pregnenolone in the presence of adrenocorticotrophic hormone (ACTH; see Fig. 5.1). Steroid hormones are bound to plasma proteins in the circulation, mainly transcortin and albumin.

Mineralocorticoids

Aldosterone is responsible for 95% of the mineralocorticoid action. Its synthesis and release are responsive to decreased extracellular fluid volume and hyperkalaemia as well as the renin–angiotensin pathway.

Renin is produced from the juxtaglomerular apparatus of the kidney in response to hypotension, reduced plasma volume, hyponatraemia, and the influence of prostaglandins. Renin converts angiotensinogen to angiotensin I. Angiotensin II is then produced by the action of angiotensin-converting enzyme in the lungs. Negative feedback is triggered by hypokalaemia and reduced ACTH.

Aldosterone promotes sodium reabsorption from the renal distal tubule at the expense of potassium and hydrogen ion loss.

Glucocorticoids

Cortisol is responsible for 95% of total glucocorticoid activity but corticosterone is also produced. Cortisol secretion follows a normal circadian rhythm with peaks in the early morning. Increased secretion is triggered by stress and ACTH from the pituitary. Cortisol has three main effects:

- *Catabolic:* protein catabolism, gluconeogenesis, glycogen storage and mobilization of fat stores.
- *Cardiovascular:* glucocorticoids allow responsiveness to catecholamines during stress.
- *Anti-inflammatory*.

Addison's disease

Addison's disease is hypoadrenalism with deficiency of mineralocorticoid and glucocorticoid hormones (Table 5.1). Secondary hypoadrenalism due to exogenous steroid medication and pituitary disease is more common, but primary disease may be due to autoimmune disease, infection (classically tuberculosis), surgery, and haemorrhage which can be associated with meningococcal sepsis.

Mineralocorticoid deficiency causes dehydration due to loss of salt and water, postural hypotension, hyperkalaemia, and metabolic acidosis. Glucocorticoid deficiency causes weight loss, muscle weakness, hypoglycaemia, nausea, and a reduced response to stress.

Addison's disease is treated with steroid replacement using hydrocortisone and fludrocortisone (50–100mcg/day). Addisonian crisis may occur in response to physiological stress and causes depressed conscious level, resistant hypotension, hypoglycaemia, and abdominal pain. Patients require high-dependency care with immediate hydrocortisone replacement (200mg initially followed by 100mg four times daily), aggressive fluid replacement and correction of glucose.

Anaesthesia and Addison's disease

Patients cannot mount a stress response to surgery. Prior to anaesthesia, hyperkalaemia and hypoglycaemia should be corrected and these should be monitored at least 4-hourly perioperatively. Hydrocortisone 50mg is given at induction to mimic the normal steroid response to stress. For major surgery 200mg is given every 24h (intermediate surgery 100mg daily) and this is continued until normal steroid regimens can be reinstituted.

Conn's syndrome

Conn's syndrome is primary hyperaldosteronism, which may occur in the presence of an adrenal adenoma, bilateral adrenal hyperplasia, or carcinoma. Secondary hyperaldosteronism commonly accompanies chronic oedematous states in which there is excess renin production, e.g. cardiac failure, cirrhosis. High levels of aldosterone cause hypertension, which is often refractory to

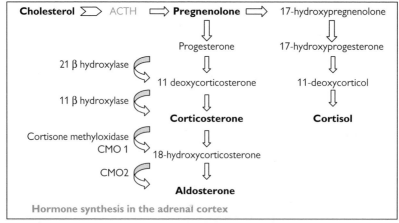

Fig. 5.1 Hormone synthesis in the adrenal cortex.

Table 5.1 Disorders of the adrenal cortex			
Syndrome	Symptoms	Signs	Anaesthesia management
Addisons disease	Fatigue, dizziness	Postural hypotension Correct potassium	
	Weight loss	Hyperkalaemia	Rehydrate
	Weakness	Metabolic acidosis	Steroid cover
	Nausea	Hypoglycaemia	
Conn's syndrome	Few	Hypertension	Control hypertension
		Hypokalaemia	Spironolactone
		Metabolic alkalosis	Correct potassium
Cushing's syndrome	Weight gain	Glucose intolerance	Metyrapone
	Muscle wasting	Hypertension	Control hypertension
	Striae	Hypokalaemia	Diabetic control
	Reflux	Sleep apnoea	

treatment, and also sodium and water retention, hypokalaemia, and metabolic alkalosis (Table 5.1). Spironolactone, an aldosterone antagonist, is an effective treatment. Adenomas are amenable to surgical removal.

Anaesthesia and Conn's syndrome

Prior to anaesthesia, blood pressure should be adequately controlled using spironolactone and antihypertensives. Hypokalaemia should be corrected.

Cushing's syndrome

Cushing's syndrome is due to excess glucocorticoid secretion by the adrenal cortex or exogenous steroids (Table 5.1). Cushing's disease is more common and is secondary to excess ACTH secretion from a pituitary adenoma. Glucocorticoid excess causes centripetal obesity with a buffalo hump and moon face, muscle wasting, and striae. Abnormal glucose tolerance and diabetes are common. Longstanding hypertension may cause end-organ damage. Hypokalaemia may occur due to the weak mineralocorticoid effect of cortisol.

Metyrapone may be used to inhibit cortisol synthesis but treatment usually involves identification and removal of the cause with pituitary or adrenal surgery.

Anaesthesia and Cushing's syndrome

Preoperatively, hypertension should be treated, with full assessment of any end-organ damage such as left ventricular hypertrophy, renal dysfunction, and ischaemic heart disease. Obese patients may need screening for obstructive sleep apnoea (see section 11.2), and oesophageal reflux is common so proton pump inhibitors may be commenced. Diabetic control perioperatively may require a sliding scale insulin infusion. Fragile skin requires extra care with positioning, blood pressure measurement, and tourniquets.

Further reading

Davies M & Hardman J (2005). Anaesthesia and adrenocortical disease. CEACCP, 5:122–6.

5.2 Diabetes mellitus

Incidence/pathogenesis

Diabetes mellitus is a multisystem disorder resulting from an absolute or relative lack of insulin, which causes disordered glucose metabolism and hyperglycaemia due to a lack of inhibition of lipolysis, proteolysis, glycogenolysis, gluconeogenesis, and ketogenesis. About 7% of the UK population has diabetes, which is categorized as type 1 or 2:

In *type 1 diabetes*, there is beta cell destruction in the pancreatic islet, causing failure of insulin secretion. These patients are reliant on insulin therapy. They typically present early in life, and are at risk of ketoacidosis.

Type 2 diabetes is due to insulin hyposecretion and resistance. This commonly presents later in life and is associated with obesity, race, and drug therapy such as corticosteroids and thiazides. Type 2 diabetes can be managed with diet, medication, and/or insulin. These patients are prone to a hyperosmotic non-ketotic state.

The WHO classification for the diagnosis of diabetes requires a random plasma glucose >11.1mmol/L or a fasting plasma glucose >7.8mmol/L.

The main concerns for the anaesthetist are the management of the long-term complications of diabetes and the perioperative control of blood glucose. Diabetic patients have increased perioperative mortality.

Complications of diabetes

Diabetes is associated with *microvascular* complications including nephropathy, retinopathy, and neuropathy, and also *macrovascular* disease from atherosclerosis. Improved glycaemic control reduces microvascular and neuropathic complications but reduction of macrovascular complications necessitates the addition of tight blood pressure control.

CVS

Diabetes may be associated with:
- Hypertension
- Ischaemic heart disease (3× incidence)
- Stroke and peripheral vascular disease
- Cardiomyopathy
- Postural hypotension and arrhythmias due to autonomic dysfunction.

Silent myocardial ischaemia is a risk in diabetes and if other risk factors are also present, screening may be advisable before major surgery.

Autonomic neuropathy may manifest as labile blood pressure, arrhythmias, and even sudden cardiac death (other features include gastroparesis and a tendency to hypothermia). It may occur in up to 40% of type 1 and 20% of type 2 diabetics and is suggested by an increase of <10bpm heart rate on deep inspiration and by the presence of postural hypotension.

Renal disease

Renal manifestations of diabetes include:
- Microalbuminuria
- Diabetic glomerulosclerosis
- End-stage renal failure.

ACEIs slow the progression of diabetic nephropathy.

Neuropathy

Features include peripheral sensory neuropathy, proximal motor myopathy, mononeuropathy, and nerve compression syndromes.

Airway

A 'stiff joint syndrome' occurs in diabetes, resulting from glycosylation of collagen, and this may affect the temporo-mandibular and atlanto-occipital joints causing an increased incidence of difficult intubation amongst patients with longstanding diabetes. Affected patients typically are unable to oppose their fingers when performing the prayer sign (hands together and wrists extended to 90°).

Decreased immunity and wound healing

Diabetic patients are at increased risk of postoperative wound infection, other hospital-acquired infections, and wound and anastomotic breakdown, particularly if diabetic control is poor.

Pre-assessment

The pre-assessment should focus on diabetic control, current management, frequency of acute complications, and on the presence of diabetic complications.

An indication of diabetic control may be derived from patients' home testing results, and from a random blood glucose, but a glycosylated haemoglobin level (HbA1c) reflects control over the preceding 6–8 weeks. HbA1c <7% indicates good control, >8.5% indicates poor control, and >12% suggests the patient will be likely to have electrolyte derangement and dehydration. If HbA1c is >8.5% it is preferable to refer for optimization of diabetic control prior to elective surgery. The frequency of hypoglycaemic episodes may influence the perioperative plan.

Assessment of cardiovascular risk and functional exercise tolerance is important as silent myocardial ischaemia may occur. As well as a resting ECG, stress testing may be appropriate. Urine testing, measurement of renal function, and postural blood pressure should be performed. Any neurological deficit should be documented.

Some diabetic patients are suitable for day surgery procedures (see section 12.3) or admission on the day of major surgery. However, prior to major surgery, most will require admission the preceding evening for blood glucose management. Type 1 diabetics may still require basal insulin, but otherwise oral hypoglycaemics and insulin may be omitted during preoperative starvation. See Box 5.1 and Table 5.2. The patient should be first on the list to minimize starving times.

Perioperative aims

- Avoid hypoglycaemia—causes irreversible cerebral damage.
- Avoid severe hyperglycaemia >14mmol/L—dehydration.
- Maintain glucose 6–10mmol/L—better glycaemic control improves perioperative morbidity and mortality.
- Prevent ketoacidosis—replace insulin.
- Prevent hypokalaemia.

The plan for perioperative blood glucose control depends on the nature of surgery, particularly the period until restoration of oral intake, whether the patient has type 1 or 2 diabetes and the quality of the blood glucose control. Minor surgery implies a short starvation period with no more than one missed meal.

Table 5.2 Oral hypoglycaemic agents and preoperative management

Drug	Action	Preop action
Sulphonylureas e.g. gliclazide	Reduce insulin resistance	Omit when NBM
	Increase beta cell sensitivity	(Glibenclamide stop 24h pre-op)
Biguanides e.g. metformin	Increase glucose utilization	Continue unless contrast used
	Decrease hepatic production	
Thiazolidinediones e.g. pioglitazone	Enhance peripheral insulin action	Continue
	Inhibit hepatic gluconeogenesis	
	? Increase MI	
Acarbose	Reduces glucose absorption	Omit when NBM
Meglitinides e.g. repaglinide	Secretagogues, stimulate insulin secretion	Omit when NBM
GLP-1 analogues e.g. exenatide	Incretin mimetic-s- Stimulate insulin production	Omit day of surgery
	Reduce glucagon secretion	
DPP IV inhibitors e.g. sitagliptin	Prevents breakdown of endogenous incretins	Omit day of surgery

The surgical stress response stimulates gluconeogenesis and reduces peripheral glucose uptake due to catecholamine, cortisol, growth hormone, and glucagon release. This may increase insulin requirements in type 1 diabetics, and necessitate insulin treatment in type 2 diabetics. The increase in insulin requirements can be unpredictable and tight metabolic control is important in both types of diabetes perioperatively.

Various insulin regimens can be used perioperatively. Although GKI (glucose, potassium, insulin) regimens are safe, variable rate IV insulin infusions (VRII) are preferred by most staff and have been shown to provide a marginal improvement in glycaemic control. Safe delivery of a VRII relies on both infusions administered via one venous access point with antireflux and antisyphon valve systems to prevent administration of one infusion alone.

Box 5.1 Insulin regimens and preoperative management

- Once daily long acting:
  - Give as normal. Check blood glucose OR reduce by 1/3.
- Twice daily mixed:
  - Give half usual dose.
- Twice daily separate long and short injection:
  - Give half total dose as long-acting insulin.
- Multiple injections:
  - Give basal long acting, omit short-acting doses.

Other anaesthetic considerations

Airway
Premedication with antacids/prokinetics, use of rapid sequence induction and avoidance of opiates in gastroparesis.

CVS
Management of hypotension and abnormal autonomic responses to general anaesthesia or neuraxial blockade.

Renal
Avoidance of nephrotoxic drugs (and avoidance of anticholinergic drugs in patients with autonomic bladder dysfunction).

Regional anaesthesia
May enable earlier postoperative oral intake but difficulty in assessing block if neuropathy present.

Further reading

McAnulty GR, Robertshaw HJ, & Hall GM (2000). Anaesthetic management of patients with diabetes. *Br J Anaesth*, 85:80–90.

NHS Diabetes (2011). *Management of Adults with Diabetes Undergoing Surgery*. London: NHS Diabetes.

Nicholson G & Hall GM (2011). Diabetes mellitus: new drugs for a new epidemic. *Br J Anaesth*, 107:65–73.

Robertshaw HJ & Hall GM (2006). Diabetes mellitus; anaesthetic management. *Anaesthesia*, 61:1187–90.

5.3 Pituitary disease and anaesthesia

The pituitary

The pituitary gland lies in the pituitary fossa of the sphenoid, just above the sphenoid sinus and below the hypothalamus and optic chiasma. It is connected to the hypothalamus via the pituitary stalk, which carries the hypophyseal portal system and allows transport of hypothalamic hormones to the pituitary. The pituitary has two distinct lobes: anterior and posterior. The posterior pituitary secretes oxytocin and vasopressin (antidiuretic hormone) and is rarely involved in disease. The hormones secreted by the anterior pituitary are detailed in Table 5.3.

Pituitary disease may present in three ways:

- Excess hormone secretion
- Mass effect (from macroadenoma)
- Underactivity (hypopituitarism).

Table 5.3 Anterior pituitary hormones			
Hormone	Positive feedback	Negative feedback	Effects
Growth hormone (GH)	GH releasing hormone (GHRH)	Somatostatin	Tissue growth
Thyroid stimulating hormone (TSH)	Thyrotrophin releasing hormone (TRH)	Thyroxine	Thyroid hormone release
Adrenocorticotrophic hormone (ACTH)	Corticotrophin releasing factor (CRF)	Cortisol	Adrenal cortisol release
Luteinizing hormone and follicle stimulating hormone (LF and FSH)	Gonadotrophin releasing hormone (GnRH)		Oestrogen release Testosterone release
Prolactin (PRL)		Dopamine	Lactation

Panhypopituitarism

Panhypopituitarism is reduced function of the anterior pituitary (see Box 5.2).

Box 5.2 Causes of panhypopituitarism
Primary
• Tumour
• Iatrogenic (post surgery or radiotherapy)
• Sarcoidosis/granulomatous disease
• Autoimmune destruction
• Ischaemic necrosis (e.g. Sheehan's syndrome post-partum).
Secondary
• Hypothalamic disease (tumour, inflammation, or head injury).

Patients present with symptoms of Addison's disease and hypothyroidism. Management is with hormone replacement, but steroid replacement may only require hydrocortisone.

These patients will always require perioperative steroid supplementation.

Pituitary adenoma

Pituitary adenomas account for 10% of intracranial tumours and 75% are secretory. Macroadenomas may cause mass effects leading to compression of the optic chiasma with bitemporal hemianopia, 3rd cranial nerve palsy, and hydrocephalus. They may also cause deficiency of the other pituitary hormones. Prolactinomas are the most common pituitary adenoma, typically causing symptoms of galactorrhoea, amenorrhoea, or impotence. Growth hormone-secreting tumours causing acromegaly and ACTH secreting tumours causing Cushing's disease also occur, and are associated with changes that are highly relevant to anaesthesia. Anaesthesia and Cushing's disease is discussed in section 5.1.

For details of the management of patients undergoing pituitary surgery, see section 22.6.

Acromegaly and anaesthesia

Airway changes

- Enlargement of the jaw
- Macroglossia
- Thickened pharyngeal and laryngeal soft tissues and vocal cords
- Decreased laryngeal aperture
- Commonly obstructive sleep apnoea
- Commonly thyroid enlargement
- Patients may have reduced central respiratory drive.

All of these factors increase the likelihood of a difficult airway in the acromegalic patient. Some authors advocate preoperative indirect laryngoscopy as part of the pre-assessment. Facemask ventilation may require a larger mask and use of oropharyngeal airways. Intubation may commonly require a long laryngoscopy blade and possibly a video-laryngoscope or fibreoptic technique.

Associated morbidity in acromegaly

Recognized comorbidities in acromegaly include:

- Hypertension (30% of patients)
- Left ventricular hypertrophy and interstitial myocardial fibrosis causing myocardial failure
- Diabetes (25% of patients)
- Increased incidence of malignancy, e.g. colorectal cancer
- Atherosclerotic disease.

Perioperative steroid replacement

Any patient who receives ≥10mg prednisolone daily, or who has received this dose in the last 3 months, requires perioperative steroid supplementation. These patients have suppression of the hypothalamic-pituitary-adrenal (HPA) axis.

Additionally, in any patient who is maintained on hydrocortisone, one should suspect adrenal or pituitary disease with failure of the HPA axis.

A suitable perioperative replacement strategy is set out in Table 5.4.

Table 5.4 Perioperative steroid replacement		
	HPA axis suppression	HPA axis failure
Minor surgery	Continue regular steroid + 25mg hydrocortisone on induction	Double normal hydro-cortisone dose
Intermediate surgery	Continue regular steroid + 50mg hydrocortisone on induction; 60mg hydrocortisone/24h until normal dose resumed	50mg hydrocortisone on induction, then 200mg/24h, halving daily until normal dose reached
Major surgery	50mg hydrocortisone on induction then 100–150mg/24h	50mg hydrocortisone on induction then 200mg/24h for 48–72h

Equivalent steroid doses

The following have equivalent glucocorticoid activity:
- Prednisolone 5mg
- Hydrocortisone 20mg
- Methylprednisolone 4mg
- Dexamethasone 0.75mg

Hydrocortisone also has weak mineralocorticoid activity.

Further reading

Menon R, Murphy PG, & Lindley AM (2011). Anaesthesia and pituitary disease. *CEACCP*, 11(4):133–7. doi:10.1093/bjaceaccp/mkr014.

Smith M & Hirsch NP (2000). Pituitary disease and anaesthesia. *Br J Anaesth*, 85(1):3–14.

5.4 Thyroid disease

Thyroid disease

Thyroid disease is common and presents as a multisystem disorder with important implications for anaesthesia. Patients with severe disorders may also present as emergencies to critical care.

Box 5.3 briefly describes the mechanism for synthesis of the thyroid hormones and their action.

Box 5.3 Synthesis and action of thyroid hormones

- The thyroid hormones are *thyroxine* (T_4) and *tri-iodothyronone* (T_3).
- Iodide ions are oxidized to iodine within the colloid of thyroid follicles.
- Tyrosine residues on thyroglobulin are iodinated to form mono and di-iodotyrosine.
- Mono and di-iodotyrosine combine to form T_3 or T_4, which are stored in combination with thyroglobulin.
- Synthesis and secretion is triggered by TSH from the pituitary.
- A negative feedback on the pituitary is exerted by the hypothalamus via TRH.
- >90% of thyroid hormone exists as T_4, which is protein bound to thyroid-binding globulin. T_3 is more potent, less protein bound and can be made in peripheral tissue from de-iodination of T_4.
- Thyroid hormones increase basal metabolic rate, increase carbohydrate and fat metabolism, and increase heart rate, contractility, and minute ventilation.

Hyperthyroidism

Hyperthyroidism is due to Graves' disease in 60–90% cases. Other causes include toxic multinodular goitre, functional thyroid adenoma, pituitary TSH secreting adenoma, and rare causes such as molar pregnancy. Hyperthyroid patients present with weight loss, heat intolerance, tremulousness, anxiety, tachycardia, and dysrhythmia. The condition may precipitate atrial fibrillation, cardiac failure, or ischaemic heart disease.

Investigation reveals raised thyroid hormones and reduced TSH. Treatment options include carbimazole or propylthiouracil, which reduce synthesis by inhibiting iodination of tyrosine, and iodine which inhibits secretion of thyroid hormones. β-blockers are often added to reduce peripheral conversion of T_4 to T_3 and block the peripheral effects of thyroid hormones. Radioactive iodine and surgery are used to destroy or remove functional tissue.

Preoperative

Preoperatively, thyroid function should be stabilized. This may require up to 8 weeks of treatment with carbimazole or propylthiouracil as well as the addition of Lugol's iodine 7–10 days prior to surgery to reduce the risk of thyroid storm and to reduce the vascularity of the thyroid gland. Resting heart rate should be below 85bpm and any dysrhythmia, ischaemia or heart failure optimized. Anaesthetic morbidity relates to excess cardiac risk and a greater risk of thyroid storm in non-euthyroid patients.

Perioperative

A major perioperative concern in hyperthyroidism is avoidance of sympathetic stimulation, which may precipitate dysrhythmia. This includes suppression of the response to laryngoscopy, using direct vasopressors instead of indirect sympathomimetic drugs and taking care with anticholinergic medication. Eye protection is very important in patients with Graves' disease who may have exophthalmos.

Thyroid storm

Thyroid storm is rare but carries a mortality of 20%. It results from excessive secretion of thyroid hormones, possibly from manipulation of thyroid tissue. It generally presents 6–24h post-op but perioperatively may present with a malignant hyperthermia-like picture (except muscle rigidity is not a feature).

Thyroid storm presents with CNS disturbance, agitation, delirium or seizures, tachycardia, hyperpyrexia and hypertension. Management requires the use of IV β-blockade, hydrocortisone (as there is an inappropriate ACTH response), antithyroid medication and supportive measures such as cooling, rehydration, and sedation.

Hypothyroidism

Hypothyroidism is primary in 95% of cases due to autoimmune disease, iatrogenic causes (postsurgery/radioactive iodine), or iodine deficiency. Secondary causes are due to pituitary disease. Hypothyroidism may be difficult to diagnose with weight gain, cold intolerance, fatigue, and lethargy as the main symptoms. Cardiovascular effects include bradycardia and reduced cardiac output. Ventilation becomes depressed. Periorbital and pretibial swelling develop. Pericardial effusions may result from hyponatraemia and fluid retention. Hypoglycaemia and anaemia are common.

Diagnosis is confirmed by low levels of thyroid hormones and raised TSH. Treatment is with thyroid hormone replacement. T_4 has a 7-day half-life so urgent replacement is instituted with T_3 (half-life 1.5 days), which requires cardiovascular monitoring as it may precipitate myocardial ischaemia.

Preoperative

Elective surgery should be avoided in severe hypothyroidism (T_4 <1mcg/dL), as there is potential for severe cardiovascular instability and myxoedema coma. Myxoedema coma is a rare condition with a high mortality, which often presents in elderly patients following a trigger such as infection or surgical stress. Conscious level is depressed and hypothermia occurs. Cardiovascular effects such as bradycardia, hypotension, and heart failure may necessitate inotropic support or even cardiac pacing. Hypoventilation may require ventilatory support. Management is largely supportive along with administration of T_3. Steroid cover is also required, since there is a poor ACTH response to stress.

Preoperatively, airway assessment is important as hypothyroid patients often have macroglossia, pharyngeal, and laryngeal oedema as well as obesity.

Perioperative

Special perioperative considerations include management of hypotension due to reduced cardiac output and intravascular volume, maintenance of normothermia, avoidance of hypoglycaemia, and avoidance of long-acting sedatives or narcotics, which may suppress conscious levels and ventilation.

Anaesthesia for thyroid surgery

Airway

There is a 6% risk of difficult intubation in patients with a goitre as compression or deviation of the trachea may occur. Symptoms of positional dyspnoea or dysphagia may increase suspicion but

Box 5.4 Complications of thyroid surgery

Difficult airway

- Caused by deviation and compression of trachea by goitre and/or mediastinal compression with a retrosternal goitre.
- Approaches to management include:
  - Induction in sitting position
  - Awake fibreoptic intubation
  - Tracheostomy under LA
  - Rigid bronchoscopy if distal tracheal compression.
  - Inhalational induction

Wound haematoma

- 0.3% incidence following thyroid surgery
- Causes direct airway compression
- Pharyngeal oedema may result from poor venous drainage
- Management:
  - Open skin clips urgently
  - Early re-intubation
  - Re-explore surgical field.

Recurrent laryngeal nerve damage

- Unilateral 4% (temporary), <1% permanent
- Unilateral palsy causes hoarse voice
- Bilateral palsy causes stridor
- NB: commonest cause post-op is laryngeal *oedema*
- Reducing the risk:
  - Using EMG tube intraoperatively
  - Check vocal cord function prior to wakening.

Tracheomalacia

- Following longstanding goitre
- Requires re-intubation.

Hypocalcaemia

- Transient hypocalcaemia occurs in up to 20% of cases
- Usually seen ±30h postoperatively
- Treatment:
  - Oral supplements if $Ca^{2+} \geq 2mmol/L$
  - IV 10% calcium gluconate if Ca^{2+} lower than 2mmol/L.

some patients may be asymptomatic. Preoperative assessment should include indirect laryngoscopy, which also assesses the vocal cord function, and CXR, starting with an AP view. Lateral thoracic inlet views may be required in suspicious cases and CT may be necessary to further delineate the extent of the goitre if CXR shows >50% narrowing, and particularly if retrosternal. Awake fibreoptic intubation or inhalational induction may be required.

Reinforced endotracheal tubes are used to prevent kinking and a smaller size may be required if significant compression is present. If a retrosternal goitre is present, the length of the tube should be predetermined from the CT scan to prevent tracheal compression worsening during surgery.

Specialized endotracheal tubes with EMG electrodes may be used. When correctly positioned at the level of the cords, they may help identification of the recurrent laryngeal nerves during surgery. A short-acting muscle relaxant is used for induction in these cases.

Positioning the patient and improving the surgical field

The neck is extended by using a sand bag between the patient's shoulder blades with the head supported in a head ring. The table should be tilted 25° head-up to assist venous drainage.

Hypotensive anaesthesia will reduce surgical blood loss and improve the field. Prior to wound closure it is important to increase the blood pressure and perform a Valsalva manoeuvre to assess haemostasis.

Extubation

Vocal cord assessment may be required prior to wakening, either with direct or fibreoptic laryngoscopy. In cases of long-standing goitre, tracheomalacia may occur and it is good practice to ensure that a cuff leak is present prior to extubation. Coughing should be avoided during extubation. Deep extubation, topical anaesthesia to the vocal cords or use of short-acting opiates may facilitate this. The patient should be extubated fully awake if there are any airway concerns as the risk of respiratory complications is higher at extubation than induction with desaturation, laryngospasm, and obstruction (Box 5.4). The patient should be recovered sitting upright to reduce oedema.

Further reading

Farling P (2000). Thyroid disease. *Br J Anaesth*. 85(1):15-28.

Malhotra S & Sodhi V (2007). Anaesthesia for thyroid and parathyroid surgery. *CEACCP*, 7(2):55–8. doi:10.1093/bjaceaccp/mkm006.

5.5 Phaeochromocytoma

The adrenal medulla synthesizes and secretes catecholamines (Fig. 5.2). The relative proportions of adrenaline and noradrenaline are 70% and 30% respectively. The catecholamines are formed from tyrosine in the chromaffin cells and stored until secretion is triggered by preganglionic sympathetic fibres in response to stress, exercise or emotion.

Phaeochromocytoma

Phaeochromocytomas are functionally active chromaffin cell tumours which secrete noradrenaline, adrenaline, or dopamine constantly or intermittently. 10% are familial, 10% bilateral, 10% malignant, and 10% extra-adrenal. There is an association with multiple endocrine neoplasia syndrome, von Hippel–Lindau syndrome, and neurofibromatosis.

Patients present with sustained hypertension, weight loss and dyspnoea, or paroxysmal hypertension with sweating, tremor, palpitations, and headache. Chronic vasoconstriction causes relative hypovolaemia. Paroxysms may be triggered by exercise, sneezing, anaesthesia, histamine-releasing drugs, metoclopramide, nicotine, and labour. Hypertensive crises may precipitate myocardial ischaemia, pulmonary oedema, cardiomyopathy, cerebrovascular accidents, and acute bleeding from the tumour. The diagnosis requires the presence of urinary metanephrine or vanillyl mandelic acid (VMA) and measurement of plasma catecholamines. Tumours may be identified on MRI scan or using MIBG scintigraphy.

Medical management

Treatment is with α-adrenergic antagonists to reverse vasoconstriction and hypertension. This restores myocardial function and normovolaemia. Phenoxybenzamine is often used: a non-selective, irreversible α antagonist started at a dose of 10mg twice daily and increased up to 200mg until blood pressure is controlled. β-adrenergic blockade is added to avoid the tachyarrhythmia that may occur through α-2 receptor antagonism. β-blockade is only initiated following α blockade due to the concern of hypertensive crisis with the unopposed vasoconstriction that may occur. Treatment should be initiated at least 2 weeks prior to surgery. Phenoxybenzamine is then stopped 24–48h preoperatively as it has a half-life of 24h.

Increasingly, selective α-1 antagonists, e.g. doxasosin or prazosin, are used, which have no risk of tachyarrhythmia and are shorter acting. β-blockade may then be unnecessary unless the tumour secretes adrenaline. This regimen may offer less cardiovascular stability perioperatively.

Preoperative assessment

Phaeochromocytomas should be operated on in specialist centres. Preoperative assessment should focus on cardiovascular evaluation and end-organ effects of hypertension. Up to 50% of patients may have hypertensive cardiomyopathy, and echocardiography should be performed if this is suspected clinically. The efficacy of medical management needs to be carefully assessed. Blood pressure control should be assessed with a 24h ambulatory recording, aiming for readings below 160/90 and heart rate below 100bpm. Postural hypotension should be measured and arrhythmias may require a 24h ECG recording. Management targets include:

- Postural hypotension >80/45
- No evidence of ECG ST segment or T-wave changes for 7 days
- Less than one ectopic every 5min
- Control of nasal congestion is a useful clinical target.

Perioperative management

The main aim perioperatively is to prevent haemodynamic compromise and arrhythmia due to catecholamine surges. Induction of anaesthesia and tracheal intubation are both times of high risk, as are laparoscopic insufflation of pneumoperitoneum, manipulation of the tumour, and ligation of the tumour's venous drainage. Preoperative medical management limits the effects of the catecholamine surges but rapid, short-acting vasodilators should be available. Phentolamine 1–5mg, labetalol 5–10mg, sodium nitroprusside, and GTN may all be used. Magnesium at doses of 2–4g/h is increasingly used, as magnesium blocks catecholamine release, blocks adrenergic receptors and provides direct vasodilatation as well as preventing arrhythmias. Tachyarrhythmias may be managed with esmolol, lidocaine, or amiodarone (see Box 5.5).

Box 5.5 Aspects of perioperative management in phaeochromocytoma

Management of catecholamine surges
- Effective preoperative medical management
- Attenuate response to laryngoscopy
- Phentolamine 1–5mg
- Labetalol 5–10mg
- Sodium nitroprusside (0.5–6mcg/kg/min)
- GTN (10–400mcg/min)
- Magnesium 2–4g/h.

Management of tachyarrhythmia
- Esmolol
- Lidocaine (1mg/kg)
- Amiodarone 300mg.

Management of hypotension
- Therapy guided by CVP, CO monitoring, ECHO
- Vasopressors and inotropes
- Consider angiotensin and steroids.

Benzodiazepine premedication is useful. Invasive blood pressure monitoring should be instituted prior to induction. Histamine-releasing drugs should be avoided for induction and the hypertensive response to laryngoscopy should be prevented with short-acting opiates. Central venous access is necessary for assessing preload and administration of vasopressors if required. Transoesophageal CO monitoring can be used to optimize fluid therapy and pressor use. If severe cardiomyopathy is present, a pulmonary artery catheter may be considered. Epidural analgesia or remifentanil infusion may be used for analgesia.

Following removal of the tumour, *hypotension* may ensue, for a number of reasons:

- Hypovolaemia
- Persistent α adrenergic blockade
- Down-regulation of adrenoceptors
- Suppression of the contralateral adrenal medulla.

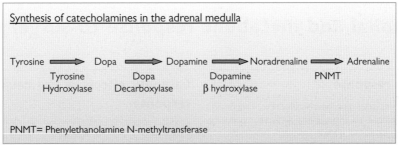

Fig. 5.2 Synthesis of catecholamines in the adrenal medulla. PNMT= phenylethanolamine N-methyltransferase.

Once central venous pressure or venous flow time is optimized, it may be necessary to commence vasopressors to correct SVR or CO. Resistance to vasopressors may be caused by the receptor down-regulation and angiotensin may be used in rare cases. Steroid replacement is required if both adrenals are removed and should also be considered for refractory hypotension.

Postoperative care

High dependency or intensive care is required postoperatively for ongoing management of cardiovascular disturbance and fluid balance. Patients are likely to develop hypoglycaemia as the α-2 mediated suppression of pancreatic β cell insulin release has been removed.

With appropriate management, the morbidity and mortality of phaeochromocytoma surgery is <2%.

Further reading

James MF and Cronje L (2004), Pheochromocytoma crisis: the use of magnesium sulfate. *Anesth Analg*, 99(3):680–6.

Pace N & Buttigieg M (2003), Phaeochromocytoma. *CEACCP*, 3(1):20. doi 10.1093/bjacepd/mkg005

5.6 Hormonal and metabolic response to surgery

Surgical stress response

The stress response includes the neuroendocrine, metabolic, and inflammatory response to tissue injury and trauma during surgery. The resulting catabolic effects maintain substrates for metabolism and retain sodium and water to maintain circulating volume. Although this response provides primitive survival advantages, it is often detrimental to recovery after modern surgery, and both anaesthetic and surgical techniques aim to attenuate the response.

The area of tissue trauma triggers both the neuroendocrine and inflammatory response. The hypothalamic–pituitary axis and sympathetic nervous system are activated by afferent nerves from the surgical site. Local tissue damage causes a cascade of cytokine-mediated inflammatory changes known as the acute phase response.

Neuroendocrine changes

Sympathetic nervous system activation

- Increased catecholamine release from adrenal medulla
- Increased noradrenaline release from presynaptic clefts.

This results in tachycardia and hypertension. There is reduced insulin secretion (via α-2 adrenergic inhibition of pancreatic β cell secretion).

Renin secretion is stimulated from the renal juxtaglomerular apparatus. This increases angiotensin II and aldosterone leading to sodium and water reabsorption from the distal convoluted tubule.

There is β-receptor mediated hepatic glycogenolysis and gluconeogenesis.

Endocrine changes

Increased ACTH and cortisol

Both an increase in hypothalamic corticotrophin-releasing hormone and antidiuretic hormone, which increases formation of an ACTH pre-cursor, cause elevated ACTH and cortisol within minutes of surgery commencing. The response peaks at 4–6h and peak levels exceed the maximum adrenocortical response as the usual negative feedback mechanism fails. The magnitude of the response is proportional to the surgical insult and it is not attenuated by administration of exogenous corticosteroids.

Increased growth hormone

Increased growth hormone secretion may have protective effects albeit with a diabetogenic action. Effects are mediated by insulin-like growth factors that reduce protein breakdown. There is also glycogenolysis, lipolysis, and reduced hepatic glucose uptake.

Increased antidiuretic hormone (vasopressin)

ADH is released from the posterior pituitary. It has both antidiuretic and vasopressor effects. ADH increases ACTH synthesis.

Reduced insulin secretion

Occurs due to increased catecholamines.

Increased glucagon

Glucagon causes increased hepatic glycogenolysis and gluconeogenesis, making a minor contribution to hyperglycaemia.

Reduced thyroid hormones

Basal metabolic rate and heat production reduces for a few days postoperatively.

Catabolic effects of the neuroendocrine response

Hyperglycaemia

- There is increased hepatic glycogenolysis and gluconeogenesis due to effects of cortisol, catecholamines, GH, and glucagon.
- Decreased insulin secretion and peripheral insulin resistance cause failure of normal glucose homeostasis.

Muscle breakdown and wasting

- Initial inhibition of protein anabolism proceeds to catabolism stimulated by cortisol and cytokines.
- May lose up to 0.5kg/day of lean muscle mass.

Lipolysis

- Increased by catecholamines, cortisol and GH.
- Produces glycerol for gluconeogenesis and ketone bodies as an alternative metabolic substrate.

Sodium and water retention

- ADH, the renin-angiotensin-aldosterone pathway and the mineralocorticoid effect of cortisol all cause reabsorption of sodium and water at the expense of potassium loss.
- There is reduced urine output and concentrated urine.

The acute phase response

Macrophages, endothelial cells, and fibroblasts at the site of tissue injury synthesize cytokines, glycoproteins including interleukins, interferons, and tumour necrosis factors. The cytokine response is proportional to the tissue damage and IL-6 has been shown to peak 12–24h post surgery. The acute phase response causes fever, systemic inflammatory response, increased acute phase proteins (e.g. CRP, fibrinogen), reduction in transport proteins (e.g. albumin, transferrin) and neutrophilia. The response promotes haemostasis, limits tissue damage, and promotes healing.

Modification of the stress response

Anaesthesia

- *Opioids:* these suppress hypothalamic and pituitary hormone secretion. Fentanyl 15mcg/kg will suppress the response to lower abdominal surgery. The high doses required to abolish the response to upper abdominal surgery (100mcg/kg fentanyl) delay recovery and spontaneous ventilation. Opioid suppression is overcome by complex major surgery.
- *Etomidate:* causes reversible inhibition of 11β hydroxylase to suppress cortisol and aldosterone synthesis for up to 8h. Concerns regarding the long-term effect on adrenocortical function limit its use.
- *Clonidine:* an α-2 agonist that attenuates the sympathetic response to surgery.
- *Regional anaesthesia:* Regional anaesthesia has been shown to abolish the neuroendocrine response to surgery if both sensory and autonomic block occurs. This cannot be completely achieved for upper abdominal and thoracic surgery. The acute phase response is unaffected.

Surgical technique

Minimally invasive surgical techniques have been shown to reduce the cytokine response but not the neuroendocrine changes that occur with surgery.

Preoperative carbohydrate loading

Preoperative oral carbohydrate solutions improve insulin resistance perioperatively, reduce the loss of lean body mass and shorten recovery time.

The principles of Enhanced Recovery are designed to reduce the stress response to surgery, see section 13.9.

Further reading

Burton D, Nicholson G, & Hall G (2004). Endocrine and metabolic response to surgery. *CEACCP*, 4(5):144–7.

Desborough JP (2000). The stress response to trauma and surgery. *Br J Anaesth*, 85:109–17

Nicholson G & Hall GM (2011). Effects of anaesthesia on the inflammatory response to injury. *Curr Opin AnaesthesioL*, 24(4):370–4. doi:10.1097/ACO.0b013e328348729e

5.7 Temperature

Thermoregulation

The normal core temperature of 37°C is maintained within a 0.5°C range by an efficient thermoregulatory system. The core compartment consists of the cranial, thoracic, abdominal, and pelvic cavities with a variable contribution from the limbs. The peripheral compartment acts as a heat sink and varies in volume depending on ambient conditions. The peripheral compartment consists of the limbs and skin, and temperature may vary from 28–36°C.

Temperature is sensed by the afferent A delta fibres which continuously sense cold. C fibres detect warmth during pyrexia only. There are more afferent signals from the core compartment than peripheral. The afferent fibres continue in the spinothalamic tract to the preoptic region of the hypothalamus. Inputs are compared to a thermoregulatory set-point. If a difference is detected the thermoregulatory mechanisms are triggered. Efferent signals via the sympathetic nerves, somatic motor centre and higher centres influence vasoconstriction, sweating, shivering, non-shivering thermogenesis in brown fat, and behavioural changes.

Hypothermia

Hypothermia is defined as a core temperature <36°C. It can occur under anaesthesia, following exposure or near drowning, and in elderly or hypothyroid patients. Basal metabolic rate decreases by 10% for every 1°C drop in core temperature. See Box 5.6 for pathophysiological effects.

Box 5.6 Pathophysiological effects of hypothermia

Cardiovascular
- Vasoconstriction, tachycardia, and hypertension
- Reduced CO and myocardial depression
- Arrhythmias and J waves on ECG at around 30°C; eventual ventricular fibrillation.

Respiratory
- Reduced oxygen delivery to tissues (↓ CO)
- Left shift of the oxyhaemoglobin dissociation curve
- Hypoxaemia
- Apnoea occurs below 24°C.

Neurological
- Reduced cerebral oxygen demand (7% per 1°C drop)
- Reduced cerebral perfusion pressure and ICP
- Confusion below 35°C
- Loss of consciousness below 30°C
- Reduced MAC for anaesthesia.

Hepatic
- Decreased blood flow and function
- Reduced drug metabolism.

Renal
- Reduced renal blood flow
- Diuresis.

Metabolic
- Metabolic acidosis (poor tissue perfusion)
- Hyperglycaemia (catecholamine release).

Haematological
- Coagulopathy (↓ clotting factor activity)
- Thrombocytopenia (sequestration)
- Raised viscosity.

Anaesthesia and hypothermia

Core temperature drops by 0.5–1.5°C in the first 30min following induction. Anaesthetic agents cause vasodilatation and core temperature is lost by heat flow to the periphery. Behavioural responses are abolished and anaesthesia also resets the hypothalamic thresholds to hypothermia by 3–4°C (and hyperthermia by 1°C). Core temperature continues to drop slowly for the next 2–3h and then stabilizes. Heat is lost by radiation (60%), convection (15%), evaporation (20% if body cavities are exposed), and conduction (5%).

Hypothermia has been shown to negatively impact on postoperative outcome. Wound infections have three times the incidence, free flaps fail to perfuse below 34°C, myocardial ischaemia is more common, and general mortality increases.

Perioperative warming strategies aim to reduce hypothermia and morbidity. Warming of patients prior to surgery and in the anaesthetic room may be used. The theatre temperature should be >24°C, and warming mattresses or blankets used for surgery of >30min duration. All IV fluids and blood products should be warmed, as should surgical irrigation fluids. Circle breathing circuits and heat and moisture exchange filters prevent respiratory heat loss. Temperature monitoring should be instituted for prolonged surgery. Warming may need to continue postoperatively in some patients.

Therapeutic hypothermia

Therapeutic hypothermia is supported to prevent post-cardiac arrest neurological dysfunction. Unconscious adult patients in whom there is return of spontaneous circulation after out-of-hospital cardiac arrest should be cooled to 32–34°C for 12–24h. The 'Hypothermia After Cardiac Arrest Study Group' showed a relative risk of 1.4 of living independently and returning to work at 6 months following therapeutic hypothermia. Mortality at 6 months was also decreased suggesting a NNT of 7. In the light of these findings, therapeutic hypothermia has been extended to all non-traumatic post-cardiac arrest patients.

Cooling is usually achieved through active external methods (cold air blowers or jackets): internal methods via a dedicated intravascular device are available, but rarely used and expensive.

Studies have shown non-significant complication rates with therapeutic hypothermia including pneumonia, hypophosphataemia, bleeding, and arrhythmia.

The cerebral metabolic uptake of oxygen reduces when temperature drops and consequently electrical activity decreases. The effect of hypothermia also plays a significant role in reperfusion injury. Suppression of free radicals, reduction in excitatory neurotransmitters and calcium shifts lead to better maintenance of the blood–brain barrier and reduced cell death.

There is also strong evidence to support therapeutic hypothermia to reduce neurological damage with severe birth asphyxia. Head cooling or total body cooling for 72h in cases of moderate–severe encephalopathy have reduced rates of death and severe disability. Further research is needed before global acceptance of this technique.

Hyperthermia

Hyperthermia is a core temperature >37.7°C. In pyrexia, the pyrogenic cytokines such as IL-6 and TNF cross the blood–brain barrier to the hypothalamus. Prostaglandins are released via the arachidonic acid pathway, e.g. PGE2, which acts via endogenous pyrogen receptors to increase temperature further. The hypothalamic thermostat is, therefore, reset and heat generating mechanisms such as shivering and rigors continue despite high core temperatures. This can be a dangerous situation and denaturation of proteins occurs at 42°C. Temperature may be lowered by:

- NSAIDs, which inhibit cyclo-oxygenase preventing the formation of prostaglandins from arachidonic acid
- Paracetamol, which prevents the synthesis of PGE2 in the hypothalamus
- Physical cooling techniques (ice packs, cool irrigation fluids, etc.).

The cause of the hyperthermia must be addressed to break the cycle. Causes include:

- Infection and systemic immune response
- Chronic immune conditions, e.g. rheumatoid disease
- Tissue destruction, e.g. pancreatitis, rhabdomyolysis
- Tumours, e.g. Hodgkin's lymphoma
- Hypermetabolic conditions, e.g. hyperthyroidism
- Status epilepticus
- Drug-induced, e.g. malignant hyperpyrexia
- Neuroleptic malignant syndrome
- Amphetamine derivatives, e.g. ecstasy, MDMA
- Hypothalamic lesions, e.g. CVA
- Exertional heatstroke.

Further reading

Hypothermia after cardiac arrest study group (2002). Mild therapeutic hypothermia to improve the neurologic outcome after cardiac arrest. *NEJM*, 346:549–56.

5.8 Obesity and malnutrition

Obesity

Obesity, defined as a BMI >30, is an increasing problem with an incidence of at least 20% in the UK. Morbid obesity, BMI >40, has reached an incidence of 4%. It presents a number of challenges for the anaesthetist and affects all body systems (see Box 5.7). Anaesthesia for bariatric surgery is discussed in section 13.8.

Box 5.7 Pathophysiological changes in obesity

Cardiovascular
- Increased oxygen consumption and CO_2 production.
- Increased blood volume.
- Increased CO.
- Hypertension: 10× incidence, often associated with left ventricular hypertrophy (or may lead to obesity cardiomyopathy if ventricular dilatation occurs).
- Ischaemic heart disease: increased atheromatous disease and increased cardiac work.
- Conduction abnormalities: fatty infiltration of conducting tissue.
- Pulmonary hypertension: may result from hypoxia and cause right ventricular failure.
- Thromboembolic disease: decreased venous return.

Respiratory
- Decreased chest wall compliance.
- Increased minute ventilation and work of breathing.
- Decreased FRC: may cause increased shunt during normal tidal ventilation when closing volume overlaps. Linear increase in A–a gradient is seen with increasing BMI.
- Obstructive sleep apnoea (OSA): upper airway obstruction during sleep causes snoring and regular hypopnoea or apnoeas with rousing. Sleep quality is poor and patients develop daytime somnolence, poor concentration and morning headaches. OSA may also affect central respiratory drive and increase opiate-related respiratory depression (see section 11.2).
- Obesity hypoventilation syndrome—hypercapnic respiratory failure which leads to cor pulmonale and may require non-invasive home ventilation.

Gastrointestinal and hepatic
- GORD and hiatus hernia—due to increased intra-abdominal pressure.
- Steatohepatitis and cirrhosis.

Endocrine
- Insulin resistance and type 2 diabetes.
- Hypercholesterolaemia.

Musculoskeletal
Osteoarthritis.

Perioperative management of the obese patient

Preoperative

Assessment should record BMI and patient weight. Comorbidities must be identified and assessed. Patients may have limited mobility making it difficult to assess cardio-respiratory function. Many standard investigations are technically difficult in the obese, e.g. echocardiography. Pharmacological stress tests with measurement of left ventricular output may yield the best results. ABGs may be necessary if oxygen saturations are below 95% in air.

Any comorbidity should be optimized. Non-invasive ventilation may decrease mortality in patients with right ventricular failure preoperatively. Antacid premedication and thromboprophylaxis may be considered prior to surgery.

In patients with morbid obesity, the risks and benefits of surgery should be discussed with the patient and surgical team. In elective surgery it may be appropriate to delay surgery to allow an attempt at weight loss.

Perioperative

Appropriate equipment for the patient weight and size should be available, e.g. trolleys, theatre tables, width extensions, and extra personnel for manual handling. Where possible, the patient should position themselves on the operating table in a semi-sitting position with leg supports to prevent slipping. Preoxygenation in a reverse Trendelenburg position increases time to desaturation. Airway maintenance may be difficult. A 'ramped' airway position reduces the difficulty of intubation. Spontaneous ventilation is often ineffective and airway pressures are often too high to allow ventilation with an LMA. Aspiration of gastric contents is also a risk.

Peripheral and central venous access may be difficult. Invasive blood pressure measurement may be necessary if non-invasive measurement is unreliable. Regional anaesthesia may be preferable, either as the primary anaesthetic or to provide analgesia. There is, however, increased difficulty with both landmark and ultrasound techniques and failure rates are high. Thromboprophylaxis and pressure area care are important.

Pharmacokinetics are altered in obesity with a higher volume of distribution for fat-soluble drugs, reduced total body water, and a higher CO. Awareness is more common and patients are slower to wake, particularly after fat-soluble drugs such as barbiturates, benzodiazepines, and more lipid-soluble volatile agents. Short-acting anaesthetic agents are desirable. In general, the dose of fat-soluble drugs should be based on ideal body weight + 20%, whilst non-lipid soluble drug doses should be based on actual body weight, e.g. suxamethonium.

Postoperative

Obese patients are prone to drowsiness, hypoventilation, and atelectasis resulting in hypoxia. High-dependency care should be considered following major surgery or in a patient with significant comorbidities. A combination of posture or early mobilization, physiotherapy, and non-invasive CPAP or ventilation may be required. Infection rates are increased.

Malnutrition

Malnutrition is also a common problem and may occur with severe chronic illness, GI disease, alcoholism, in the elderly and socially deprived, and in those with eating disorders such as anorexia nervosa. The effects on body systems have important implications for anaesthesia (see Box 5.8).

Box 5.8 Pathophysiological consequences of malnutrition

Cardiovascular

- Bradycardia and hypotension: due to decreased BMR.
- ECG abnormalities: AV block, ST depression, T wave inversion, QT interval prolongation—due to hypocalcaemia and hypomagnesaemia with starvation.
- Arrhythmias: sinus arrest, SVT, VT—about 20% incidence under anaesthesia in anorexia nervosa.
- Left ventricular dysfunction: with starvation and as a direct effect of purging drugs in eating disorders.

Respiratory

- Persistent vomiting may cause metabolic acidosis and bradypnoea or pneumothoraces and pneumomediastinum.

Gastrointestinal

- Prolonged gastric emptying time in starvation.
- Persistent vomiting may cause oesophagitis and strictures.

Endocrine

- Hypothalamic function is altered by malnutrition and patients may display features of panhypopituitarism.

Renal/metabolic

- Proteinuria.
- Electrolyte disorders and dehydration.

Neurological

- Thermoregulation is impaired and shivering response inadequate. Core temperature often <36.3°C.
- Cognitive function impairment with reduction in grey matter.
- Seizures or coma: secondary to electrolyte disturbances or hypoglycaemia.

Perioperative management of the malnourished patient

Preoperative

Electrolyte blood levels should be checked including phosphate, magnesium, and calcium, as well as blood glucose. An ECG should be performed to assess abnormalities and the potential for developing arrhythmias. Antacid premedication and a prokinetic to enhance gastric emptying may be considered. It may be appropriate to postpone elective surgery if good nutrition can be established by enteral or parenteral means. Patients may be susceptible to refeeding syndrome which can cause rebound hypokalaemia, hypophosphataemia, and hypomagnesaemia, increased oxygen consumption, extracellular fluid, and cardiac work. They should be supervised by a nutrition specialist.

Perioperative

In starvation, gastric emptying may be delayed and rapid sequence induction should be considered. Careful positioning and padding of pressure areas is required as patients are susceptible to neuronal injury and fractures. Temperature monitoring and patient warming are essential.

Pharmacokinetics are altered with reduced albumin, reduced protein binding of drugs, and therefore increased free drug concentrations. In the presence of hypokalaemia and hypocalcaemia, neuromuscular blocking agents have a prolonged duration of action.

Further reading

AAGBI Guidelines (2007). *Perioperative Management of the Morbidly Obese*. London: AAGBI.

Denner AM & Townley SA (2009). Anorexia nervosa: perioperative implications. *CEACCP*, 9(2):61–4. doi:10.1093/bjaceaccp/mkp004.

Lotia S & Bellamy MC (2008). Anaesthesia and morbid obesity. *CCEACCP*, 8(5):151–6. doi:10.1093/bjaceaccp/mkn030.

Chapter 6

Nervous and musculoskeletal systems

6.1 Consciousness and sleep

Consciousness

Consciousness can be defined as being 'awake and aware of one's surroundings'. An individual's state of consciousness exists on a spectrum from fully conscious to comatose. When in a comatose state an individual can be considered in an unrousable state of unconsciousness. There is ongoing philosophical debate as to the precise definition of human consciousness but as medical professionals our primary concern is the comparison of the current level of consciousness with a patient's baseline conscious level (see Box 6.1).

Box 6.1 Causes of delayed recovery of consciousness after anaesthesia

- *Patent factors:* age, pre-existing hepatic/renal disease, pharmacogenetic variation
- *Neurological factors:* seizures, ischaemia, haemorrhage, hypoxia
- *Respiratory factors:* reduced respiratory drive, muscular weakness, pulmonary pathology
- *Metabolic factors:* hypo/hypernatraemia, hypo/hyperglycaemia, hypothermia, hypothyroidism, sepsis
- *Surgical factors:* prolonged duration of surgery, regional/local techniques, degree of tissue trauma/pain
- *Drug factors:* anaesthetic dose, pharmacokinetic interaction (absorption, distribution, metabolism), pharmacodynamic interaction (synergism, potentiation).

Sleep

Sleep is a natural and recurring state of unconsciousness. It is characterized by reduced consciousness with decreased response to external stimuli. A sleeping subject is usually easily roused. Sleep deprivation may have important consequences (Box 6.2).

Sleep architecture

Initially standardized in 1968 by the 'Rechtschaffen and Kales Sleep Scoring Manual', sleep can be divided into two types: non-rapid eye movement sleep (NREM) and rapid eye movement sleep (REM).

NREM sleep was traditionally split into four stages (1–4), describing progressively deepening sleep. In 2007, the American Academy of Sleep Medicine (AASM) amalgamated stages 3 and 4 so more recent texts describe only NREM 1, 2, and 3.

The types and stages of sleep are differentiated by electroencephalograph (EEG) waveforms (Table 6.1), muscle tone, and eye movements. Sleep EEG demonstrates persistently altering waveforms, and does not resemble unconsciousness resulting from brain damage. Sleep should, therefore, be considered an active state.

In health, sleep has a circadian rhythm and normally occurs in cycles (5–6 per night) with rapid oscillations between stages. On entering sleep (N1), it typically deepens through N2 and N3, and is subsequently followed by cyclical patterns of REM sleep. Typically NREM sleep accounts for 75% of the total, and REM 25%. The first cycle of NREM: REM sleep lasts 70–100min, and this time period lengthens to 90–120min with increased periods of REM sleep.

NREM stage 1

Primarily the initial stage of sleep, N1 lasts between 2% to 5% of the total sleep period. EEG demonstrates transition of alpha waves (8–13Hz) to low voltage, mixed frequency waves. In this stage sleep may easily be disrupted. People may wake and may experience myoclonic jerks or hypnagogic hallucinations.

NREM stage 2

Normally lasting 10–25min in the first sleep cycle, this time period lengthens as sleep continues to contribute to 45–55% of the total sleep period. EEG demonstrates low-voltage, mixed frequency activity characterized by the presence of sleep spindles (11–16Hz) and K-complexes. Sleep spindles are generated by bursts of hyperpolarizing GABAnergic neurons in the reticular nucleus of the thalamus, which in turn inhibit thalamocortical projection neurons. K complexes are described as a brief negative peak, usually greater than 100μV, followed by a slower positive complex and a subsequent negative peak.

NREM stage 3

Also known as slow wave sleep (SWS), N3 usually occurs during the first third of a night's sleep. It represents 5–15% of the total sleep period. Somniloquy, sleepwalking and parasomnias occur in this stage of sleep, as does a fall in muscle tone, reflex activity, cerebral activity, blood pressure, and heart rate. The EEG is characterized by high-voltage, slow activity delta waves (0.5–3Hz).

REM sleep

Initially brief in the first sleep cycle, REM sleep lengthens as the total sleep period progresses. With 5–6 episodes a night it represents 20–25% of the total sleep period. REM sleep is associated with dreaming, and descending muscle atonia is present (except respiratory, extra-ocular and inner ear muscles), which plays an important role in the prevention of acting out dreams.

The EEG demonstrates low-voltage, mixed frequency, desynchronized cortical activity with sawtooth waveforms and theta activity (4–7Hz; see Fig. 6.1). In this stage, the eyes fluctuate back and forth, and generalized autonomic excitation occurs (Table 6.2). Due to the EEG resembling that recorded in the aroused state, and the increased sympathetic activity associated with REM sleep, it is also known as paradoxical sleep.

Table 6.1 Frequencies of EEG waveforms

Wave	Frequency
Alpha	8–13Hz
Beta	>13Hz
Theta	4–7Hz
Delta	0.5–3Hz

Table 6.2 Physiological changes during sleep

	NREM	REM
Heart rate	Decreases	Increases
Blood pressure	Decreases	Increases
Respiratory rate	Decreases	Increases & irregular
Muscle tone	Decreases	Increases
Cerebral activity	Decreases	Increases
Cerebral blood flow	Decreases	Increases
Cerebral metabolism	Decreases	Increases
Sympathetic activity	Decreases	Increases

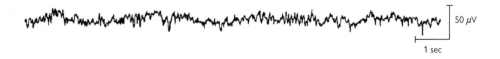

Drowsy – 8 to 12 cps – alpha waves

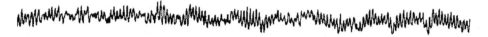

Stage 1 – 3 to 7 cps – theta waves

Theta Waves

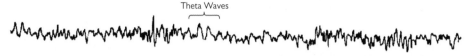

Stage 2 – 12 to 14 cps – sleep spindles and K complexes

Sleep Spindles   K Complex —

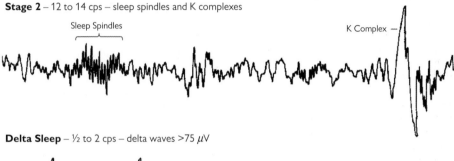

Delta Sleep – ½ to 2 cps – delta waves >75 μV

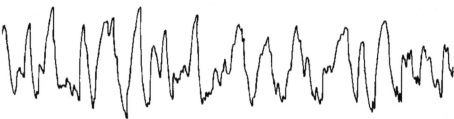

REM Sleep – low voltage – random, fast with sawtooth waves

Sawtooth Waves   Sawtooth Waves

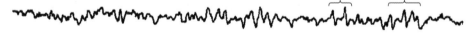

Fig. 6.1 EEG traces during the different stages of sleep. Reproduced from Schupp M and Hanning CD, 'Physiology of Sleep', *Continuing Education in Anaesthesia Critical Care and Pain*, 2003, 3, 3, pp. 69–74, by permission of The Board of Management Trustees of the British Journal of Anaesthesia and Oxford University Press.

Sleep regulation

Sleep is regulated by the reticular formation (RF). Given the RF's fundamental importance in maintaining consciousness, it is of particular note that it is not the absence of input to the RF that allows for sleep, but rather an active inhibitory process. The preoptic region, between the anterior commissure and the optic chiasma, has substantial efferent projections to the midbrain and is known to induce the EEG signs of sleep and inhibit the conscious processes. The suprachiasmatic nucleus acts as the sleep pacemaker, and controls cycles of slow wave sleep. Neurotransmitters associated with sleep include serotonin, noradrenaline, and acetylcholine.

Sleep changes with age

Sleep patterns alter considerably through life in respect of how sleep is initiated and maintained, and the periods of time spent in each of the different stages. The total period spent sleeping decreases from an average of 18h in newborns to 8h in adults. The total period of REM sleep also decreases (50% vs 25% respectively). Newborns experience disrupted sleep throughout the day, with no regular rhythm or concentration of a sleep wake cycle. By 3 months the circadian rhythm has evolved, and with social interaction, sleep becomes more regular and lengthens. In the elderly, as the percentage of REM sleep declines further, and their ability to maintain N3 diminishes, disturbed sleep is a common feature.

Effect of surgery and anaesthesia on sleep

Surgical stress has a profound effect on the sleep cycle for the first 2–5 nights postoperatively. The effect is proportional to the surgical insult. A considerable reduction in N3 and REM sleep occurs, with frequent awakenings during the immediate postoperative period. The rebound recovery of REM sleep on nights 2–5 may increase oxygen demands and cause hypoxia after major surgery (see Box 6.3).

Box 6.2 Effects of sleep deprivation

- Decreased cerebral function and cognitive dysfunction
- Decreased immunity
- Decreased thermal regulation
- Depression
- Hallucinations
- Tremors.

Box 6.3 Respiratory changes during sleep

NREM sleep
- Reduced hypercarbic and hypoxic ventilatory drive
- Reduced muscle tone of upper airway
- Leading to decreased minute ventilation by 25%, increased respiratory rate by 50%.

REM sleep
- Further reduction in ventilatory drive
- Reduction in chest wall skeletal muscle tone
- Leading to irregular breathing with increased V/Q mismatch.

Common sleep disorders

Some of the more common sleep disorders are presented in Box 6.4.

Box 6.4 Sleep disorders

- *Insomnia*: difficulty in falling asleep or staying asleep.
- *Parasomnia*: abnormal sleep behaviour such as sleepwalking (complex automatic behaviour during N3) and night terrors.
- *Narcolepsy*: affects 0.05% population: a disorder of the normal sleep–wake cycle where REM sleep may occur rapidly. Causes disturbed sleep, excessive daytime sleepiness, cataplexy, sleep paralysis, and hypnogogic hallucinations.
- *Sleep paralysis*: temporary paralysis shortly before or after sleep.
- *Periodic limb movement disorder*: limbs move involuntarily during NREM sleep.
- *Restless leg syndrome*: occurs whilst awake with a voluntary response to an uncomfortable feeling in the legs. Involuntary movements also occur during sleep.
- *Fatal familial insomnia*: a very rare, autosomal dominant inherited prion disease.
- *Obstructive sleep apnoea*—see section 11.2.

Sleep deprivation in ITUs

Sleep deprivation is very common in critically ill patients (Box 6.5). In the ITU, a patient will sleep for an average of <2h/day with <6% in REM sleep. The consequences of this sleep disruption may lead to slow weaning from mechanical ventilation, increased catabolism, and predispose to ITU psychosis.

Box 6.5 Causes of sleep deprivation on ITUs

- *Pre-existing disease*: patients with sleep apnoea and chronic obstructive airways disease have reduced total sleep and REM sleep times.
- *Surgical stress response*: anxiety, pain, sympathetic stimulation and fever can decrease the time spent in NREM and REM sleep.
- *Pharmacological*: benzodiazepines reduce periods of deep sleep, Catecholamines increase wakefulness, Barbiturates and amphetamines cause inhibition of REM sleep.
- *Environmental factors*: noise, bright lighting, high/low ambient temperature.

The Glasgow Coma Scale (GCS)

First described in 1974 by Teasdale and Jennett, the Glasgow Coma Scale (Table 6.3) is a widely used scoring system for assessing CNS function in patients with a reduced level of consciousness. It describes conscious level according to three domains; eye opening, verbal response, and motor response. Originally described in the assessment of head injury, it is now more widely applied to CNS evaluation. It can be used to dynamically chart a patient's conscious level, prognosticate severity of injury, and is also used for therapeutic decision-making (e.g. intubation of a patient if GCS <8).

Table 6.3 The Glasgow Coma Scale

Best motor response	Follows commands	6
	Localizes pain	5
	Withdraws from pain	4
	Flexion response to pain	3
	Extension response to pain	2
	No response	1
Best verbal response	Fully orientated	5
	Confused	4
	Inappropriate words	3
	Incomprehensible sounds	2
	No response	1
Best eye response	Eyes spontaneously open	4
	Eyes open to voice	3
	Eyes open to pain	2
	Eyes remain closed	1

Reprinted from *The Lancet*, 304, 7872, Teasdale G and Jennett B, 'Assessment of coma and impaired consciousness: a practical scale', pp. 81–84, copyright 1974, with permission from Elsevier.

Further reading

Iber C, Ancoli-Israel S, Chesson A, *et al.* (2007). *The AASM Manual for the Scoring of Sleep and Associated Events: Rules, Terminology and Technical Specifications* (1st edn). Darien, IL: American Academy of Sleep Medicine.

Teasdale G & Jennett B (1974). Assessment of coma and impaired consciousness: a practical scale. *Lancet*, 2(7872):81–4.

6.2 Assessment of anaesthetic depth and avoidance of awareness

Assessing anaesthetic depth

Clinical signs

Monitoring autonomic parameters such as heart rate, blood pressure, pupillary dilatation, and the presence of lacrimation and sweating gives an indication of the state of sympathetic nervous system activation. Whilst this may reflect anaesthetic depth, many factors can render these parameters unreliable (Table 6.4). EEG monitors have also shown changes consistent with awareness minutes before changes in autonomic parameters are observed.

Table 6.4 Clinical signs of awareness—and factors that may impair their use as a marker of anaesthetic depth

Sign of awareness	Factors impairing the sign
Tachycardia	Heart block, β-blockers, hypothyroidism, autonomic neuropathy (e.g. diabetes, renal failure)
Hypertension	Heart block, β-blockers, hypothyroidism, vasodilators, epidural analgesia, blood loss, autonomic neuropathy
Sweating	Antimuscarinic drugs (e.g. atropine, glycopyrrolate)
Tear production	Antimuscarinic drugs, eye tape/ointment
Movement/grimacing	Neuromuscular blocking agents (NMBAs), sheets covering the patient
Tachypnoea	NMBAs
Pupillary dilatation/reactivity to light	Antimuscarinic drugs, opioids, ocular pathology, eye tape/ointment

End-tidal agent monitoring

The minimum alveolar concentration (MAC) of a volatile agent is the minimum concentration at an ambient pressure of 1 atmosphere to prevent movement in 50% of non-premedicated subjects to a standard painful stimulus. It should be noted that this definition makes no mention of awareness or recall. Increasing the MAC of an agent requires an increased dose of the agent and therefore does bear some correlation with anaesthetic depth (see Box 6.6 for factors which alter the MAC).

Box 6.6 Factors altering the MAC of a volatile agent

Increased MAC
Pyrexia, hyperthyroidism, obesity, anxiety, young age, tobacco smoking, chronic alcohol abuse, recreational drug abuse (e.g. opioids, amphetamines, cocaine), chronic sedative use (e.g. temazepam), and previous and repeated exposure to anaesthetic agents.

Decreased MAC
Hypocapnia, pregnancy, hypothyroidism, hypothermia, hypotension, old age.

Pharmacological modelling of IV agent concentration

Pharmacokinetic models incorporated into IV infusion devices provide an indication of the plasma concentration of the infused drug. The algorithms are continually being refined however, there

remains a high degree of inter-individual pharmacokinetic variability. The clinical effect of a particular plasma drug concentration also varies between individuals.

EEG monitoring

Changes in cortical activity with altered depth of anaesthesia are observed on EEG recording. The unprocessed EEG is impractical for monitoring depth of anaesthesia as it produces vast quantities of data that require specialist analysis. There is an increasing range of technology available which is can process the EEG into a quantitative marker of anaesthetic depth. The early monitors compared changes in compound EEG voltages over time, but these have largely been superseded by monitors, which perform fast *Fourier analysis* on the EEG thus allowing analysis of the component sine waves. Further analysis is then possible based on (1) frequency distribution; (2) power contained within different frequencies (a function of wave amplitude); and (3) phase relationships between waves of different frequencies. The degree of disorder (*entropy*) in the EEG is seen to decrease with increased anaesthetic depth and may also be used as a monitoring tool.

Bispectral index monitor (BIS)

BIS monitoring combines EEG power spectral analysis with comparison of the phase relationships between component waves of differing frequencies. It also incorporates other EEG subparameters as part of its proprietary algorithm. The monitor generates a dimensionless number on a scale of 0–100 and also displays a real-time frontal EEG recording (see Boxes 6.7 and 6.8).

Box 6.7 Suggested interpretation of BIS values

- 100–85: awake, aware, capable of memory processing and explicit recall
- 85–60: increasing sedation and impairment of memory processing. Rousable in response to stimulation
- 60–40: surgical anaesthesia. Decreasing probability of postoperative recall. Auditory processing and reflex movement still occurs
- 40–0: increasing frequency of burst suppression. BIS of 0 indicates cortical electrical silence.

Box 6.8 Limitations of BIS

- Interindividual variability in depth of sedation/anaesthesia for a given BIS value.
- Minimally affected by opioids therefore may not reflect a 'balanced' anaesthetic regimen.
- Changes in consciousness from ketamine and nitrous oxide are not faithfully represented.
- Electrical interference from muscle activity.

Evoked potentials (EPs)

Monitoring electrical potentials in specific brain areas in response to stimulation of selected neural pathways may indicate depth of anaesthesia. Examples include somatosensory, visual and auditory EPs of which auditory EPs (AEPs) have shown greatest correlation with anaesthetic depth. The 8th cranial nerve is stimulated by a 6–10Hz auditory stimulus whilst cortical activity is monitored by an electrode placed over the mastoid process. Increasing anaesthetic depth causes a fall in amplitude and increased latency of the mid-cortical AEP. By comparing changes in AEPs the monitor displays an index on which >80 is considered awake and <50 anaesthetized. Inter-individual variability means that neither sensitive nor specific 'cut-off' values for awareness are available.

Techniques of limited significance

Respiratory sinus arrhythmia and RR interval variation

This method reflects the decrease in autonomic function with increasing depth of anaesthesia. Its use is limited in patients with autonomic dysfunction (e.g. elderly, diabetes mellitus, sepsis), cardiac conduction abnormalities or β-blocker therapy.

Isolated forearm technique

During general anaesthesia, a tourniquet is applied to the upper arm and inflated to above systolic blood pressure before the administration of muscle relaxant. This enables the subject able to signal wakefulness or awareness with the 'unparalysed' forearm. Its use is limited by ischaemic paralysis from the tourniquet and by the high degree of cooperation required by the subject.

Oesophageal contractility

Spontaneous and provoked oesophageal contraction is seen to reduce in frequency and amplitude with increased depth of anaesthesia. This technique is limited by the high degree of false positive and false negative results.

Frontalis electromyogram (EMG)

The scalp EMG is seen to reduce in amplitude with increased depth of anaesthesia. It cannot be used in patients who have received muscle relaxants.

Awareness

Awareness is the formation of explicit or implicit memories during general anaesthesia. Explicit memories are able to be recalled either spontaneously or on direct questioning. Implicit memories are not able to be consciously recalled but may have effects on behaviour or cognition. The sequelae of awareness are most commonly psychological and may present as a post-traumatic stress syndrome with features such as sleep disturbance, anxiety, and personality change. It is the subject of the latest National Audit Project (NAP 5) undertaken by the RCoA.

Incidence of awareness

Awareness is an uncommon event and is likely to be under-reorted. The RCoA patient information leaflet quotes an incidence of awareness of 0.1–0.2% of patients undergoing a GA. The incidence is higher in certain types of surgery (e.g. emergency caesarean section under GA (0.4%) and cardiac surgery (1.5%))

Causes of awareness

- Inadequate induction agent dose.
- Prolonged or difficult airway manoeuvres without further doses of hypnotic agent.
- Omission or late commencement of maintenance anaesthetic after induction of anaesthesia.

- Reduced dose of anaesthetic agent to maintain arterial pressure during episodes of hypotension or blood loss.
- Physiological resistance to anaesthetic agents (see Box 6.6).
- Equipment failure, e.g. breathing system leaks, vaporizer malfunction, disconnection/occlusion of TIVA systems.
- Monitoring failure, e.g. failure to monitor volatile agent concentration within a circle breathing system.

Avoiding awareness

Perioperative management

Benzodiazepine administration at induction may reduce the likelihood of awareness particularly if airway instrumentation is expected to be prolonged.

Titration of volatile agent dose to >0.8 MAC has been shown to decrease the incidence of awareness. Consideration of appropriate MAC value for a specific patient is also important, e.g. a fit and well 25-year-old will require an increased anaesthetic dose compared to a 90-year-old with hypothermia.

Treat intraoperative hypotension with IV fluids/vasopressors rather than reduction in anaesthetic agent dose below what is appropriate for that patient.

The use of NMBAs may increase the incidence of awareness. Their use should be carefully considered dependent on the procedure being undertaken.

Depth of anaesthesia monitoring remains controversial as a tool for reducing awareness.

Management of awareness

Intraoperative

Clinical signs consistent with potential awareness should be treated immediately by deepening anaesthesia. Whilst benzodiazepine administration (e.g. midazolam 5mg) has not been shown to cause retrograde amnesia it may reduce postoperative recall.

Postoperative

The responsible anaesthetist should visit the patient and obtain a thorough history of events. This should be documented in the patient's notes. Relating the timing of events to the procedure may help in distinguishing between dreaming and awareness. Specific events recalled by the patient (e.g. the moment of incision, overheard conversation) should also be recorded. Be sympathetic and apologize where appropriate. Direct denial of events without logical explanation may worsen the psychological outcome for the patient. The patient should be offered psychological support and counselling.

Meticulous note keeping and liaison with the hospital legal team will be helpful in the event of ensuing litigation. This will be a stressful event for the responsible anaesthetist who should seek the support and advice of colleagues.

Further reading

Aitkenhead AR & Hardman JG (2005). Awareness during anaesthesia. *CEACCP*, 5(6):183–6.

Kent CD & Domino KB (2009). Depth of anesthesia. *Curr Opin Anaesthesiol*. 22:782–7.

6.3 Control of convulsions

Seizures are periods of abnormal and excessive electrical brain activity. Seizures can be described as partial or generalized (Box 6.9). A seizure may commence as a partial seizure and become generalized. During a partial seizure, focal brain areas are affected. Consciousness may be lost (complex partial seizure) or maintained (simple partial seizure). Generalized seizures involve bilateral electrical brain activity. They may present as transient disturbances of consciousness (absence/petit-mal) seizures or with generalized muscular activity (tonic, clonic, tonic–clonic or grand mal). The term 'convulsion' (see Box 6.11) commonly refers to tonic–clonic seizures.

Approximately 1 in 50 people will experience a seizure during their lifetime with 1 in 200 diagnosed with epilepsy. For a diagnosis of epilepsy to be established, there must be recurrent (two or more) seizures without an immediately identifiable cause. A single non-recurring seizure is not considered epileptic.

Box 6.9 Classification of epileptic seizures

Partial seizures
- Simple
- Complex
- Partial onset with generalization.

Generalized seizures
- Inhibitory:
  - Absence
  - Atonic.
- Excitatory:
  - Myoclonic
  - Tonic
  - Clonic.

Pseudoseizures

Non-epileptic seizures

Mechanism of epilepsy

The mechanism of epilepsy may be related to:
- Loss of postsynaptic inhibition with loss of inhibitory γ-aminobutyric acid (GABA) activity.
- New excitatory synaptic connections with increased release of glutamate (an excitatory amino acid).
- Appearance of pacemaker neurons with abnormal voltage mediated calcium currents, triggering abnormal neuronal firing.

Box 6.10 Causes of convulsions

- Genetic determination, e.g. juvenile myoclonic epilepsy
- Trauma
- Tumour—more common with slow growing tumour
- Infection—meningitis/encephalitis
- Cerebral degeneration
- Cerebrovascular disease
- Multiple sclerosis
- Alcohol—reduced seizure threshold. Seizures may occur with acute intoxication or withdrawal
- Metabolic disorders—hypo/hypercalcaemia, hypo/hypernatraemia, hypomagnesaemia, hypoglycaemia
- Hepatic/renal impairment
- Eclampsia
- Local anaesthetic toxicity.

Differential diagnosis of seizures

- Syncope—multifocal myoclonic muscular activity can be observed after loss of consciousness:
  - Cardiac—reduced cardiac output leads to cerebral hypoperfusion and syncope. Causes include heart block, bradyarrhythmia, supraventricular tachycardia and carotid sinus pressure.
  - Autonomic failure and postural hypotension.
  - Micturition and cough syncope.
- Transient ischaemic attacks—may present with impaired consciousness and abnormal limb movement.
- Migraine—loss of consciousness is observed in basilar migraine although tonic–clonic seizure activity is rare.
- Hyperventilation—associated with dizziness, impaired consciousness and limb weakness.
- Narcolepsy and cataplexy—narcolepsy is characterized by excessive daytime somnolence. Cataplexy is precipitated by arousal and manifests with a sudden loss in muscle tone leading to a fall.
- Myoclonus induced by anaesthetic agents—e.g. propofol.
- Non-epileptic seizures—often occur in patients with a psychiatric history. More common in women. Attacks tend to occur in the presence of a witness. Vocalization is common and incontinence uncommon. Pupillary reflexes are maintained and plasma prolactin levels remain unchanged 20min after the event.

Investigations

A specific cause for convulsions (see Box 6.10) is absent in up to 66% of cases.

- EEG—abnormalities seen in up to 50% of epileptics. 4% of individuals who have never had a seizure show epileptiform discharges on EEG.
- CT—may indicate a structural abnormality as a cause of the seizures.
- MRI—more sensitive and specific for identifying structural brain lesions than CT.
- Single photon-emission computed tomography (SPECT) and positron emission tomography (PET)—allow measurement of cerebral blood flow and glucose metabolism (PET only). Epileptiform areas may show a reduced blood flow/glucose metabolism.

Antiepileptic drugs (AEDs)

The choice of agent (Table 6.5) depends on seizure type and frequency, patient age, and drug side effect profile. Treatment is commonly commenced with a single agent titrated to an appropriate plasma level. Continuing seizures or intolerable side effects may require a change of AED or addition of second/third-line agent.

Anaesthetic considerations

Preoperative

History—epilepsy aetiology, seizure type, frequency and control, AED medication and side effects.

LFT, FBC, and coagulation screen in patients on valproate and carbamazepine. Consider measuring and optimizing plasma levels of AED.

Continue AED up to time of surgery and aim to restart as soon as possible postoperatively. AED half-life tends to be long so a delayed or missed dose is usually well tolerated. Many

Table 6.5 Commonly used AEDs		
Drug	Mechanism of action	Side effects
Phenytoin	Na+ channel blocker	Enzyme induction, megaloblastic anaemia, haemolysis (G6PD def.)
Valproate	Na+ and Ca2+ blockers	Enzyme induction, thrombocytopenia, hepatotoxicity
Carbamazepine	Na+ channel blocker	Enzyme induction, blood dyscrasias, hepatotoxicity
Phenobarbital	GABA agonist	Enzyme induction, sedation, megaloblastic anaemia
Clonazepam	GABA agonist	Sedation, CNS depression
Vigabatrine	Augments GABA	Irritability/aggression, ↓ phenytoin levels
Lamotrigine	Na+ channel blocker	GI upset, sedation, dizziness

AEDs are available only as oral preparations—hence a perioperative AED plan (in consultation with neurological specialists) should be established if a prolonged period of nil-by-mouth is anticipated.

General or regional anaesthesia

Regional anaesthesia can be considered in cooperative patients with well-controlled epilepsy. The benefits of regional anaesthesia must be weighed against the possibility of an intraoperative seizure in an awake patient. The seizure threshold may be reduced by hypocapnia secondary to anxiety-induced hyperventilation.

Induction

Propofol and thiopentone are considered safe to use in epilepsy. Low doses of propofol may cause epileptogenic changes in the EEG but at induction doses it causes EEG suppression (Table 6.6). Sevoflurane also causes epileptiform EEG changes however this risk may be balanced by it being the most appropriate agent to use in an inhalational induction for an uncooperative child.

Neuromuscular blockade

Resistance to non-depolarizing NMBAs may occur due to liver enzyme induction by AEDs. An increased dose or frequency of dosing of NMB may be required and neuromuscular function should be monitored with a peripheral nerve stimulator.

Maintenance of anaesthesia

Hepatic enzyme induction by AEDs may cause increased metabolism of halogenated volatile agents, increasing the risk of halothane hepatitis. This may also increase the metabolism of opioids resulting in an increased analgesic requirement. Agents with epileptogenic potential such as ketamine and alfentanil should be avoided.

Post operative

Restart AED medication as soon as possible, consider checking plasma levels if significant delay.

Table 6.6 EEG effects of anaesthetic drugs	
EEG activation	EEG suppression
Propofol (low dose)	Propofol (clinical dose)
Ketamine	Thiopentone
Etomidate (low dose)	Etomidate (high dose)
Sevoflurane	Isoflurane
Alfentanil	Desflurane
Fentanyl (15–35mcg/kg)	Fentanyl (<5mcg/kg)
Morphine (high dose—animal studies)	

Postoperative pseudo-epileptic seizures

Shivering and shaking is common after general anaesthesia with volatile anaesthetic agents and may be confused with seizure activity. Some anaesthetic drugs may also cause dystonic movements.

Pseudo-seizures may also occur postoperatively. These resemble tonic–clonic seizures but are not associated with abnormal cortical electrical activity. They may be associated with a history of convulsion and/or psychosomatic illness. Characteristically the movements are asynchronous and flamboyant with eye closure that is resistant to eye opening. Incontinence and tongue biting may be present but without cyanosis or post-ictal period. The plasma prolactin level (raised after epileptic seizures) is often normal and pupillary reflexes are maintained during the seizure. The seizures are terminated with time and reassurance. It is possible for epileptic and pseudo-epileptic seizures to coexist.

Status epilepticus

This is defined as continuous seizure activity of at least 30min duration or intermittent seizure activity of at least 30min duration during which consciousness is not regained. Generalized convulsive status epilepticus (GCSE) is the most common form but seizures may also be non-convulsive or partial. GCSE is characterized by tonic–clonic seizures, loss of consciousness, tongue biting and incontinence. After 30min of seizure, increased ICP, hypotension, and failed auto-regulation result in decreased cerebral perfusion. Failure of central breathing control causes hypoxia, pulmonary hypertension, and cardiac failure.

Management is to ensure maintenance of airway breathing and circulation whilst pharmacologically terminating the seizure. Endotracheal intubation may be necessary to protect against aspiration of gastric contents. If NMBAs are to be continued beyond intubation then EEG monitoring must be instituted to monitor seizure activity. Send blood for FBC, U&E, LFT, glucose, ABG, toxicology, and AED levels. Consider 50mL 50% dextrose with thiamine 100mg if alcoholism/malnutrition is present.

Drug therapy

- Lorazepam 0.1mg/kg (up to 4mg)—repeat if seizures continue for 10min.
- Phenytoin 15mg/kg at <50mg/min or fosphenytoin at <100–150mg/min.
- Induction of anaesthesia with thiopentone 4–5mg/kg with 3–5mg/kg/h infusion.

Seizures under general anaesthesia

These may be difficult to diagnose especially if a NMB has been used. Signs are hypermetabolic in nature but are also subtle and non-specific. Unexplained tachycardia, hypertension, increased muscle tone, rising end-tidal CO_2, pupillary dilatation, and raised oxygen consumption may indicate underlying seizure activity. Diagnosis relies on the EEG, which is often not available in theatre. Treatment involves 100% oxygen, deepening of anaesthesia, administration of an anticonvulsant such as propofol or thiopentone, and removal of precipitating factors (e.g. hypoxia, hypoglycaemia, electrolyte imbalance).

Further reading

Barakat AR & Mallory S (2011). Anaesthesia and childhood epilepsy. *CEACCP*, 11(4):1–6.

Gratrix AP & Enright SM (2005). Epilepsy in anaesthesia and intensive care. *CEACCP*, 5(4):118–21.

6.4 Control of cerebral circulation, intracranial, and intraocular pressures

Failure of adequate cerebral circulation results rapidly in neuronal cell death. Multiple mechanisms maintain homeostasis keeping cerebral blood flow (CBF) constant in health.

Determinants of intracranial pressure (ICP) and intraocular pressure (IOP) share many common themes.

Control of cerebral circulation

Anatomy
The brain receives a dual arterial supply comprising 70% from the internal carotid arteries and 30% from the vertebral arteries. These arteries anastomose in the circle of Willis at the base of the brain (Fig 6.2). Venous drainage occurs via the superficial cerebral veins flowing into the dural sinuses and thence into the jugular bulb. Intracranial venous pressure is usually 2–4mmHg higher than ICP to ensure forward flow.

Normal cerebral circulation
In normal circumstances the brain receives 15% of the cardiac output which corresponds to a CBF of 50mL/min/100g of brain tissue or 600mL/min. Cerebral perfusion pressure (CPP) = MAP – ICP. Normally ICP is 5–15mmHg, but in disease states may be considerably higher.

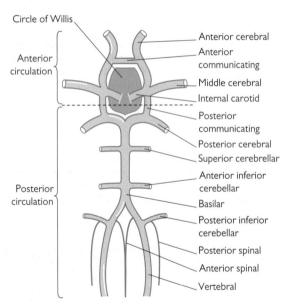

Fig. 6.2 The cerebral circulation. Reproduced from Catherine Spoors and Kevin Kiff, *Training in Anaesthesia*, 2010, Figure 7.26, page 157, with permission from Oxford University Press.

Factors affecting cerebral blood flow

Autoregulation
Cerebral blood flow is maintained at a constant level despite changing blood pressures by myogenic and metabolic mechanisms. In response to increasing MAP the arteries contract to reduce their calibre and conversely when blood pressure falls they dilate. This keeps CBF constant between MAP of 50–150mmHg (Fig. 6.3). Above and below these limits or in the traumatized brain autoregulation is lost. In chronic hypertension

the autoregulation curve is shifted to the right and therefore these patients tolerate hypotension poorly. Autoregulation usually normalizes in the stable treated hypertensive patient. Metabolic control is especially important at low CPP causing vessel dilation in metabolically active areas of brain.

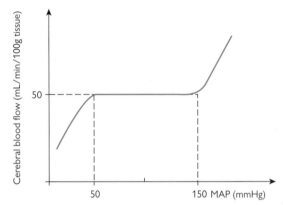

Fig. 6.3 Autoregulation of cerebral blood flow. Reproduced from Catherine Spoors and Kevin Kiff, *Training in Anaesthesia*, 2010, Figure 7.29, page 157, with permission from Oxford University Press.

Chemical control
CBF is altered in response to changes in hydrogen ion concentration, $PaCO_2$, and PaO_2. Changes in $PaCO_2$ results in a linear alteration in CBF in the physiological range (Fig. 6.4). An increase from a $PaCO_2$ of 4kPa to 8kPa results in a doubling of CBF. Above a $PaCO_2$ of 10.6kPa there is no further increase in flow as the blood vessels are maximally dilated. Below $PaCO_2$ of 3.5kPa the response is non-linear and at $PaCO_2$ of 2.6kPa the blood vessels are maximally constricted.

PO_2 has little effect on CBF above a PaO_2 of 8kPa. Below this value there is a pronounced effect resulting in a doubling of CBF if PO_2 falls from 8kPa to 4 kPa (Fig. 6.5).

Cerebral metabolism
Alteration in cerebral metabolic rate result in changes in CBF. This is usually more relevant for regional changes in blood flow,

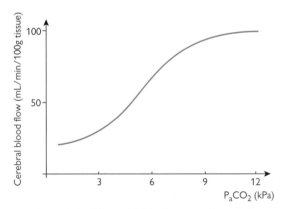

Fig. 6.4 Cerebral blood flow and $PaCO_2$. Reproduced from Catherine Spoors and Kevin Kiff, *Training in Anaesthesia*, 2010, Figure 7.30, page 157, with permission from Oxford University Press.

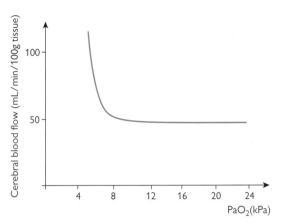

Fig. 6.5 Cerebral blood flow and PaO_2. Reproduced from Catherine Spoors and Kevin Kiff, *Training in Anaesthesia*, 2010, Figure 7.31, page 157, with permission from Oxford University Press.

but in situations where global cerebral metabolic rate is altered, large changes in total CBF can be seen. Examples of this would include increases associated with seizures and the fall in CBF seen in brainstem death.

Neurogenic control
Cerebral blood vessels have extensive innervation from the autonomic nervous system. Sympathetic fibres from the superior cervical and stellate ganglia cause vasoconstriction. This protects the cerebral circulation form the hypertension associated with sympathetic stimulation. Conversely parasympathetic fibres from the sphenopalatine and otic ganglia cause vasodilatation.

Control of intracranial pressure

Basic anatomy
The adult skull is often thought of as a fixed box with three main constituents, brain (85%), CSF (10%), and blood (5%). Should an alteration occur in the volume of one of the three components the others attempt to accommodate this change and hence avoid a raise in ICP. For example, if brain volume increases the CSF volume will fall. This is the Monro–Kellie doctrine. If a critical volume is reached the ICP will rise sharply as the ability to compensate has been exceeded (Fig. 6.6).

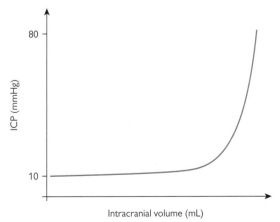

Fig. 6.6 Intracranial pressure–volume relationship. Reproduced from Catherine Spoors and Kevin Kiff, *Training in Anaesthesia*, 2010, Figure 7.32, page 159, with permission from Oxford University Press.

Normal ICP is 5–15mmHg in the supine position. ICP is closely related to intrathoracic pressure and a respiratory swing in ICP is normally seen. When ICP exceeds 20mmHg focal ischaemia occurs and above 50mmHg global ischaemia is seen.

Factors affecting intracranial pressure
These include factors that alter the volume of the intracranial contents:

Cerebral arterial blood volume
This is affected by changes in $PaCO_2$ and PaO_2, by altered cerebral metabolism, and by neurogenic mechanisms. Increased blood volume is seen in intracranial haemorrhage.

Cerebral venous blood volume
Any factor impeding venous drainage will increase cerebral venous blood volume.
Factors include patient positioning, coughing, straining, neck lines and the use of PEEP.

CSF volume
CSF is produced at a constant rate of 0.35mL/min (500mL/day) mainly by active secretion from the choroid plexus in the lateral ventricles. From here it flows to the 3rd and 4th ventricles and then to the cerebellar cisterns. The total CSF volume is 150mL. Any impedance to this flow may result in raised ICP. Venous engorgement causes dilation of the valveless Batson's plexus in the epidural space causing a displacement of CSF into the cranium.

Brain volume
Cerebral oedema, contusions, and masses cause an increase in brain volume. If too severe for compensatory mechanisms these will result in raised ICP.

Control of intraocular pressure

The globe is essentially a fixed sphere encircled in tough connective tissue within a rigid bony orbit. Normal IOP is 10–20mmHg. In open eye injuries a rise in IOP may cause extrusion of globe contents. See Box 6.11.

Determinants of IOP

Aqueous humour volume
Aqueous humour occupies the anterior chamber of the eye. It is the main compensatory mechanism for alteration in volume of other components within the globe as vitrous humour volume is relatively fixed. It is produced in the ciliary bodies via active secretion (80%) and ultrafiltration (20%). Rate of secretion is independent of IOP. Reabsorption in the trabecular network

---

Box 6.11 Anaesthetic implications of raised IOP

Induction
Thiopentone and propofol reduce IOP. Suxamethonium increases IOP and use should be based on risk vs benefit in open eye injury.

Pressor response to laryngoscopy
If unattenuated, laryngoscopy results in a 10–20mmHg rise in IOP: use high-dose opiates, deep extubation, or LMA.

Coughing and vomiting
Can cause 30–40mmHg rise in IOP. Use muscle relaxation or deep plane of anaesthesia. Avoid emesis.

Positioning
Promote venous drainage with head-up position.

Chemical control
Maintain low normal $PaCO_2$, avoid hypoxia.

and canal of Schlemm (at angle between cornea and iris) occurs directly into the episcleral veins and therefore down a pressure gradient. Hence raised IOP results in increased aqueous drainage.

Venous drainage

Episcleral venous plexuses are usually only 1–2mmHg below IOP, therefore raised CVP results in reduced aqueous humour drainage.

Arterial blood volume

Factors influencing arterial flow are analogous to CBF covered above. Of note, choroidal blood vessels do not display myogenic autoregulation.

External pressure

Pressure on the globe due to pathology such as a retrobulbar haemorrhage or local anaesthetic injection can cause a rapid increase in IOP.

Further reading

Moss E (2001). The cerebral circulation. *CEACCP*, 1(3):67–71.

Murgatroyd H & Bembridge J (2008). Intraocular pressure. *CEACCP*, 8(3):100–3.

6.5 Disorders of the autonomic nervous system

Overview of the autonomic nervous system

The ANS encompasses the neural and humoral mechanisms that control involuntary body systems. These include cardiac rate and force of contraction, vascular tone, gut motility, bladder and bronchial tone, pupillary reflexes, and glandular secretion. The ANS is controlled by centres in the CNS including the spinal cord, brainstem, and hypothalamus. The two limbs of the ANS are the parasympathetic and sympathetic systems which are tonically active and act to balance each other.

The parasympathetic nervous system (PNS) is cranio-sacral in origin and has synapses in close proximity to the effector organs. This means that the first-order neuron is long, and the second has a shorter course. Acetylcholine is the neurotransmitter at the pre- and postganglionic nerve endings. Physiological effects of PNS activation include bradycardia, reduced blood pressure, and increased gastric motility. It is the system of 'rest and digest'.

The outflow from the sympathetic nervous system (SNS) occurs from T1-L2 of the spinal cord with the majority of fibres synapsing in the paravertebral sympathetic chain. Preganglionic neurotransmission is mediated by acetylcholine whereas noradrenaline is secreted at the postganglionic nerve endings. The sympathetic second-order neurons are long since the sympathetic ganglia are distant from the effector organs. SNS stimulation increases cardiovascular activity and reduces GI motility and perfusion resulting in the 'fight or flight response'.

Primary disorders of the ANS are uncommon: however, symptomatic autonomic neuropathy is frequently seen in association with general medical conditions.

Symptoms and signs of autonomic dysfunction

See Box 6.12.

Box 6.12 Autonomic dysfunction
Symptoms
• Dizziness
• Constipation
• Fainting
• GORD
• Nocturia
• Disordered sweating
• Impotence.
Signs
• Postural hypotension
• Episodic hypertension
• Cardiac conduction defects.

Testing the autonomic nervous system

Bedside tests

Lying/standing blood pressure and pulse

A postural systolic blood pressure drop of <20mmHg from lying to standing in a euvolaemic patient suggests autonomic dysfunction.

Loss of sinus arrhythmia on palpation of the pulse (or on ECG) is abnormal.

Sustained tonic muscular activity

A sustained hand grip should, in an intact ANS, result in an increase heart rate and a rise in diastolic blood pressure of 15mmHg.

Laboratory tests

The Valsalva manoeuvre involves a forced expiration against a closed glottis, resulting in increased intrathoracic pressure of 40mmHg held for 10sec. This normally results in a characteristic cardiovascular response (Fig. 6.7) whereby blood pressure initially increased due to the transmission of intrathoracic pressure onto the aorta (phase I). Decrease venous return then activates the SNS causing tachycardia and vasoconstriction returning blood pressure to normal (phase II). With termination of the manoeuvre intrathoracic pressure falls and blood pressure falls (phase III). Restoration of venous return results in an increased cardiac output into a vasoconstricted arterial tree resulting in an overshoot of blood pressure (phase IV).

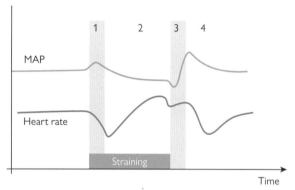

Fig. 6.7 Normal Valsalva response. Reproduced from Catherine Spoors and Kevin Kiff, *Training in Anaesthesia*, 2010, Figure 10.24, page 259, with permission from Oxford University Press.

In autonomic dysfunction the heart rate remains unchanged and the blood pressure consistently falls as compensatory mechanisms are lost (Fig. 6.8).

Tilt table testing involves close monitoring of ECG and blood pressure whilst the patient's posture is altered by adjusting the angle of the table on which they are lying (from 0° up to 80°). Postural hypotension and arrhythmias are common in autonomic dysfunction.

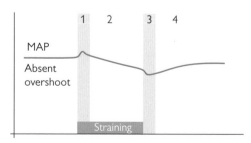

Fig. 6.8 Valsalva response in autonomic dysfunction. Reproduced from Catherine Spoors and Kevin Kiff, *Training in Anaesthesia*, 2010, Figure 10.26, page 259, with permission from Oxford University Press.

Diseases of the autonomic nervous system

Autonomic disorders have important implications for anaesthesia: see Box 6.13.

Familial dysautonomia

Familial dysautonomia is a congenital disorder in subgroup III of the hereditary sensory and autonomic neuropathies. It results from an autosomal recessive mutation on chromosome 9. It presents with vomiting, hypertension, tachycardia, sweating, and altered personality. There is a 50% mortality by 30 years of age: death occurs from aspiration or autonomic crisis.

Multisystem atrophy (Shy–Drager syndrome)

Multisystem atrophy presents in late middle age with ataxia, Parkinsonism, and progressive autonomic dysfunction. 80% of patients become disabled within 5 years, and life expectancy is <10 years post diagnosis.

Secondary acquired disorders

Diabetes mellitus, chronic alcoholism (a direct toxic effect of alcohol and associated nutritional deficiencies), Guillain–Barré syndrome, and Parkinson's disease are all associated with autonomic dysfunction. Infectious diseases such as Lyme disease, botulism, diphtheria, and leprosy may cause autonomic neuropathy.

Box 6.13 Anaesthesia in patients with autonomic dysfunction

- Premedicate with H_2 antagonists/proton pump inhibitors/metoclopramide to reduce the risk of gastric aspiration.
- Consider invasive arterial monitoring pre induction; a CVP line may aide optimization of volaemic status.
- Neuraxial blocks are controversial: they may be well tolerated since sympathetic tone may already be reduced or they can cause severe hypotension.
- Direct-acting vasopressors and atropine should be readily available. Atropine can cause a paradoxical bradycardia.
- Rapid sequence induction if at risk of aspiration. Patients with autonomic neuropathy may tolerate IPPV poorly resulting in hypotension if not adequately fluid loaded.
- Cardiovascular instability can occur including bradyarrhythmias and cardiac arrest. Laparoscopic surgery may cause greater haemodynamic disturbance when compared to open surgery.
- Slow, staged intraoperative positioning should be used to minimize haemodynamic instability.

6.6 Consequences of spinal cord injury and deafferentation

Mechanisms of cord injury

Spinal cord injuries result in motor, sensory, or autonomic disturbances, which may be temporary or permanent. Trauma is the most common mechanism for cord injury, typically affecting young adults (60% of cases occur in those <30 years of age), and are often associated with bony or ligamentous damage to the spinal column. This most frequently occurs as a result of road traffic incidents, falls, or sports injuries. Cord injury can occur at any level, but the lower cervical spine and thoracolumbar junction are particularly vulnerable.

Other mechanisms include compression by bone fragments, discs, haematoma, tumours, or spinal cord ischaemia.

Phases of injury

Immediate
Brief episode of mass sympathetic outflow at time of primary injury associated with tachycardia and hypertension. Followed by hypotension.

Acute (1–2 days)
Spinal shock, hypotension, relative or true hypovolaemia, evolving cord damage with associated flaccid paralysis.

Tonic phase (2 days to up to 12 weeks)
Return of spinal reflexes, spinal shock resolution results in spasticity, autonomic hyper-reflexia is possible.

Initial management

All trauma patients with an appropriate mechanism of injury should be presumed to have injury to the axial skeleton and should be treated with spinal precautions to prevent exacerbation of spinal injury. Initial management should be based upon ATLS guidelines so that associated injuries are not missed and life-threatening injuries are treated first.

Initial management should involve resuscitation based on an ABC approach. The patient should be immobilized on a spinal board with a hard collar to maintain alignment of the cervical spine.

Secondary cord injury should be minimized (primary injury occurs at the time of trauma–it can be prevented but not treated).

Maintaining an adequate spinal cord perfusion pressure is of great importance. The determinants of this are similar to those for cerebral perfusion pressure (see section 6.4).

Important measures therefore include:

Avoid hypotension
Spinal cord perfusion pressure should be optimized by ensuring an acceptable MAP.

Optimize respiration
Avoid hypoxia both to regulate blood flow and to ensure appropriate oxygen carriage.

Control CO_2 aiming for a $PaCO_2$ of 4–4.5kPa to prevent vasoconstriction or dilatation.

Control blood sugar
Hypo- and hyperglycaemia are associated with worse outcomes after neurological injury.

Steroids
High-dose methylprednisolone may improve long-term neurological outcome.

Temperature control
Hyperthermia is associated with a worse neurological outcome.

CSF drainage
Spinal drainage of CSF may improve cord perfusion by lowering CSF pressure around the cord.

Implications of cord injury

Airway
Should intubation be required, it should be performed with minimal movement of the cervical spine either with the collar still *in situ* or with manual in-line stabilization to maintain the neck in a neutral position. A difficult laryngoscopic view should be expected. Where difficult intubation is encountered an intubating LMA (and/or videolarnygoscope) is helpful. It is safe to use suxamethonium during the first 48–72h after spinal injury without the risk of hyperkalaemia.

An awake fibreoptic intubation with the neck immobilized in a hard collar may be the optimal management if time and expertise allow. This allows for neurology to be checked post-intubation, prior to the administration of general anaesthesia.

Respiratory
Injury at C1–C3 results in complete paralysis of respiratory muscles. Diaphragmatic function is retained with lesions below C5. If the lesion occurs between C3 and C5, diaphragmatic function may be affected.

Paralysis of intercostal muscles causes marked changes in respiratory mechanics. The chest wall is drawn inward on diaphragmatic contraction rather than moving upwards and outwards as it does in health. Respiratory efficacy is greatly reduced resulting in seesaw respiration. Loss of abdominal muscle tone results in poor cough and an inability to clear secretions. These factors result in atelectasis, alveolar hypoventilation, and respiratory failure.

Cardiovascular
Lesions above T6 result in hypotension as a result of vasodilatation due to traumatic sympathectomy and unopposed parasympathetic neural outflow, and bradycardia due to loss of cardioaccelerator fibres. A fixed heart rate results in a cardiac output, which is very dependent on stroke volume. Changes in posture or commencement of positive pressure ventilation can result in cardiovascular instability due to a fall in venous return. Neurogenic shock, therefore, should be initially managed with fluid loading. Once volaemic status has been optimized, vasopressors should be started to maintain a MAP of >80mmHg to ensure adequate spinal cord perfusion pressure. Atropine and glycopyrrolate can be given for bradycardia.

Autonomic hyper-reflexia
Autonomic hyper-reflexia can occur typically 4–6 weeks after injury, and classically is due to stimulus from visceral stretch of bladder or bowel. It can occur following somatic stimulation. Clinically, the patient exhibits profound vasoconstriction below the level of the spinal cord lesion due to unopposed sympathetic

outflow, since loss of the normal descending inhibitory pathways has occurred. The resultant hypertension and reflex, vagally-mediated, bradycardia is often associated with flushing above the lesion, headache, and sweating. Initial management involves removal of the stimulus and pharmacological treatment of the hypertension with α-blocking vasodilators.

Thromboembolism
Due to paralysis and venous stasis, DVT is very common. It should be prevented with TED stockings and LMWH.

Constipation
Constipation must be avoided due to the risk of autonomic hyper-reflexia. The combination of reduced mobility and loss of bowel sensation make bowel impaction common.

Patterns of cord injury

Level of injury
Neurological level of injury is the most distal uninvolved spinal cord segment, not necessarily the level of bony trauma.

An incomplete cord lesion will have partial preservation of neurological function at a level below the cord injury. A complete lesion results in paralysis and loss of sensation below the lesion.

Brown–Sequard syndrome
This occurs following hemisection of the spinal cord. It results in ipsilateral loss of modalities carried in the dorsal columns (fine touch and proprioception) and corticospinal tracts (motor function) as these decussate above the level of the lesion. There is contralateral loss of afferent input from the spinothalamic tracts (pain and temperature).

Anterior spinal cord syndrome
This is due to anterior spinal cord ischaemia and results in loss of motor function, pain, and temperature sensory loss below the level of the lesion. Dorsal column function is preserved (proprioception and fine touch).

Cauda equina syndrome
This represents damage to the leash of nerves below the conus medullaris (L1–S5 roots). Symptoms include leg weakness, saddle anaesthesia, bladder and sexual dysfunction, and decreased anal tone.

Prognosis

Prognosis after spinal cord injury depends on the level and completeness of the lesion. Patients with complete cord injury have very little chance of recovery, especially if paralysis is present after >72h. Incomplete lesions have a much better outlook.

Further reading

Denton M & McKinlay J (2009). Cervical cord injury and critical care. *CEACCP*, 9(3):82–6.

Veale P & Lamb J (2002). Anaesthesia and acute spinal cord injury. *CEACCP*, 2(5):139–42.

6.7 Neuromuscular blocking drugs

History

Tubocurare alkaloids, the precursor of the modern non-depolarizing NMBAs, were prepared from the *Chrondrodendrum tomentosum* vine and used as hunting poisons by the Macoushi Indians in South America. Charles Waterton discovered them early in the 19th century, but they were not introduced into clinical practice until 1952 when Griffiths and Johnson marketed introcostrin.

Structure–activity relationship

All neuromuscular blocking drugs have at least two charged nitrogen atoms. The distance between the nitrogen atoms (the intraonium distance) that gives the highest affinity is 12.5A (Amstrong units) and the potency of the drug falls if this distance is increased or reduced.

For a nicotinic receptor on the postsynaptic membrane to open, two acetylcholine (ACh) molecules must bind with the ACh binding site on the two α subunits simultaneously. This causes a conformational change in the nicotinic receptor which results in a localized miniature end-plate potential in the muscle cell membrane. If enough nicotinic receptors are activated at the same time, a threshold potential is reached, the muscle cell membrane will depolarize, and an action potential will spread along the muscle cell membrane. Calcium ions then enter the muscle cytoplasm resulting in contraction of the muscle cell.

Non-depolarizing drugs probably work by competitively binding with the ACh binding sites on the α subunit of the nicotinic receptor. One theory is that one of the nitrogen atoms on the drug molecule binds with a high affinity to an accessory binding site on the α subunit a short distance from the ACh binding site, holding the drug molecule on the receptor. The second nitrogen atom then competes with ACh for the binding site.

Depolarizing agents may work by an agonist effect on the nicotinic receptor, although they may have other actions such as inhibiting the acetylcholinesterase enzyme in the synaptic cleft, potentiating the duration of action of ACh or they may have presynaptic actions.

Pharmacokinetics

Empirically it has been observed that the most potent neuromuscular blocking drugs have a slow onset and a long duration, but weak drugs have a fast onset and short duration. With a 2× ED95 dose the duration of action is typically about 7× the onset time. Attempts to introduce weak drugs into clinical practice have been unsuccessful as weak agents have a high incidence of side effects.

Depolarizing drugs

Suxamethonium is the only depolarizing drug that is commonly used (Fig. 6.9).

Suxamethonium

This drug has a fast onset, a paralysing dose typically acting within 45sec. In most people it is rapidly broken down by plasma cholinesterase with a short duration of action of about 5min. However, in people with reduced levels of plasma cholinesterase (genetic predisposition, liver failure, pregnancy) it has a longer duration of action and may result in significant paralysis for up to 4h.

Two molecules of ACh

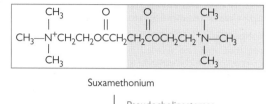

Suxamethonium

Pseudocholinesterase

Choline + Succinylmonocholine

Pseudocholinesterase

Choline + Succinic acid

Fig. 6.9 Structure of suxamethonium. Reproduced from Catherine Spoors and Kevin Kiff, *Training in Anaesthesia*, 2010, Figure 8.13, page 217, with permission from Oxford University Press.

Suxamethonium has a high incidence of side effects that include muscle pains, arrhythmias (particularly bradycardia following multiple doses), raised intraocular and intracranial pressure, hyperkalaemia (especially with severe burns, paraplegia, extensive muscle damage, and peripheral neuropathies), histamine release, and anaphylactoid reactions. It is also a trigger for malignant hyperpyrexia.

Non-depolarizing drugs

Steroid molecules

Pancuronium

This was the first steroid non-depolarizing muscle relaxant introduced. It is potent (intubating dose 0.05mg/kg) with a slow onset (5min) and long duration (45min) and is highly protein bound. It is associated with a small degree of vagal blockade which results in some tachycardia.

Vecuronium

This has an intermediate potency (intubating dose 0.1mg/kg), onset (3min) and duration (25min) with few side effects. It is metabolized in the liver and excreted unchanged in urine and faeces. .

Rocuronium

This is an intermediate potency drug (intubating dose 1mg/kg), with an intermediate duration (25min), but an unusually fast onset (1min). As such is does not fit the onset/offset relationship seen with most other agents. About 30% is protein bound and it is excreted unchanged in bile and urine.

Benzylisoquinolium molecules

Atracurium

This is an intermediate potency (intubating dose 0.6mg/kg) non-depolarizing drug with intermediate onset (4min) and duration (25min). It was designed to undergo Hofmann elimination (spontaneous degradation of the molecule at high pH and temperature), although redistribution and metabolism by cholinesterases also contribute to recovery. It has 16 potential isomers, 12 of which are found in the clinical preparation. A purified isomer, cisatracurium, is available. Laudanosine, a by-product of Hofmann elimination, is associated with epileptic activity, but this is not normally clinically relevant as laudanosine is eliminated rapidly.

Mivacurium

This is an intermediate potency (intubating dose 0.2mg/kg) drug with an intermediate onset (3min) and duration (15min). It undergoes metabolism by liver cholinesterases and so may be the agent of choice where reversal with neostigmine is undesirable. It potentially has a prolonged duration in patients with liver failure. It has three possible isomers.

Non-depolarizing drugs no longer in use

Tubocurarine was the first muscle relaxant drug in clinical use. It has a high incidence of histamine release and is associated with ganglion blockade.

Gallamine is unusual in that it has 3 charged nitrogen atoms and depends on renal excretion for elimination.

Alcuronium is a slow-onset, long-acting agent.

Rapacuronium is a weak steroid muscle relaxant with a fast onset (1.5min) and short duration (15min). It was introduced in 2001, but withdrawn because of a high incidence of side effects, notably bronchospasm.

Reversal techniques

Non-drug techniques

The effects of all neuromuscular blocking drugs will wear off if given enough time. They may be metabolized to an inactive form, excreted unchanged in urine or bile or redistributed to other tissues.

Anticholinesterase drugs

These drugs prevent ACh breakdown by anticholinesterase and therefore increase ACh activity at the neuromuscular junction.

Neostigmine

An intermediate-acting anticholinesterase drug used to reverse non-depolarizing neuromuscular blockade. It causes bradycardia by potentiation of ACh activity on the heart and so is commonly administered with a cholinergic agent such as glycopyrrolate.

Physostigmine

A long-acting anticholinesterase normally used in the treatment of myasthenia gravis.

Chelating agents

Sugammadex

This is a cyclodextrin–a toroid (doughnut shaped) structure with 8 linked sugar molecules (Fig. 6.10). It is hydrophilic on the outside and so it is water soluble, but its core is lipophilic. This structure facilitates the chelation of steroid molecules, with the steroid molecule bound with high affinity in the centre of the complex. The sugammadex/steroid complex is inactive and excreted unchanged in the urine (Box 6.14). Sugammadex has a high affinity for rocuronium and may reverse an intubating dose of rocuronium within 3min, which allows a rocuronium/sugammadex technique to be used for rapid sequence induction. Sugammadex binds with and reverses the effects of all the steroid muscle relaxants, but not the non-steroid muscle relaxants. It has a faster action than neostigmine with low risk of residual block and has few side effects.

> **Box 6.14 Properties of sugammadex**
> - Volume of distribution 10–15L
> - Half-life 2.5h
> - > 90% excreted within 24h
> - 2mg/kg for reversal of shallow block–effect in 1–1.5min
> - 4mg/kg for reversal of profound block—effect in 2–3min
> - 16mg/kg for immediate reversal—effect in 3.5–5min

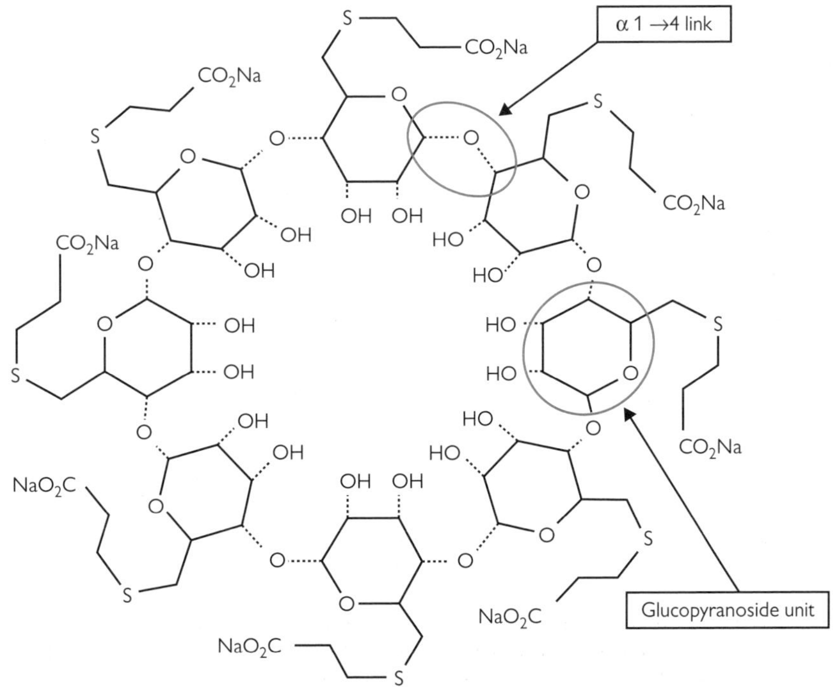

Fig. 6.10 Structure of sugammadex. Reproduced from Welliver M, 'Update for nurse anesthetists. Part 3. Cyclodextrin introduction to anesthesia practice: form, function, and application', *AANA Journal*, 75, pp. 289–296, Copyright 2007 American Association of Nurse Anaesthetists, with permission.

Muscle relaxants and neuromuscular disorders

Depolarizing muscle relaxants

In neuromuscular disorders where muscle is denervated or prolonged disuse has occurred, extrajunctional nicotinic ACh receptors may develop. If suxamethonium is administered in this situation, a potentially life-threatening hyperkalaemia can occur.

In myotonic conditions, suxamethonium can precipitate severe muscle spasm and this may also affect the masseter muscles impacting on airway management.

Myasthenic conditions may actually show resistance to suxamethonium and require twice the usual dose.

Non depolarizing neuromuscular blockers

Most patients with neuromuscular disorders will show increased sensitivity to these drugs and may only require 10–20% of the usual dose. Prolonged block and inadequate reversal may lead to respiratory failure and bulbar weakness.

Reversal of muscle relaxation

Anticholinesterases may cause hyperkalaemia by the same mechanism as suxamethonium in neuromuscular disorders. They may precipitate a cholinergic crisis in myasthenia.

Sugammadex has increasingly been used with success to reverse aminosteroids adequately in these patients.

Further reading

Srivaslava A & Hunter JM (2009). Reversal of neuromuscular block. *Br J Anaesth,* 103(1):115–29.

6.8 Monitoring neuromuscular blockade

Clinical tests

Bedside tests can be subjective, e.g. head lift, or objective, e.g. changes in FEV$_1$. They can only be done on conscious patients.

Supramaximal stimulation

During the 19th century, scientists discovered that electrical stimuli applied to a nerve cause the muscle it supplies to contract. As the nerve stimulus increases so does the muscle response as more nerve axons are recruited. The muscle response plateaus when all the nerve axons have been recruited. Further increases in nerve stimulus cause some axons to be recruited for a second time, even further increasing the muscle response. The 'supramaximal stimulus' was developed to give a standard response, with a stimulus large enough (50–80mA) to recruit all the axons, but short enough (0.1–0.2msec) to recruit them only once.

Muscle response

Measurement of muscle response may be by:
- Mechanomyography—measures the force of contraction.
- Accelerography—measures movement caused by muscle contraction.
- Electromyography—measures electrical activity in the muscle.

As these measure different responses, direct comparisons between studies using different modalities are inappropriate.

Methods of stimulation

Repeated T1 twitch
Repeated supramaximal stimuli are administered to a nerve at low rates (0.1Hz) of stimulation. The magnitude of muscle response falls with increasing blockade until there is no response.

Advantages
- It measures depolarizing and non-depolarizing blockade.

Disadvantages
- A baseline response is required before paralysis.
- A wandering baseline affects results and 'recovery' may be to a greater or lesser response than the initial baseline response.
- Stimuli at different rates of stimulation give different results.

Tetanic stimulation
Repeated supramaximal stimuli are applied to the nerve at high (50Hz) rates of stimulation. The magnitude of fade in muscle response reflects the degree of non-depolarizing blockade.

Advantages
- It gives a more 'physiological' response than T1.
- The baseline is established shortly before the degree of fade is assessed, so wandering baseline is not a problem.

Disadvantages
- The stimulus is painful in conscious patients.
- It is not useful for assessing onset of blockade.
- A single tetanic stimulus affects subsequent responses.

- Repeated tetanic stimuli result in a faster recovery from blockade in that motor unit, but not in other muscle groups giving a false appearance of early recovery.
- It does not measure depolarizing blockade.

Train of Four (ToF) fade
It was empirically found that significant fade occurs during non-depolarizing blockade with intermediate rates of stimulation. If four supramaximal stimuli are given at 2Hz, the height of the 4th twitch can be compared with the first, giving the ToF ratio.

Advantages
- A ToF stimulus can be repeated every 10sec without affecting subsequent stimuli.
- Repeated ToF stimuli can be used to monitor onset of and recovery from blockade.
- Minor degrees of block can be identified and quantified.
- The baseline (T1 twitch) is only 1.5sec before the assessed (T4 twitch) so a wandering baseline is not an issue.

Disadvantages
- It does not measure deep levels of blockade.
- It does not measure depolarizing blockade.

Post-tetanic count
Following a 50Hz tetanic stimulus supramaximal twitches at 1Hz are administered and the number of responses counted. In non-depolarizing block there is potentiation of the T1 twitch following a titanic stimulus but this does not occur during depolarizing block. The lower the post-tetanic count the greater the degree of blockade.

Advantages
- It assesses deep levels of blockade.

Disadvantages
- It does not assess depolarizing block.

Double burst suppression
Two 50Hz tetanic bursts lasting 750msec separated by 500msec are administered. The presence of fade in the second tetanic stimulus indicates a small residual degree of blockade.

Advantages
- It assesses minor degrees of blockade.

Disadvantages
- It does not measure depolarizing blockade.

Features of neuromuscular blockade

Total paralysis
- There is no response to any mode of stimulation.

Partial depolarizing blockade
- Depression of T1 twitch.
- Depression of tetanic response, but no fade.
- No post tetanic potentiation.
- No ToF fade.
- No fade with double burst stimulation.

Partial non-depolarizing blockade

- Depression of T1 twitch.
- Depression of tetanic response with fade.
- Post tetanic potentiation.
- ToF fade.
- Fade with double burst stimulation.

Neuromuscular responses

Fig. 6.11 demonstrates the neuromuscular responses in non-paralysed, completely paralysed, and partial depolarizing and non-depolarizing block.

The figure shows the response to repeat T1 twitch, tetanic stimulation and post tetanic response, train of four fade, and response to double burst suppression.

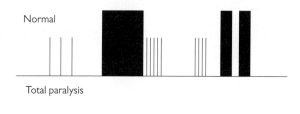

Normal

Total paralysis

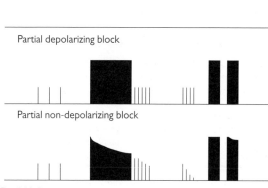

Partial depolarizing block

Partial non-depolarizing block

Fig. 6.11 Response patterns in neuromuscular block.

Chapter 7

General therapeutics

161

7.1 Drug toxicity in anaesthesia

Patients undergoing anaesthesia are exposed to a wide variety of drugs. Important examples of potential toxicity from amongst these many and disparate agents are discussed in this section. Local anaesthetic toxicity is discussed in section 19.2.

Propofol

Propofol became available in its current lipid emulsion formulation some 30 years ago. It gained rapid popularity owing to several advantages—most especially rapid recovery characteristics and laryngeal reflex suppression. As an intravenous induction agent, it has an excellent safety record, and its use has been successfully extended both to anaesthesia maintenance and to (usually short-term) sedation in ITU.

In longer-term use (>72h), however, especially at high doses, propofol has been associated with a range of toxic reactions, including metabolic acidosis, rhabdomyolysis, cardiac failure, and death. The term 'propofol infusion syndrome' (PRIS) was first used in the context of *paediatric* patients in 1998, but more recently, similar cases have been described in adult patients (Box 7.1).

Box 7.1 Clinical features of possible propofol infusion syndrome
• Prolonged, high infusion rates (>5mg/kg/h for >48h) • Metabolic acidosis and hyperkalaemia • Raised creatine kinase/rhabdomyolysis/haematuria • Bradyarrhythmias/depressed myocardial function • Absence of other obvious clinical cause

The clinical features of PRIS are similar to those of the mitochondrial myopathies in which there is a disturbance of lipid metabolism in cardiac and skeletal muscle. It has been suggested that diversion from carbohydrate to fat metabolism may trigger PRIS, possibly in patients with a genetic susceptibility, and that there is a failure of mitochondrial free fatty acid metabolism in these patients. Children have smaller carbohydrate stores than adults. They also require relatively larger doses of propofol for sedation, and may therefore be more susceptible. Additionally, ensuring adequate carbohydrate intake may help prevent PRIS (see Box 7.2).

Box 7.2 Treatment and prevention of propofol infusion syndrome
Treatment: • Stop the infusion • Consider haemofiltration to remove propofol • Consider cardiac pacing if refractory bradycardia • Maintain ionized calcium >1.0mmol/L. *Prevention:* • Avoid prolonged infusions above 5mg/kg/h • Avoid use of propofol as sole sedative agent • Aggressive early feeding.

Hyperlipidaemia has been reported in patients receiving prolonged propofol ITU sedation, even in doses well below those recommended for TPN in critically ill patients.

Additionally, infective complications have been reported, and an aseptic technique is recommended when handling propofol. Unused propofol should be discarded 6h after opening.

Volatile anaesthetic agents

The toxic potential of volatile halogenated anaesthetic agents derives from their hepatic or renal metabolism. The degree of metabolism of a volatile agent depends partly on the amount absorbed, and therefore correlates quite well with solubility in blood and other tissues (see Table 7.1).

Table 7.1 Blood-gas partition coefficients and rates of metabolism of volatile agents		
	Blood-gas partition coefficient	Rate of metabolism
Halothane	2.30	20%
Enflurane	1.80	2%
Isoflurane	1.41	0.2%
Desflurane	0.42	0.01%
Sevoflurane	0.69	3–5%

The liver is the major organ for metabolism, and up to one-third of inhaled halothane undergoes oxidative metabolism by cytochrome p450 enzymes. Trifluoroacetyl chloride is formed as an intermediate, and has a high ability to acetylate liver proteins. The degree of metabolism of enflurane, isoflurane, and desflurane is much lower than that of halothane, and severe hepatic injury from these agents is rare. Sevoflurane is also metabolized by cytochrome p450 enzymes, but trifluoroacetyl compounds are not formed: one of the important degradation products is inorganic fluoride.

The major organs affected by volatile agent toxicity are the liver and kidney. An association between halothane exposure and severe liver dysfunction became apparent shortly after its clinical introduction in the late 1950s. Two forms of injury are recognized: a rare, but often fatal hepatic necrosis with an estimated incidence of 1:35 000, contrasting with a mild, but much more common, form of hepatocellular injury that can be observed in up to 20% of exposed patients.

In the mild form of halothane-induced injury, there is acetylation of liver proteins usually manifest as a transient elevation of liver enzymes. The severe form is *immune-mediated* in susceptible individuals—antibodies form against these acetylated neo-antigens. Enflurane, isoflurane, and desflurane may also trigger fulminant hepatic injury through the same mechanism, but much less commonly.

The vast majority of patients with severe hepatic damage have a history of one or more halothane anaesthetics, sometimes many years previously. The risk is higher in females and in obese patients, and lower in children. Cross-sensitization between volatile agents can occur in susceptible patients, and it is recommended that no other halogenated agent be used in patients who have experienced hepatic dysfunction after exposure to any one of them. Sevoflurane might possibly be safe because of its different metabolic pathway, but there are no clinical data to support this.

Sevoflurane has been the subject of concern in respect of possible nephrotoxicity from inorganic fluoride and compound A.

Inorganic fluoride was thought to be nephrotoxic when methoxyflurane was found to cause renal dysfunction. Methoxyflurane is metabolized to inorganic fluoride, and levels correlated with the degree of renal injury. It was concluded that circulating inorganic fluoride was nephrotoxic at serum concentrations in excess of 50µmol/L.

Sevoflurane undergoes liver metabolism to inorganic fluoride and hexafluoroisopropanol. Concentrations of inorganic fluoride often exceed 50µmol/l after prolonged sevoflurane anaesthesia and yet there are no reports of renal toxicity. The assumption is that it is not, in fact, circulating inorganic fluoride that is the nephrotoxin, but actually that methoxyflurane nephrotoxicity results from local cytochrome p450 enzyme activity *within the kidney* causing defluorination of the parent molecule. This local enzyme activity has a tenfold higher affinity for methoxyflurane than for sevoflurane.

Compound A is a vinyl ether that forms within circle systems, as a degradation product from sevoflurane within CO_2 absorbers, especially at low fresh gas flows. Nephrotoxicity is clearly demonstrable in rats, according to the levels of compound A present and the duration of the exposure.

To date, there are no robust data to suggest that compound A is capable of causing renal toxicity in humans, nor indeed, in any species other than rodents.

Nitrous oxide

Nitrous oxide (N_2O) has been in continuous clinical use for 150 years. In the 1950s, a case series was published reporting megaloblastic changes in the bone marrow following prolonged exposure. Subsequent work confirmed that an interaction with vitamin B_{12} and folate metabolism was the underlying mechanism for N_2O toxicity.

Vitamin B_{12} serves as a co-enzyme for methionine synthetase. Methionine plays a crucial role as a methyl-group donor in several synthetic pathways, including DNA synthesis. In addition to vitamin B_{12}, methionine synthetase also requires 5-methyl-tetrahydrofolate as a co-enzyme.

Only the *reduced* form of vitamin B_{12} serves as a co-enzyme for methionine synthetase. N_2O causes rapid oxidation of B_{12} and thus inhibits methionine synthetase activity. Enzyme activity is reduced by half within 1h exposure to 70% N_2O, and takes 3–4 days to recover, suggesting that B_{12} inactivation may be irreversible and that *de novo* vitamin B_{12} is required.

Exposures of 6h or less appear to have no effect on bone marrow morphology or function, but more prolonged exposure has been demonstrated to cause megaloblastic changes and impaired bone marrow function. Shorter exposures may be significant in patients with pre-existing deficiencies of vitamin B_{12} or folate.

In addition, long-term N_2O exposure has been linked with neurological symptoms, the commonest of which are numbness or tingling in the extremities, with improvement following folic acid therapy.

The case is unproven in respect of a potential adverse effect on healthcare personnel of trace exposure to N_2O or other anaesthetic agents—there is no clear evidence of teratogenicity or organ toxicity, following initial studies suggesting reduced fertility and increased rates of abortion in healthcare workers exposed to trace levels of N_2O. Nonetheless, low-flow techniques and scavenging should routinely be used to reduce exposure.

Opioid toxicity

Central nervous system
The most serious, and potentially fatal, effect of opioids is respiratory depression, which is the usual cause of death in accidental or intended overdose. The risk is increased at extremes of age, when there is coexistent respiratory disease or sleep apnoea, and in the presence of other sedatives, particularly benzodiazepines.

Other CNS manifestations of opioid toxicity include:
- Nausea and vomiting: direct chemoreceptor trigger zone (CTZ) stimulation.
- Serotonin syndrome: pethidine and tramadol interact with MAOIs and SSRIs.
- Opioid-induced neurotoxicity (OIN): has been described with high-dose opioid use in palliative care, presenting with myoclonus and seizures.
- Seizures: have been linked with *tramadol* but unlikely in the absence of additional risk factors (history of epilepsy or additional drug therapies that lower the seizure threshold).

Cardiovascular system
Most opioids cause a relative bradycardia from a vagomimetic action combined with reduced central sympathetic outflow. Hypotension may be seen, typically with morphine, due to histamine release causing vasodilatation. High-dose opioid therapy is associated with pulmonary oedema, which is thought more likely to represent increased capillary permeability, rather than direct myocardial depression.

Gastrointestinal system
In terms of the symptomatic burden on patients, GI side effects are an important consideration in respect of opioid therapy. Constipation is a particular problem when opioid therapy accompanies a postoperative ileus, and also during long-term use for chronic pain. Opioids also cause delayed gastric emptying, and contraction of the sphincter of Oddi and distal common bile duct.

Muscle relaxants

Until the advent of mechanical ventilation, all neuromuscular blocking drugs (NMBs) could be considered lethal toxins.

Clinical studies of NMB toxicity are difficult to design, because of the requirement for mechanical ventilation and anaesthesia. In clinical doses, there appear to be no teratogenic effects, but high and repetitive doses during LSCS may cause fetal muscle weakness, especially if the fetus is hypoxic and/or acidotic.

Clinically, the most important side-effects of NMBs relate to perioperative anaphylaxis (see section 7.4); the benzylisoquinoline agents (e.g. atracurium) cause direct histamine release from mast cells, in addition to potential IgE-mediated reactions.

Long-term administration of muscle relaxants in ITU is associated with persistent weakness. Appropriate sedation practices (see section 20.5) should be designed to minimize NMB exposure.

Suxamethonium is associated with a number of important reactions, including:
- Potent trigger for malignant hyperpyrexia (MH) in susceptible individuals
- Hyperkalaemia, rhabdomyolysis, and MH-like reactions in patients with muscle disorders
- Bradycardia (and even asystole)—especially after repeated doses.

Further reading

Best Practice & Research Clinical Anesthesiology [Whole issue], 2003; 17(1):1–161.

7.2 Initial management of acute poisoning

Drug poisoning or overdose—both accidental and intentional—is an important cause of mortality and morbidity, especially amongst the young. Approximately 2000 deaths occur in the UK each year through intentional self-poisoning, and a further 1000 deaths occur following accidental ingestion.

Evaluation of the poisoned patient

A systematic approach is important in evaluation and management. A brief initial examination is required to assess vital signs. In the seriously ill patient, resuscitation should proceed along an ABC approach. Self-evidently, critically ill patients with CNS depression will require airway protection.

Toxidromes

Several classes of toxin produce characteristic constellations of signs and symptoms, known as 'toxidromes' (Table 7.2). There may be overlapping features between them, and concomitant medications (e.g. β-blockade) may obtund typical responses. Nonetheless, eliciting a toxidrome may help narrow the differential diagnosis in the case of a critically ill patient with an unknown overdose.

Hyperthermic syndromes

Several toxic syndromes are recognized in which hyperthermia is a particular feature:

- *Sympathomimetics*: drugs such as cocaine and amphetamines produce cause thermal deregulation through excess serotonin and dopamine. Treatment is predominantly supportive, including active cooling ± benzodiazepines
- *Uncoupling syndrome*: disruption of oxidative phosphorylation generates heat, and may occur in severe salicylate poisoning
- *Serotonin syndrome*: presents with rigidity, hyper-reflexia and hyperthermia—may be seen with MAOI interactions (e.g. with pethidine)
- *Neuroleptic malignant syndrome*: associated with dopamine receptor antagonists or withdrawal of L-DOPA therapy. Dantrolene has been used in therapy.
- *Malignant hyperthermia*: occurs during exposure to volatile agents or depolarizing neuromuscular blockers in genetically susceptible individuals.

ECG abnormalities

An ECG should routinely be performed, and may provide both diagnostic and prognostic information (see Box 7.3).

Box 7.3 ECG changes in poisoning

Bradycardia or AV block
β-blockers, calcium antagonists, digoxin, opioids, organophosphates.

Tachyarrhythmias
Sympathomimetics (cocaine, amphetamine, theophylline), anticholinergics (e.g. tricyclics), thyroid hormones.

Prolonged QT interval
Tricyclics, phenothiazines, antihistamines (e.g. terfenadine), antiarrhythmics (e.g. quinidine, procainamide, amiodarone, disopyramide).

Laboratory screens

- *Routine in all patients*: urea and electrolytes, creatinine, and glucose.
- *Toxic screens*: measurement of paracetamol and salicylate levels is strongly recommended for patients with an uncertain history or those with intentional poisoning—even lethal doses may produce few clinical signs, and specific treatment instituted early may be lifesaving.
- Inexpensive immunoassay screens are now readily available to provide rapid detection in urine of numerous agents including opioids, benzodiazepines, cocaine metabolites, and tricyclics. Interpretation requires caution, however, and, whether positive or negative, the results may not provide reliable information on the nature, timing or amount of exposure.
- *Serum osmolal gap*: this is the difference between measured serum osmolality (Osm_M) and the calculated osmolality (Osm_C), where $Osm_C = (2[Na^+] + [urea] + [glucose])$. The normal osmolal gap ($Osm_M - Osm_C$) is ≤10mOsm/kg. A high serum osmolal gap is typical of alcohol poisoning (e.g. ethanol, methanol, ethylene glycol).
- *Arterial blood gases and anion gap*: the presence of a metabolic acidosis with a raised anion gap ($[Na^+] + [Cl^- + HCO_3^-]$) indicates an excess of unmeasured anions—either endogenous (e.g. lactate) or exogenous (e.g. salicylates). The normal anion gap is 8–16mmol/L. A worsening anion gap acidosis in a poisoned patient should prompt a search for acidic toxins or metabolites (e.g. salicylates, ethanol, ibuprofen) or for toxins that cause a lactic acidosis (e.g. cyanide, iron). Many mnemonics are used to recall the causes of a high anion gap acidosis: perhaps the most complete is 'cute dimples' (Box 7.4).

Table 7.2 Toxidromes					
Toxidrome	Mental status	Pupils	Vital signs	Other features	Examples
Opioid	Sedation, coma	Miosis	Low RR, HR, BP	Pulmonary oedema, needle marks, hypore-flexia	Diamorphine Morphine Oxycodone
Anticholinergic	Agitation, delirium. hallucinations, coma	Mydriasis	High RR, HR, BP Hyperthermia	Dry, flushed skin	Antihistamines Tricyclic antide-pressants
Sympathomimetic	Agitation, hallucinations, paranoia	Mydriasis	High RR, HR, BP Hyperthermia	Sweating, hyperreflexia, seizures	Cocaine Am-phetamines Theophylline
Cholinergic	Confusion, coma	Miosis	Bradycardia High or low BP + RR	Salivation, sweating, diarrhoea, seizures	Organophos-phates Nicotine
Sedative-hypnotic	CNS depression: Confusion, stupor, coma	Normal or miosis	Low RR Usually low HR + BP Hypothermia	Hyporeflexia	Benzodiazepines Barbiturates Alcohol
Serotonin syndrome	Confusion, agitation Coma	Mydriasis	High RR, HR, BP Hyperthermia	Tremor, clonus, hyper-reflexia	MAOIs alone or with SSRIs

Box 7.4 Causes of a high anion gap metabolic acidosis		
C	cyanide	D	diabetic ketoacidosis
U	uraemia	I	isoniazid, ibuprofen, iron
T	toluene	M	methanol
E	ethanol	P	propylene glycol
		L	lactic acidosis
		E	ethylene glycol
		S	salicylates

General approach to treatment

Treatment will always include supportive care, supported by techniques to reduce absorption ('decontamination') or enhance elimination. Specific antidotes may be available, depending on the poison(s) involved.

Supportive care

In addition to an ABC approach to resuscitation, the following problems may require immediate attention:

Hypotension

The initial approach should be treatment with IV fluids ± vasopressors. Refractory hypotension will require invasive monitoring to guide further treatment. Inotropes should be used with caution, and may precipitate arrhythmias. When a specific aetiology is suspected, antidotes may be used to treat hypotension, e.g. naloxone (opioids), glucagon (β-blockers), digoxin-specific antibodies (digoxin). Hypotension with bradycardia is strongly suggestive of poisoning with β-blockers, digoxin, or calcium antagonists.

Arrhythmias

Arrhythmias associated with poisoning should, in most instances, *not* be treated with standard antiarrhythmic agents as first-line therapy. Aggravating factors such as hypoxia, acidosis, hypokalaemia, or hypomagnesaemia should initially be corrected.

Bradyarrhythmias associated with hypotension may require atropine or temporary pacing but calcium, glucagon, or digoxin-specific antibodies may obviate the need for further measures in cases of calcium antagonist, β-blocker, or digoxin poisoning respectively.

QRS widening and tachyarrhythmias in the context of *tricyclic* overdose should be treated with sodium bicarbonate as first-line therapy. DC cardioversion may produce asystole.

Torsades de pointes (polymorphic VT) may be seen following poisoning with agents that prolong the QT interval and should be treated with magnesium sulphate (2g over 2–5min); overdrive pacing may also be used.

Narrow complex tachycardias and hypertension usually reflect hyperadrenergic states (e.g. cocaine or amphetamine poisoning) and treatment consists primarily of benzodiazepines. β-blockers should be avoided, and DC cardioversion is rarely effective.

Seizures

Seizures are common in poisoning or withdrawal states. After supportive measures and correction of hypoglycaemia, benzodiazepines are first-line therapy for toxin-induced seizures. Propofol has emerged as second-line therapy for refractory seizures. Phenytoin should generally be avoided, as it may aggravate the overall picture in poisoning cases. In the rare instance of seizures due to isoniazid overdose, pyridoxine (vitamin B_6) is required.

Hyperthermia

A core temperature of >39.0°C requires active cooling to lessen the risk of complications such as rhabdomyolysis, acute renal failure and DIC. In hyperadrenergic states, intravenous benzodiazepines are the drugs of choice. In patients with resistant hyperthermia, a discussion should take place with a clinical toxicologist—therapy with dantrolene or cyproheptadine (a serotonin antagonist) may be advised in selected cases.

Decontamination

Whilst no controlled trials have confirmed an actual reduction in mortality or morbidity from GI decontamination, it is believed to help some poisoned patients. Activated charcoal (AC) has emerged as the preferred technique: other methods include gastric lavage, induced emesis and whole bowel irrigation.

Activated charcoal is an insoluble, fine carbon powder capable of adsorbing toxin molecules, thereby reducing absorption. Of the various methods of GI decontamination, AC is likely to be most effective. It is best administered within an hour of toxin ingestion. The usual dose is 1g/kg, administered orally or via an orogastric tube. It is contraindicated in patients with an unprotected airway. Endotracheal intubation for the *sole* indication of AC administration is usually not recommended. The commonest serious complication is aspiration.

Gastric lavage is no longer recommended for routine use in the majority of poisoned patients. It is less effective than AC in reducing toxin absorption, and is associated with a higher incidence of aspiration, endotracheal intubation and ITU admission.

Similarly, there is no evidence that use of ipecacuana for *induced emesis* improves outcome, and it has been superseded by activated charcoal.

Whole bowel irrigation involves enteral administration of a polyethylene glycol balanced electrolyte solution, and may be effective for agents not well adsorbed by AC (e.g. lithium). In other instances, AC remains the preferred agent.

Enhanced elimination

In the severely poisoned patient, enhancing toxin elimination may improve outcome for some poisonings.

Urine alkalinization with $NaHCO_3$ favours excretion of toxins that are excreted as weak acids in the urine. The reaction

$$HA \leftrightarrow H^+ + A^-$$

is shifted to the right by alkalinization, favouring an increase in charged salt (A^-), which is more readily excreted. The technique is most commonly used in salicylate and phenobarbital poisoning.

Haemodialysis or haemofiltration may be considered in severe poisoning: generally, toxins should be of low molecular weight, minimally protein-bound and with a low volume of distribution, e.g. salicylates, lithium, and toxic alcohols.

Antidote therapy

Several specific antidotes may be employed in individual poisoning cases (see Box 7.5 and section 7.3).

Box 7.5 Major antidotes
• N-acetylcysteine (paracetamol)
• Glucagon (β-blockers)
• Digoxin-specific abs (digoxin)
• Naloxone (opioids)
• Flumazenil (benzodiazepines)
• Desferrioxamine (iron)
• $NaHCO_3$ (tricyclics)
• EDTA (heavy metals)
• Dicobalt edetate/hydroxycobalamin (cyanide)
• Atropine + pralidoxime (organophosphates)
• Ethanol (ethylene glycol / methanol).

7.3 Management of specific poisons

Paracetamol remains the most common drug taken in overdose in the UK (see Box 7.6 for other examples), accounting for some 50% of cases.

Box 7.6 Drugs commonly involved in UK poisoning cases

- Paracetamol
- Aspirin and NSAIDs
- Benzodiazepines
- Cocaine, ecstasy and other 'social' drugs
- Alcohol
- Antidepressants (tricyclics and SSRIs)
- Opioids
- Aminophylline
- Digoxin.

Paracetamol

Paracetamol poisoning causes about 150–200 deaths a year through acute liver failure and is also a common indication for super-urgent liver transplantation.

At therapeutic doses, 90% of paracetamol undergoes conjugation with glucuronide and sulphide in the liver before renal excretion. About 2% is excreted unchanged in the urine. The remainder is metabolized via hepatic cytochrome p450 enzymes into a highly reactive intermediate, N-acetyl-p-benzoquinone mine, which is normally rapidly and harmlessly conjugated with hepatic glutathione, forming products that are excreted in the urine. In overdose, however, the glucuronide and sulphide pathways become saturated, leading to a greater proportion being metabolized via the cytochrome p450 pathway. Injury begins when hepatic glutathione stores become 70–80% depleted. N-acetyl-p-benzoquinone mine binds irreversibly to cysteine groups on liver macromolecules, causing oxidative injury and hepatocellular necrosis.

Acting as a glutathione donor, intravenous *N-acetylcysteine* (NAC) is almost 100% effective as an antidote if administered within 8h of ingestion.

The hepatotoxic dose of paracetamol is generally accepted as 150mg/kg. Two groups of factors have been identified as potentially putting patients at 'high risk' of liver injury following paracetamol overdose:

- *Conditions that decrease hepatic glutathione stores*: malnutrition, anorexia or bulimia, HIV, cystic fibrosis.
- *Chronic therapy with cytochrome p450 enzyme inducers*: phenytoin, carbamazepine, rifampicin, phenobarbitone.

It remains uncertain as to whether chronic alcohol ingestion constitutes a risk factor for increased hepatotoxicity.

Management depends on time of presentation after ingestion, and on whether the ingestion took place within a short space of time or was staggered over a more prolonged period:

- *Early (<15h) presentation (non-staggered ingestion)*: management is guided by the paracetamol level taken at presentation (see Fig. 7.1), or 4h after ingestion (whichever is the later). If patients present >8h after ingestion (>150mg/kg or >75mg/kg in a high-risk group), NAC should be started empirically until paracetamol levels become available.

- *Late (>15h) presentation (non-staggered ingestion)*: these patients are at higher risk and should immediately receive NAC. Paracetamol levels >15h may be unreliable. The decision to stop NAC is more usefully guided by clinical and other biochemical markers (INR, HCO_3^-, creatinine, and LFTs)

- *Staggered paracetamol poisoning*: patients who have ingested >150mg/kg in any 24h period (>75mg/kg in high-risk groups) should receive NAC.

The INR, HCO_3^-, creatinine, and LFTs should be monitored during and after completion of the course of NAC to determine whether or not NAC should be continued, and whether discussions should be had with a regional liver unit (Box 7.7).

Box 7.7 Criteria for liver unit referral after paracetamol overdose

- PT (sec) greater than number of hours since ingestion
- INR >2 at 24h, >4 at 48h, >6 at 72h
- Metabolic acidosis (pH <7.35 and/or lactate >3mmol/L)
- Renal impairment (creatinine >200µmol/L)
- Hypoglycaemia
- Encephalopathy.

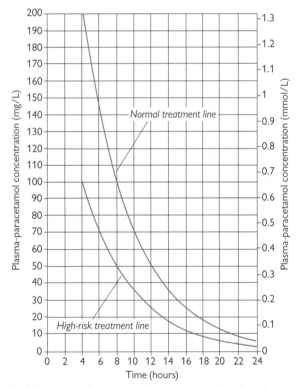

Fig. 7.1 Paracetamol normogram. Reproduced from Punit Ramraka and Kevin Moore, *Oxford Handbook of Acute Medicine*, Second edition, 2004, Figure on page 831, with permission from Oxford University Press.

Aspirin

Whilst the incidence of salicylate poisoning has declined in the UK and elsewhere, it remains an important clinical problem with potentially fatal consequences.

The clinical features and management relate to the amount ingested:

- >150mg/kg: mild toxicity with nausea, vomiting, tinnitus; respiratory alkalosis due to direct respiratory centre stimulation (may progress to acidosis or a mixed picture as part of uncoupling syndrome—see section 7.2); acidosis reduces renal salicylate elimination.
- >250mg/kg: peripheral vasodilatation, sweating, agitation, petechial haemorrhage.
- >500mg/kg: severe poisoning results in metabolic acidosis, seizures, renal failure and eventual coma and cardiovascular collapse.

Patients who have ingested >125mg/kg of salicylate should receive activated charcoal, preferably in repeated doses until plasma salicylate levels stabilize. Early salicylate levels may be an unreliable guide to the severity of poisoning, especially with enteric-coated preparations. The actual levels should not be taken in isolation as a correlate of clinical severity—the presence of a metabolic acidosis is an important negative predictor of outcome.

Urinary alkalinization with IV $NaHCO_3$ increases renal excretion of salicylates and should be undertaken in moderate to severe cases, even if there is significant respiratory alkalosis. Potassium supplementation helps to promote an alkaline urine (hypokalaemia promotes K^+ reabsorption and H^+ secretion in the distal tubule).

Patients with severe poisoning should receive haemodialysis or haemodiafiltration; conventional haemofiltration is likely to be much less efficient.

Opioids

Deliberate or accidental opioid overdose is common: most deaths occur before hospital presentation. The typical clinical picture is a reduced level of consciousness, with miosis and respiratory depression. Naloxone is a specific opioid antagonist and is ideally administered intravenously in small incremental doses, titrated against conscious level and other vital signs. Naloxone has a short half-life, and repeated doses, or an infusion, may be required.

Opioids may be taken in overdose as part of a compound analgesic preparation, and plasma paracetamol levels should be measured. Dextropropoxyphene (as part of co-proxamol) has membrane-stabilizing effects and may produce QRS prolongation and cardiovascular compromise that may respond to IV $NaHCO_3$.

Aminophylline

As safer therapies for asthma have developed, the use of theophylline and its IV equivalent, aminophylline (80% theophylline + ethylenediamine) has declined dramatically. Theophylline has a narrow therapeutic index and, when toxicity occurs, the clinical consequences can be severe.

The important clinical features are persistent vomiting, seizures, agitation, and tachyarrhythmias (ventricular in adults, supraventricular in children); these are frequently accompanied by hypokalaemia and hyperglycaemia.

Digoxin

Digoxin toxicity manifests as arrhythmias and should be suspected in any patient who is receiving the drug and shows signs of increased automaticity and decreased conduction. Ventricular bigeminy is highly suggestive, but almost any arrhythmia can occur. Toxicity is exacerbated by hypokalaemia. Extracardiac manifestations include nausea, and visual symptoms such as xanthopsia. Treatment involves K^+ supplementation and administration of digoxin-specific F(ab) fragments, which have provided an effective therapy for a potentially life-threatening disturbance.

Antidepressants (TCAs and SSRIs)

Classically, tricyclic antidepressants (TCAs) were the most common cause of poison-related ICU admission. TCAs typically produce anticholinergic effects, but in overdose, Na^+ channel blockade leads to life-threatening cardiac conduction abnormalities. QRS prolongation in excess of 120ms is an adverse prognostic factor.

8.4% $NaHCO_3$ is the mainstay of treatment, reducing TCA toxicity both through systemic alkalinization *and* hypertonic sodium loading.

SSRIs have largely superseded TCAs in terms of numbers treated. Overdose of some agents (e.g. citalopram) may produce QRS and QT prolongation, and also the *serotonin syndrome*, characterized by altered mentation, neuromuscular excitability and autonomic instability. Treatment involves supportive care ± benzodiazepines. Rarely, serotonin antagonists (e.g. cyproheptadine) may be used on specialist advice.

Cocaine

Cocaine is a sympathomimetic and increases myocardial oxygen demands. It also causes direct coronary vasoconstriction and increases platelet aggregation. Cocaine-related acute coronary syndrome (ACS) is unrelated to the ingested dose and can occur in both occasional and habitual users. Some aspects of management differ from those of 'classical' ACS: β-blockers are contraindicated since they produce unopposed α-receptor stimulation and increased coronary vasospasm. Thrombolytic therapy is associated with a significant risk of intracranial haemorrhage from hypertension. First-line therapies are oxygen, benzodiazepines, nitrates, and aspirin.

Ecstasy (3,4 methylenedioxymethamphetamine)

Ecstasy or MDMA has become established as a dance drug, popular at 'rave' parties. Its immediate effects vary from the minor to the life threatening. Severe effects include sudden death, hyperpyrexia, rhabdomyolysis and multiorgan failure, serotonin syndrome, and hyponatraemia with cerebral oedema. Treatment is supportive with aggressive cooling ± dantrolene therapy. Careful correction of fluid and electrolyte imbalance is crucial (see section 3.2).

Further reading

Boyle JS, Bechtel LK, & Holstege CP (2009). Management of the critically poisoned patient. *Scand J Trauma Resusc Emerg Med*, 17(1):29. doi:10.1186/1757-7241-17-29.

Greene SL, Dargan PI, & Jones AL (2005). Acute poisoning: understanding 90% of cases in a nutshell. *Postgrad Med J*, 81(954):204–16. doi:10.1136/pgmj.2004.024794.

Hall AP & Henry JA (2006). Acute toxic effects of 'Ecstasy' (MDMA) and related compounds: overview of pathophysiology and clinical management. *Br J Anaesth*, 96(6):678–85. doi:10.1093/bja/ael078.

7.4 Perioperative anaphylaxis

The reported incidence of perioperative anaphylaxis varies from 1:6000 to 1:20 000 anaesthetics.

Anaesthetists are more likely than their non-theatre colleagues to encounter allergic reactions amongst their patients. During anaesthesia, patients routinely receive multiple drugs in rapid succession. The theatre environment also contains numerous potential non-drug triggers, for example, latex and skin preparation solutions.

Mechanisms of anaphylaxis: allergic and non-allergic

The term 'anaphylaxis' denotes a severe, life-threatening, generalized or systemic hypersensitivity reaction. Minor, localized, or non-systemic reactions lie outside the definition of anaphylaxis.

Anaphylaxis is subdivided into 'allergic' and 'non-allergic' forms, the clinical features of which may be identical.

'Allergic' anaphylaxis is medicated by an immunological mechanism, such as IgE, IgG, or complement activation by immune complexes (e.g. dextrans).

Most commonly, the allergen interacts with specific IgE antibodies. In sensitized individuals, these bind to high-affinity Fc receptors within the plasma membrane of mast cells and basophils (and to low-affinity Fc receptors on lymphocytes, eosinophils, and platelets). These interactions cause cellular release of both preformed and newly synthesized inflammatory mediators such as:

- Phospholipid-derived mediators (leukotrienes, prostaglandins, thromboxane A2, and platelet-activating factor)
- Histamine and tryptase
- Chemokines and cytokines.

Non IgE-mediated reactions are sometimes referred to as 'anaphylactoid', although use of this term is now discouraged, and the term 'non-allergic anaphylaxis' is preferred. In the context of perioperative anaphylaxis, common causes for non-allergic anaphylaxis include opioids and NSAIDs. The mechanism is less well understood than is the case for IgE-mediated reactions.

Clinical recognition of anaphylaxis

Anaesthesia-related anaphylaxis usually results from *IV* drug administration, but exposure through other routes (cutaneous, mucosal, intra-articular, peritoneal, etc.) may also be responsible. The IV route tends to produce sudden reactions, whereas mucous membrane or skin exposure tends to lead to reactions of slower onset.

The clinical presentation of anaphylaxis is a spectrum, which can vary from a barely discernible reaction to overwhelming collapse.

Anaphylaxis is, of course, generally unanticipated. The signs during anaesthesia differ in some respects to those that occur in other circumstances, and a high level of vigilance is essential.

Early signs that may be observed in, or reported by, the awake patient (such as malaise, itching, or breathlessness) will be absent. Cutaneous signs may be difficult to elicit when the patient is covered, whilst cardiorespiratory changes may initially be misinterpreted as occurring secondary to anaesthesia (general and/or neuraxial) or surgery.

In essence, there are three important groups of manifestations: cardiovascular, respiratory and cutaneous (see Table 7.3). IgE-mediated reactions are usually more severe than non-IgE-mediated reactions. 90% of reactions appear within minutes of

Table 7.3 Clinical signs of anaphylaxis (% reactions)		
	IgE	Non-IgE
Cardiovascular:	78.6%	31.7%
Tachycardia and hypotension		
Cardiovascular collapse		
Bradycardia/cardiac arrest		
Cutaneous:	66.4%	93.6%
Erythema		
Urticaria		
Oedema		
Respiratory:	39.9%	19.5%
Bronchospasm		

Reprinted from *Immunology and Allergy Clinics of North America*, 29, 3, Mertes PM et al., 'Perioperative anaphylaxis', pp. 429–451, Copyright 2009, with permission from Elsevier. doi:10.1016/j.iac.2009.04.004.

induction, and typically represent allergy to a neuromuscular blocker or antibiotic. Signs appearing later suggest an allergy to latex, volume expanders or dyes.

Patient factors influence the clinical picture of a reaction:
- Patients with asthma are more likely to exhibit bronchospasm.
- Patients with significant cardiac disease (and/or receiving β-blocker therapy) are likely to be less tolerant, and more susceptible to profound cardiovascular collapse.

In practice, commonly reported initial features or anaphylaxis occurring during anaesthesia include reduced pulse volume, difficulty in ventilation, and desaturation. A decreased end-tidal CO_2 is an important sign. Cutaneous symptoms are common, especially in non-IgE-mediated reactions, and it is important to look for them. An absence of cutaneous signs, however, does *not* exclude anaphylaxis.

There is, of course, a wide differential diagnosis for many of the signs of anaphylaxis (see Box 7.8), but that does not diminish the importance of keeping anaphylaxis firmly in the frame as a possible cause of sudden patient deterioration.

Box 7.8 Differential diagnosis of perioperative anaphylaxis
• Overdose of vasoactive substance
• Asthma/bronchospasm of any cause
• Pneumothorax
• Tracheal tube obstruction or misplacement/breathing system obstruction
• Arrhythmia/MI/tamponade/PE
• Sepsis
• Thromboembolism
• Malignant hyperthermia/myotonia/masseter spasm
• Hereditary angioedema/mastocytosis.

Initial management of perioperative anaphylaxis

Initiating specific treatment at an *early* stage appears to improve outcome. All drug (and colloid) administration should be stopped, and anaesthesia maintained, if necessary, with a volatile agent.

Resuscitation should proceed along an ABC approach. An immediate assessment of the airway and breathing is essential—upper airway oedema may occur as the reaction develops, hence the patient should usually be intubated, and the lungs ventilated with 100% oxygen.

There is consensus that adrenaline should be given as early as possible, in an initial dose in adults of 50mcg (0.5mL of 1:10 000 solution). Several doses may be required if there is severe hypotension or bronchospasm.

Intravascular volume should be maintained with IV Hartmann's solution or saline, avoiding colloids if these were running prior to the event.

When hypotension is resistant to adrenaline, early use of a vasoconstrictor such as metaraminol is recommended, possibly culminating in a noradrenaline infusion.

Persistent bronchospasm may respond to salbutamol (administered intravenously or nebulized). Magnesium or aminophylline should also be considered.

Once the patient becomes more stable, an H_1-receptor antagonist (chlorpheniramine) and hydrocortisone should be given intravenously. If surgery cannot be postponed, then ongoing haemodynamic instability should be anticipated and managed.

Blood should be taken for mast cell tryptase analysis as soon as practically possible. Three samples will be required: one at time zero, the second at 1-2h after the start of symptoms, followed by a third sample at 24 h (to provide an indication of the patient's normal baseline).

Notes on individual triggering agents

Muscle relaxants

Approximately 60% of cases of perioperative anaphylaxis are thought to be due to neuromuscular blocking agents (NMBAs).

Atracurium and mivacurium are most commonly associated with non-allergic anaphylaxis, clinically indistinguishable from allergic anaphylaxis, and caused by direct release of histamine and other mediators from mast cells.

Suxamethonium is the NMBA most likely to cause allergic anaphylaxis.

An excess of cases involving rocuronium was previously reported in Norway and France, but not in other countries. Statistical limitations of previous data mean that further large epidemiological studies will be required to establish the true situation.

In >50% of cases of NMBA anaphylaxis, there is no history of previous exposure. The allergenic epitope in NMBAs is the quaternary ammonium ion, and this is shared amongst common environmental chemicals, such as toothpastes, shampoos and, notably, cough syrups containing pholcodine.

Patients who have suffered NMBA allergy should be skin prick tested for all agents in common use. Ideally, they should avoid all future exposure, but if it becomes necessary in the future, an agent with a negative skin response should be used, albeit with no guarantee that anaphylaxis will not occur. There is highly variable cross-sensitivity among the different NMBAs (averaging 60–70%). Cross-reactivity to *all* agents is relatively unusual.

Latex

This is commonly quoted as the second most common trigger for perioperative anaphylaxis, although the incidence may be falling, at least in part due to changes in policy and reduced exposure.

There are several potential routes of exposure to natural rubber latex during anaesthesia (via the airway, mucus membranes,

surgical field, or via parenteral injection) and reactions may take one of three forms:

- *Type I hypersensitivity reaction*: most severe but least frequent. Symptoms and signs are those of anaphylaxis but generally less severe than with NMBAs. A proportion of individuals also react to certain fruits cross-reacting with latex proteins (banana/chestnut/avocado).
- *Contact dermatitis*: a T-cell-mediated, delayed hypersensitivity reaction that is non-life-threatening (eczematous reaction after repeated skin or mucosal contact) but which may predispose to more severe reactions.
- *Non-immune mediated dermatitis*: the commonest reaction—an *irritant* dermatitis limited to the contact area, characterized by itching, irritation, and blistering.

Certain groups of patients are at increased risk of latex allergy (see Box 7.9).

> **Box 7.9 Risk factors for latex allergy**
> - Atopic individuals/patients with severe contact dermatitis
> - Multiple surgical procedures/surgery at a young age, e.g. spina bifida
> - Healthcare professionals
> - Allergy to nuts and fruits: especially banana, chestnut, and avocado
> - Occupational exposure to latex.

Antibiotics

These account for about 15% of anaesthesia-related anaphylaxis, and of these, some 70% are in response to penicillins or first-generation cephalosporins (which share the beta-lactam ring). The incidence appears to have increased in recent years. Anaphylaxis to IV antibiotics may be catastrophic, and a history of previous reactions should be taken seriously.

Colloids

These account for about 4% of perioperative reactions, and the vast majority are linked to gelatins.

Antiseptics

Reactions to chlorhexidine range from contact dermatitis to life-threatening anaphylaxis. Some reactions have occurred in response to chlorhexidine-bonded central venous catheters.

Dyes

Patent blue is used as a tracer to map lymphatics during sentinel lymph node biopsy. 2–3% of such patients experience allergic reactions, even anaphylaxis. They may have become sensitized from the widespread use of such dyes in cosmetics and other products. Methylene blue is rarely implicated in anaphylactic reactions and may be a safer alternative.

Further reading

Harper NJN, Dixon T, Dugué P, et al. (2009). Suspected anaphylactic reactions associated with anaesthesia. *Anaesthesia*, 64(2):199–211. doi:10.1111/j.1365-2044.2008.05733.x.

Mertes P M, Lambert M, Guéant-Rodriguez RM, et al. (2009). Perioperative anaphylaxis. *Immunol Allergy Clin North Am*, 29(3), 429–451. doi:10.1016/j.iac.2009.04.004.

Nel L & Eren E (2011). Peri-operative anaphylaxis. *Br J Clin Pharmacol*, 71(5), 647–658. doi:10.1111/j.1365-2125.2011.03913.x.

7.5 Problems of substance abuse and dependency

According to the *Diagnostic and Statistical Manual of Mental Disorders* (DSM), *substance abuse* is defined as 'a maladaptive pattern of substance use leading to clinically significant impairment or distress'.

Dependence can sometimes occur after repeated use. This is characterized by an increasing *tolerance* to the effects of the substance and *withdrawal symptoms* following a reduction in use.

A wide range of substances can be abused. In some cases, these will be drugs obtained legitimately from healthcare professionals (e.g. benzodiazepines and opioids), but other drugs will be obtained by illegal means (e.g. cannabis and cocaine).

Illicit substance abuse is common: according to the 2011/12 Crime Survey of England and Wales (CSEW), an estimated 36.5% of adults had taken an illicit drug in their lifetime, with 8.9% having consumed one or more within the previous year, and 5.2% in the past month.

It is in the nature of drug misuse that many users become patients. Anaesthetists—and indeed all clinicians—require an understanding of how illicit drugs exert their effects, of the complications associated with their use, and of practical approaches to management.

Overview of common drugs of abuse

Opioids

Diamorphine (diacetylmorphine or heroin) is the most widely abused opioid. Its pharmacokinetic properties allow it to cross the blood–brain barrier extremely rapidly, to produce a rapid onset of euphoria. It is taken most commonly by IV injection, but may be smoked or snorted. Addiction and its consequences (tolerance and withdrawal symptoms) follow very rapidly, after just a week or two of regular use.

Tolerance may be lost after just a few days' abstinence, increasing the risk of potentially fatal overdose after repeat administration.

The opioid withdrawal syndrome is unpleasant, but not life threatening, and commences within 24h of abstinence from the drug. Symptoms resemble those of a 'flu-like illness, with sweating, anxiety, piloerection, and rhinorrhoea.

Cocaine

Cocaine inhibits neuronal re-uptake of catecholamines. This explains both the perceived benefits of the drug, and the serious complications associated with its use:

- Blocking re-uptake of dopamine (and of serotonin) produces a euphoric 'high'.
- Blocking noradrenaline uptake has important cardiovascular effects, causing hypertension and coronary vasospasm.

In addition, as a local anaesthetic agent, it causes Na^+ channel blockade, which may provoke arrhythmias. Cocaine is frequently snorted, and sometimes smoked in its freebase form ('crack').

Amphetamines and related drugs

Amphetamines have a profound sympathomimetic effect and produce tachycardia, CNS stimulation and euphoria. The potential for addiction is less than in the case of heroin or cocaine.

Recreational use of 3,4-methylenedioxy-N-methylamphetamine (MDMA or 'Ecstasy'), typically amongst young people, has been widely publicized during recent years. It causes release of serotonin, dopamine, and noradrenaline within the central nervous system. The behavioural effects are summarized as the '3

E's'—namely, energy, empathy, and euphoria. There are potentially very serious effects associated with its use (Box 7.10).

> **Box 7.10 Serious potential adverse effects of 'Ecstasy'**
>
> - Exertional hyperpyrexia (leading to rhabdomyolysis and multiple organ failure)
> - Hyponatraemia and cerebral oedema
> - Serotonin syndrome
> - Cerebrovascular accident
> - Anxiety and panic disorder.

The syndrome of hyperpyrexia with rhabdomyolysis and multiorgan failure appears to be associated with inadequate fluid replacement in the face of excessive exertion. Awareness of the danger of hyperthermia led to the practice of drinking large volumes of water to combat dehydration. This, in turn, has led to a second potentially lethal syndrome associated with Ecstasy use, that of hyponatraemia and cerebral oedema. This is compounded by a serotoninergic stimulation of antidiuretic hormone production.

Ketamine

Ketamine causes dissociative anaesthesia, and has hypnotic, analgesic, hallucinogenic, and amnesic effects. Its dissociative effect produces a trance-like state in abusers, who may sense an out-of-body experience. Users may present with altered consciousness, confusion or apparent psychosis.

Perioperative issues associated with substance abuse

Patients who abuse drugs may present acutely with a complication related to their drug abuse, or they may require treatment for an entirely unrelated issue.

Diagnostic clues to drug misuse

It is important to be alert to possible signs of drug abuse, since patients often do not disclose their habit.

Unusual presentations—such as cardiovascular pathology in a young person, behavioural disturbances, or unexplained coma or collapse, may be pointers to an underlying drug problem. Near-patient urine testing strips are available for most commonly abused agents.

Physical clues may include injection 'track-marks', phlebitis, or abscesses.

Perioperative problems

A variety of problems may be encountered in addition to the acute effects related to any particular drug. These include:

- Difficult venous access
- Arterial injury ± distal ischaemia
- DVT
- Abscess formation ± gas gangrene
- High prevalence of blood-borne infections (HIV, hepatitis, etc.)
- Severe COPD in cannabis users.

Acute pain management in opioid users

This is an especially challenging area of practice. Opioid users may display both tolerance and physical dependence, and these combine to make assessment of analgesic needs extremely difficult. A multidisciplinary approach is required.

If patients are currently using opioids, or are on a methadone programme, their present dosing regimen should be identified. PCA opioids are commonly used, but not without problems.

In recovered addicts, there is a danger of re-introducing drug-carving behaviour if opioids are administered by IV bolus dosing.

If the situation permits, it is preferable to provide additional analgesia using non-opioid techniques: paracetamol, NSAIDs, and local, regional, or neuraxial anaesthesia.

Substance abuse amongst anaesthetists and other doctors

Drug and alcohol abuse is relatively common in the general population, and increasing in prevalence.

In respect of alcohol, studies suggest that the prevalence of abuse amongst doctors mirrors that of the general population. Amongst anaesthetists, alcohol dependence is more common in older practitioners, but less common than in other specialties.

Anaesthetists, psychiatrists, and emergency physicians are up to three times more likely to require treatment for substance abuse than other specialty groups. Anaesthetists are more likely to abuse opioids, and to be addicted to more than one drug. Amongst anaesthetists, drug abuse is more common in those under the age of 40 years, and 80% of users are male.

Anaesthetists are at greatly increased risk of suicide and drug-related death compared to matched controls in the general population. The risk is maximal in the first 5 years following graduation.

Aside from commonly abused drugs, abuses of propofol and of volatile agents are well described. Propofol abuse has been reported since the 1990s and carries a mortality approaching 30%. Inhalational agents are often used in conjunction with other substances, sometimes to ease the symptoms of opioid withdrawal.

Factors influencing substance abuse

Many factors are involved, many of them not exclusive to doctors:
- Genetic factors: some individuals may have an inherent susceptibility to addiction.
- Stress: the anaesthetist's role is a demanding one, with high levels of responsibility and the potential for errors to have serious consequences.
- Psychological factors: mental illness—predominantly anxiety or depression—will affect about a third of the population at some point during their lives. In some people, this may lead to abuse of drugs and/or alcohol.
- Availability: anaesthetists have relatively easy access to a wide range of psychotropic drugs.

Warning signs of possible substance abuse

If a doctor is working under the influence of drugs or alcohol, there is a risk of harm—both to patients, in respect of impaired decision-making, risk-taking behaviour, and slower reactions in urgent situations, and also to the doctor, in relation to his or her mental and physical health, personal relationships, and career. See Box 7.11 for warning signs.

Box 7.11 Warning signs of substance abuse

Warning signs of alcohol abuse
- Subtle personality change
- Mood swings or anxiety
- Getting drunk easily at departmental events
- Dishevelled appearance/smelling of alcohol
- Lateness for work/socially isolated or secretive
- Marital/relationship problems.

Warning signs of drug abuse
- Behavioural changes
- Needle marks/long sleeves
- Volunteering to draw up drugs for others
- Over-anxious to give breaks
- Failure to discard waste.

Interventions in cases of actual or suspected substance abuse by a colleague

Concerns should normally be reported to the clinical director in the first instance, although junior doctors may find it easier to approach their educational supervisor. Efforts should be made to obtain objective evidence.

If clear evidence exists, then urgent intervention is required, especially if there is evidence of real or potential harm to patients. The doctor should be interviewed by the medical director and clinical director. Plans must immediately be put in place to offer the doctor support and treatment—there is a very real possibility of self-harm.

Advice from the GMC must be sought at an early stage when there is any suspicion of danger to patients from doctors who are abusing alcohol and drugs.

The GMC will arrange for medical assessment and then decide whether a Fitness to Practice hearing is required to decide whether or not restrictions upon a doctor's registration should be imposed.

Treatment may require inpatient detoxification and rehabilitation and subsequent long-term support. The goal for a substance-dependent doctor should be lifelong abstinence from all mood altering substances, and the ultimate objective, though challenging, should be for the doctor to be able to resume a normal personal and professional life.

Further reading

AAGBI (2011). *Drug and Alcohol Abuse amongst Anaesthetists: Guidance on Identification and Management*. London: AAGBI.

Hall AP & Henry JA (2006). Acute toxic effects of 'Ecstasy' (MDMA) and related compounds: overview of pathophysiology and clinical management. *Brit J Anaesth*, 96(6):678–85. doi:10.1093/bja/ael078.

Hall AP & Henry JA (2007). Illicit drugs and surgery. *Int J Surg*, 5(5):365–70. doi:10.1016/j.ijsu.2006.06.006.

7.6 Anaesthesia and the environment

It is now widely accepted that rising concentrations of man-made gases are having an adverse effect upon our environment.

Halogenated gases deplete the layer of ozone contained within the stratosphere resulting in an increase in UV light and damage to organisms.

'Greenhouse gases' such as carbon dioxide, methane, and nitrous oxide prevent infrared light from escaping the troposphere and exacerbate the phenomenon known as 'global warming'.

The NHS is responsible for the production of 19 million tonnes of carbon dioxide each year.

When using desflurane at 1 MAC and a fresh gas flow of 1–2L/min, an anaesthetist's contribution to daily greenhouse gas production would equate to 58–116 days of car emissions.

The anaesthetist must be aware of the wider environmental impact of his or her practice and seek out ways to become more 'environmentally friendly' whilst maintaining the highest standards of patient care.

Anaesthetic waste

On average, 2300kg of anaesthetic waste and 230kg of sharps waste are produced annually by each operating theatre in the UK. This has enormous financial and environmental implications.

90% of anaesthetic waste is either incinerated (£750 per tonne) or buried in landfill (£80 per tonne).

Since 'greenhouse gases' are a common by-product of the manufacturing process this approach will only to lead to further environmental damage.

In order to address this, the Association of Anaesthetists of Great Britain and Ireland (AAGBI) has advocated using a 5 R's approach:

- Waste should be *reduced* wherever possible.
- Appropriate items should be *reused* and/or *recycled*.
- Current methods should undergo a careful *rethink*.
- *Research* should aim at developing long term strategies that transform the way we manage waste.

Environmental impact of volatile agents

Volatile agents have the potential to cause environmental damage in two ways:

Ozone layer depletion

Chlorine and bromine are cleaved from volatile agents by UV radiation and react with ozone (O_3) to produce chlorine oxide (ClO), or bromine oxide (BrO), and oxygen (O_2). Depletion of the ozone layer in the stratosphere allows concentrations of UV light to penetrate the atmosphere and damage living organisms.

The effect of a volatile agent upon the ozone layer depends upon its molecular weight, number and type of halogen atoms, and its atmospheric lifetime.

Atmospheric lifetime is defined as the time taken to neutralize 63% (1/e) of the gas.

Bromine destroys 35–50 times more ozone than chlorine. Fluoride has minimal effect.

Halothane, therefore, is more hazardous than isoflurane, whilst sevoflurane and desflurane have little, or no, impact upon the ozone layer.

Halothane is estimated to have caused 1% of ozone layer depletion.

The ozone depletion potential (ODP) compares the potential depleting effects of the different volatile agents against those of chlorofluorocarbon-12 (see Table 7.4).

Table 7.4 Environmental impact of anaesthetic gases and volatile agents			
Compound	Lifetime (yrs)	ODP	GWP
CFC-12	100	1	10900
CO_2	5–200	0	1
N_2O	114	0.02	298
Halothane	7	0.36	–
Isoflurane	3–6	0.01	510–571
Sevoflurane	1–4	0	141–298
Desflurane	9–21	0	1525–1746

CFC-12 = chlorofluorocarbon-12; GWP = global warming potential; ODP = ozone depletion potential.
Reproduced from Table 1 in *Southern African Journal of Anaesthesia and Analgesia*, 17, 5, 'Anaesthetic gases: environmental impact and alternatives', Bosenberg, M, pp. 345–348, Copyright 2011, with permission from South African Society of Anaesthesiologists. Data from Ryan SM, Nielsen CJ. Global warming potential of inhaled anesthetics: application to clinical use. *Anesth Analg*. 2010;111:92–98; Langbein T, Sonntag H, Trapp D, et al. Volatile anaesthetics and the atmosphere: atmospheric lifetimes and atmospheric effects of halothane, enflurane, isoflurane, desflurane and sevoflurane. *Br J Anaesth*. 1999;82:66–73; Sulbaek Andersen MP, Sander SP, Nielsen OJ, et al. Inhalational anaesthesia and climate change. *Br J Anaesth*. 2010;105:760–766; Brown AC, Canosa-Mas CE, Parr AD, et al. Tropospheric lifetimes of halogenated anaesthetics. *Nature* 1989;341: 635–637.

Global warming

Halogens absorb the infra-red radiation that is emitted by the sun and reflected off the earth's surface. As a result, heat is retained within the troposphere.

The contribution of a gas towards 'global warming' can be calculated by multiplying the atmospheric lifetime of the gas by its global warming potential (GWP) (Table 7.4).

The GWP describes the ratio of how much heat is trapped by a given gas to that of the same mass of carbon dioxide (CO_2).

Whilst desflurane has the lowest ODP and has little impact upon the ozone layer, its long lifetime and high GWP makes it the most hazardous volatile agent to the environment. This is exacerbated by the fact that more is required to deliver the same anaesthetic effect than other volatile agents.

Nitrous oxide is a highly stable gas with an atmospheric lifetime of 114 years. Therefore despite its low ODP and GWP, its longevity means that the gas plays a considerable part in ozone depletion and global warming.

Since between 1% and 3% of nitrous oxide emissions are the result of medical practices, reducing nitrous oxide use by anaesthetists may have a positive effect upon our environment.

Potential strategies to reduce use of volatiles

Reducing fresh gas flow

Compared to 'open' systems, 'semi closed' and 'closed' breathing circuits can reduce volatile agent use by up to 90%. Further savings can also be made if a 'low-flow' technique is also implemented.

By reducing fresh gas flow (FGF) from 2L/min to 1L/min, an anaesthetist can prevent as much as 18 900L of isoflurane from entering the atmosphere in the course of his or her working lifetime.

It is of course mandatory to measure O_2 and volatile concentrations during low-flow circle system anaesthesia in order to ensure appropriate levels are maintained.

During maintenance, oxygen flow can be reduced in 50mL increments until the inspired oxygen concentration begins to fall. This can be performed manually or by using automated tools such as the Zeus Anaesthetic Delivery System (GE Healthcare) which allows users to set a minimum FGF and target concentrations of oxygen and volatile agent which are then managed automatically.

Scavenging volatile agents
When inserted into the scavenging line of an anaesthetic circuit, devices such as the silica zeolyte (Deltazite™) filter can absorb volatile agents for up to 8h.

The volatile agents contained in these filters can be reclaimed and the gases used again.

The 'Anaesthetic Conserving Device' (ACD) is a circle system that is closed to volatile agents but open to other gases. In ACDs the volatile agent is added through a syringe pump. This has been shown to reduce use by up to 75%.

Novel anaesthetic agents
Xenon has several properties that make it a highly effective anaesthetic agent. Unlike nitrous oxide, xenon occurs naturally in the earth's atmosphere and therefore presents no threat to the environment.

Xenon is, however, manufactured from the fractional distillation of air, a process that consumes enormous amounts of energy. It is more than 200 times more expensive to obtain than nitrous oxide and therefore difficult to justify on environmental grounds.

TIVA and regional anaesthesia
Using total intravenous anaesthesia (TIVA) with or without regional anaesthesia obviously eradicates volatile agent use.

Environmental costs still occur. However, in respect of production, transport and so on, and thus contribute to ozone depletion and greenhouse gas production.

Personal actions to reduce climate change

In 2008, the *British Medical Journal* cited a number of practical actions that doctors could take to combat climate change. These included:
- Becoming informed about the basic science of climate change, the health benefits of taking action, and the urgency to do so.
- Informing patients that a better diet and more exercise (walking, cycling, etc.) will not only improve personal health but also have a positive impact upon climate change.
- Adopting energy efficiency measures at home and at work, such as improving home insulation and turning off electrical appliances when not in use.
- Fly and drive less. Use teleconferencing wherever possible.
- Eat more local produce and less processed food. Drink tap water.
- Agitate for personal carbon entitlements and financial incentives in order to reduce carbon costs.
- Advocate population stabilization, by promoting literacy and women's access to birth control (e.g. via the International Planned Parenthood Federation (<http://www.ippf.org>).
- Put climate change on the agenda during meetings with clinical teams and managers.
- Ally with other health professionals by joining the Climate and Health Council or the Health and Sustainability Network/Centre for Sustainable Healthcare.

Further reading

Climate and Health Council website: <http://www.climateandhealth.org>

Griffiths J, Hill A, Spilby J, *et al.* (2008). Ten practical steps for doctors to fight climate change. *BMJ*, 336:1507.

Health and Sustainability Network/Centre for Sustainable Healthcare website: <http://sustainablehealthcare.org.uk/>.

Sneyd JR, Montgomery H, & Pencheon D (2010). The anaesthetist and the environment. *Anaesthesia*, 65(5):435–7. doi:10.1111/j.1365-2044.2010.06332.x.

7.7 Antimicrobial agents

Mechanisms of action of antibiotics

Antibiotics are either *bactericidal* (killing micro-organisms directly), or *bacteriostatic* (slowing down micro-organism reproduction, allowing host defences to kill them).

Current antibacterial agents employ one of four principal mechanisms of action to achieve selective toxicity:

Inhibition of bacterial wall synthesis

β-lactam antibiotics (penicillins and cephalosporins) bind to transpeptidase preventing cross-linkage of peptidoglycans, weakening the cell wall. Some bacteria produce β-lactamase hindering β-lactam. Addition of a β-lactamase inhibitor to the antibiotic (e.g. as in co-amoxiclav) restores its efficacy.

Glycopeptides (e.g. vancomycin and teicoplanin) bind to amino acids in peptidoglycan, preventing its formation in the cell wall.

Inhibition of bacterial DNA synthesis

These antibiotics tend to be bactericidal and include quinolones (e.g. ciprofloxacin) as well as metronidazole and rifampicin.

Inhibition of bacterial protein synthesis

Macrolides (e.g. erythromycin) inhibit bacterial ribosomes responsible for protein synthesis. Aminoglycosides (e.g. gentamicin and amikacin) are bactericidal and cause misreading of messenger RNA resulting in dysfunctional protein. Tetracyclines work by blocking transfer RNA.

Inhibition of bacterial folic acid synthesis

This group includes sulphonamides and trimethoprim. Acting separately, these are bacteriostatic but combined as co-trimoxazole are bactericidal and work synergistically.

Choosing a bactericidal or bacteriostatic agent is most relevant when managing neutropenic patients. Here, bactericidal agents are necessary because host defences cannot eliminate non-replicating pathogens, thus rendering bacteriostatic agents ineffective. They are also indicated in bacterial meningitis or when treating infective endocarditis.

Pharmacodynamics and pharmacokinetics

Pharmacokinetic antibiotic parameters most commonly measured include the peak serum concentration, minimum inhibitory concentration (MIC—the lowest concentration of antibiotic that inhibits the growth of the micro-organisms in vitro), and the area under the serum concentration–time curve (AUC).

Antibiotic effectiveness is dependent either on concentration or time at the infective site. Concentration-dependent killing (as exhibited by aminoglycosides and quinolones) is where higher concentrations make the antibiotic more bactericidal but this effect is limited by drug toxicity. The index for efficacy is shown by peak concentration/MIC. Time-dependent killing (as exhibited by β-lactams and macrolides), where the proportion of time above the MIC is the best indicator of efficacy, shows that raised concentrations are more effective than intermittent high peaks. This is shown by the AUC:MIC ratio or the time:MIC ratio.

Antibiotics are mainly excreted via the kidneys by glomerular filtration or tubular secretion so should be used cautiously in patients with impaired renal function to prevent accumulation. Particular caution is required with aminoglycosides, as toxic effects closely relate to intracellular concentration and elimination parallels creatinine clearance.

Antibiotic resistance

Resistance is either intrinsic (e.g. vancomycin against Gram-negative organisms) or acquired by mutation/transfer of genetic material from resistant to susceptible organisms. Factors influencing microbial resistance include excess antibiotic usage, incorrect use of broad-spectrum agents, incorrect dosing, and non-compliance.

Choice of drug

Most antibiotics have a mode of action that is more effective against either Gram-positive (Table 7.5) or Gram-negative bacteria (Table 7.6). The difference is due to the possession of different structured cell walls, distinguished under microscopy by Gram-staining. They are either aerobic or anaerobic depending on whether or not they grow in the presence of oxygen and are either generally spherical (cocci) or rod-shaped (bacilli). Different antibiotics are used to target the different types of organisms.

Table 7.5 Gram-positive microorganisms			
Cocci		**Bacilli**	
Aerobic	Anaerobic	Aerobic	Anaerobic
Streptococcus spp. *Staphylococcus* spp.	*Peptostreptococcus*	*Bacillus* spp. *Listeria monocytogenes*	*Clostridium* spp. *Acintomyces* *Lactobacillus*

Table 7.6 Gram-negative microorganisms			
Cocci		**Bacilli**	
Aerobic	Anaerobic	Aerobic	Anaerobic
Neisseria spp. *Moraxella*	*Veillonella* spp.	*Pseudomonas* *Proteus* spp. *Salmonella* *Shigella* *Escherichia coli* *Enterobacter* *Klebsiella* *Legionella* *Haemophilus* *Helicobacter pylori*	*Bacteroides*

Adverse effects

Most side effects such as diarrhoea, vomiting and headaches are relatively minor. Clindamycin, the quinolones and macrolides may cause pseudomembranous colitis by aiding the development of *Clostridium difficile*. Aminoglycosides can cause permanent nephrotoxicity and ototoxicity.

Allergic reactions are most common with penicillins. This reaction can range from mild urticaria and rashes to fatal anaphylaxis. The incidence of cross-reactivity to other beta-lactams (cephalosporins and carbapenems) is 6.5–10% so these should be avoided in patients with known immediate hypersensitivity to penicillin.

Prophylaxis against surgical infection

The need for antibiotic prophylaxis depends on the type of operation being performed. Several categories of surgery are described:

- *Clean*: surgery that does not open body cavities namely respiratory, gastrointestinal (GI) or genitourinary tracts (GU) and is not associated with inflamed tissue.
- *Clean-contaminated*: involving the oropharynx or opening of body cavities.
- *Contaminated*: involving acute inflammation, infected bilious or urinary secretions or bowel and wound contamination.
- *Dirty*: surgery performed where an established infection exists, in the presence of pus, or open injuries that are >4h old.

The NICE 2008 guidelines recommend giving antibiotic prophylaxis to patients before clean surgery involving the placement of a prosthesis or implant, clean-contaminated surgery, or contaminated surgery. Antibiotics are not required routinely for clean, non-prosthetic, uncomplicated surgery. Antibiotic treatment in addition to prophylaxis is required for surgery on a dirty or infected wound.

A single antibiotic dose, in accordance with the national and local policies and formulary, should be given intravenously on starting anaesthesia, or earlier for operations in which a tourniquet is used. A repeat prophylactic dose is required when the operation is longer than the half-life of the antibiotic given.

It has been shown that surgical wound infection rate is lowest if antibiotics are administered within 30min of skin incision with the likelihood of infection doubling if given after the start of surgery or >60min before.

Prophylaxis against infective endocarditis
Patients with the following cardiac conditions should be regarded as being at risk of developing infective endocarditis:

- Acquired valvular disease with stenosis or regurgitation
- Valve replacement
- Structural congenital heart disease (excluding isolated atrial septal defects, a fully repaired ventricular septal defect, or a fully repaired patent ductus arteriosus)
- Previous infective endocarditis
- Hypertrophic cardiomyopathy.

2008 NICE guidelines on prophylaxis against infective endocarditis state that routine antibiotic cover is no longer recommended for dental procedures or procedures of the upper and lower GI tract, urogenital tract (including childbirth and obstetric operations), and upper and lower respiratory tracts (including bronchoscopy, and ENToperations).

At-risk patients undergoing a GI or urogenital procedure *at a site where there is a suspected infection* should receive antibiotics, chosen to cover organisms that cause infective endocarditis.

Therapy of bacterial infection

Anaesthetists are involved in treating established bacterial infection when working on critical care. This includes the management of severe community-acquired pneumonia, hospital-acquired and ventilator-associated pneumonia, meningococcal septicaemia, necrotizing fasciitis, catheter-related bloodstream infections, severe sepsis, or septic shock.

Broad-spectrum antibiotics, for example, cephalosporins, quinolones, carbapenems and β-lactam/β-lactamase inhibitor combinations (co-amoxiclav and tazocin) are useful for empirical treatment in critically ill, septic patients (Box 7.12). They cover a wide range of pathogens but should be changed to a more targeted therapy once culture and sensitivity reports are available.

Other than in exceptional circumstances (e.g. suspected meningitis), cultures should always be taken prior to initial administration of antibiotics.

Box 7.12 Antibiotics commonly prescribed in critical care

- Amoxicillin—enterococcal infection. 90% staphylococcal resistance (less as co-amoxiclav).
- Flucloxacillin—staphylococcal infection.
- Benzylpenicillin—streptococcal, *Neisseria*, and *Clostridia* infection.
- Piperacillin—broad-spectrum sepsis cover on ICU (as Tazocin®). Treatment of pseudomonal infection.
- Cefuroxime—2nd-generation cephalosporin used in general and orthopaedic surgical prophylaxis, and to treat pneumonia, peritonitis, joint infection, and urinary sepsis.
- Cefotaxime—3rd-generation cephalosporin used to treat meningitis, nosocomial pneumonia, and wound sepsis. Less Gram-positive effect than cefuroxime (no *Enterococcus* cover), and excellent Gram-negative cover (except *Pseudomonas*)
- Imipenem—used in neutropenic sepsis, and severe sepsis on ICU. Broad antimicrobial spectrum.
- Erythromycin—Gram-positive infection if penicillin allergic and of *Legionella* and *Mycoplasma*.
- Gentamicin—Gram-negative sepsis and surgical prophylaxis. Anaerobes and streptococcus are resistant.
- Ciprofloxacin—Gram-negative sepsis, biliary sepsis, and enteric fever. Excellent tissue penetration.
- Vancomycin—MRSA, other Gram-positive infection, pseudomembranous colitis.
- Clindamycin—staphylococcal, streptococcal, and anaerobic infection. Good bone penetration.
- Metronidazole—exclusively anaerobic and parasitic (*Giardia* and *Trichomonas*) cover.
- Teicoplanin—treatment and prophylaxis of serious Gram-positive infection.

Therapy of viral infection

Antivirals act upon various stages of the viral replication process, primarily by targeting reverse transcriptase.

Acyclovir is used to treat infection caused by herpes simplex and varicella zoster. Dose reduction is required in renal failure and it may cause thrombophlebitis or CNS symptoms (tremor, confusion, and seizures.)

Zidovudine is used to treat HIV in combination with other antivirals. Side effects include renal impairment, GI upset, anaemia, neutropenia, and hyperpigmentation.

Therapy of fungal infection

Fungal and human cells are similar at the molecular level therefore many antifungals cause serious side effects.

The azoles (e.g. fluconazole and itraconazole) are active against yeast and fungi including *Candida* spp., *Cryptococcus* spp., and *Histoplasma* spp. Itraconazole also covers *Aspergillus* spp. Side effects include GI upset, hepatitis, and enhancement of warfarin.

Amphotericin is used in the treatment of severe systemic infections including *Candida* and *Aspergillus*. It is only administered intravenously and may cause renal and liver impairment, blood dyscrasias, visual disturbances, and GI upset.

Chapter 8

Nutrition

8.1 Nutritional assessment

Nutritional assessment should in the first instance be differentiated from nutritional screening. Screening is a rapid technique used by nursing staff/medical staff on first contact with a patient to identify patients at risk of malnutrition. Nutritional assessment is a much more detailed evaluation of an individual's nutritional state:

- Anthropometric assessment
- Biochemical assessment
- Clinical evaluation
- Dietary assessment.

Anthropometric assessment

The World Health Organization (WHO) provides guidelines (WHO, 1995) for anthropometric assessment in adults and children within different population groups. The WHO state: 'Anthropometry provides the single most portable, universally applicable, inexpensive and non-invasive technique for assessing the size, proportions and composition of the human body'.

Anthropometric assessment includes:

- Body weight (including % weight change)
- Height (in relation to body weight)
- Adiposity (body mass index (BMI), waist circumference, waist-to-hip ratio, skinfold thickness)
- Muscle mass (mid-arm circumference, grip strength)
- Body water content and body composition such as impedance measures (opposition of flow of electric current through tissues) and sophisticated techniques such as dual-energy X-ray absorptiometry (DEXA) scanning.

Body weight

Serial body weight measurements are used to determine weight change and to calculate percentage increase or decrease (Table 8.1).

$$\text{Weight change}(\%) = \frac{(\text{usual weight} - \text{actual weight})}{\text{usual weight} \times 100}$$

Percentage weight loss could be used to determine when nutrition support should be instigated. Malnourished patients are identified as:

- BMI <18.5kg/m^2
- Unintentional weight loss of >10% over 3–6 months
- Unintentional weight loss of >5% in a patient with a BMI <20kg/m^2 over 3–6 months (NICE 2006)

A single body weight measurement could be used to determine BMI:

$$\text{BMI} = \frac{\text{weight}(kg)}{(\text{height}(m))^2}$$

Daily weights will give an indication of fluid balance.

When weighing patients consider the presence of oedema or ascites, whether patients are wearing bulky clothing or shoes, if they have casts, splints, or amputations, and also consider the accuracy of the scales.

Detailed guidance on the technique of anthropometric measurement can be obtained in the WHO report (1995).

Table 8.1 Measurements of body composition (techniques in italics are mostly used in clinical research)

Protein stores	Fat stores	Body water
Mid-arm muscle circumference (MAMC)	Waist circumference	Bioelectrical impedance
Grip strength	Waist to hip ratio	Biochemistry (electrolytes)
Nitrogen balance	BMI	Fluid balance charts
Plasma proteins	Skinfold thickness	Daily weight
Muscle ultrasound	Bioelectrical impedance	Abdominal circumference (ascites)
Protein turnover studies	*DEXA*	Pitting of ankles and lower limbs (oedema)
DEXA	*MRI/CT*	*DEXA*
MRI/CT		*Dilution methods*
Underwater weighing or densitometry	*Underwater weighing or densitometry*	
Total body potassium		

Biochemical assessment

Biochemical data can provide information on the nutritional status of a patient and can also be used to monitor nutrition support (Table 8.2).

Table 8.2 Biochemical assessment of nutritional status

Parameter	Assessment
Urea & creatinine	Renal function 24h urinary urea (N$_2$ balance), 24h urinary creatinine (muscle mass loss)
Potassium, phosphate, magnesium	Electrolyte and metabolic abnormalities, monitoring of rRefeeding syndrome
Proteins: Albumin	Long half- life (14--20 days) → *poor* marker of nutritional status
Pre-albumin	Short half- life (< 2 days) → sensitive marker of response to nutritional support
Serum transferrin Retinol binding protein	8–10 day half- life, affected by stress and iron status 12hour half- life, sensitive to protein depletion
C-reactive protein	Acute phase response protein, albumin should be interpreted alongside CRP
White cell count	Infection and inflammation

Clinical evaluation

This should consist of:

- Assessment of physical appearance
- Past medical history
- Medication history
- Current diagnosis.

Physical appearance

An initial subjective assessment should be used to see if a patient is underweight or overweight in the first instance. Evidence of muscle wasting or subcutaneous fat loss or gain should be assessed. Sunken eyes, fragile skin, and dry mouth could indicate dehydration. Patient's mobility, mood, psychosocial condition, presence of oedema, and/or evidence of poor wound healing could briefly be assessed.

Dietary assessment

Dietary evaluation should assess:
- Current diet and fluid intake (24h recall method)
- Presence of appetite change or change in oral intake
- Factors affecting food and fluid intake (e.g. confusion)
- Consideration of individual requirements.

Monitoring

Monitoring should occur regularly by a trained healthcare professional in the hospital environment or by the patient in their home environment (Table 8.3). This will ensure that treatment is appropriate and should help to minimize complications that may occur due to nutritional support.

Table 8.3 Monitoring of nutritional status		
Parameter	Rationale	Frequency
Weight	Mass, fluid balance	Initial weight, then weekly Daily for fluid balance
Height	BMI	Once
Anthropometry	Body composition change	Initial assessment, then weekly or as required
Medications	Intake, metabolism, interactions	Initial assessment, every few days
Diet	Intake (under or over)	Initial assessment, as required thereafter
Biochemistry	See Table 8.1	Daily initially and if critically ill, twice weekly once stable

Refeeding syndrome

Refeeding syndrome is characterized by severe fluid and electrolyte shifts and occurs when undernourished patients are fed and the metabolism shifts from a previously starved or semi-starved state to that of carbohydrate metabolism. Once patients are fed carbohydrate or glucose, insulin is released and the electrolytes shift into the cells. A rapid reduction in the levels of serum potassium, phosphate, and magnesium might follow with clinical consequences associated with significant morbidity and mortality. Characterized by:

- Hypophosphatemia
- Hypokalaemia
- Hypomagnesaemia
- Altered glucose metabolism
- Fluid abnormalities
- Vitamin deficiency.

At-risk patients should be identified and treated with very slow initiation of nutrition support, electrolyte supplementation as required, and supplementation of vitamins, in particular thiamine and vitamin B compound or intravenous equivalents. Please refer to NICE guidelines (*Nutrition support in adults*) (2006) for detailed guidance.

Requirements

NICE guidelines (2006) suggest that nutritional prescription should include:
- Energy (kcal/day)
- Protein/nitrogen (g/day)
- Fluid (mL/day)
- Electrolytes, i.e. potassium (mmol/L)
- Micronutrients (vitamins and trace elements)
- Minerals (magnesium, phosphate)
- Fibre.

The underlying clinical condition as well as patient activity levels should be considered when working out requirements.

Nutritional prescription

In patients that are not critically ill and in whom refeeding syndrome is not expected the following prescription should be considered:
- 25–35kcal/kg/day total energy
- 0.8–1.5g protein/kg/day (0.13–0.24g nitrogen/kg/day)
- 30–35mL/kg fluid per day
- Electrolytes, vitamins, minerals, and fibre as required.

Further reading

Ellis KJ (2000). Human body composition: in vivo techniques. *Physiol Rev*, 80:649–80.

National Institute for Health and Clinical Excellence (2006). *Nutrition Support in Adults*. London: NICE.

Thomas B & Bishop J (eds) (2007). Manual of Dietetic Practice (4th edn). London: British Dietetic Association.

World Health Organization Report (1995). Physical Status: The Use and Interpretation of Anthropometry. Geneva: WHO.

8.2 Nutrition and outcome

Hospital patients

A number of studies have demonstrated that hospitalized patients benefit from some form of nutrition support. Meta-analysis and systematic reviews consistently recommend oral nutrition supplements (ONS) for a variety of patient groups, showing a reduction in infectious complications, mortality, and hospital re-admission rates.

Elderly hospitalized patients

In elderly hospitalized patients, high-protein oral nutrition support may reduce overall complications along with hospital readmissions. Improvements in grip strength and protein and energy intakes were seen without improvement in body weight per se.

Malnourished medical patients

Malnourished medical patients benefit from individualized nutrition support according to a recent study. Reductions in complications, antibiotic use and readmissions to hospital were observed along with an increase in body weight (Starke et al., 2011).

Malnourished surgical patients

Some studies recommend immune-modulating enteral feeds in the postoperative period for malnourished patients. A recent study found a reduction in hospital length of stay, reduced infection rates, and reduced morbidity and mortality of patients on immunonutrient enteral feeds (Klek et al., 2011); however, data from other studies are inconsistent.

Major elective surgical patients

A recent meta-analysis indicates that immune-modulating feeds (with arginine and fish oils) should be used in high-risk surgical patients. This study observed reductions in acquired infections, wound complications, and a shorter hospital length of stay for elective surgical patients (Marik & Zaloga, 2010).

Cancer patients

In patients undergoing radiotherapy, meta-analysis showed that ONS significantly increased dietary intake compared to routine care. In patients undergoing surgery, meta-analyses showed that enteral tube feeding (ETF) resulted in a significantly shorter length of hospital stay, lower incidence of complications (including infectious complications), and lower sepsis scores. No difference in mortality was observed when ETF was compared to parenteral nutrition. No difference in mortality was found between ONS or ETF vs routine care in patients undergoing chemotherapy/radiotherapy or surgery (Elia et al., 2006).

Pressure ulcers

A systematic review and meta-analysis of pressure ulcer prevention and treatment showed a significant reduction in the development of pressure ulcers (by 25%) with high-protein ONS (250–500kcal for up to 26 weeks) when compared to routine care. A trend towards healing of existing ulcers was seen with the use of high-protein enteral formulae; however, future research would need to confirm these results (Stratton et al., 2005).

Critically ill patients

Nutritional studies assessing mortality and morbidity outcomes in the ICU setting are challenging and results remain conflicting.

Infectious complications

There are a multitude of studies assessing infectious complications with the use of immune-enhancing feeds and controversy remains in this area of research. Key nutrients that have been studied include glutamine, arginine, selenium, fish oils, and nucleotides. A recent RCT looking at the use of IV glutamine or IV selenium or both demonstrated a reduction in new infections with IV selenium supplementation for >5 days (no mortality effect) whereas IV glutamine showed no effect on either infection rate/mortality (Andrews et al., 2011). Decades of earlier research into glutamine supplementation seemed to show the opposite, with improvements found in infectious and overall outcomes for ICU patients (Griffiths et al., 1997).

Mechanical ventilation

Alberda et al. (2009) showed an increase in number of ventilator-free days with increased provision of energy and protein intakes in ICU patients with a BMI <25 or ≥35.

Length of stay

A multicentre, cluster randomized study demonstrated a significant reduction in mean hospital length of stay (25 vs 35 days; p = 0.003) by using evidence-based algorithms to improve nutritional support in the ICU (Martin et al., 2004). The mean ICU length of stay did not differ between groups in this study.

Mortality

Alberda et al. (2009) observed a lower mortality in ICU patients with increased provision of energy and protein in patients with a BMI <25 or ≥35. No benefit was seen in patients with a BMI of 25–35. Martin et al. (2004) found a trend towards a reduction in mortality with evidence-based algorithms and early enteral feeding. Singer et al. (2011) showed a trend towards reduced hospital mortality by providing actively supervised individualized nutrition support and calorie provision based on repeated energy measurements for ICU patients.

Further reading

Alberda C, Gramlich L, Jones N, et al. (2009). The relationship between nutritional intake and clinical outcomes in critically ill patients: results of an international multicenter observational study. *Intensive Care Med*, 35:1728–37.

Elia M, Van Bokhorst-de van der Schueren MA, Garvey J, et al. (2006). Enteral nutrition support and eicosapentaenoic acid in patients with cancer: a systematic review. *Int J Oncol*, 28(1):5-23.

Stratton RJ & Elia M. (2010). Encouraging appropriate evidence based use of oral nutritional supplements. *Proc Nutr Soc*, 69(4):477–87.

Stratton RJ, Ek AC, Engfer M, et al. (2005). Enteral nutrition support in the treatment and prevention of pressure ulcers: a systematic review and meta-analysis. *Ageing Res Rev*, 4(3):422–50.

8.3 Enteral and parenteral nutrition

Nutrition support

Nutrition can be provided as oral, enteral (EN), or parenteral nutrition (PN) support or a combination of these methods. Artificial nutrition support should be considered when patients are either malnourished or at risk of developing malnutrition. Risk factors for malnutrition include:

- Poor oral intake for past 5 days and expected to continue
- Poor absorptive capacity, high losses of nutrients, or increased demands (catabolic and hypermetabolic patients).

Nutrition support teams consisting of gastroenterologists, intensivists, nutrition support nurses, dietitians, pharmacists, and other trained healthcare professionals could provide effective treatment of in-patients requiring nutrition support. This team will play a vital role in minimizing complications that may arise from either EN or PN.

Enteral nutrition

Consider enteral tube feeding when patients with a functional GI tract are either:

- Malnourished or at risk
- Have an inadequate or unsafe oral intake
- Patients with increased requirements due to a disease process.

Enteral access routes

- Naso-gastric feeding tubes (NGTs) for short-term feeding (up to 4 weeks)
- Oro-gastric feeding tubes (OGTs) for patients with a base of skull fracture or facial trauma where NGTs cannot be passed
- Post-pyloric feeding (duodenal or jejunal) for upper GI obstruction or dysfunction
- Gastrostomy for longer-term enteral feeding (4 weeks or longer).
  Gastrostomies can be placed either via:
- Surgical placement (less common)
- Endoscopic placement: percutaneous endoscopic gastroscopy (PEG)
- Radiological placement: radiological inserted gastrostomy (RIG) mostly in head and neck cancer patients.

Management

Trained healthcare professionals should insert feeding tubes. The National Patient Safety Agency advises that NGTs should be checked after placement and daily before use with pH paper (pH <5.5) to ensure correct stomach placement (or with X-ray if required).

Administration

Bolus or continuous delivery of EN could be provided and this should be discussed with patients to fit in with their needs. Drug administration may also determine timing of feeding. Continuous feeding may vary between 16–24h.

Formulae

Feeds can mainly be categorized into whole protein feeds or peptide based (semi-elemental) feeds.
Whole protein feeds could further be divided into standard (1kcal/mL) formulae, high-energy formulae (1.2–2.0kcal/mL), high-protein formulae, and disease-specific feeds (renal, respiratory, low sodium, immune formulae).
Peptide-based feeds are mostly used in patients with severe gut impairment.

Monitoring of nutritional status

It is important to monitor patients receiving nutritional support on a number of levels (Table 8.4).

Table 8.4	Monitoring of enteral nutrition	
Parameter	Rationale	Frequency
Weight	Mass, fluid balance	Initial weight, then weekly. Daily for fluid balance
Fluid status	Fluid balance	Daily; twice weekly once stable
Anthropometry	Mid arm circumference	Initial then monthly
Medications	Interactions	Initial assessment, every few days
Feed volume	Adequacy and tolerance of feed	Daily then twice weekly once stable
GI tract (nausea, vomiting, diarrhoea, distention)	Feed tolerance, other factors causing vomiting and diarrhoea	Daily, then twice weekly once stable
Tube position, (e.g. nasal fixation if NGT) Stoma site	Correct placement Infection	Daily (if NGT with pH paper) Daily
Biochemistry	See section 8.1, Table 8.2	Daily initially and if critically ill, twice weekly once stable
Phosphate, magnesium, potassium	Refeeding syndrome risk	Daily until stable
Blood glucose	To detect abnormal blood glucose levels or overfeeding	Daily; twice weekly once stable
Temperature	Monitor for presence of infection	Daily

Parenteral nutrition

Consider parenteral nutrition (PN or TPN) in patients:

- Who do not have a functioning GI tract
- Who cannot tolerate full volumes of EN due to poor absorption or prolonged ileus
- With proximal high output or enterocutaneous fistulae
- With short bowel syndrome
- With oral mucositis
- Prolonged intestinal failure, i.e. radiation enteritis, necrotic bowel
- PN can also be used as 'top-up' nutrition support where enteral feeding is not deemed adequate.

The potential risk outweighs any perceived benefit if PN is provided for <5 days (NICE, 2006).

Parenteral access routes

Central access routes:

- Subclavian or internal jugular vein access for shorter-term PN
- A free dedicated lumen in a multilumen central line

- A dedicated peripherally inserted central catheter (PICC line) for medium-term access
- Tunnelled lines for long-term access (e.g. Hickman or Portacath).
  Peripheral access routes:
- Only used in institutions where nutrition team/nursing staff are able to monitor access sites.

Management
Trained healthcare professionals that are competent in catheter placement should place catheters. Adequately trained professionals should not only monitor access sites but also monitor the administration of PN.

Administration
Continuous administration is the preferred method when PN is initiated and when patients are critically ill. Once a patient is stable, and particularly if they are mobile, cyclical delivery of PN could be considered.

Unless contraindicated some trophic enteral feed (10–30mL/h) should be administered to maintain GI integrity (reducing villous atrophy). PN should not be disconnected if patients leave the ward for investigations as this increases the likelihood of line infections.

PN should be weaned gradually to avoid rebound hypoglycaemia. Patients should have approximately 50% of their requirements met by EN before PN is discontinued. It is prudent to monitor blood glucose levels whilst PN is weaned and once it is discontinued.

Formulae
PN is usually provided as an all-in-one preparation (1.5–3L) consisting of amino acids, lipids and glucose. Hospitals either purchase compounded PN, or make up compound PN in the aseptics unit in pharmacy for each patient. Here the lipid, glucose, and amino acid components are mixed together and additions (electrolytes, vitamins, and minerals) are added under aseptic conditions.

Complications
Careful monitoring detects most complications associated with PN.

Catheter/insertion related complications
- Pneumothorax
- Air embolism
- Thrombophlebitis
- Catheter occlusion
- Central venous thrombosis
- Catheter-related sepsis.

Nutritional/metabolic complications
- Hyperglycaemia
- Hypoglycaemia
- Refeeding syndrome
- Liver dysfunction
- Lipaemia
- Electrolyte imbalance.

Monitoring (Table 8.5)

Table 8.5 Monitoring of parenteral nutrition		
Parameter	Rationale	Frequency
Weight	Mass, fluid balance	Baseline, then weekly Daily: fluid balance
Fluid status	Fluid balance	Daily
Anthropometry	Mid arm circumference	Initial then monthly
Medications and IV fluids	Interactions, monitor electrolyte content of PN	Daily
PN rate	Adequacy, volume delivered	Daily
Catheter exit site	Signs of infection or phlebitis	Daily
Biochemistry	See section 8.1, Table 8.2 (nutritional assessment chapter)	Daily until stable
Phosphate, magnesium, potassium	Refeeding sSyndrome risk	Daily until stable
LFTs	Overfeeding PN	Daily initially then 3 ×x/week
Blood glucose	To detect hyper-or hypoglycaemia	4- hourly initially then twice daily once stable
Trace elements	To detect deficiencies	Baseline, then as required
Lipids (triglycerides)	To detect imbalances/ overfeeding	Baseline, then as required
Temperature	Monitor for presence of infection	Daily

Further reading
Cano NJM, Aparicio M, Brunori G, *et al.* (2009). ESPEN guidelines for adult parenteral nutrition. *Clin Nutr*, 28:359–479.

National Institute for Health and Clinical Excellence (2006). *Nutrition Support in Adults*. London: NICE.

Thomas B & Bishop J (eds) (2007). *Manual of Dietetic Practice* (4th edn). London: British Dietetic Association.

8.4 Nutrition in critical illness

Critically ill patients are typically hypermetabolic and hypercatabolic. Losses of muscle mass are estimated to be between 1% and 2% per day. Patients are unlikely to become anabolic until they are in a recovery phase. Preservation of muscle mass is vital in this population. The aims of nutrition support during a period of critical illness are to minimize losses and to provide nutrition in a safe and timely manner.

Nutritional assessment

Assessment of the nutritional status of the ICU patient is challenging. Many of the assessment techniques discussed in section 8.1 are of limited value in the ICU setting. Anthropometric assessment is greatly influenced by oedema and dietary assessment may be limited depending on the available history. Daily biochemical and clinical assessments are, however, central to planning and monitoring of nutrition support on the ICU.

Requirements

Energy requirements
Estimating the energy needs of critically ill patients remain one of the biggest nutritional challenges in this population. Indirect calorimetry is deemed the gold standard method; however, it is mostly used in the research arena.

Various predictive equations are used, each with their own inherent limitations. Commonly used equations or formulae include:

- 20–25kcal/kg (American College of Chest Physicians)
- 25–30kcal/kg (European Society of Enteral and Parenteral Nutrition (ESPEN))
- *Schofield equation* (1985) with additional stress factor (age, gender, and weight-specific requirement)
- *Ireton Jones* equation (1992; age, gender, weight, presence of trauma or burn information required)
- *Penn State* equation (2009; age, gender, weight, max. body temperature and minute ventilation required)
- *Harris Benedict* equation (age, gender, ideal body weight, and height-specific equation)

One should be mindful that these provide *estimated* energy requirements only. Sedation, paralysis, hypothermia, and mandatory ventilation may decrease requirements whereas pyrexia, disease state, surgery, pain, and physiotherapy may increase energy expenditure. Monitoring therefore becomes crucial to avoid overfeeding and underfeeding.

Protein requirements
Critically ill patients are unlikely to be in a positive nitrogen balance, the breakdown of protein and muscle far exceeds any muscle protein synthesis. Determining adequate protein intake for patients may again be difficult to assess.

Protein recommendations:
- 1.2g/kg/day in the general ICU population
- 1.5–2.5g/kg/day for patients on CRRT
- 1.3–1.5g/kg ideal body weight for parenteral feeding (Singer et al., 2009)
- 1.2–2.0g/kg/day—likely higher in burns or multiple trauma (Society of Critical Care Medicine (SCCM) and the American Society for Parenteral and Enteral Nutrition (ASPEN)).

Carbohydrate requirements and glucose control
Hyperglycaemia and insulin resistance is common during a period of critical illness. Excessive carbohydrate intake may cause hyperglycaemia, hypertriglyceridaemia, fatty liver, and hypercapnia. To avoid excess CO_2 production from surplus carbohydrate the glucose oxidation rate can be calculated:

$$\text{Glucose oxidation rate} = 4-7\text{mg/kg body weight/min/day}$$

Recent studies have focused on glycaemic control in the ICU patient. Tight glycaemic control was initially advocated (4.4–6.1mmol/L) after better outcomes were seen in cardiac surgical ICU patients. Many subsequent studies failed to replicate the original study findings. The NICE-SUGAR study (2009) reported an increased mortality in tight glycaemic control patients when compared to conventional blood sugar levels of 10mmol/L. Most ICUs are now using a more relaxed approach to glucose monitoring with upper limits of 10–11mol/L being accepted.

Overfeeding
Carbohydrate overfeeding has been discussed in the previous paragraph and this could potentially prolong mechanical ventilation. Overfeeding of protein or nitrogen can lead to azotemia and metabolic acidosis with renal insufficiency but this may be rare.

Lipid requirements
Usually 0.8–1.0g/kg/day.

Hypocaloric feeding
A further challenge to the calculation of energy requirements is the increase in the number of obese patients that are admitted to ICUs. Very little is currently known on how to best feed these patients. Permissive hypocaloric feeding has been recommended by some groups.

For patients with BMI >30, the SCCM and ASPEN recommend:
- 11–14kcal/kg actual body weight
- 22–25kcal/kg ideal body weight.

Fluid requirements
Fluid balance on the ICU is highly complex with fluid retention commonly being observed. Nutrition support aims should clearly fit in with the clinical condition and daily overall fluid balance aim for each individual patient.

Vitamin and mineral requirements
Although studies are lacking as to the optimum vitamin and mineral requirements it is thought that most enteral and parenteral formulae should provide sufficient micronutrient cover for the general ICU population. Patients on a burns ICU tend to receive additional vitamin and mineral supplementation.

Route of nutrition support

Enteral versus parenteral nutrition
EN is deemed the route of choice by American, Canadian, and European Critical Care groups. Equally, with conflicting evidence appearing, various international multicentre studies are currently under way to determine whether EN or indeed PN might be the best way to feed ICU patients.

Underfeeding may occur if patients rely on EN alone. Many institutions advocate the use of combined EN and PN to optimize nutrient intake. Consensus has not been reached yet regarding when to commence PN once EN has failed.

Timing

Early nutrition support is recommended, 24–48h after ICU admission once a patient has been sufficiently resuscitated. Early EN has been associated with a trend towards reduced mortality and infectious complications. No difference in ICU length of stay has been observed.

Protocols

The use of evidence-based protocols is strongly encouraged to ensure that nutrition support is initiated, increased, and monitored appropriately.

Protocols should:
- Promote early feeding
- Indicate gradual increases in EN
- Suggest a gastric residual volume cut off, typically 250–500mL (no evidence to suggest a specific value)
- Encourage the use of prokinetic agents if gastric feed is not tolerated
- Advocate the use of post-pyloric feeding tubes for feeding intolerance.

Immunonutrition

This popular area of ICU research remains somewhat controversial. Many enteral and parenteral formulations with the aim of enhancing immune function have been studied; however, methodological issues make some of the studies hard to interpret. Current 'hot topic nutrients' include glutamine, selenium, nucleotides, omega-3 fatty acids, and arginine supplementation to name only a few.

The role of probiotic agents in the ICU population remains unclear with some studies demonstrating harm and others showing improved outcomes.

Key points

- Optimum macro- and micronutrient requirements for ICU patients are still not known.
- It remains unclear whether meeting requirements of these nutrients would lead to improved ICU outcomes.

- Both over- and underfeeding should be avoided.
- Approximately 25kcal/kg/day would be appropriate for most general ICU patients.
- 1.2g/kg/day protein should be provided.
- Early nutrition support should be considered (24–48h after ICU admission).
- Feeding protocols may allow for a more optimum nutrient delivery.

Further reading

Frankenfield DC, Coleman A, Alam S, *et al.* (2009). Analysis of estimation of resting metabolic rates in critically ill adults. *JPEN*, 33(1):27–36.

Heyland DK et al. (2003). Canadian practice guidelines for nutrition support in mechanically ventilated, critically ill adult patients. *JPEN*, 27 (5):355–73. Guidelines updated: 2009.

Kreymann KG, Berger MM, Deutz NE, *et al.* (2006). European Society for Enteral and Parenteral Nutrition. Guidelines on enteral nutrition: intensive care. *Clin Nutr*, 25:210–23.

Martindale RG, McClave SA, Vanek VW, *et al.* (2009). Guidelines for the provision and assessment of nutrition support therapy in the adult critically ill patient: Society of Critical Care Medicine and American Society of Parenteral and Enteral Nutrition: Executive Summary. *Crit Care Med*, 37(5):1757–61.

National Institute for Clinical Excellence (2006). *Nutrition Support in Adults*. London: NICE.

NICE-SUGAR Study Investigators, Finfer S, Chittock DR, *et al.* (2009). Intensive versus conventional glucose control in critically ill patients. *NEJM*, 360(13):1283–97.

Reid CL, Campbell IT, Little RA (2004). Muscle wasting and energy balance in critical illness. *Clin Nutr*, 23:273–80.

Singer P, Berger MM, Van den Berghe G, *et al.* (2009). European Society for Enteral and Parenteral Nutrition. Guidelines on parenteral nutrition: intensive care. *Clin Nutr*, 28:387–400.

Thomas B & Bishop J (eds) (2007). *Manual of Dietetic Practice* (4th edn). London: British Dietetic Association.

Chapter 9

Statistical basis of clinical trials

9.1 Study designs

A study is the detailed examination of a phenomenon, which involves the collection and analysis of data in order to address a specific hypothesis. The research conducted during a study needs to be systematic, following rigorous methodology in order for the results to be valid, meaningful, and reproducible by other investigators. Poor study design will threaten the validity of findings and conclusions.

There are many different ways in which a study can be performed and the choice of design will depend upon the question being asked, available resources, and the feasibility of different models. When reading published studies it is important to take note of study design and reflect upon its limitations when determining the value of its results. Most commonly in medicine we seek to determine whether cause and effect are related (e.g. smoking and lung cancer) or whether treatment A is more effective than treatment B.

Observational studies

These studies seek new information about treatment effects based upon studying non-randomly selected individuals or groups who have been exposed to a particular condition (e.g. smoking) or intervention (e.g. a drug). The investigator does not interfere with the normal management of patients but merely observes outcomes in different selected cohorts. Control populations can be concurrent (patients with similar characteristics, but clearly differing in some respects as they have not been exposed to the condition or intervention) or historical. Controls may be matched or unmatched in terms of certain specific characteristics such as age and gender. However, bias cannot be excluded and confounding is likely. Results from observational studies can be used to inform the design of future randomized controlled trials (RCTs).

Cohort studies

This type of study tends to follow different cohorts of non-randomized groups to determine the effect of a difference, such as exposure to potentially noxious agent (e.g. smoking). After a period of time, the exposed and non-exposed participants can be compared. See Box 9.1.

Cohort studies are usually but not exclusively prospective.

Box 9.1 Features of cohort studies

- Outcome is measured after the exposure
- Yields true incidence rates and relative risks
- They may uncover unanticipated associations with outcome
- Best suited for common outcomes
- Can be expensive
- Require large numbers of subjects
- Takes a long time to complete
- Prone to attrition bias
- Prone to the bias of change in methods over time.

Case–control studies

This type of study (see Box 9.2) compares the characteristics of a known group of patients with a specific disease (the cases) to a group of patients in whom the disease is absent (the controls). Comparison is then made between the two groups to identify factors that occur with different frequency in the groups. These factors may represent risk factors for the disease. It is clearly important

that the control group is selected carefully, otherwise results may be subject to bias. Many case–control studies use demographic matching in order to create a similar control group. Here the control group is selected to match specific criteria, e.g. age, gender, ethnicity, that will match the participants in the case group.

Case–control studies are usually but not exclusively retrospective.

Box 9.2 Features of case–control studies

- Outcome is measured before exposure
- Controls are selected on the basis of not having the outcome
- Good for rare outcomes
- Relatively inexpensive
- Smaller numbers of subjects required
- Quicker to complete
- Prone to selection bias
- Prone to recall/retrospective bias.

Prospective studies

A prospective study observes for outcomes, such as the development of a disease, during the study period and relates this to other factors such as suspected risk factors. The study usually involves taking a cohort of subjects and watching them over a long period. The outcome of interest should be common; otherwise, the number of outcomes observed will be too small to be statistically meaningful. Bias can be introduced by the loss of patients to follow-up over time. Prospective studies usually have fewer potential sources of bias and confounding than retrospective studies. Prospective investigation is required to make precise estimates of either the incidence of an outcome or the relative risk of an outcome based on exposure.

Retrospective studies

A retrospective study looks backwards in time and examines exposures to suspected risk factors in relation to an outcome that is already know at the commencement of the study. Temporal relationships are less easy to determine in retrospective studies and bias is greater than in prospective studies. For this reason, retrospective investigations are often criticized. However, retrospective studies have the advantage of generally being easier and less costly to conduct. Also, they can be specifically designed to look at rare diseases: that is much more challenging prospectively as it requires very large numbers of participants.

Cross-sectional (longitudinal) study

This design of study involves the collection of data in a population at a single defined time point. They are frequently used to measure the prevalence of a disease and investigate possible causative factors. They are not particularly suited to the study of rare diseases but have been performed in ICUs across the world to gather information about common disorders such as sepsis and acute lung injury. Such studies tend to be relatively inexpensive and yield large quantities of data to analyse.

Interventional studies

Also called experimental studies, these involve alteration of a patient's management in order to observe a measurable outcome. The clinical trial (section 9.2) is the commonest and most robust example of an interventional study. Other examples include early phase drug trials (phase I and II) in which a small group of volunteers is given a drug to test its safety and efficacy profile, without a comparison control group.

Sample size calculations

Studies of any design can be limited by incorrect sample size, typically insufficient participants in the study. It is neither ethical, efficient, nor economical to conduct a study that is too large or too small. If a study is too large, an excessive number of patients may be exposed to an ineffective or harmful treatment; if too small, there is a risk that a successful treatment effect may be missed (type 2 error).

Four factors are generally required to calculate sample size:

Sample variation
The expected degree of variability (usually standard deviation) of the measured outcome in the population, usually estimated from previous work in the field. Greater variation will require a larger sample size to reach a desired power.

Effect size
This is the desired clinical effect as determined by the investigators, e.g. 10% improvement in survival.

Significance
This is the probability of a type I error (α) i.e. rejection of the null hypothesis when it is true (false positive) and is commonly set at 0.05 (a 5% chance of this occurring by chance).

Power
Power is a calculation of how likely it is that that an effect will be detected for a given sample size, effect size, and significance. Power increases with increasing sample size, meaning that large studies are more likely to detect real differences than small ones. It can be referred to as type II error (β) or likelihood of false negative results. β is commonly set at 10 or 20%.

The effect of altering these variables can be seen in Fig. 9.1.

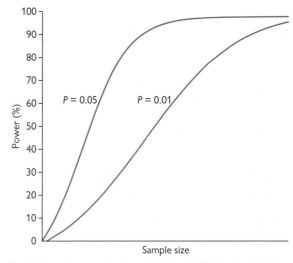

Fig. 9.1 Power curve graph. Reproduced from McCluskey A and Lalkhen AG, 'Statistics IV: Interpreting the results of statistical tests', *Continuing Education in Anaesthesia, Critical Care and Pain*, 2007, 7, 6, figure 3, p. 211, by permission of The Board of Management and Trustees of the British Journal of Anaesthesia and Oxford University Press.

Further reading

Petrie A & Sabin C (2001). *Medical Statistics at a Glance*. Oxford: Blackwell Science.

9.2 Design and conduct of clinical trials

Medicine frequently advances due to the pragmatic adoption of practices deemed beneficial to patients. The move towards an evidence-based approach, however, requires the design and conduct of robust clinical experiments (clinical trials) to create the evidence base. Clinical trials come in a variety of guises but the 'gold standard' has become the randomized controlled trial (RCT).

The purpose of a clinical trial is to assess the effectiveness of a treatment, drug, medical device, or complex intervention in the management of disease. The new treatment is usually compared against either a placebo or an 'active' control, which may be best available conventional therapy. Thus clinical trials are interventional (as opposed to observational) studies, as the process of the study requires alteration of a patient's management.

Best practice in the conduct of clinical trials is paramount, both for the patients directly involved in the trials and society as a whole, if the conclusions are acted upon. The design of each trial will depend on the nature and complexity of the proposed scientific question and the constraints imposed by logistical, financial and ethical considerations.

Design of clinical trials

The most robust design for a clinical trial is an RCT. Its validity lies in the fact that patients are randomly allocated to treatment groups without interference from clinicians or researchers. This minimizes selection (allocation) bias that may otherwise be caused by non-random allocation of the intervention.

The commonest type of RCT is the parallel group trial, where two groups receiving different treatments are directly compared. In a cross-over trial each participant receives both treatments being studied, one after another and the order of allocation is randomized; providing a robust comparison of the treatments within the same individuals. Cluster randomized trials look at the effect of interventions on groups of individuals randomly assigned to a treatment, for example allocation of a whole hospital to one treatment or another. In factorial studies two or more experimental interventions are not only evaluated separately but also in combination and against a control. Commonly a '2×2' study design is constructed in which two treatments are being evaluated (A & B) and the cohorts consist of: (1) neither treatment A nor B (double control), (2) treatment A + control, (3) treatment B + control, and (4) both treatments A & B.

Robust study design is imperative if resulting data are to be believed. Errors in the design phase of a study can render the data uninterruptable and therefore the study results meaningless. A clear hypothesis should be stated from the outset and commonly a single primary outcome measure should be selected (e.g. survival, blood pressure, length of hospital stay). The statistical methodology should be pre-determined for clinical trials to avoid selective analysis post data collection. This can now be confirmed through the registration of all high-quality randomized trials in order to ensure that the methods reported are the originally intended methods (e.g. <http://clinicaltrials.gov>).

Drug trials

Trials of pharmaceutical agents go through a number of stages from the development of the drug in a laboratory to accepted use in patients. These stages are referred to as phases (I to IV).

- *Phase I:* first human trials in small numbers of healthy volunteers to explore the pharmacokinetics, and pharmacodynamics of the drug along with some safety data.

- *Phase II:* if safe, the drug is given to groups of patients to define dosage levels, obtain pilot data on efficacy, and to gain further information about pharmacokinetics, and pharmacodynamics. This is a common phase at which unsuccessful drugs fail.

- *Phase III:* randomized controlled trials on large numbers of patients to ascertain whether the new drug is clinically effective.

- *Phase IV:* post-marketing surveillance of the successfully implement drug, so-called pharmovigilance, including testing of the drug for new cohorts of patients previously not studied.

Ethics approval

All research studies need to undergo a number of formal approvals prior to commencement; an independent ethics committee, a sponsor (usually a hospital, university, or drug company), and the local hospital research and development (R&D) team. The study may only commence on completion of all three of these approvals.

All studies on NHS patients in the UK are coordinated through the Integrated Research Approval System (IRAS) and completion of the application leads to review by a research ethics committee (REC) under the umbrella of the National Research Ethics Service (NRES). The sponsor is the body responsible for guaranteeing the value of the study and ensuring its safe and ethical conduct. Studies of investigational medicinal products (IMPs) also require approval from the Medicines and Healthcare products Regulatory Agency (MHRA) prior to commencement. Unexpected and adverse events that occur during the study must be reported to the sponsor. In large trials an independent data monitoring committee will be formed to periodically assess the trial and, if necessary, halt it if there are safety concerns.

Bias

Bias is a preconceived preference, conscious or unconscious, or an inclination that precludes the impartial conduct of a trial. Bias results in systematic error within the study and in general results in overestimation of the true effect of the intervention being assessed. Interpreting the results of a clinical trial not only requires an understanding of the statistical methods presented but the reader must also spend some time assessing the methodology behind the results. Poorly constructed studies lead to bias that may not be immediately obvious. There are a number of key components to consider when evaluating the risk of bias in a study.

Randomization

This is the process of assigning trial participants to different treatment groups and should give each participant an equal likelihood of being assigned to each group. A proper process of randomization is crucial if selection bias in clinical trials is to be eliminated. Without it, investigators may consciously (or subconsciously) allocate patients into favoured treatment groups and affect the ultimate outcome of the trial. Non-randomized studies overestimate treatment effects, presumably because of the underlying biases held by the investigators. The method of randomization does not matter, as long as it is truly random. Allocation by date of birth, day of the week, and medical record number is *not* truly random and should be avoided. Typically computer programs perform the randomization selection.

Blinding (allocation concealment)

Following randomization, blinding is the process through which the allocation of groupings within a trial (e.g. treatment or placebo) is withheld from specific persons. These persons might be the participants, care providers, or data assessors and withholding treatment allocation information from them aims to reduce bias that may be introduced by knowing which arm of the trial participants are in. Ideally, as many people as possible involved with the study should be blinded to allocation, although in some studies this will be impossible, e.g. blinding care givers and patients following allocation to ECMO or traditional mechanical ventilation.

Single-blinding tends to mean that one of the three categories of individuals (usually the participant) remains unaware of intervention allocations throughout the trial. In a double-blind trial, participants, and investigator assessors of outcome remain unaware of the intervention allocation throughout the trial. The allocation of participants should only be unblinded after all data has been analysed.

Control groups

Particular thought should be given to the nature of control (i.e. non-treatment or placebo) groups in clinical trials. Many large-scale trials have been criticized for having inappropriate control arms, e.g. the ARDSnet trial of low tidal volumes in the mechanical ventilation of patients with ARDS; in this case the control group was deemed to have been administered excessively high tidal volumes, compared with perceived standard of care, thus questioning the value of the study's findings.

Follow-up

Participants lost to follow-up during clinical trials may be non-random and result in a systematic bias, thereby affecting study results. Therefore studies with significant loss to follow-up should be interpreted cautiously.

Other limitations of a study that should be considered include the number of sites involved in a trial (single or multi-centre), because the results of single-centre studies may reflect unique local conditions and therefore not be generalizable to other centres, and the unavoidable fact that positive studies have traditionally been preferred for publication by journals, thus creating publication bias.

Hawthorne effect

It has been demonstrated that the conduct of experiments involving people, including clinical trials, leads to an overall improvement in outcomes regardless of the effectiveness of the treatment or whether the subject is in the intervention or placebo group. Named the Hawthorne effect (after experiments conducted in the Hawthorne Works of the Western Electric Company in Chicago in the 1920s), it describes the modification of behaviour within subjects when they are aware of being studied. Today, this effect may also encompass the change in behaviour of healthcare providers within the context of a study.

Levels for grading evidence and recommendations

A number of grading systems for evidence and recommendations are currently in use; it is important, however, to remember that they relate to the strength of the literature (quality of methods and data) but not necessarily its clinical importance. Two systems are commonly employed (see Boxes 9.3 and 9.4).

Box 9.3 Grading of evidence

Ia: systematic review or meta-analysis of RCTs.

Ib: at least one RCT.

IIa: at least one well-designed controlled study without randomization.

IIb: at least one well-designed quasi-experimental study, such as a cohort study.

III: well-designed non-experimental descriptive studies, such as comparative studies, correlation studies, case-control studies and case series.

IV: expert committee reports, opinions and/or clinical experience of respected authorities.

Reproduced with permission from *Acute Pain Management: Operative or Medical Procedures and Trauma. AHCPR Clinical Practice Guidelines, No. 1.* Acute Pain Management Guideline Panel. Rockville (MD): Agency for Health Care Policy and Research (AHCPR); 1992 Feb, Available from: http://www.ncbi.nlm.nih.gov/books/NBK52152.

Box 9.4 Grading of recommendations

A: based on hierarchy I evidence.

B: based on hierarchy II evidence or extrapolated from hierarchy I evidence.

C: based on hierarchy II evidence or extrapolated from hierarchy I or II evidence.

D: directly based on hierarchy IV evidence or extrapolated from hierarchy I, II or III evidence.

Reproduced with permission from Jacox A, Carr DB, Payne R. *Management of Cancer Pain.* Rockville (MD): Agency for Health Care Policy and Research (AHCPR); 1994 Mar. (AHCPR Clinical Practice Guidelines, No. 9.). Available from: http://www.ncbi.nlm.nih.gov/books/NBK52301.

Altering clinical practice based upon one RCT may not always be in a patient's best interest as the findings may have arisen by chance or due to bias. In general, results should be corroborated by similar trials and proven to be of value through systematic review and meta-analysis.

Systematic review

This is a methodologically unbiased review of studies in a particular field that aims to answer a specific question. Systematic reviews (SRs) are conducted using a rigorous methodology, as for any scientific experiment. SRs are unlike narrative reviews, which are subjective descriptive overviews of a particular topic, in that it they explicitly seek to avoid bias. The search for relevant studies must be exhaustive to avoid publication bias. This may involve contacting the investigators of unpublished trials and the translation of trials from other languages. The Cochrane Collaboration has helped to formalize this method of interpreting multiple clinical trial outcomes (<http://www.cochrane.org>).

SRs seek to provide a definitive answer about a particular clinical issue and this is often achieved by meta-analysis. This is a statistical process that combines the results of multiple studies (by regression analysis models) to calculate an overall likelihood of the effectiveness of the treatment under scrutiny. The validity of the overall result is dependent on the quality and heterogeneity of the studies used in the calculation.

Further reading

Petrie A & Sabin C (2009). *Medical Statistics at a Glance* (3rd edn). Oxford: Wiley-Blackwell.

9.3 Common statistical techniques

It is important to have an understanding of the common statistical methods used in research in order to interpret results presented in manuscripts and determine the clinical relevance of data. The meaning of data may be either obscured or clarified by statistics and the true message needs to be carefully sought by the reader. Authors may choose to use specific methods to generate a greater impact for their study thus statistical methodology must be considered when assessing all outcomes. It is important to have an understanding of some of the common terms and methods that are used in scientific reports.

Measures of proportion for binary data

Event rate
When considering clinical trials, an event rate is the number of people experiencing an event (i.e. disease, complication, or death depending on the study) expressed as a proportion of the relevant population.

Absolute risk
Absolute risk (AR) is the arithmetic difference between two event rates, i.e. the risk of an event in the control group minus the risk of an event in the treated group; usually expressed as a percentage. Clinically, the term absolute risk reduction (ARR) tends to be used in reference to the effectiveness of new treatments.

Relative risk
Relative risk (RR) is the ratio of probability of two events, with an event being the measured outcome of interest, e.g. developing a disease or death from a disease. It expresses the risk of the outcome in one group compared with another group and is expressed as the risk ratio in cohort studies and clinical trials. RR and risk ratio are therefore frequently used interchangeably. RR is particularly useful when describing the outcome of a clinical trial data, when it is used to compare the risk of developing a disease in patients not receiving a treatment against those that are on a new treatment for that disease.
- *RR = 1.0*: no difference in risk between the two groups
- *RR <1.0*: event is less likely to occur in the experimental group than in the control group
- *RR >1.0*: event is more likely to occur in the experimental group than in the control group.

In clinical trials, relative risk reduction (RRR) describes the proportion of the risk removed by a treatment. It is calculated by dividing absolute risk reduction by the event rate in the control group and is usually expressed as a percentage.

Odds ratio
The odds ratio (OR) is the ratio of the odds of an event occurring in one group to the odds of it occurring in another group calculated by dividing the odds in the treated or exposed by the odds in the control group. An OR >1.0 implies that the event is more likely whilst an OR <1.0 implies that it is less likely.

Whilst ORs and RRs are both relative measure of risk and the values may be similar, they are not equivalent. The value of RR approaches that of OR as diseases become increasingly rare.

It should be remembered that the OR is a ratio of the odds whilst the RR is a ratio of percentages. OR describes how much more likely it is that someone who is exposed to the factor under study (e.g. the risk or drug) will develop the outcome (event) as compared to someone who is not exposed. In clinical research, OR is commonly used for case-control studies whilst RR tends to be used in randomized controlled trials and cohort studies. RR tends to be of greater clinical value than OR (as it is a more intuitive measure), however, OR is much more widely use in statistics than RR as logistic regression calculations use the log of the OR.

Number needed to treat
Number needed to treat (NNT) is a commonly used measure that provides an easy to understand indication of the effectiveness of a treatment. It tells us the average number of patients that will require a new treatment in order to prevent a negative outcome. It is the inverse of absolute risk reduction and the higher the number the less effective a treatment is; with the ideal NNT being 1.

Example
A clinical trial of the anti-sepsis drug Xylanox against placebo, in 340 patients with sepsis; the outcome variable is sepsis/no sepsis after treatment with Xylanox (Table 9.1).

Table 9.1 Results of example trial		
	Sepsis	No Sepsis
Xylanox	45	120
Placebo	90	85

Xylanox event rate for sepsis: 45/165 = 0.375 (37.5%)
Placebo event rate (ER) for sepsis: 90/175 = 0.514 (51.4%)

For Xylanox treatment vs placebo
- *ARR*: 51.4% − 37.5% = 13.9%
- *RR*: 37.5%/51.4% = 73.0% or 0.73
- *OR* = (45/120)/(90/85) = 0.375/1.059 = 0.354
- *NNT* = 1/ARR = 1/0.139 = 7.19

Thus Xylanox appears effective in reducing sepsis (OR 0.354) with a NNT of 7.19 patients.

Measures of statistical significance

Whilst measures such as RR, OR, and NNT provide an indication of the magnitude of difference between specified groups, we also require a measure of the likelihood that this difference did not occur by chance The difference presented in a study needs to be considered in the context of the wider population and clinicians need to know if this difference is likely to be repeated in their own patients. Perhaps the difference arose purely due to chance; confidence intervals and p-values attempt provide some information about how likely this is.

p-values
Most clinicians are familiar with the emphasis placed on p-values and the doctrine that a p-value <0.05 equates with statistical (but not necessarily clinical) significance. A p-value is in reference to the null hypothesis, which states that there is no true difference in the selected measure between groups in a study. The p-value is the probability that we would observe the effects demonstrated in the study if there was truly no difference between the treatments i.e. the chance of a false positive. If the calculated p-value is small, the findings are unlikely to have arisen by chance; the null hypothesis is rejected and assumes that there is a real difference between two treatments. Arbitrarily it is common to accept the chance of false positive finding as one in 20, i.e. a p-value of 0.05. This value is universally accepted to be a relevant threshold for clinical trials but still means that the result has a one in

20 possibility of occurring by chance. A further limitation of the p-value is that is gives a binary indication of reliability (significant vs. not significant) and fails to provide a range of values within which any true effect is likely to reside.

Confidence intervals

An alternative and more informative way of expressing the reliability of presented differences is the use of a confidence interval (CI). CIs give a clearer indication of the range within which a true difference is likely to lie. They describe the range within which a result for the whole population would occur for a specified proportion of times a survey or test was repeated among a sample of the population. If the measured difference has a high error level, the corresponding CI will be wide, and therefore we would be less certain that the trial results would apply to the rest of the population. On the whole, larger sample sizes tend to reduce the magnitude of the CI. As with the threshold of 0.05 for p-values, it is common practice to report the 95% CI, which means there is a 95% chance that the quoted range includes the reported difference. The value of 95% is connected to the fact that is the range of results is normally distributed; approximately 95% of them will lie within 2 standard deviations of the mean.

If the range of the CI crosses zero then a finding is not statistically significant. Also, when a study result is positive (i.e. the CI does not cross zero), it is possible to ascertain whether the sample size was adequate by checking the lower boundary of the CI. If this value is smaller than the smallest difference your patients would consider important, the sample size could be inadequate. For example, if mortality in sepsis was reduced from 15.5% to 10.0% with Xylanox: ARR is 5% and is RRR 33.3%, an impressive finding. However, if the 95% CI for the RRR was 14.3–52.3 %, whilst still statistically significant, the range is wide and a possible true RRR of only 14.3% may be unacceptable when the side effects and costs of this treatment are taken into consideration. A larger trial would then need to be conducted in order to reduce the size of the CI and ascertain whether the effects of Xylanox were really as good as the original trial suggested. CIs therefore greatly aid our interpretation of clinical trial data by putting upper and lower bounds on the likely size of any true effect.

What does significance mean?

When considering both p-values and CIs it is worth emphasizing that a finding of no statistical significance does not mean absence of a clinical effect. Small studies might report non-significant results, when important real effects exist that a larger study would have detected (a type II error). Conversely, statistical significance does not necessarily mean that the observed effect is either real or relevant. There is a possibility that it occurred by chance alone (type I error). Finally, statistical significance gives no guarantee of clinical significance, which requires interpretation of the magnitude of the result in the context of clinical knowledge of the underlying condition.

Receiver operating characteristic curve

This is a method used to assess the ability of a diagnostic test to discriminate between healthy and diseased individuals. It is applied to tests for which there is a variable cut off (e.g. anaerobic threshold for preoperative fitness) and graphically represents the relationship between sensitivity, specificity and the selected cut off (e.g. 11mL/kg/min).

- The *sensitivity* of a diagnostic test is the proportion of patients for whom the outcome is positive that are correctly identified by the test.
- The *specificity* is the proportion of patients for whom the outcome is negative that are correctly identified by the test.

For any diagnostic test there must always be a trade-off between sensitivity and specificity.

The receiver operator characteristic (ROC) curve displays true positive rate on the y-axis (sensitivity) and false positive rate on the x-axis (1 − specificity). When plotted, the area below the curve represents a measure of the validity of the test, an ideal test would have an area of 1.0, and as the value declines the test becomes less effective until 0.5 is reached, which indicates the test result is equivalent to a random number generator (see Fig. 9.2).

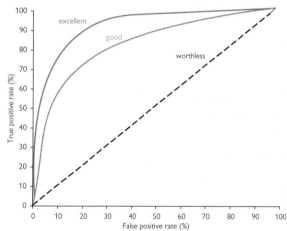

Fig. 9.2 Receiver operator characteristic curves.

Further reading

Norman GR & Streiner DL (2008). *Biostatistics: The Bare Essentials* (3rd edn). New York: McGraw-Hill Medical.

Chapter 10

Physics and clinical measurement

195

10.1 Interpretation of laboratory test results

It is fundamentally important when requesting and interpreting laboratory tests to have an understanding of the processes by which results are generated, and of the potential sources of error.

Reasons for performing laboratory tests

There are four principal *clinical* reasons to perform laboratory investigations:

Diagnosis

The cornerstone of the diagnostic process in medicine remains the history and clinical examination, by which the clinician usually formulates a differential diagnosis. Laboratory tests may be used to confirm or refute a particular diagnosis.

Prognosis

Tests may be used to predict the risk of developing a particular condition: for example, a lipid profile as an indicator of coronary artery disease risk.

Monitoring

Laboratory investigations are frequently used to monitor the progress of a disease or the effects of treatment—for example, HbA_{1C} levels in diabetes, or the INR in patients on warfarin therapy.

Screening

It has become increasingly common over recent decades to use investigations to detect disease at a subclinical stage, on the assumption that earlier diagnosis and treatment will improve prognosis. Screening can be implemented at several levels:

- Population: e.g. Guthrie test in babies for phenylketonuria.
- Selective: e.g. PSA screening in men over a certain age.
- Individual: for example, lipid profile in a well-man clinic.
- Opportunistic: when people attend with something else e.g. fasting glucose in a newly-diagnosed hypertensive.

Collection of specimens

In the UK, Clinical Pathology Accreditation (CPA) regulations specify that the laboratory will carefully stipulate the necessary 'Standard Operating Procedure' (SOP) for sample collection, handling and transport to the laboratory.

The process begins with the clinician making a request, either on paper or electronically. Sufficient identifying details should be given (patient name, hospital number, and date of birth, together with the destination for the report and contact details). Adequate clinical information (and, in some cases concurrent drug therapy) is necessary in order for the results to be interpreted in context.

It may be necessary to standardize the conditions under which the specimen is taken—for example, morning cortisol or fasting glucose.

It is readily apparent that samples must be collected into the correct container (and also in the correct order, to avoid possible contamination of 'plain' samples with anticoagulant). In terms of sampling itself, care should be taken to avoid haemolysis, and to avoid saline contamination of the sample from IV infusions or from pressure-transducer lines.

Analysis of results

The ideal analytical method will be:
- *Accurate:* gives a correct result.

- *Precise:* gives the same result if repeated.
- *Sensitive:* able to measure low concentrations of the substance.
- *Specific:* unaffected by presence of other substances.

Analytical methods are subject to strict quality control procedures, but the potential for some imprecision remains ever-present. Such *analytical variation* can be expressed mathematically as a coefficient of variation (standard deviation/mean) when repeated analyses are made on the same sample.

Sources of error

For any result to be valuable, it must not only be accurate and relevant, but also communicated to, and understood by, the clinician who has made the request.

Errors may arise at any stage during the processes of specimen gathering, laboratory analysis and communication of results, although robust procedures exist in every recognized institution in order that these be minimized.

Errors are typically classified as:
- *Pre-analytical:* those arising on account of the manner by which samples are obtained, labelled, handled, or stored until they arrive at the laboratory.
- *Analytical:* errors occurring *within* the laboratory, and arising from human or instrumental failure.
- *Post-analytical:* a correct result is generated, but an error occurs subsequently in recording, communicating, interpreting or responding to the result.

Pre-analytical errors occur most commonly (about 60% of the total). The commonest pre-analytical errors are:
- Specimen tube empty or not properly filled
- Wrong specimen tube or container
- Error in patient identification (actual or recorded)
- Sample contamination (drip arm/heparin flush etc.).

Analytical errors are the least common category (15% of the total). Most modern analysers are automated to a high degree and will not report results if an analytical channel or electrode have not passed stringent quality assurance and control procedures.

Interpretation of results

Is the result normal or abnormal?

Statistically, the term 'normal' refers to the common Gaussian distribution of many biological variables. If the variable being measured has a normal distribution within a population, then 95.5% of values will lie within the range mean ±2 standard deviations (SD), and 99.7% will lie within the mean ±3SD range.

In statistical terms, mean ±2SD is the normal range. This has several important implications:
- 5% of healthy individuals will have results outside the normal range.
- The statistical term 'normal' may not correlate with what the term might more generally imply—for example, a cholesterol level within the normal range for apparently healthy men may still be associated with increased cardiovascular risk: many laboratories prefer instead to use the term *reference range* to avoid any assumptions being made in respect of what is 'normal'.

In essence, a normal result does not always exclude a pathological process, neither does an abnormal one confirm it.

Comparing results

When a test is repeated (for example, when monitoring a chronic condition such as renal impairment), it is important to determine whether or not observed differences are significant. Factors affecting this are:

- Analytical variation: the precision of the assay
- Biological variation: the natural variation of values within individuals at different times.

How useful is the result?

Various properties of a test result enable the clinician to appreciate its importance in context. Amongst the most important are:

- Specificity and sensitivity and ROC curves
- Predictive values.

Specificity and sensitivity

The *specificity* of a test is a measure of the incidence of true negatives (TN) i.e. negative results in people truly without the disease (Box 10.1).

Box 10.1 Calculating specificity and sensitivity

$$\text{Specificity} = \frac{TN}{\text{all without disease (TN + FP)}} \times 100$$

$$\text{Sensitivity} = \frac{TP}{\text{all with disease (TP + FN)}} \times 100$$

FP = false positives
FN = false negatives

The *sensitivity* is a measure of the incidence of true positives (TP) i.e. positive results in people who are known to have the disease (Box 10.1).

The ideal test would have 100% sensitivity (gives a positive result in all patients with a particular disease) and 100% specificity (gives a negative result in all patients free of a disease). This is rarely the case: in general, when specificity rises, sensitivity falls, and vice versa. The relative importance of sensitivity and specificity of a test depends to some extent on the nature of the disease being tested for: a screening test for a potentially serious disease, for example, absolutely requires a highly sensitive test. A lack of specificity will entail anxiety and further investigations for the patients whose results are false positives.

ROCs are a useful graphical representation of sensitivity and specificity (see section 9.3).

Predictive values

Even if a test is both highly sensitive and specific, it may not perform well in a clinical context, which is dependent upon the prevalence of the disease within the population. If a condition has a low prevalence and the test is less than 100% specific, then many false positives will result, i.e. the *predictive value* of a positive result is low.

In respect of screening tests, it is important that cases of a disease are not missed. The predictive value of a negative result should, therefore, be high (see Box 10.2).

Box 10.2 Predictive values of positive and negative test results

$$PV_{+ve} = \frac{TP}{TP + FP} \times 100$$

$$PV_{-ve} = \frac{TN}{TN + FN} \times 100$$

Point of care testing

An increasingly common means of carrying out pathology testing is to bring the analyser as near to the patient or group of patients as possible. The collection and handling of samples should be as rigorous as if they are being sent to the pathology laboratory.

The point of care testing (POCT) analyser should be run and maintained by scientific staff from the pathology department, or dedicated and suitably qualified staff from the host department who will carry out the same quality control and assurance checks to ensure that the results from the analysers are consistent with those from the central laboratory, thus minimizing analytical errors.

There is a common misconception that results from POCT instruments are in some way inferior to those from the main pathology laboratory (the so called 'formal' results). This is absolutely not the case - provided that professionally accountable staff, having undergone appropriate training, are doing the tests. If this cannot consistently be achieved, then point of care testing becomes potentially dangerous.

Further reading

Marshall WJ & Bangert SK (2008). Biochemical investigations in clinical medicine. In Marshall WJ & Bangert SK (eds) *Clinical Chemistry* (6th edn), pp. 1–14. London: Elsevier Ltd.

Wians FH (2009). Clinical laboratory tests: which, why, and what do the results mean? *Lab Med*, 40(2):105–13. doi:10.1309/LM4O4L0HHUTWWUDD.

10.2 Measurement of blood coagulation and interpretation of data

Evolution of theories of coagulation

The coagulation system represents a balance between procoagulant and anticoagulant mechanisms, requiring that haemostasis be maintained without causing widespread vascular occlusion and restriction of normal blood flow.

Historically, the phenomenon of blood clotting was thought to represent cooling of the blood upon exposure to air, through the observations of both Hippocrates and Aristotle.

During the 20th century, a 'classical' theory of coagulation emerged, describing the conversion of prothrombin to thrombin in the presence of calcium. Thrombin was then able to convert fibrinogen into solid fibrin.

By the 1940s and 1950s, many other coagulation factors, upstream from thrombin, were discovered and woven into an explanation of the process in terms of a *cascade*. Newly identified factors were named either after their discoverer, or after a patient deficient in them, and numbered (Roman numerals) in order of their discovery.

The *cascade model* comprises a series of steps in which pro-enzyme substrates are cleaved, predominantly on phospholipid membranes and in the presence of calcium, to generate the next enzyme in the cascade.

The model was subdivided into *extrinsic* and *intrinsic* pathways:

- Extrinsic: located *outside* the blood, and comprising tissue factor (TF) and factor VIIa.
- Intrinsic: localized within the blood, and initiated through contact activation of factor XII.

Either pathway could activate a *common pathway* in which factor Xa, in the presence of factor Va, could activate prothrombin (II) to thrombin (IIa), thence fibrinogen to fibrin.

The cascade model was very useful in understanding the enzymatic processes involved in plasma-based *in vitro* coagulation, and formed the basis of laboratory tests such as the prothrombin time (PT), to identify deficiencies in the extrinsic or common pathways, and the activated partial thromboplastin time (aPTT), whose prolongation reflects deficiencies in the intrinsic or common pathways.

It became apparent, however, that the model does *not* adequately explain the haemostatic process such as it occurs *in vivo*. Clinical manifestations of clotting factor deficiencies clearly contradict the concept—for example:

- Factor XII deficiency causes marked aPTT prolongation, but is not associated with a bleeding tendency in mice or humans.
- In situations in which the INR is markedly prolonged, there may be no clinical evidence of a bleeding diathesis.
- Deficiency of factor VIII or IX (haemophilia A or B) results in a marked bleeding tendency, despite an intact extrinsic pathway.

A new understanding of haemostasis incorporates the role of *cells*. Four overlapping phases are described in an integrated *cell-based model of coagulation*, in which the participation of two different cell types is required: platelets and a TF-bearing cell.

The cell-based model of coagulation

The four phases of clot development can overlap and coexist as the clot is forming.

Initiation

TF is the sole relevant initiator of coagulation *in vivo*. Cells expressing TF are generally located outside the vasculature—thus initiation of coagulation is prevented under normal circumstances with an intact endothelium. When an injury occurs, circulating factor VIIa (the only circulating *active* clotting factor) rapidly binds to an exposed TF-bearing cell. The TF-factor VIIa complex activates additional factor VII to factor VIIa, resulting in further TF-factor VIIa activity, and activation of factor X.

The factor Xa generated by TF-factor VIIa binds to a fewcofactor (Va) molecules to form a *prothrombinase* complex. This cleaves prothrombin and generates a small amount of thrombin.

Amplification

The small amount of thrombin generated on the surface of a TF-bearing cell during the initiation phase is then available to activate *platelets* that have leaked from the vasculature at the site of injury. Thrombin binds to platelet surface receptors causing granule release. These contain the raw materials for coagulation processes, and also factors that promote further platelet activation. Thrombin also causes cleavage of the factor VIII–vWF (von Willebrand factor) complex. vWF promotes further platelet adhesion and aggregation, whilst the released factor VIII is activated to factor VIIIa.

Propagation

Propagation occurs as large numbers of platelets become activated and more and more glycoprotein receptor sites on the platelet surface become available for platelet binding. This leads to a *burst* of thrombin generation, which in turn activates more platelets and cleaves fibrinogen to fibrin, which forms a solid localized matrix with activated platelets.

Termination

Once the fibrin/platelet clot is formed at the site of injury, the progression of its formation must be limited to prevent harmful thrombotic occlusion of surrounding vasculature. Three naturally occurring anticoagulants limit the propagation of the clot—antithrombin III and proteins S and C.

The activity of these anticoagulant proteins relies on the presence of an intact glycocalyx, the endothelial cells of which express *heparinoids*, which activate antithrombin III, *thrombomodulin*, which binds to thrombin, causing activation of protein C, and *tissue factor pathway inhibitor* (TFPI).

Until relatively recently the role of the vascular endothelium was given little prominence but it is in fact fundamental in the clotting process: where it is damaged, clot forms; when intact, it exerts essential anticoagulant activity.

Point of care coagulation testing

There has been a huge interest in recent years in point of care coagulation testing, owing to a number of factors:

- The long turnaround time of conventional laboratory tests.
- A desire to reduce inappropriate transfusion (of red cells or clotting factors).
- Wide acceptance of the cell-based model of coagulation (its emphasis on the pivotal role of platelets has caused interest to move away from *plasma-based* laboratory tests to tests on *whole blood*)

- An increasing realization that conventional tests of coagulation (INR and aPTT) provide only limited insights, reflecting only small elements of the coagulation process—they were never intended to be relevant markers of *in vivo* haemostasis or predictors of perioperative bleeding risk.

Viscoelastic tests of haemostasis: TEG® and ROTEM®

The cell-based model of coagulation emphasizes the role of *platelets* in thrombin generation. There are several pre-requisites for effective haemostasis:

- Sufficient thrombin generation (via clotting factors and platelets)
- Adequate substrate (fibrinogen)
- Clot stability.

Thromboelastography (TEG®) and thromboelastometry (ROTEM®) give dynamic information in respect of all these factors.

Both methods measure the shear elastance of the clot as it forms over time. Both employ a vertical pin placed in a blood sample held in a cup or cuvette. In the TEG® the cup is slowly oscillated clockwise and anticlockwise through 4°. As the clot forms in the cup, it starts to move the pin, and as the strength of the clot increases (propagation phase), the pin is moved more. In the ROTEM®, a variant of the original TEG®, the cup is held still, and the *pin* oscillates. Both techniques measure the viscoelastic properties of the clot as it forms or lyses.

Each technique provides—both visually and numerically—a complete picture of clot initiation, formation, and stability. TEG® and ROTEM® parameters have a different nomenclature, but refer to identical stages of clot formation.

In respect of the TEG®, the five important parameters are the R-time, the K-time, the α-angle, the maximum amplitude (MA), and the LY30 (lysis at 30min)—see Box 10.3 and Figs. 10.1 and 10.2.

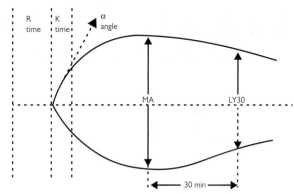

Fig. 10.1 Schematic of important TEG® parameters. Reproduced from Srivastava A and Kelleher A, 'Point-of-care coagulation testing', *Continuing Education in Anaesthesia, Critical Care and Pain*, 2012, 13, 1, pp. 12–16, by permission of The Board of Management and Trustees of the British Journal of Anaesthesia and Oxford University Press, doi:10.1093/bjaceaccp/mks049.

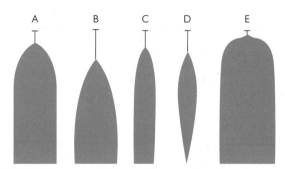

Fig. 10.2 Characteristic TEG® traces. A = normal trace. B = haemophilia: marked prolongation of r and K times. Decreased alpha angle, C = thrombocytopenia: normal r and rK times, decreased MA (< 40 mm). D = fibrinolysis: CLI <85%. E = hypercoagulability: short r time, increased MA and steep clot formation rate. Reproduced from SV Mallett and DJA Cox, 'Thrombelastography', *British Journal of Anaesthesia*, 1992, 69, pp. 307–313, by permission of The Board of Management and Trustees of the British Journal of Anaesthesia and Oxford University Press.

Additional applications of thromboelastography

TEG® Platelet Mapping provides a percentage platelet inhibition relative to the patient's baseline viscoelastic profile. Selective platelet agonists are used (arachidonic acid for aspirin, and ADP for thienopyridines or GPIIb/IIIa antagonists—see section 1.20). This may have widespread clinical applications in cardiology, and in assessing patients presenting for surgery who are receiving single or dual antiplatelet therapy.

The TEG® functional fibrinogen assay measures the contribution of fibrin to the overall platelet/fibrin by blocking platelet GpIIb/IIIa receptors. Clot initiation is by tissue factor rather than thrombin.

Further reading

Mallett SV & Cox D (1992). Thrombelastography. *Br J Anaesth*, 69(3):307–13.

Mallett SV, Chowdary P, & Burroughs AK (2013). Clinical utility of viscoelastic tests of coagulation in patients with liver disease. *Liver Int*, 33(7):961–74. doi:10.1111/liv.12158.

Smith SA (2009). The cell-based model of coagulation. *J Vet Emerg Crit Care*, 19(1):3–10. doi:10.1111/j.1476.Srivastava A & Kelleher A (2012). Point-of-care coagulation testing. *CEACCP*, 13:12–16. doi:10.1093/bjaceaccp/mks049.

> **Box 10.3 The five important TEG® parameters**
>
> *R-time (reaction time)*
> - Corresponds to initial fibrin formation.
> - Prolonged by anticoagulants, factor deficiencies, and hypofibrinogenaemia.
> - Shortened in hypercoagulable states.
>
> *K-time (clot formation time)*
> - Measures the kinetics of clot formation.
> - Prolonged by anticoagulants, hypofibrinogenaemia, and thrombocytopenia.
>
> *α-angle*
> - Represents the speed at which solid clot forms.
> - Decreased by anticoagulants or factor deficiencies, hypofibrinogenaemia and thrombocytopenia.
> - Increased in prothrombotic and hypercoagulable states.
>
> *MA (maximum amplitude)*
> - Represents maximum clot strength (platelets + fibrin).
> - Predominantly reflects *platelet* number or function.
>
> *LY30 (% lysis 30min after MA is reached)*
> - Reflects fibrinolysis.

10.3 Radiation protection

The importance of radiation protection

The applications of radiation in medicine – and, in particular, the scope of interventional radiology – continue to increase. Medical procedures utilising radiation constitute the most rapidly increasing source of radiation worldwide. There is an inherent obligation on the part of those involved to understand the risks for both patients and staff, and the strategies to minimize harm.

Three major categories of medical procedure utilise radiation:

- Nuclear medicine: administration of unsealed radioactive pharmaceuticals for diagnosis or treatment
- Radiotherapy: using either external radiation or internal radioactive sources, principally in the treatment of cancer
- Diagnostic and interventional radiology: simple X-rays, CT and fluoroscopically-guided interventional procedures

Levels of radiation exposure

The International Commission on Radiological Protection (ICRP) specifies safe radiation exposure limits in terms of *equivalent* doses for individual organs or tissues, and an *effective dose* for whole-body exposure (see Box 10.4).

Data on safe levels of exposure derive largely from follow-up of those exposed to the nuclear bombs of 1945, and from a collaborative study across 15 countries of workers in the nuclear industry. Gamma rays and X-rays have similar carcinogenic potential.

Box 10.4 Recommended dose limits for occupational radiation exposure	
Effective dose:	20mSv / year (averaged over 5 years) Maximum 50 mSv in any single year
Equivalent doses:	
Lens:	150 mSv / year
Skin:	500 mSv / year
Hands + feet:	500 mSv / year

Members of the public receive on average about 6 mSv per year, half of which derives from background radiation, and the remainder from medical and other sources.

Levels of *occupational* exposure associated with radiological procedures are highly variable, ranging from almost negligible in respect of a simple chest X-ray, to quite significant in the case of complex interventional procedures. In simple terms, there are two potential sources of occupational exposure:

- From the X-ray beam: either from the primary beam, or from other areas of the beam (so-called leakage X-rays) – in practice, both should be minimal
- From the patient: the X-ray beam interacts with the patient's body surface and produces *scattered radiation*, which emanates from the patient in all directions

Scattered radiation is the main determinant of occupational exposure, which in turn, therefore, relates to the proximity of personnel to the patient when exposures are being made. Since the level of scatter is determined largely by the dose that the patient receives, it follows that steps to minimize the patient's dose will also reduce occupational exposure.

Effects of ionizing radiation

Two categories of effect are described:

- *Stochastic effects:* these refer to the development of cancer (and possible hereditary effects) occurring secondary to DNA damage
- *Deterministic effects:* these produce cell death at the tissue level, after high absorbed doses. Skin erythema is a typical manifestation, but sometimes more severe deterministic injuries may occur (during radiotherapy, of course, radiation is administered at a dose *intended* to cause local deterministic effects)

Stochastic effects are cumulative and have a long latency period. There is no "safe" dose below which induced neoplasia does not occur. A linear relationship exists between excess cancer risk and radiation dose.

Ocular effects of radiation exposure

The eye may be the organ most sensitive to radiation damage, principally from scatter radiation. In practice, damage to the eye may be more important than cardiogenic or teratogenic effects of radiation exposure. During interventional procedures, the radiation dose to the anaesthetist's eye may be up to three times greater than to the radiologist's.

Radiation damage causes posterior lens opacification (as seen in diabetes and steroid-induced cataracts). It is considered a deterministic effect (i.e. occurring at a dose above a minimum threshold for injury), but recent data suggest that radiation-induced cataracts may be a stochastic effect, and that there is no safe threshold.

Teratogenic effects of occupational exposure

The recommended lower limit for fetal occupational radiation exposure is 1–5 mSv. The potential effects at higher doses are deterministic. Standard radiation protection measures result in negligible fetal risk, since the threshold dose is well above that which would be received beneath a protective apron. Nonetheless, in-utero exposure to ionizing radiation *at any dose* is associated with an increased risk of childhood malignancy. The risk of childhood leukaemia is estimated to be in excess of 6% at doses above 0.5 Gy.

Determinants of the level of occupational exposure

As discussed, the primary determinant for occupational exposure is the proximity of personnel to the patient.

In many situations – typically general X-ray and CT – there is no need for attendant personnel to be physically close to the patient. This reduces exposure to scattered radiation since radiation intensity falls off rapidly with distance, according to the so-called "inverse-square law". In addition, structural shielding may be placed between the patient and personnel (for example, within the wall and window of the control room), which should ensure that occupational exposure is essentially zero in these situations.

In other situations, however—typically during fluoroscopy and image-guided interventional procedures—it will be necessary to maintain close physical contact with the patient. In the absence of the protection afforded through distance and structural barriers, measures are necessary to attenuate exposure to scattered radiation. These include protective clothing (aprons, spectacles and thyroid shields) and protective screens that can be wheeled between the patient and personnel. Protective eyewear reduces lens exposure to scatter by 90%.

Implications of novel imaging techniques

New technologies have allowed more complex diagnostic and interventional procedures to be performed, often with the advantage that more hazardous open surgical intervention can be avoided (for example, in the treatment of aortic and intracranial aneurysms). However, there are important implications in terms of the safety of attendant personnel.

Many procedures utilizing fluoroscopy are performed outside the radiology suite—typically in the vascular or urology theatre—and fluoroscopy times may be very long indeed (perhaps in excess of one hour in the treatment of a complex aneurysm). Many units have dedicated interventional theatres, in which the procedures are, at least in part, being performed by radiologists. Nonetheless, other staff may be involved who fall outside the umbrella of the radiology department, and who may have received less training in the use of the equipment and in radiation protection.

Strategies for effective radiation protection

Robust policies and protocols are essential in order to deliver effective and appropriate radiation protection.

There are five modifiable risk factors for radiation exposure (see Box 10.5). For the anaesthetist, the two most important factors in reducing radiation exposure are *distance* and *shielding*.

Box 10.5 Modifiable risk factors for radiation exposure
Duration of the procedure
Distance from the radiation source
Barriers and shielding: structural and personal
Education and training
Monitoring

Procedure duration

The total duration of radiation exposure during an intervention is, of course, predominantly a function of the complexity of the procedure and the experience of the operator, and the anaesthetist will have relatively less control over this.

Distance from the radiation source

Increasing distance from the radiation source is of fundamental importance in reducing radiation exposure. Complex interventions, however, frequently require the anaesthetist to remain in close proximity to the patient. In addition, the operating theatre environment is frequently cramped, limiting the ability of the anaesthetist to position him- or herself at an adequately safe distance.

Barriers and shielding

These are areas in which the anaesthetist does have control, both for corporate and individual protection.

Structural shielding comprises material embedded into the walls of the radiology suite, in addition to mobile shields that can be positioned as required.

The important components of personal shielding are aprons, thyroid shields and protective eyewear. The latter is particularly important, and most often neglected. Lateral C-arms are typically orientated such that the X-ray source is on the anaesthesia side, pointing towards the radiologist and patient. Scatter therefore reflects back towards the anaesthesia personnel. Lightweight leaded spectacles offer in excess of 98% radiation reduction, and their use should become part of standard practice.

Education and training

Education of medical professionals in respect of radiation protection is a continuing challenge. It is not a subject that receives prominence either at undergraduate or postgraduate level. International initiatives exist to rectify this through, for example, courses run by the International Atomic Energy Agency.

Monitoring

Fluoroscopy devices record both the peak skin dose and the total screening time. In addition, all personnel who are regularly exposed should wear dosimeters. These should be worn outside personal protective shielding. They are obviously specific to the individual, and must not be shared. Exposure is typically monitored over a 3 month period, but more frequently if recorded exposures reach 10% of acceptable limits.

Further Reading

Anastasian, Z. H., Strozyk, D., Meyers, P. M., Wang, S., & Berman, M. F. (2011). Radiation exposure of the anesthesiologist in the neuro-interventional suite. *Anesthesiology, 114*(3), 512–520. doi:10.1097/ALN.0b013e31820c2b81

Dagal, A. (2011). Radiation safety for anesthesiologists. *Current Opinion in Anaesthesiology, 24*(4), 445–450. doi:10.1097/ACO.0b013e328347f984

International Commission on Radiological Protection. The 2007 recommendations of the International commission on Radiological Protection. ICRP Publication 103. Ann ICRP 2007: 37: 1-332.

Ismail, S., Khan, F., Sultan, N., & Naqvi, M. (2010). Radiation exposure to anaesthetists during interventional radiology. *Anaesthesia, 65*(1), 54–60. doi:10.1111/j.1365-2044.2009.06166.x

Le Heron, J., Padovani, R., Smith, I., & Czarwinski, R. (2010). Radiation protection of medical staff. *European Journal of Radiology, 76*(1), 20–23. doi:10.1016/j.ejrad.2010.06.034

Taylor, J., Chandramohan, M., & Simpson, K. H. (2013). Radiation safety for anaesthetists. *BJA CEPD Reviews, 13*(2), 59–62. doi:10.1093/bjaceaccp/mks055

Part 2

Clinical anaesthesia

Chapter 11

Airway management and anaesthesia for ENT, maxillofacial, and dental surgery

11.1 Airway assessment

Preoperative assessment

One of the objectives of the preoperative visit is to identify patients at increased risk of difficult face mask ventilation and/or direct laryngoscopy. Recognition of these patients will hopefully prevent the unexpected difficult airway and enable the anaesthetist to plan an appropriate individualized technique. It has been shown that a well-documented airway plan decreases the risk of the 'can't intubate can't ventilate' (CICV) scenario. However, there remains no definitive means of recognizing a difficult airway and occasionally the previously unrecognized difficult airway will present itself. In this situation the airway plan becomes integral to patient safety.

Airway history

Preoperative evaluation should include a history of previous anaesthesia and any problems that occurred. Patients will hopefully have been informed if airway difficulties were encountered and may have been given full details to aid future airway management. Further information may be acquired from previous anaesthetic charts. A previously documented difficult airway should always be taken seriously irrespective of the grade/experience of the anaesthetist involved and an appropriate plan made. A previously easy airway may become more difficult with time due to progression of medical conditions (Box 11.1).

The patient should be questioned specifically on signs or symptoms of potential airway obstruction (Box 11.2). This is particularly important for patients presenting for ear, nose, and throat (ENT) or maxillofacial surgery. The presence of symptoms may increase the chances of a difficult airway.

Box 11.1 Medical conditions associated with airway difficulty
• Obesity
• OSA
• Diabetes
• Rheumatoid arthritis
• Ankylosing spondylitis
• Pituitary tumours (acromegaly)
• Scleroderma
• Thyroid disease
• Previous cervical spine surgery.

Box 11.2 Signs and symptoms suggestive of a difficult airway
• Change in voice, hoarseness
• Previous head and neck surgery or radiotherapy
• Dysphagia
• Drooling
• Inability to lie flat
• Spitting
• Dyspnoea
• Stridor (may only be present on exertion as patients may learn to control ventilation and overcome obstruction.)

ENT/head and neck patients will frequently have undergone an outpatient nasendoscopy. A description of the view obtained, any abnormal pathology, and pictures may be available.

Airway examination

Examination of the airway should add to any information obtained from the history. In patients with known airway pathology the aims of the assessment should be to establish a good knowledge of the location, type, and impact of the pathology on the airway.

An initial examination of the gross anatomy including body habitus, neck circumference, dentition, gross facial abnormalities, presence of facial hair, micrognathia, and nasal bone shape may help predict difficult facemask ventilation. Once complete, bedside airway tests should be performed.

Over 20 bedside tests have been developed as predictors of difficult intubation. The number of tests available illustrates that each of these, on their own, may lack the sensitivity and specificity to accurately diagnose difficult laryngoscopy. However, by combining a number of these tests, the likelihood of detecting airway difficulty is increased.

The most commonly used tests are Mallampati grading, measurement of thyromental distance, and mandibular subluxation.

Mallampati grading

This is the view obtained by maximal mouth opening and tongue protrusion while sat upright. Whilst the test has 4 grades in the clinical setting it indicates a potential difficulty if the posterior pharyngeal wall is not seen. This test has a poor predictive value and poor inter-observer variability when used in isolation.

Thyromental distance

With the patient's neck maximally extended, the distance from the tip of the chin to the thyroid cartilage is measured. A distance <6.5cm is associated with difficult laryngoscopy.

Mandibular subluxation

The patient is asked to move the lower teeth in front of the upper teeth. It is scored in 3 grades. Clinically an inability to do this increases the risk of difficult intubation.

Airway investigations

Nasendoscopy

Special investigations are often not performed prior to routine surgery. Patients presenting for head and neck cancer or major ENT surgery will commonly have had an outpatient nasendoscopy. A picture or description should be present in the notes (Fig. 11.1). This simple, relatively non-invasive investigation is extremely useful in the patient with airway pathology. Information is available about the position, size of the lesion, airway anatomy, and visualization of the vocal cords. If a significant period of time has passed since the endoscopy it may be useful to repeat the procedure. It can be performed with a flexible fibreoptic bronchoscope with some topical anaesthetic to the nasal passages.

Flow–volume loops

This investigation is a plot of airflow against lung volume during inspiration and forced expiration (Fig. 11.2). Characteristic patterns provide information on intra- and extra-thoracic pathology. Evidence of upper or lower airway obstruction can be seen.

Lateral cervical spine X-ray

Several features on a cervical spine X-ray have been associated with a difficult intubation:

• Reduced distance between the occiput and spinous process of C1

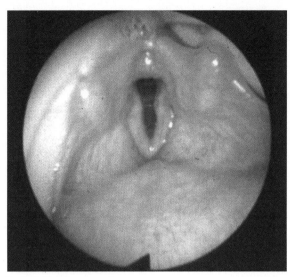

Fig. 11.1 View from nasendoscopy.

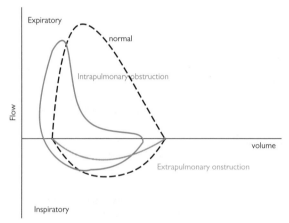

Fig. 11.2 Flow–volume loops in airway obstruction.

- Reduced distance between spinous process of C1 and C2
- Ratio of mandibular length to posterior mandibular depth >3.6
- Bamboo spine
- Atlanto-occipital restriction in flexion and extension views.

Chest X-ray

CXRs are not usually performed preoperatively but may reveal the following:

- Tracheal deviation
- Tracheal narrowing
- Intrathoracic tumours
- Goitres.

CT/MRI

CT or MRI may be performed to investigate the upper airway. These will often assist the anaesthetist in formulating an airway plan. It should also be noted that these investigations are performed in the awake patient so may bear little resemblance to the anaesthetised and paralysed airway.

Interpreting these images can be difficult and requires multi-disciplinary input. Information that is relevant to airway management includes:

- Tumour extension and invasion
- Airway impingement and level
- Tumour size
- Tracheal size, compression, level of obstruction.

Airway planning

The combination of airway history and assessment should allow an individualised plan for airway management. Several important questions must be considered—see Box 11.3.

Box 11.3 Airway planning
• Is mask ventilation feasible?
• Is supraglottic airway insertion feasible?
• Is laryngoscopy feasible?
• Is the patient suitable for awake fibreoptic intubation?
• Is the trachea easily accessible for a surgical airway should intubation or ventilation fail?

Finally, as in most clinical situations, good communication both within and between teams is important. The WHO safe surgery check should highlight any concerns regarding the airway. The close proximity of a surgical colleague in the event of a 'can't intubate, can't ventilate' scenario may be lifesaving.

Obstructive sleep apnoea

OSA occurs in 2% of women and 4% of men. It is largely associated with obesity, particularly if neck circumference is >40cm in men, but may be associated with diabetes, hypothyroidism, acromegaly, and neuromuscular disorders. OSA also occurs in children in association with adenotonsillar hypertrophy or craniofacial abnormality. OSA is a disorder in which intermittent and repeated upper airway collapse occurs during sleep, causing airway obstruction. This results in a cyclical pattern of loud snoring, apnoeas, oxygen desaturation, and arousal from deep sleep.

Pathophysiology

A patent upper airway depends on contraction of the oropharyngeal dilator and abductor muscles overcoming the negative pressure generated during inspiration. Patients with OSA have narrow airways surrounded by adipose tissue and require increased muscle tone during wakefulness to maintain airway patency.

During anaesthesia or sleep (especially REM sleep) there is profound muscle relaxation resulting in partial or complete airway obstruction. The Bernoulli effect further accentuates the airway collapse during inspiration. Partial airway obstruction causes snoring but as obstruction worsens oxygen saturation reduces and $PaCO_2$ increases. There is an increase in inspiratory effort with marked diaphragmatic movement leading to arousal from sleep. Airway tone restores on arousal and a large inspiratory effort follows with an increased arterial blood pressure and a period of hyperventilation. The cycle repeats as sleep deepens again.

These events can happen hundreds of times throughout the night and the resultant sleep disturbance may cause daytime somnolence and poor health. In addition, patients with OSA have an increased risk of road traffic collisions and work-related injury due to fatigue.

A number of medical conditions have been associated with untreated OSA. Notably arterial hypertension, pulmonary hypertension, right heart failure, ischaemic heart disease, and an increased incidence of cerebrovascular events.

For symptoms and signs associated with sleep apnoea see Boxes 11.4 and 11.5.

Box 11.4 Symptoms associated with OSA

Children present with:
- Snoring
- Restless or disturbed sleep with odd sleeping postures
- Daytime somnolence or hyperactivity
- Behavioural problems
- Frequent respiratory tract infections.

Adults present with:
- Heavy snoring
- Witnessed nocturnal apnoeas
- Waking with 'choking'
- Daytime somnolence, poor concentration, and memory
- Morning headaches
- Mood and personality changes
- Accidents related to somnolence.

Box 11.5 Signs associated with OSA
- Oedematous soft palate or uvula
- Long soft palate and uvula
- Decreased oropharyngeal dimensions
- Nasal obstruction
- Maxillary hypoplasia
- Retrognathia
- Central obesity and increased neck circumference
- Hypertension and cardiovascular disease.

Investigations

Overnight oximetry
Observing the oximetry readings during sleep is a simple way of screening for OSA. There are practical difficulties with movement artefact.

Polysomnography (PSG)
A full overnight PSG is regarded as the gold standard for diagnosis of OSA. The stages of sleep are recorded from EEG, submental electromyogram (EMG) and electro-oculogram. Respiratory patterns are assessed by oronasal airflow, respiratory movement (measured by inductance/impedance pneumography or diaphragmatic EMG) and oxyhaemoglobin saturation by pulse oximetry (Fig. 11.3). Other measurements taken include ECG and sound recordings. The data is analysed in 30sec epochs when the stage of sleep is correlated with the respiratory pattern and arousals.

Apnoeic spells are defined as a cessation of airflow lasting a minimum of 10sec. If the patient has airway obstruction repeatedly for >10sec with continued diaphragmatic movements and a desaturation of 4% from baseline then a diagnosis of OSA is made. The severity of OSA is related to the extent of desaturation and the apnoea/hypopnoea index (AHI), which equates to the frequency of events per hour.

Nasendoscopy
Direct visualization of the upper airway under sedation is widely used by ENT surgeons to confirm OSA and to identify those who may benefit from a surgical treatment.

Treatment

This depends on the severity of the condition but may include behavioural, non-surgical, or surgical interventions.

Behavioural interventions
Weight reduction strategies can have a significant impact in OSA but are often difficult to achieve and maintain. Smoking cessation and alcohol reduction are other lifestyle changes that have shown improvement in OSA. Sedative drugs should be avoided.

Non-surgical interventions
The gold standard treatment is nasal CPAP. There is good evidence for reduction in AHI, improved quality of life, and reversal of many of the associated cardiac and cerebrovascular conditions. Patients require support and education to improve compliance. CPAP levels may be adjusted from 5–20cmH$_2$O.

Patients with mild OSA can be managed with mandibular advancement splints. Patients are most likely to benefit if retrognathic, and the device relies on partial dislocation of the temporomandibular joint.

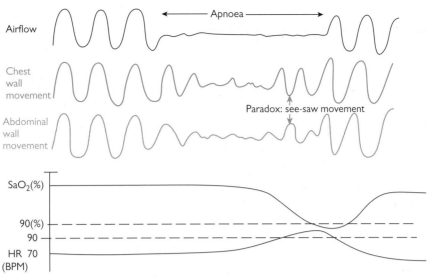

Fig. 11.3 Sleep study demonstrating airway obstruction. Reproduced from Catherine Spoors and Kevin Kiff, *Training in Anaesthesia*, 2010, Figure 13.8, page 339, with permission from Oxford University Press.

Surgical interventions

Tonsillectomy

Tonsillar enlargement may cause OSA in children and may contribute to symptoms in adult patients. Tonsillectomy may improve, reduce, or relieve obstruction.

Uvulopalatoplasty and laser-assisted uvuloplasty (LAUP)

Palatal surgery includes uvulo-palato-pharyngoplasty (UPPP), which involves removal of the uvula, pharyngeal arches, and partial removal of the soft palate; and LAUP, which involves vaporizing the free edge of the soft palate and uvula. These procedures can improve snoring but there is little evidence to demonstrate improvement in OSA. There is a significant complication rate for these procedures including nasopharyngeal reflux, voice change, palatal dryness, and loss of taste. This has decreased the popularity of these procedures for OSA.

Maxillofacial surgery

This is the most invasive surgery for OSA and is used when patients with craniofacial abnormality are not tolerant of CPAP. Procedures include genioplasty and Le Fort osteotomies.

Nasal surgery

There is no evidence that nasal surgery improves OSA, but it may improve compliance and benefit from nasal CPAP.

Tracheostomy

This is reserved for very severe and life-threatening scenarios when non-invasive techniques are not tolerated.

Bariatric surgery

Weight loss surgery can improve or resolve OSA.

Anaesthetic management

This group of patients represents a challenge to the anaesthetist as OSA is associated with increased perioperative morbidity. Obese patients, or patients with other risk factors, should be specifically screened for undiagnosed OSA with questions relating to snoring, sleep, and daytime somnolence (see Box 11.6). If history is suggestive of OSA, further investigation may be required and surgery deferred pending management. Patients diagnosed with OSA and established on treatment must continue with this in the perioperative period.

Box 11.6 Screening for OSA—the 'STOP BANG' questionnaire

Yes to more than three questions indicates risk of OSA.

• Snoring	Do you snore loudly?
• Tiredness	Are you tired in the day?
• Observed	Do you stop breathing during at night?
• Pressure	Have you had high blood pressure?
• BMI	BMI >35
• Age	Age >50 years
• Neck	Neck circumference >40cm
• Gender	Male

Reproduced from Chung F et al., 'STOP Questionnaire: A Tool to Screen Patients for Obstructive Sleep Apnea', Anaesthesiology, 108, 5, pp. 812–821, copyright 2009, with permission from The American Society of Anaesthesiologists and Wolters Kluwer.

Patients with known OSA

It is important in these patients to have a complete peri-operative anaesthetic plan including planning of postoperative care and high-dependency needs.

OSA is associated with difficult facemask ventilation and difficult intubation especially if the patient is obese. Patients also have an increased central respiratory depressant effect to opioids and other sedative drugs. Regional anaesthesia is preferable where possible. Where GA is necessary, a difficult airway should be anticipated and appropriate equipment and personnel available. Regional analgesia or short-acting opiates should be used and neuromuscular blockade carefully reversed at the end of surgery. Patients should be extubated when fully alert. Patients on home CPAP should bring their machines with them to theatres for use in the recovery ward.

Postsurgical high-dependency care should be considered following major surgery with opiate use, thoracic surgery, or airway surgery particularly if this prevents use of CPAP. Patients should be continued on oxygen therapy with oximetry monitoring.

The use of regional anaesthesia decreases the use of opiates and likelihood of postoperative respiratory complications.

Further reading

Loadsman JA & Hillman DR (2001). Anaesthesia and sleep apnoea. *Br J Aneasthesia*, 86(2), 254–266.

11.3 Management of the difficult airway

Techniques to deal with the difficult airway depend on whether the problem is anticipated and whether airway obstruction is present. As with all areas of anaesthetic practice, there is often more than one technique for management. The important aspect of airway management is to form an individualized plan A for the specific situation. Plan B is the technique for use should plan A fail, and a back-up plan is necessary should both plan A and B fail.

The anticipated difficult airway

Recognition of the difficult airway could be straightforward due to congenital or acquired abnormalities, or may be detected only by careful history and examination. Once recognized, a careful planned strategy will result in a better outcome. In view of this, several guidelines have been published over the last 15 years. The commonly used guidelines are from the Difficult Airway Society (DAS) (Figs. 11.4–11.7).

The first assessment needs to differentiate airway obstruction from a non-obstructed airway.

Unobstructed airway

In a patient who presents for surgery with a difficult but unobstructed airway several options need to be considered. It may be possible to perform the surgery under local or regional anaesthesia.

If facemask ventilation is predicted to be easy, then airway management can occur under anaesthesia. There are two opposing views as to best practice:

1. A gas induction may be used to maintain spontaneous ventilation and allow more immediate reversal.
2. An IV induction with neuromuscular blockade may be used to optimize airway maintenance via facemask.

If facemask ventilation may be difficult, an awake fibreoptic intubation is the safest approach (see section 11.4). If the patient is unsuitable for this (paediatric, learning difficulties) then an alternative technique is considered.

Difficult airway equipment should be available and it is prudent to have a plan B. The surgical team and equipment for a surgical airway should also be available.

Difficulties with managing an airway can occur at any stage of the procedure. A high percentage of complications occur in the recovery ward. It is therefore imperative to have a plan for induction, maintenance, and extubation and the recovery phase. This is particularly important if the surgery is to be on or around the airway. A plan for re-intubation in the event of complications (haemorrhage, oedema) and in the face of increased airway difficulty should be made prior to the extubation. This plan should be discussed with the surgical and recovery team.

The patient should be closely monitored until fully conscious and self-ventilating adequately.

The obstructed airway

The obstructed airway by definition is a compromised airway. The initial priority is to maintain ventilation, and assess the site, nature, and speed of development of the obstruction. This will alter the management plan.

Upper airway obstruction causes stridor when the diameter is reduced by >50%. Rapidly increasing airway obstruction causes respiratory distress and anxiety and the airway must be secured early. More chronic airway obstruction allows time for planning and the airway can be secured electively. The obstruction may be assessed with nasendoscopy. This can be performed without any laryngeal preparation or contact, avoiding the risk of precipitating complete obstruction. Nasendoscopy may allow assessment of cause and extent of obstruction as well as identifying cases where distorted anatomy will make oral intubation impossible.

Box 11.7 Causes of stridor and initial management

Causes
- Infection:
  - Epiglottitis
  - Retropharyngeal abscess
  - Croup
- Malignancy: supraglottic/glottis tumours
- Oedema:
  - Anaphylaxis
  - Post airway instrumentation
- Foreign bodies
- Subglottic stenosis.

Initial management
- Sit upright, 100% oxygen
- Nebulized adrenaline 1mg (every 30min)
- Dexamethasone IV 0.1mg/kg
- Consider Heliox.

In life-threatening compromise an emergent action is required (Box 11.7) with resuscitation guidelines being followed. Even when an airway is becoming rapidly compromised there is time to make a basic assessment of the situation and assemble necessary equipment and personnel. It is imperative that an assessment of ease of mask ventilation is made. If this is not considered possible then the situation may require a surgical airway as plan A. If it is felt that mask ventilation and laryngoscopy are achievable this can be carried out after pre-oxygenation with an IV or inhalational induction. There is conflict of opinion as to the best method. One school of thought is that the easiest airway to manage is a paralysed airway; the other, that an inhalational induction with a spontaneously breathing patient, in theory, allows a more immediate reversal of the situation.

Gas induction

A gas induction in an adult patient with airway obstruction is a difficult procedure. Safety relies on maintenance of spontaneous ventilation. The obstruction will increase as conscious level reduces and airway tone is lost. If complete obstruction occurs, anaesthesia lightens and airway tone returns.

Gas induction in these cases should be performed within the theatre with full monitoring and an experienced ENT surgeon present. Difficult airway equipment should be available as well as facilities for surgical tracheostomy and rigid bronchoscopy.

Gas induction is performed with sevoflurane in 100% oxygen. Nasopharyngeal airways may be helpful (after topical preparation of the nose to prevent bleeding), but oropharyngeal airways may precipitate laryngeal spasm. If apnoea occurs, rather than support ventilation, the CO_2 should be allowed to rise and spontaneous ventilation will resume. The blood pressure and heart rate will decrease with depth of anaesthesia. Pupil size

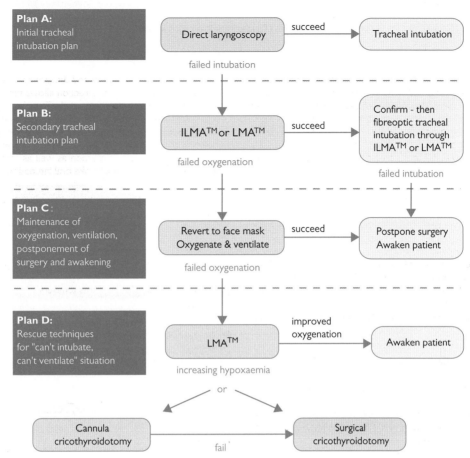

Fig. 11.4 Overall scheme for the difficult airway. Reproduced from Henderson JJ, Popat MT, Latto IP, Pearce AC. Difficult Airway Society guidelines for management of the unanticipated difficult intubation. *Anaesthesia* 2004; 59:675–94, with permission from Blackwell Publishing Ltd.

and position will also suggest adequate depth. It can be difficult with adults to achieve adequate depth of anaesthesia using sevoflurane whilst maintaining spontaneous breathing. Halothane may be used in these situations.

Laryngoscopy can be attempted during deep volatile anaesthesia. There should be limited attempts at intubation to avoid bleeding or oedema. If intubation is not possible, asleep tracheostomy can be performed whilst the patient continues to self-ventilate.

Intravenous induction
Many ENT anaesthetists would support using an IV induction in the event of airway obstruction in adults. An inhalation induction reduces intraluminal airway pressure and increases obstruction. The resultant reduction in tidal volume and high dead space fraction may cause slow and ineffective induction of anaesthesia. Positive pressure bag mask ventilation can reduce obstruction by increasing intraluminal pressure. Neuromuscular blockade further optimizes the airway by causing vocal cord relaxation. If an IV induction is used, the aim should be to provide muscle relaxation simultaneously with onset of loss of consciousness.

The importance of the level of obstruction
The patient requiring urgent, but not emergency, intervention allows time to consider options and plans more carefully. It is important to assess the level of obstruction.

Supraglottic obstruction
Causes of airway obstruction above the glottis include naso-pharyngeal tumours, effects of previous surgery, or anatomical deformity. Although the pathology may cause deviation of the larynx, the glottis should be patent with normal anatomy. In this instance an awake fibreoptic intubation would be the method of choice, with a plan B of a supraglottic device or direct laryngoscopy.

Glottic obstruction
These cases require planning with an ENT surgeon. Lesions in or around the glottis need to be assessed by nasendoscopy. If the nasendoscopy can visualize the vocal cords and there is sufficient space for an endotracheal tube (ETT) to pass, then an IV induction and either laryngoscopy or asleep fibreoptic intubation may be performed. Inhalational induction may also be considered. If direct laryngoscopy is planned, a needle cricothyrotomy can be performed electively prior to induction and used to oxygenate the patient if intubation fails while a surgical airway is inserted. Awake fibreoptic intubation is usually avoided as the glottis may become completely obstructed during the procedure. This is intolerable to a conscious patient. If the glottis space is considered too small for an ETT to pass, then a surgical airway is performed on the awake patient.

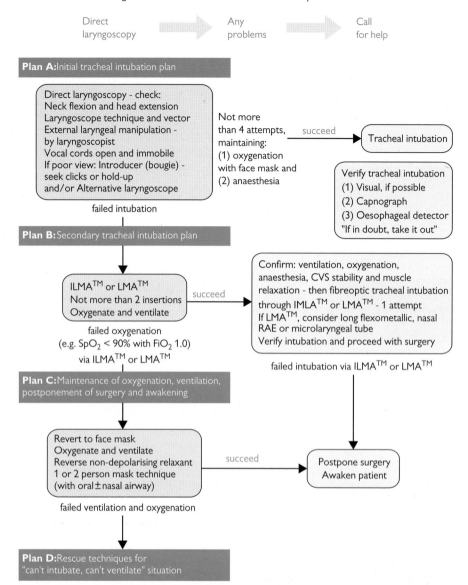

Fig. 11.5 Unexpected difficult intubation (elective). Reproduced from Henderson JJ, Popat MT, Latto IP, Pearce AC. Difficult Airway Society guidelines for management of the unanticipated difficult intubation. *Anaesthesia* 2004; 59:675–94, with permission from Blackwell Publishing Ltd.

Subglottic obstruction

It is important to differentiate intrathoracic from extrathoracic obstruction. Intrathoracic obstruction is extremely difficult to manage once the patient is anaesthetized and may result in complete collapse of the airway and cardiac arrest. These cases should be managed in a cardiothoracic centre with cardiopulmonary bypass facilities.

Extrathoracic obstruction can be due to tracheal abnormalities, either tumours or tracheomalacia. External compression can occur due to enlargement of the thyroid or postsurgical bleeding from carotid or thyroid surgery. Management of these patients is commonly with IV induction and direct laryngoscopy. The main consideration is difficulty passing the ETT through the obstruction. An array of sizes of ETT should be present along with facilities to

jet ventilate and perform rigid bronchoscopy. Jet ventilation from above the level of obstruction may be possible through the ETT. This should only be performed by skilled personnel as there is a high risk of barotrauma and pneumomediastinum.

Tracheostomy under local anaesthesia

This is an important option which should not be forgotten. In cases of severe airway obstruction with hypoxaemia, or cases where difficult face mask ventilation is anticipated, tracheostomy should be performed under local anaesthesia by an experienced ENT surgeon. Patients will often not manage a supine position for preparation, or even surgery. The procedure is surprisingly well tolerated.

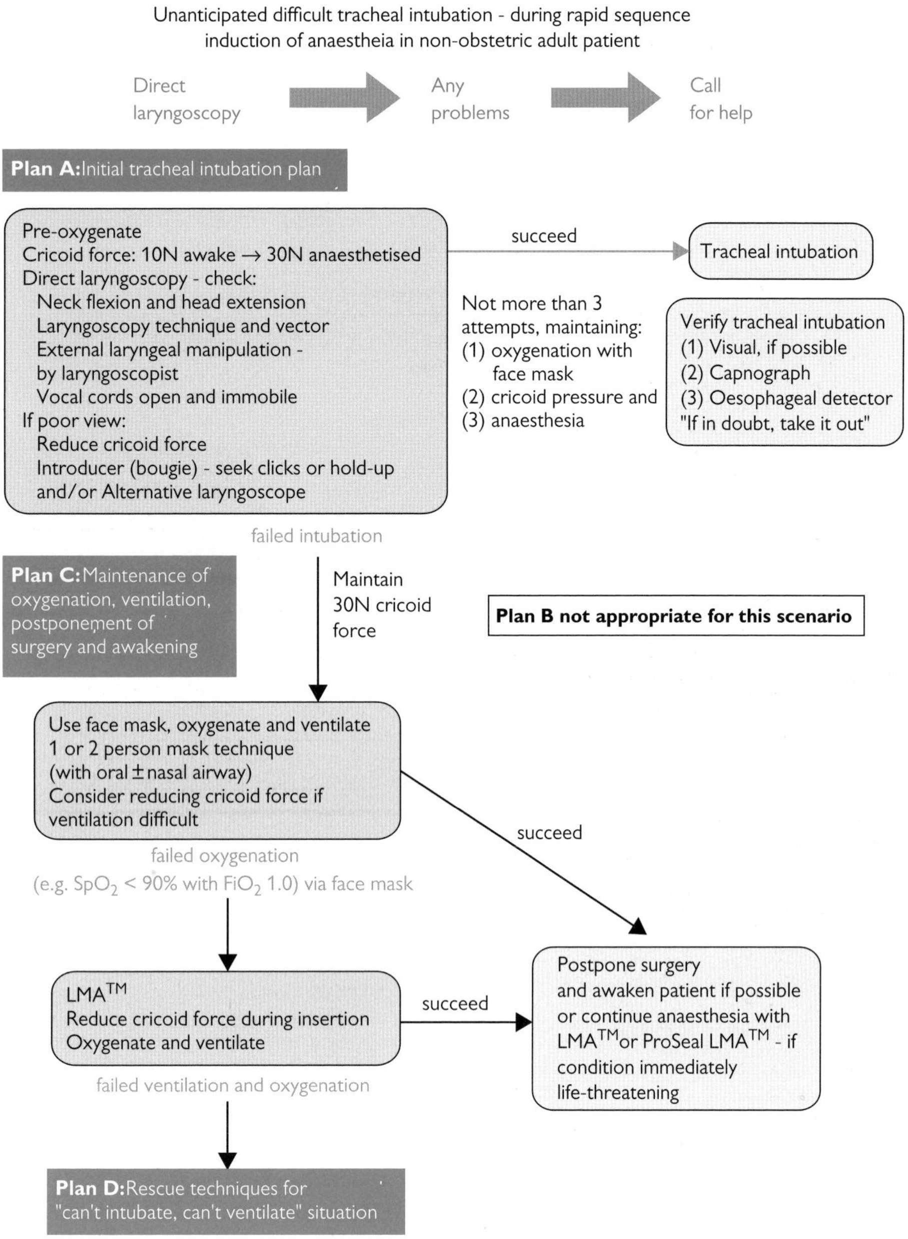

Unanticipated difficult tracheal intubation - during rapid sequence
induction of anaesthesia in non-obstetric adult patient

Direct
laryngoscopy → Any
problems → Call
for help

Plan A: Initial tracheal intubation plan

Pre-oxygenate
Cricoid force: 10N awake → 30N anaesthetised
Direct laryngoscopy - check:
  Neck flexion and head extension
  Laryngoscopy technique and vector
  External laryngeal manipulation -
  by laryngoscopist
  Vocal cords open and immobile
If poor view:
  Reduce cricoid force
  Introducer (bougie) - seek clicks or hold-up
  and/ or Alternative laryngoscope

— succeed → Tracheal intubation

Not more than 3
attempts, maintaining:
(1) oxygenation with
    face mask
(2) cricoid pressure and
(3) anaesthesia

Verify tracheal intubation
(1) Visual, if possible
(2) Capnograph
(3) Oesophageal detector
"If in doubt, take it out"

failed intubation

Plan C: Maintenance of oxygenation, ventilation, postponement of surgery and awakening

Maintain
30N cricoid
force

Plan B not appropriate for this scenario

Use face mask, oxygenate and ventilate
1 or 2 person mask technique
(with oral ± nasal airway)
Consider reducing cricoid force if
ventilation difficult

— succeed →

failed oxygenation
(e.g. $SpO_2 < 90\%$ with FiO_2 1.0) via face mask

LMA™
Reduce cricoid force during insertion
Oxygenate and ventilate

— succeed →

Postpone surgery
and awaken patient if possible
or continue anaesthesia with
LMA™ or ProSeal LMA™ - if
condition immediately
life-threatening

failed ventilation and oxygenation

Plan D: Rescue techniques for
"can't intubate, can't ventilate" situation

Fig. 11.6 Unexpected difficult intubation (RSI). Reproduced from Henderson JJ, Popat MT, Latto IP, Pearce AC. Difficult Airway Society guidelines for management of the unanticipated difficult intubation. *Anaesthesia* 2004; 59:675–94, with permission from Blackwell Publishing Ltd.

Needle cricothyroidotomy

See section 11.5.

The unexpected difficult airway

The *unexpected* difficult airway is the main cause of hypoxia, brain damage, and death in anaesthesia. Unfortunately this occurs despite good airway assessment due to the poor sensitivity of the tests used.

This is a rare event, which requires well-practised emergency management. Knowledge and simulated practice of the DAS guidelines prepare us for this event. The DAS guidelines represent a simple, stepwise plan with focus on oxygenation of the

patient. The equipment used should be familiar to every anaesthetist and regular training with the equipment may be required.

If the unexpected difficult airway arises during a rapid sequence induction the guidelines vary, as it is important to prevent aspiration during the airway rescue (Fig. 11.6).

Follow-up after unanticipated difficult airway

Once a patient has been diagnosed with a difficult airway it is important to follow-up the patient and inform them. Any underlying pathology may need further investigation and referral to ENT surgeons. An airway alert form can be found on the DAS

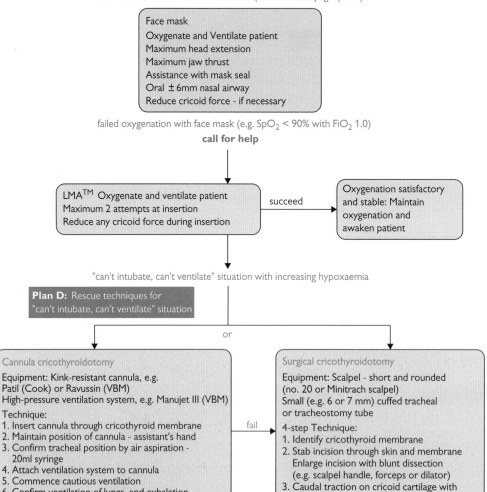

Failed intubation, increasing hypoxaemia and difficult ventilation in the paralysed anaesthetized patient: Rescue techniques for the "can't intubate, can't ventilate" situation

failed intubation and difficult ventilation (other than laryngospasm)

Face mask
Oxygenate and Ventilate patient
Maximum head extension
Maximum jaw thrust
Assistance with mask seal
Oral ± 6mm nasal airway
Reduce cricoid force - if necessary

failed oxygenation with face mask (e.g. SpO$_2$ < 90% with FiO$_2$ 1.0)

call for help

LMA^{TM} Oxygenate and ventilate patient
Maximum 2 attempts at insertion
Reduce any cricoid force during insertion

succeed →

Oxygenation satisfactory and stable: Maintain oxygenation and awaken patient

"can't intubate, can't ventilate" situation with increasing hypoxaemia

Plan D: Rescue techniques for "can't intubate, can't ventilate" situation

or

Cannula cricothyroidotomy

Equipment: Kink-resistant cannula, e.g.
Patil (Cook) or Ravussin (VBM)
High-pressure ventilation system, e.g. Manujet III (VBM)
Technique:
1. Insert cannula through cricothyroid membrane
2. Maintain position of cannula - assistant's hand
3. Confirm tracheal position by air aspiration - 20ml syringe
4. Attach ventilation system to cannula
5. Commence cautious ventilation
6. Confirm ventilation of lungs, and exhalation through upper airway
7. If ventilation fails, or surgical emphysema or any other complication develops - convert immediately to surgical cricothyroidotomy

fail →

Surgical cricothyroidotomy

Equipment: Scalpel - short and rounded (no. 20 or Minitrach scalpel)
Small (e.g. 6 or 7 mm) cuffed tracheal or tracheostomy tube
4-step Technique:
1. Identify cricothyroid membrane
2. Stab incision through skin and membrane
   Enlarge incision with blunt dissection (e.g. scalpel handle, forceps or dilator)
3. Caudal traction on cricoid cartilage with tracheal hook
4. Insert tube and inflate cuff
Ventilate with low-pressure source
Verify tube position and pulmonary ventilation

Notes:
1. These techniques can have serious complications - use only in life-threatening situations
2. Convert to definitive airway as soon as possible
3. Postoperative management - see other difficult airway guidelines and flow-charts
4. 4mm cannula with low-pressure ventilation may be successful in patient breathing spontaneously

Fig. 11.7 Can't intubate, can't ventilate. Reproduced from Henderson JJ, Popat MT, Latto IP, Pearce AC. Difficult Airway Society guidelines for management of the unanticipated difficult intubation. *Anaesthesia* 2004; 59:675–94, with permission from Blackwell Publishing Ltd.

website (see Further reading). A copy should be filed in the notes, a copy should be sent to the GP, and in some circumstances a medi-alert bracelet can be issued. A letter should be given to the patient highlighting the issue and outlining difficulties and management. This is helpful should the patient require any further surgery.

Further reading

Difficult Airway Society website: <http://www.das.uk.com>.

Henderson JJ, Popat MT, Latto IP, *et al.* (2004). Difficult Airway Society guidelines for management of the unanticipated difficult intubation. *Anaesthesia*, 59:675–94.

11.4 Awake fibreoptic intubation

Awake fibreoptic intubation

Awake fibreoptic intubation (AFOI) is commonly performed on patients when it is thought that face mask ventilation and/or direct laryngoscopy will be impossible. A successful AFOI requires careful planning.

Patient preparation

It is vital that the procedure is explained to the patient in such a way that they understand every step of the process. Consent for the AFOI should be taken verbally. It is particularly important for patients who will not receive sedation and in those patients who may require multiple AFOI in the future.

Premedication

The purpose of this is to reduce secretions using glycopyrrolate, producing a dry mouth to improve the effect of the local anaesthetic and the view via the scope. If required, prophylaxis for aspiration should also be administered.

Theatre personnel

To improve safety, two anaesthetists should be present at AFOI. Whilst one performs the topical anaesthesia and intubation, assisted by the ODP, the other monitors the patient and administers sedation if used. The second anaesthetist is also required to deliver the induction agents once the ETT is in place and secure.

Equipment

Assembling all the equipment and checking it is functional is imperative. If a 'spray as you go' technique is used, the catheter needs to be inserted down the injection port of the scope. The ETT is mounted onto the fibreoptic scope. Suction equipment must be readily available.

Routine monitoring, anaesthetic, and emergency drugs are essential. The airway equipment necessary for plan B and surgical airway equipment should also be readily available.

Back-up plan

AFOI is not always successful and a back-up plan is required. What this is will depend on the circumstances, but in most cases may have to be an awake tracheostomy.

Sedation

Once the procedure has been clearly explained and the patient consented, conscious sedation can be given. This is to relieve anxiety, produce amnesia, and relieve any pain or discomfort experienced during the procedure. This results in a smoother AFOI for patient and operator. However, these patients may have a critically compromised airway so it is essential that the patient remains conscious and rapidly reversible drugs are desirable. Commonly used drugs are:
- Midazolam and fentanyl
- Propofol infusion (target controlled)
- Remifentanil infusion
- α-2 agonists, e.g. dexmedetomidine.

The drug with which the operator is most familiar should be used with careful titration. It can take up to 20min to establish a safe level of conscious sedation in some patients: patience is essential.

Local anaesthesia for AFOI

There are two techniques for anaesthetizing the airway:
- Direct application of local anaesthetic: numerous techniques and pieces of equipment exist for doing this.
- Nerve blocks: these are less popular and often less effective than topical anaesthesia.

Whichever technique is employed it is important to anaesthetize the whole airway from nose to subglottis.

Topical anaesthesia

Nasal topicalization

Initially the nasal mucosa is vasoconstricted with a mixture of phenylephrine 0.5% and lidocaine 5%. This prevents bleeding and allows easier access through the nasal passage. Lidocaine is then applied either via a ribbon and gauze pack or by application of lidocaine gel to a nasopharyngeal airway which is gently inserted. The airway can either be cut longitudinally and the scope passed through or removed just prior to insertion of the scope.

Oropharynx

Lidocaine 4% is sprayed via an atomizer onto the mucosa. Posterior application can sometimes cause coughing. Alternatively the patient can be asked to gargle lidocaine gel until the oropharynx feels numb.

Supraglottic, glottis, and subglottic region

Anaesthesia can be provided by the 'spray as you go' technique. A 16G epidural catheter is placed in the suction port of the scope. A single end hole is desirable. A 2mL syringe can be attached via the Luer lock connector. The catheter can be directed by the scope and more accurate placement of local anaesthetic achieved if the catheter is pushed out of the scope by 1cm. This should be retracted before the scope is progressed as it can irritate the airway and create discomfort. As the scope advances, the process is repeated anaesthetizing the airway 'as you go'.

Nerve blocks for AFOI

The glossopharyngeal nerve supplies sensory innervation to the posterior third of the tongue (with facial and vagus nerves) and the posterior and lateral pharyngeal walls, the vallecula, and anterior epiglottic surface via its lingual branch. The glossopharyngeal nerve can be blocked by injection into the palatoglossal fold.

The superior laryngeal nerve (a branch of the vagus nerve) divides into the external and internal laryngeal nerves. The internal laryngeal nerve provides sensory innervation to the tongue base, vallecula, epiglottis, arytenoids, and mucosa above the vocal cords. The superior laryngeal nerve can be blocked by bilateral injections between the superior cornu of the hyoid and thyroid cartilages through the thyrohyoid membrane.

Nerve blocks may be associated with complications such as haematoma, intravascular injection, and airway obstruction (e.g. vocal cord paralysis with superior laryngeal nerve block).

Translaryngeal local anaesthesia may be delivered via a cricothyroid cannula. Lidocaine is delivered at the end of expiration to anaesthetize topically below the vocal cords to the carina. This will cause coughing.

Patient position

Traditionally AFOI has been taught with the patient supine and the operator standing behind the patient. The advantage of this position is the view of the larynx seen is identical to that seen on direct laryngoscopy, improving orientation.

During AFOI patients may have compromised ventilation due to airway pathology and lying flat is not possible. A better technique is to keep the patient sitting upright with the operator approaching from the front. Apart from requiring some re-orientation of the anatomy, this has the advantage of the operator being able to observe the patient and can be less frightening for the patient.

Anatomy

Nasendoscopy

As the scope is placed into the nasal cavity the septum, floor of the nose, and inferior turbinate should be identified. The scope is advanced through the turbinate space to enter the posterior nasal space. The soft palate can then be seen below and the nasopharyngeal wall ahead. The scope should pass between the soft palate and pharyngeal wall allowing visualization of the epiglottis. If at any stage the structures are not recognizable or the view is unclear, the scope should be withdrawn until the anatomy is again recognized. If the scope is blindly inserted there is a risk of mucosal bleeding and also perforation.

Epiglottis to intubation

Once the epiglottis is seen the 'spray as you go' technique can be used and the scope gently advanced. If the patient appears uncomfortable at any stage the scope can be withdrawn slightly and the area sprayed again. Maximum dose is 9mL/kg lidocaine as a large amount is swallowed rather than being absorbed.

Before the ETT is inserted, the vocal cords and subglottic region are topically anaesthetized. The ETT is gently advanced along the scope. If the ETT tip gets caught on the epiglottis, the whole scope and ETT are withdrawn a few mm, then rotated in a clockwise direction and together re-inserted. When using a reinforced ETT it may be easier to rotate the tube constantly on insertion in a 'screwdriver' fashion.

Complications

AFOI in the right hands is a safe, highly successful technique and is regarded as the 'gold standard' for patients with a predictably difficult airway. However it is not a panacea for every difficult airway as it requires a compliant patient, an air space to work within, and may lead to complete airway obstruction in glottic lesions. Blood and secretions can render the visual field absent, resulting in failure or further damage.

It is a relatively slow procedure so if rapid airway management is needed it may be an inappropriate technique.

Further reading

Heidegger T (2011). Fiberoptic intubation. *NEJM*, 364(20):e42.

Xue F-S, Cheng Y, & Li R-P (2013). Awake intubation with video laryngoscope and fiberoptic bronchoscope in difficult airway patients. *Anesthesiology*, 118(2):462–3. doi:10.1097/ALN.0b013e31827bd357.

11.5 Cricothyroidotomy and jet ventilation

Emergency airway management

Failure to *oxygenate* rather than *ventilate* is the cause of morbidity and mortality associated with the 'can't intubate, can't ventilate' (CICV) situation. Airway access to deliver oxygen is required to buy time until either the definitive airway is established or adequate spontaneous respiration is resumed. The DAS guidelines for management of CICV, state that if it is not possible to maintain SaO_2 >90% with airway manoeuvres and adjuncts, a cricothyroidotomy should be performed immediately as a life-saving procedure. It is the *decision* to establish emergency airway access and local knowledge of the available equipment along with practice and training that are the key determinants to outcome. Simulator or mannequin-based training is useful to prepare for this scenario. Regular retraining is required as CICV is rare in clinical practice.

Emergency airway access can be obtained by needle cricothyroidotomy or surgical techniques. Needle cricothyroidotomy cannulae have a small internal diameter allowing oxygen delivery but not reliable ventilation. When jet ventilation is used, barotrauma may occur due to lack of expiratory pathway. A definitive surgical airway is still required for ongoing management. Surgical cricothyroidotomy results in placement of a cuffed, small tracheostomy tube (6–6.5mm internal diameter). This provides a definitive airway, allowing oxygenation and ventilation. It is compatible with conventional breathing circuits and ventilation systems. Success rates may be higher with surgical airways than with needle techniques.

Relevant anatomy

The cricothyroid membrane is a median, fibroelastic membrane extending from the inferior surface of the thyroid cartilage to the superior surface of the cricoid cartilage. On average, it is 8mm deep to the skin, 1–1.5cm in height, and 2–2.5cm in width.

When palpating in the midline down from the chin, the cricothyroid ligament can be felt just below the prominence of the thyroid cartilage, although it may be difficult to feel in obese people or in people with a short neck and limited neck extension. The vocal cords lie approximately 1cm above the cricothyroid membrane.

The patient is positioned supine with extension of the neck if possible. The cricothyroid membrane is identified by palpation between the thyroid and cricoid cartilages and the larynx is stabilized in the midline with the non-dominant hand.

Needle cricothyroidotomy

Equipment
Kink-resistant cannula with needle stylet (e.g. VBM Ravussin 13G cannula and Patil-Cook cannula), 5mL syringe filled with 2–3mL saline, high-pressure jet ventilating system (e.g. Manujet III). Seldinger wire-guided equipment is used less commonly as the procedure is less rapid.

In an emergency, any large-bore (14G or 16G) IV cannula can be used but extra precautions must be taken to prevent it from kinking. The new percutaneous cricothyroidotomy devices (e.g. Portex, Cook, VBM) have larger internal diameter (4–4.5mm) and are cuffed which offers distinct advantages over the conventional small-bore cannulae.

Technique
The cricothyroid membrane is punctured with the cannula and the stylet attached to a saline-filled syringe. The cannula is directed 45° caudally and constant negative pressure is applied while advancing through the tissues. Entry into the trachea is confirmed by aspiration of air freely into the syringe. The stylet needle is stabilized at this level and the cannula is fully advanced over the stylet. The stylet is removed and cannula is secured in place. Aspiration of air through the cannula must be verified before commencing jet ventilation.

Post-procedure
Manual jet ventilation is started through the cannula with inspiratory and expiratory times of 1sec and 4sec respectively to ensure complete expiration with each breath (see 'Low-frequency jet ventilation').

If a jet ventilator is not available, an oxygen flow meter giving set at 10–15L/min is attached to the cannula via a three-way tap. The open end of the three-way tap is manually occluded intermittently in order to provide inspiration.

The new larger-bore cricothyroidotomy devices have a connector to allow the use of a standard ventilation circuit.

Surgical cricothyroidotomy

Equipment
Scalpel (short and round tip), size ≥6mm internal diameter cuffed tracheostomy tube, tracheal hook.

Technique
A vertical incision is made through the skin and the cricothyroid membrane followed by blunt dissection to widen the incision with the handle of the scalpel. Caudal traction on the cricoid cartilage with a tracheal hook may help retract further. A tracheostomy tube is inserted and cuff inflated.

Post procedure
When position is confirmed, a conventional ventilator is attached allowing oxygenation, ventilation, and anaesthesia.

Precautions

The neck and upper airway are very vascular and bleeding must be minimized by careful, blunt dissection and avoiding direct incision over the visible veins. Tributaries from the anterior jugular and inferior thyroid veins are often found in the midline which can cause significant bleeding.

After needle cricothyroidotomy, care must be taken to prevent kinking and displacement of the cannula. The patient must be watched closely for signs of barotrauma and pneumothorax, especially with the use of a jet ventilator in the presence of potential upper airway obstruction. Depth of anaesthesia must be safely maintained with IV agents.

If the needle cricothyroidotomy fails, a surgical cricothyroidotomy must be undertaken immediately.

The Portex Minitrach II is used for tracheal toileting and is not suitable as an emergency airway device.

Complications

Early complications

- Failure to improve oxygenation (This may result from alveolar distension increasing intrathoracic pressure and RV afterload worsening V/Q mismatch. Often due to lack of expiratory pathway.)
- Kinking or dislodgement of the cannula
- Subcutaneous emphysema—misplacement
- Barotrauma (pneumothorax/mediastinum)
- Bleeding
- Oesophageal and posterior tracheal perforation, laryngeal trauma.

Late complications

- Tracheal or subglottic stenosis
- Tracheo-oesophageal fistula
- Infection.

Jet ventilation indications

Low-frequency jet ventilation (LFJV) may be used in the emergency situation to oxygenate the patient via a cricothyroid cannula.

Electively, HFJV may be used to optimize surgical access for airway surgery, e.g. vocal cord surgery, surgical laryngosopy, tracheal resection, or reconstruction; and as an alternative to one-lung ventilation for lung resection or surgical access to thoracic structures.

Advantages as compared to IPPV are:

- Improved CVS stability
- Better surgical field and access
- Avoidance of double-lumen tube
- Avoidance of one-lung ventilation.

Disadvantages may include:

- Barotrauma if expiration is obstructed
- Gastric insufflation with supraglottic ventilation
- Difficulty in assessing adequacy of ventilation and airway pressure
- Airway is unprotected from soiling
- Little control of temperature and humidification
- TIVA maintenance is required.

Jet ventilation can be delivered via a cricothyroid cannula, ETT, surgical laryngoscope, or bronchoscope. Some of the jet-specific equipment has double lumens allowing a ventilation lumen and a monitoring lumen for airway pressure or CO_2, e.g. Portex gas monitoring ETT, Mallinkrodt 'Hi-Lo' ETT.

Low-frequency jet ventilation

Sanders described the first jet ventilation system in 1967. The Sanders injector and the Manujet systems are used to provide LFJV.

Jet ventilation systems are powered by pipeline oxygen at 4 bar which passes through a pressure regulating valve with pressure gauge. A hand operated trigger stops and starts the gas flow and may also allow pressure outlet alteration. Ventilation is initiated with a low driving pressure of 1 bar. The operator controls frequency of jet ventilation and can change pressure outlet to achieve the desired chest wall movement. The oxygen jet entrains air into the system to form the tidal volume. This 'jet mixing' is similar to the Venturi principle and typically FiO_2 becomes 0.8–0.9. Following jet delivery (about 1sec), a pause allows passive expiration (4sec) due to lung and chest wall recoil. An expiratory pathway is essential and the upper airway should be cleared with jaw thrust and an oropharyngeal or laryngeal mask airway.

High-frequency jet ventilation

High-frequency jet ventilators are now available to deliver time-cycled, pressure-limited ventilation. These systems also allow warming and humidification of delivered gas flow. Pressure can be limited to preset levels and pressure-measurement occurs between cycles (pause pressure). A frequency of 60–600 cycles/min is possible. The tidal volume created is dependent on driving pressure, inspiratory time, air entrainment, and resistance to flow. Typical tidal volumes generated are around 150mL whilst peak airway pressures remain low at about 5cmH2O. This system allows continuous expiratory flow.

HFJV delivers a tidal volume less than the dead space volume. The physiological mechanisms to explain gas exchange with HFJV include:

- Taylor-type dispersion: increased velocity at the centre of parabolic airflow waveform during laminar flow with jet ventilation. Airway gradients establish between the fast central flow and the slower radial flow leading to gas mixing.
- Pendelluft ventilation: variable time-constants of alveolar units create gas flow between neighbouring units. Low tidal volumes with higher mean airway pressures increase Pendelluft ventilation during HFJV.
- Coaxial flow: due to changes in the velocity profiles, central tracheal flow is directed inwards and forwards. Expiratory flow occurs along the lumen periphery and is directed outwards.
- Bulk flow: this is one of the main mechanisms responsible for gas exchange in proximal alveoli and minimizes dead space ventilation.
- Augmented molecular diffusion: this takes place at the level of the distal alveoli.

Monitoring of jet ventilation

It is difficult to monitor adequacy of ventilation during LFJV and its use is restricted to short procedures such as surgical laryngoscopy or bronchoscopy. The patient may require intermittent ventilation via a supraglottic airway.

HFJV may allow monitoring of airway pressure between cycles if a specialized dual-lumen catheter or ETT is used. $ETCO_2$ monitoring may be used intermittently, i.e. single-breath $ETCO_2$ when the ventilator is switched to manual mode. ABG analysis is required to assess adequacy of ventilation during prolonged surgery.

Further reading

Evans E, Biro P, & Bedforth N (2007). Jet ventilation. *CEACCP*, 7:2–5.

Patel B & Frerk C (2008). Large bore cricothyroidotomy devices. *CEACCP*, 8(5):157–60.

11.6 Tracheostomy

Tracheostomy

Tracheostomy was first documented in the 1700s for upper airway obstruction, but evidence of tracheostomies has been found on Egyptian hieroglyphs dating as far back as 3600BC.

The expanding use of tracheostomies means the anaesthetist will commonly be required to manage such patients in theatres or intensive care. This will include anaesthetic management during insertion and management of complications such as the blocked or misplaced tracheostomy.

Indications for tracheostomy

To maintain airway patency
- Reduced consciousness
- Upper airway obstruction (tumour, infection, burns, oedema)
- Intubation difficulties
- Post upper airway surgery/laryngectomy.

Airway protection
- Neurological disease, e.g. bulbar palsy
- Cervical spine injury
- Severe obstructive sleep apnoea.

Bronchial toileting
- Excessive secretions
- Inadequate cough.

Weaning from IPPV
- Patient comfort
- Reduced sedation requirements
- Reduced dead space and work of breathing.

Contraindications to tracheostomy

Absolute
- Localized sepsis
- Uncontrollable coagulopathy.

Relative
- Difficult anatomy
- Moderate coagulopathy
- Proximity to recent trauma site or surgery
- Potential aggravated morbidity, e.g. unstable intracranial pressure
- Severe gas exchange problems
- Age <12 years old (increasing use in neonatal population).

Management of a patient for surgical tracheostomy

The procedure may be performed under LA or GA. Consent is required as with any surgical procedure. In the ICU or emergency setting this may be informed assent. Preprocedure management includes:
- Consent checked.
- Preoperative visit: airway assessed including documented grade of laryngoscopy, current mode of ventilation mode, and FiO$_2$/PEEP requirements. Ideally the procedure should be performed when FiO2 <0.5 and PEEP <10cmH$_2$O. Relevant medical history should be recorded, including allergies, blood results (INR <1.5, platelet count >50), and evidence of a "group and save" sample having been received in the laboratory. Anticoagulant drugs should be discontinued. Starvation time confirmed.
- Preparation of emergency airway equipment and drugs.
- Assembly of experienced personnel.
- Transfer to theatres if required.

The principles for anaesthetizing patients for a tracheostomy are as for any shared airway procedure. The patient should be positioned to promote neck extension and improve surgical access. This may require padding below the shoulders and a head ring to stabilize the head. The patient should be anaesthetized and muscle relaxation provided. High FiO$_2$ is used and PEEP maintained to preoxygenate the patient. The ETT is withdrawn into the upper trachea under vision by direct laryngoscopy. The cuff should be just below the vocal cords. As the trachea is incised, the cuff is deflated but the ETT left in position. During formation of the tracheostomy ventilation via the ETT may fail due to leak and it is important to maintain adequate levels of anaesthesia to avoid awareness. When the tracheostomy is inserted, checked (ETCO$_2$, auscultation) and satisfactory, the ETT is removed.

Emergency airway equipment should be available prior to starting the case. Often a laryngeal mask will be an appropriate rescue device should the airway be lost during the procedure.

Percutaneous tracheostomy

Percutaneous tracheostomy may be performed as an alternative to elective surgical tracheostomy and is commonly performed in the ICU. Patients with difficult anatomy or bleeding disorders may be better managed surgically. Two anaesthetists and a skilled assistant are required. The procedure is commonly monitored with fibreoptic bronchoscopy. Percutaneous tracheostomy techniques include:
- Single tapered dilation system
- Serial dilators
- Guidewire dilator forceps technique
- Balloon dilatational techniques.

Assessment of the anatomy may include ultrasound examination. The same preprocedure management is required as for a surgical procedure. The patient is sedated, preoxygenated, and positioned with the neck extended. Anatomical landmarks are identified, the tracheal rings are palpated where possible, and the approach chosen. A low approach between 2nd and 3rd tracheal rings may reduce tracheal stenosis but the space between the 1st and 2nd tracheal rings may also be used. The 2nd tracheal ring is normally the midpoint between cricoid and suprasternal notch.

After local anaesthetic infiltration (lidocaine with adrenaline), a 2cm horizontal incision is made and dilated with a blunt instrument until the tracheal rings are visualized. The ETT is withdrawn until the cuff is near the level of the cords. The trachea is located with the introducer needle and cannula between tracheal rings aiming slightly caudad to prevent damage to the posterior wall. The cannula is fed over the needle and air is aspirated to confirm position. A Seldinger wire is fed into the trachea through the cannula, which can then be removed. The tracheal dilator system is then used over the guide-wire. Finally, the tracheostomy tube can

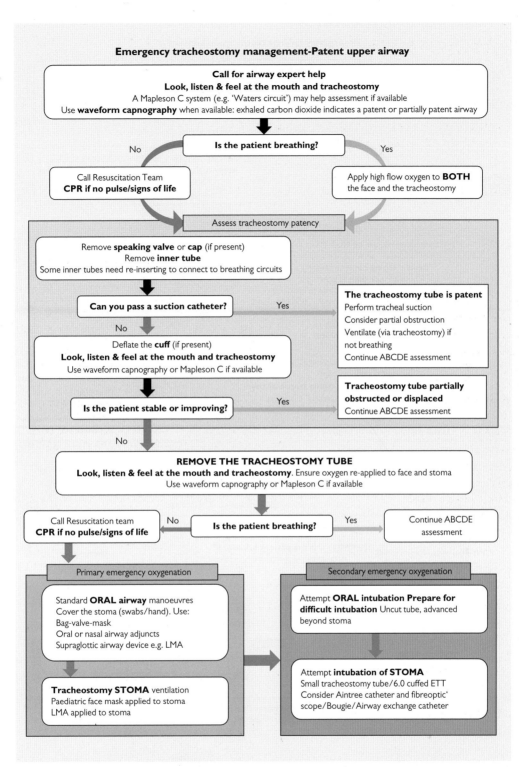

Fig. 11.8 Emergency tracheostomy management algorithm. Reproduced from McGrath BA et al., 'Multidisciplinary guidelines for the management of tracheostomy and laryngectomy airway emergencies', *Anaesthesia*, figure 1, pp. 1025–1041, © 2012 The Association of Anaesthetists of Great Britain and Ireland and Wiley, with permission.

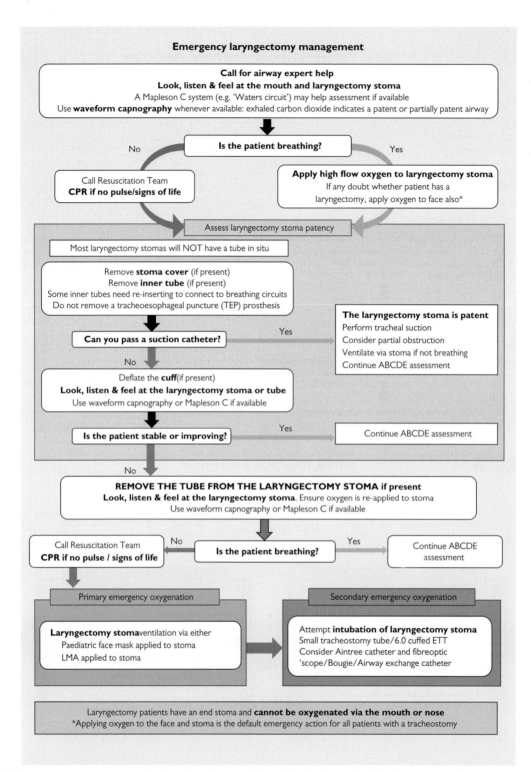

Emergency laryngectomy management

Call for airway expert help
Look, listen & feel at the mouth and laryngectomy stoma
A Mapleson C system (e.g. 'Waters circuit') may help assessment if available
Use **waveform capnography** whenever available: exhaled carbon dioxide indicates a patent or partially patent airway

Is the patient breathing?

No — Call Resuscitation Team
CPR if no pulse/signs of life

Yes — **Apply high flow oxygen to laryngectomy stoma**
If any doubt whether patient has a
laryngectomy, apply oxygen to face also*

Assess laryngectomy stoma patency

Most laryngectomy stomas will NOT have a tube in situ

Remove **stoma cover** (if present)
Remove **inner tube** (if present)
Some inner tubes need re-inserting to connect to breathing circuits
Do not remove a tracheoesophageal puncture (TEP) prosthesis

Can you pass a suction catheter?

Yes — **The laryngectomy stoma is patent**
Perform tracheal suction
Consider partial obstruction
Ventilate via stoma if not breathing
Continue ABCDE assessment

No — Deflate the **cuff**(if present)
Look, listen & feel at the laryngectomy stoma or tube
Use waveform capnography or Mapleson C if available

Is the patient stable or improving?

Yes — Continue ABCDE assessment

No — **REMOVE THE TUBE FROM THE LARYNGECTOMY STOMA if present**
Look, listen & feel at the laryngectomy stoma. Ensure oxygen is re-applied to stoma
Use waveform capnography or Mapleson C if available

Is the patient breathing?

No — Call Resuscitation Team
CPR if no pulse / signs of life

Yes — Continue ABCDE assessment

Primary emergency oxygenation

Laryngectomy stomaventilation via either
Paediatric face mask applied to stoma
LMA applied to stoma

Secondary emergency oxygenation

Attempt **intubation of laryngectomy stoma**
Small tracheostomy tube/6.0 cuffed ETT
Consider Aintree catheter and fibreoptic
'scope/Bougie/Airway exchange catheter

Laryngectomy patients have an end stoma and **cannot be oxygenated via the mouth or nose**
*Applying oxygen to the face and stoma is the default emergency action for all patients with a tracheostomy

Fig. 11.9 Emergency laryngectomy management algorithm. Reproduced from McGrath BA et al., 'Multidisciplinary guidelines for the management of tracheostomy and laryngectomy airway emergencies', *Anaesthesia*, figure 2, pp. 1025–1041, © 2012 The Association of Anaesthetists of Great Britain and Ireland and Wiley, with permission.

be inserted over a loading dilator and the guide-wire removed. The process can be monitored at each stage with bronchoscopy to prevent false passage. Following cuff inflation, ventilation and $ETCO_2$ is confirmed and the final position is further confirmed by CXR.

Early complications include:

- bleeding
- creation of false passage and surgical emphysema
- oesophageal perforation
- infection.

Late complications include:

- granuloma
- tracheo arterial/oesophageal fistula
- persistent stoma
- subglottic stenosis.

If accidental decannulation occurs within 5 days, orotracheal tube placement may be required as the tract can be difficult to re-establish.

Management of the blocked or misplaced tracheostomy tube

Blocked or misplaced tubes are life-threatening complications of tracheostomy. The tracheostomy tube can become dislodged or blocked for a number of reasons and hence it is important to have a strategy for dealing with this. Most departments will have guidelines to help manage these scenarios.

The National Tracheostomy Safety Project was initiated in response to a number of adverse incidents relating to tracheostomies and laryngectomies. Even if a problem occurred in a critical care area, NAP4 (the 4th National Audit Project of the RCoA) found that 50% of patients died from early complications such as haemorrhage, tube displacement, or blockage. The algorithms produced aim to guide management. The tracheostomy algorithm assumes a potentially patent upper airway (see Figs. 11.8 and 11.9). Further information can be obtained from <http://www.tracheostomy.org.uk>.

Only experienced personnel should attempt to replace the tube. There is a risk of making a false passage, which can lead to the development of surgical emphysema in the ventilated patient. This may make airway management extremely difficult. An even more serious complication of mal-insertion is haemorrhage from the great vessels. Multiple attempts should be avoided and if the tube cannot be reinserted, the airway should be established by the orotracheal route using direct laryngoscopy after anaesthesia and muscle relaxation.

If the tube is occluded a suction catheter can be passed in an attempt to clear the blockage. This should not be forced.

Further reading

McGrath BA, Bates L, Arkinson D, et al. (2012). Multidisciplinary guidelines for the management of tracheostomy and laryngectomy airway emergencies. *Anaesthesia*, 67(9):1025–41. doi:10.111/j.1365-2044.2012.07217.

11.7 ENT anaesthesia

ENT

ENT procedures vary from minor surgery to major head and neck surgery. Patients are commonly at the extremes of age and most minor procedures are performed as day surgery cases. Paediatric patients may have obstructive sleep apnoea related to tonsillar size and frequent respiratory tract infections. Patients with ENT malignancy may have smoking or alcohol-related comorbidities. Preoperative evaluation should include a comprehensive airway examination and prediction of difficult facemask ventilation (FMV) and/or intubation (see section 11.1).

Airway planning
The shared airway means that good planning and communication between surgeon and anaesthetist are vital. For cases with airway obstruction, a shared understanding of the algorithms (Plans A, B, and C) will allow rapid decisions in the event of a CICV scenario (see section 11.3). Tracheostomy or needle cricothyroid puncture may need to be performed electively under LA. An ENT surgeon should be present at induction where there are airway concerns. The patient's head is remote from the anaesthetic machine necessitating a long coaxial breathing system and secure connections. Patients must be warned that teeth and caps are at risk if rigid laryngoscopes or gags are used.

Choice of airway (and nerve monitoring)
Many procedures are possible using a reinforced LMA. If an ETT is used, vocal cords are sprayed with lidocaine and it is often changed to an LMA at the end of surgery (under deep anaesthesia) because of the improved recovery profile. The patient is able to wake sitting up with less coughing (reducing venous pressure) and the airway is protected from bleeding from the oro/nasopharynx.

ENT procedures may require monitoring of the recurrent laryngeal nerve. Specialized ETTs are used with a nerve stimulator positioned proximal to the cuff. The facial nerve may be monitored for ear/parotid surgery. Short-acting muscle relaxants may be used at induction (or avoided with high-dose opioid techniques). Maintenance of low-normal CO_2 and use of remifentanil obtunds respiratory effort.

Perioperative positioning
To improve venous drainage the head is tilted upwards 30° and the airway taped rather than tied. Procedure-specific positioning is also required.

Vigilance for airway obstruction
Airway obstruction may occur during repositioning of the head and particularly during insertion of surgical gags. Disconnection is also common during repositioning.

Hypotensive techniques
Systolic blood pressure, hyperdynamic circulation, and venous congestion all contribute to surgical bleeding. Hypotensive anaesthetic techniques can be employed to minimize bleeding and improve the surgical field but are not without risk. The morbidity associated with maintenance of systolic pressures <80mmHg has encouraged an individualized approach dependent on the surgery and patient comorbidity. Invasive blood pressure monitoring should be used to allow continuous monitoring and avoid precipitous drops in pressure. Risks from hypotensive anaesthesia include:

- Myocardial ischaemia from reduced coronary blood flow. This is compounded with techniques that allow reflex tachycardia.
- Cerebral hypoperfusion.
- Reduced renal blood flow and acute kidney injury.

Agents used should be easy to titrate and rapidly reversible:

- Remifentanil is commonly used to provide analgesia, and to reduce heart rate and systolic pressure.
- β-blockers such as esmolol (β1 antagonist with a half-life of 9min) or labetalol.
- GTN provides venodilation to reduce preload whilst decreasing myocardial oxygen consumption. Onset within 1–2min and offset in 3–5min allows for easy titration.
- Hydralazine, a direct vasodilator, may also be used but causes reflex tachycardia.

Ear surgery

Cases range from simple grommet insertion to cochlear implants. Communication difficulties may be caused by hearing loss or congenital deafness (which may be associated with other congenital syndromes).

Anaesthetic considerations
- Nitrous oxide expands in the middle ear, contributes to PONV, and should be avoided.
- The facial nerve may be monitored.
- Reinforced LMA used for most procedures (superior wake up profile and avoidance of paralysis).
- Simple analgesics are usually adequate.
- Multimodal antiemesis is routinely used.

Nausea, vomiting, and dizziness can be problematic despite multimodal prophylaxis and may delay hospital discharge.

Nose

Includes endoscopic sinus surgery and septorhinoplasty.

Anaesthetic considerations
The LMA has a number of benefits for nasal surgery including the mask acting as a roof shielding the glottis from blood, avoidance of the complications of intubation, and a superior recovery profile.

Throat packs are often used in conjunction with an LMA or ETT to absorb blood. It is important to label that there is a pack *in situ* and document that it has been removed after surgery (as per NPSA guidelines). Good suctioning is vital at the end of the case (see Box 11.8).

> **Box 11.8 The coroner's clot**
>
> It is good practice after all types of nose surgery (and tonsillectomy) to suction the nasopharynx under direct vision after removal of the throat pack to ensure there are no clots retained behind the uvula. This is commonly known as the 'coroner's clot' as it can cause potentially fatal airway obstruction during emergence from anaesthesia.

Preparation of the nose
The nose is prepared to provide topical anaesthesia and vasoconstriction. Some surgeons prefer to perform this themselves. The head is extended, tilted down, and the eyes protected with swabs before nasal preparation.

Moffat's solution consists of a mixture of 2mL 10% cocaine, 2mL 1% bicarbonate, and 1mL of 1:1000 adrenaline. This mixture is highly dangerous if given IV and also has a number of complications topically such as hypertension and tachycardia. It should be avoided or diluted in patients with a history of cardiovascular disease. Other nasal preparations include co-phenylcaine or xylometazoline.

Postoperatively

Head-up nursing, blood pressure control, and vigilance for bleeding (remembering much may be swallowed).

Throat

Throat surgery usually presents a significant anaesthetic challenge. Patients may present with voice change, stridor, dysphagia, or dyspnoea and will commonly have smoking/alcohol-related comorbidity. Previous radiotherapy or radical surgery can make airway management more difficult. Pulmonary flow volume loops can be useful in assessing airway obstruction.

Up-to-date imaging provides information on the size and location of lesion in relation to the glottis which guides airway management, i.e. supraglottic, glottic, or infraglottic (endo- or extratracheal, with or without tracheal deviation). The airway plan, made in conjunction with the surgeon, should consider induction with laryngoscopy and intubation, maintenance and ventilation, and emergence.

Airway and induction

If there is any doubt concerning FMV after induction, an awake technique should be considered. A transtracheal device may be used as a primary airway or pre-emptive plan B should FMV be impossible. It may be left *in situ* if postoperative oedema is a risk.

Supraglottic lesions may be approached with fibreoptic intubation. In glottic lesions, fibreoptic intubation may create complete airway obstruction ('cork in bottle'), may be technically difficult due to limited airspace and anatomical disruption and may result in contact bleeding. In glottic lesions, either a supraglottic approach with surgical laryngoscopy and jet techniques, or an infraglottic surgical airway are employed. Many glottic lesions can be managed conventionally with intubation. Infraglottic lesions can be approached by supraglottic jet ventilation. Tracheal compression may require rigid bronchoscopy and endotracheal jet ventilation if standard intubation fails.

Postoperative

For the major types of throat surgery, HDU or a specialized ward familiar with airway/tracheostomy care is mandatory for patient safety. Complications such as oedema, bleeding, and stridor are common. Early warning and clear management plans can save lives. IV steroids and nebulized adrenaline can be useful in temporizing airway swelling but regular anaesthetic review is required.

Specific procedures

Tonsillectomy

Commonly performed in children and young adults. Reinforced LMAs confer a number of advantages but in laser surgery a specific ETT is required. The time of Boyle Davis gag insertion is highly stimulating to the patient and may cause airway obstruction. It is a painful operation which requires multimodal analgesia with paracetamol, NSAIDs, and opioids. Blood loss should be monitored carefully, particularly in children. Tonsillectomy may be performed as day surgery but a 6h stay is required to detect early postoperative bleeding.

Laryngectomy

Patients with carcinoma of the larynx often have smoking- and alcohol-related comorbidities. Airway examination may include nasoendoscopy to assess the patency of the airway and, in conjunction with radiology and surgical discussion, should allow airway planning. Options such as elective tracheostomy or elective wide-bore cricothyroid puncture should be considered. Repeated attempts at intubation can cause bleeding and oedema leading to CICV.

During laryngectomy, a stoma is formed and a laryngectomy tube is inserted by the surgeon and sutured to the skin. At the end of the procedure a tracheostomy tube is inserted. Postoperative airway intervention requires specialist input.

Radical neck surgery can involve laryngectomy, glossectomy, or pharyngectomy. The procedures can be lengthy and require blood transfusion, full haemodynamic monitoring, and HDU/ITU postoperatively.

Parotid surgery

Because of the route of the facial nerve through the parotid gland, the nerve is tested by stimulus during dissection.

Thyroid surgery

Airway obstruction is rare electively but tracheal deviation may create difficulty with laryngoscopy, and tracheal compression may necessitate a smaller-sized ETT. The recurrent laryngeal nerve can be monitored using a specialized ETT. Cord function may be assessed fibreoptically at the end of the case. Tracheomalacia may be associated with retrosternal goitres (see also section 5.4).

Pharyngoscopy and endoscopic pouch surgery

A microlaryngoscopy tube allows best surgical access to the pharynx. In external approaches, a reinforced ETT can be used. Food debris can be problematic.

Microlaryngoscopy

Surgical preference often dictates the airway required. Microlaryngoscopy tubes may be acceptable and allow conventional IPPV. The procedure is short and therefore a short-acting muscle relaxant should be used or a longer-acting relaxant with sugammadex reversal. The cords are sprayed with lidocaine.

A supraglottic jet technique may be required (see section 11.5). The jet catheter is inserted and taped securely to the left of the mouth. An LMA is also inserted to ventilate the patient until the time of surgical laryngoscopy. Maintenance of anaesthesia requires TIVA using propofol and remifentanil at adequate depth for this very stimulating procedure. On insertion of the rigid laryngoscope, jet ventilation commences and the laryngoscope provides an expiratory pathway.

Further reading

Difficult Airway Society: Algorithms for difficult airway management. <http://www.das.uk.com/guidelines/downloads.html>.

Popat M (2009). *Difficult Airway Management*. Oxford: Oxford University Press.

11.8 ENT emergencies

Bleeding tonsils

Bleeding post tonsillectomy occurs in about 3% of cases. Primary haemorrhage occurs within 24h postoperatively, secondary haemorrhage within 28 days. About 0.8% of patients will require operative intervention.

Problems

Hypovolaemia

Blood loss is difficult to quantify and much is swallowed although excessive bleeding may cause the patient to spit. Hypovolaemia may be evident from clinical assessment and IV access should be established to allow fluid resuscitation and blood transfusion if indicated. Adequate resuscitation will improve cardiovascular stability on induction.

Airway

Laryngoscopic view may be very difficult in the presence of brisk tonsillar bleeding, and two suction devices should be available for simultaneous use. Intubation may also be difficult due to airway oedema secondary to recent airway instrumentation. ETT sizes smaller than expected should be immediately available. Patients are also at risk of aspiration, both of blood and gastric contents, since they will usually not be starved.

Anxiety

Patients will often be distressed and anxious especially if paediatric cases.

Anaesthetic technique

The anaesthetic technique of choice is a rapid sequence induction. This familiar technique allows rapid control of the airway and prevention of aspiration, particularly if a slight head-down position is used. However, there is a risk of difficult laryngoscopic view and difficult intubation.

An alternative technique involves performing a gas induction in the left lateral, head-down position and deep intubation. Many anaesthetists now have little experience of intubating in this position and cardiovascular compromise may occur in the presence of hypovolaemia.

Perioperatively, fluid resuscitation should continue and a wide-bore NGT should be inserted to empty the stomach. This is removed prior to waking the patient. Extubation should be performed with the patient in the left lateral, head-down position and with the patient wide awake. The patient requires close monitoring for further bleeding.

Epiglottitis

Epiglottitis (Fig. 11.10) typically presents in children aged 2–5 years but can occur in adults. The incidence has been dramatically decreased by routine vaccination against *Haemophilus influenzae*. Streptococcal infection is now commonly responsible. Patients present with symptoms of systemic infection and rapidly developing upper airway obstruction with stridor and drooling. Early detection and management are vital as the condition can progress rapidly to complete airway obstruction.

Initial management is aimed at keeping the child calm, giving oxygen if possible and assembling the necessary senior personnel. The child should be kept in a sitting position. IV access may cause distress and worsen symptoms of airway obstruction. An experienced anaesthetist and ENT surgeon should be present. Airway equipment should include a variety of ETTs, in smaller sizes than anticipated and emergency cricothyroid/tracheostomy equipment.

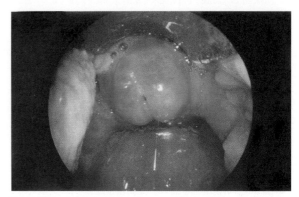

Fig. 11.10 Laryngoscopic view of acute epiglottitis. Reproduced with permission from: Calder I, Pearce A, *Core Topics in Airway Management* second edition, Fig 21.6, p. 200, 2011, Cambridge University Press.

The airway should be secured early. A gas induction with oxygen and sevoflurane in the sitting position is the most appropriate technique. Monitoring and IV access are established when asleep and intubation is performed deep. A smaller ETT will be necessary and the intubation is often difficult due to oedematous, distorted anatomy. Air bubbles may help to identify the glottis.

In adult patients, a gas induction for impending airway obstruction may be more difficult. Halothane may be useful for providing deep anaesthesia to allow intubation. Alternative strategies in adults include IV induction with neuromuscular blockade or fibreoptic techniques.

Ventilation will be required on ICU until antibiotic therapy (e.g. cefotaxime) has reduced airway inflammation and oedema. Extubation may be attempted, usually after 24–48h, when a leak around the ETT can be demonstrated.

Croup

Croup or laryngotracheobronchitis is a very common cause of winter-time upper airway obstruction in infants. It is caused by respiratory syncytial virus, parainfluenza, or influenza. It is associated with a gradual onset, a typical barking cough but little systemic upset.

Assessment of stridor, respiratory distress, oxygenation, and conscious level help to determine severity. Severe croup will cause respiratory distress with tachypnoea and recession, reduced air entry, saturations <93% on oxygen, tachycardia, and depressed levels of consciousness. Initial management of croup is aimed at reducing airway inflammation using adrenaline and steroid nebulizers (Box 11.9).

Box 11.9 Medical management of croup

- Humidified oxygen.
- Hydration.
- Adrenaline nebulizer. 0.5mL/kg. Max. 5mL. Repeat after 30min. Requires ECG monitoring and dosing may be limited by tachycardia.
- Budesonide nebulizer 2mg. *Or* oral dexamethasone 0.6mg/kg (max. 8mg).

The child should be carefully assessed for response but many respond well to medical management. Intubation may be required if airway obstruction is worsening or if the child is exhausted. The conduct of anaesthesia is as for epiglottitis.

Inhaled foreign bodies

Inhaled foreign bodies are a relatively common problem in younger children. They can present in a variety of ways depending on the size and position of the object. Large objects may require emergency management of complete upper airway obstruction with back blows or Heimlich manoeuvre. More typically, objects have passed through the larynx to the lower airways and may be asymptomatic.

The clinical assessment should include examination for:
• Reduced air entry
• Wheeze
• Hyperinflation.

These may all be signs of an inhaled foreign body. A CXR may confirm the diagnosis by demonstrating hyperinflation of the airways beyond the obstruction. Some foreign bodies may also be easily identifiable. Organic matter such as peanuts may also cause an inflammatory reaction with airway oedema and obstruction, which can also be visualized on CXR within a few hours.

The urgency of the situation will depend on the clinical condition of the child and the nature of the foreign body, i.e. organic matter. Rigid bronchoscopy is required to remove the foreign body.

Anaesthetic technique
Positive pressure ventilation during anaesthesia is often avoided for two reasons:
• It may cause distal migration of the foreign body to less accessible airways.
• It may cause a ball-valve effect leading to distal gas trapping.

To maintain spontaneous ventilation a gas induction is typically the technique of choice. Premedication with atropine (20mcg/kg up to 600mcg) may be used to reduce airway secretions and bradycardia associated with laryngoscopy. Sevoflurane in oxygen is suitable. Nitrous oxide should be avoided to prevent increasing the distal air trapping. Induction may be slow in the face of airway obstruction.

Two surgical techniques may be used to retrieve the foreign body:
• The ventilating bronchoscope
• Rigid bronchoscopy.

The ventilating bronchoscope is preferable as anaesthesia can be delivered via the side arm of the scope using a T-piece system. It is therefore possible to maintain volatile anaesthesia at adequate depth throughout the stimulating procedure. The rigid bronchoscope does not allow attachment of an anaesthetic breathing system and requires IV anaesthesia for maintenance. A jet ventilator system may be used to oxygenate the child during use. This may dislodge the foreign body and can cause barotrauma.

In practice, it may be very difficult to maintain adequate spontaneous ventilation throughout the procedure and hypercapnia may necessitate positive pressure ventilation.

Dexamethasone is administered to reduce airway oedema. Oedema may continue for 48h and the child should be closely monitored for this time and continued on humidified oxygen if tolerated.

Further reading

Children's Acute transport Service. CATS guidelines for croup management: http://site.cats.nhs.uk/in-a-hurry/cats-clinical-guidelines/.

Makepeace J & Patel A (2011). ENT Emergencies. *Anaesth Intens Care Med*, 12(7):306–8.

11.9 Lasers in ENT surgery

Types of lasers

Laser or 'light amplification by stimulated emission of radiation' is commonly used for ENT/head and neck surgery. A variety of laser types are used including:

The CO_2 laser

The CO_2 laser is the most commonly used in practice. It produces infrared radiation which is absorbed by water in tissues, causing vaporization and tissue destruction. As it is so well absorbed by water, the energy remains concentrated at the target tissue with little dissipation to surrounding tissue. It is used for precise cutting and coagulation and is associated with less postoperative tissue oedema and pain. The CO_2 laser is commonly used for tonsillectomy, uvulopalatoplasty, sinus surgery, and sublottic stenoses.

The Nd:YAG laser

The Nd:YAG (neodymium:yttrium-aluminium garnet) laser produces radiation in the near infrared spectrum. The smaller wavelength is less well absorbed in water and penetrates tissue deeply. It acts on pigmented or vascular tissue and can be delivered by flexible fibres (unlike the CO_2 laser) so may be used for lesions of the tracheobronchial tree.

The KTP 'greenlight' laser

The KTP or 'greenlight' laser involves directing the beam of a Nd:YAG laser through a potassium titanyl phosphate crystal. This is used for photoablation and photocoagulation as in the Nd:YAG laser, but with a much more superficial effect. It is commonly used for prostatic surgery.

Photodynamic therapy (PDT)

PDT is used to target malignant or diseased cells. A light-sensitive compound is administered to the patient. When selected diseased tissue areas are exposed to laser the compound becomes toxic and causes tissue destruction.

Considerations for laser use

Staff safety

All staff should be familiar with local laser safety protocols. Laser-specific goggles should be worn by all staff during the case as the non-divergent beam loses no power and is a danger to the retina. Each different laser wavelength requires specific goggles. Normal prescription glasses are not considered adequate protection.

Fine particulate matter is released by laser tissue destruction and inhalation causes alveolar deposition with the potential for chronic lung disease and malignancy.

Theatre doors should remain locked whilst the laser is in use, with signs placed outside to prevent flow of staff during the procedure.

Patient safety

Laser use creates the potential for operating room fires. The combination of heat produced by the laser, an oxygen-enriched atmosphere, and available fuel (drapes, alcohol-based preparation solutions) makes fire safety a high priority. Care must be taken to use non-flammable preparation solutions and to ensure adequate drying prior to laser use. Drapes should be positioned carefully to prevent pockets of oxygen-enriched air.

Risk of airway fire

Laser use in the airway creates a risk of fire in the presence of:
- Oxygen-enriched atmosphere
- Flammable anaesthetic agents
- Nitrous oxide which supports combustion
- Flammable ETTs which support combustion.
  The risk of airway fire is reduced by the following precautions:
- Using the lowest possible concentration of oxygen with air, ideally FiO_2 0.25.
- Using TIVA maintenance.
- Specialized laser ETTs that are generally made of flexible stainless steel or have a metallic powder coating. ETT cuffs are inflated with saline instead of air or methylene blue to allow early detection of cuff rupture. Some specialized ETTs have double cuffs. Even specialized ETTs will not withstand a direct laser beam for long periods.
- Laser-safe jet catheters are also available to allow glottic procedures. As this is an open system, the FiO_2 must be kept very low.

Surrounding tissue damage

Reflective damage to the tissues surrounding the area of direct laser is reduced by using black instruments and covering with wet swabs.

Management of airway fires

There should be a 'Fire Drill' protocol in every unit using lasers for the emergency management of airway fires (Box 11.10).

> **Box 11.10 Laser 'fire drill' procedure**
>
> - Remove the source—turn the laser off.
> - Stop oxygen—disconnect the circuit and extubate.
> - Flood the site with saline (a 50mL syringe of saline should be prepared for this reason during the conduct of laser airway surgery).
> - Maintain ventilation via a facemask and maintain anaesthesia with TIVA.
> - Bronchoscopic evaluation of damage, removal of debris with lavage.
> - Reintubation and CXR.
> - Supportive management on ITU.

Anaesthetic techniques for laser airway surgery

Non-intubated techniques

Apnoeic oxygenation where surgical laser intervention occurs during periods of patient apnoea under anaesthesia may be performed. This provides a low risk of fire and good surgical conditions with no movement of field but obviously limits the surgical time and provides no monitoring of ventilation.

Jet ventilation techniques may be used in the same way but require TIVA maintenance and may have the added risk of barotrauma.

Self-ventilating techniques create a moving surgical field and depth of anaesthesia may be inconsistent with volatile maintenance.

Intubation

Intubation with laser specialized ETTs allows controlled ventilation during the procedure and full monitoring of ventilation. However, the ETT may disturb the surgical field and the risk of airway fire is increased.

Further reading

Dhar P & Malik A (2011). Anesthesia for laser surgery in ENT and the various ventilatory techniques. *Trends Anaesth Criti Care*, 1(2):60–6. doi:10.1016/j.tacc.2011.01.011.

Maxillofacial trauma, infection, and orthognathic surgery require careful management of a potentially difficult 'supraglottic' airway. Management necessitates good airway assessment, planning, and team communication. Maxillofacial surgery involves a shared airway and a variety of surgical access requirements specific to each operation.

Maxillofacial trauma

Facial trauma occurs most frequently in young men following assault or accidental injury (sports, road traffic incidents). It may be associated with soft tissue, brain, and cervical spine injury. Assessment includes mechanism of injury and a careful examination for associated injuries.

Acutely, these patients require management as per ATLS guidelines and occasionally, definitive airway control may be necessary early. Airway obstruction can result from anatomical disruption, oedema, bleeding, and dental damage. This may be indicated by hypoxia, stridor, dyspnoea, drooling, trismus, voice change, and surgical emphysema. During management of the airway in acute maxillofacial trauma, other considerations include:

- Poor patient cooperation—hypoxia, intoxication, brain injury.
- Need for cervical spine immobilization.
- Aspiration risk from full stomach.
- Facemask ventilation may be difficult due to anatomical distortion.
- Nasal airway adjuncts or route for intubation may be contra-indicated if basal skull fracture is suspected.

Awake intubation techniques require a cooperative patient. A rapid sequence induction following careful preoxygenation is often the preferred technique. Due to a high incidence of difficult intubation associated with these injuries, a careful airway plan should be made, a full range of difficult airway equipment available and the procedure should be performed by the most experienced personnel available. Equipment for emergency cricothyroidotomy must be available. Alternatively, a surgical airway may be established under LA.

Scheduled maxillofacial trauma surgery

Many patients with isolated maxillofacial trauma can await surgery at home, allowing swelling to subside. Ambulatory surgery may be scheduled within a few days on dedicated maxillofacial trauma operating lists.

Preoperative considerations

The site of the fracture and route of repair will affect intubation options and should be discussed with the surgeon. A thorough airway assessment should include nasal patency, mouth opening, protrusion of the mandible, and interdental distance. Trismus should be discussed with the surgeon as well as plans for throat/nasal packing, facial nerve monitoring, and intermaxillary fixation for malocclusion.

Perioperative

Awake fibreoptic intubation, IV induction, or gaseous induction may be considered as per difficult airway management (see section 11.3). An airway strategy including intubation and extubation phases should be discussed with the whole team to ensure emergency airway access can be provided swiftly.

Tracheal tubes need to be well secured intraoperatively with tape or even by suture. Eye tapes and pads are needed to protect the eyes in lower facial surgery. Eye lubricant (e.g. Viscotears® or Lacrilube®) is needed, if the eyes are left uncovered during surgery, to reduce the risk of corneal damage.

Postoperative

Throat pack vigilance is of upmost importance in line with NPSA guidance (stickers, two-person check, records on swab board). Oropharyngeal and posterior nasal space suctioning under direct vision prior to extubation ensure no debris or clot is left in the airway. Extubation is best performed awake.

Airway oedema can worsen in the first 48h after surgery and dexamethasone is used to reduce this. Pain is often decreased after fixation of fractures. Infiltration of LA intraoperatively by the surgeon helps reduce early postoperative pain. Simple analgesics such as paracetamol and NSAIDs are used, with opioids titrated to effect. Adequate analgesia reduces patient agitation and postoperative haematoma or bleeding.

HDU care should be considered if ongoing airway oedema or bleeding may cause airway compromise.

Lower face fractures

The lower third of the face is made up by the mandible which forms a ring with the temporomandibular joint (TMJ) and the base of the skull. Mandibular fractures only impact on the airway when complex.

Trismus associated with mandibular fractures will relax post induction as it is a response to pain. TMJ fractures or zygomatic bone impingement into the TMJ may continue to affect mouth opening post induction. The surgeon's opinion is needed to ascertain this possibility.

Nasal intubation is often the most appropriate airway management. This allows full surgical access to the mouth and allows the surgeon to place teeth in occlusion if required. Nasal intubation can be performed via the blind method or using a fibreoptic scope (asleep or awake) but there is rarely a difficulty in visualizing the vocal cords with laryngoscopy in mandibular fractures. It is important to minimize nasal bleeding with vasoconstrictors, full cuff deflation, and lubrication.

Midface fractures

The midface is made up of the maxilla, zygoma, and lower half of the naso-orbital-ethmoidal complex.

Midface fractures include Le Fort, nasal, orbital, and zygoma fractures. 'True' Le Fort fractures are rare as they are bilateral and create an unstable midface. This can bleed heavily and cause airway obstruction when supine as the midface falls back and occludes the nasal and upper airway. Le Fort fractures in vivo are often unilateral and more stable. Access to repair fractures is via the mouth and lower eyelid to minimize scarring.

Anaesthetic considerations in midface fractures

Airway management requires consultation with the surgeon. Nasal intubation will allow access to the mouth and dental occlusion if required. A south-facing RAE (Ring, Adair, and Elwyn) orotracheal tube is used for orbital, zygomatic, or other fractures where dental occlusion is not needed. A reinforced LMA can be used in place of a RAE tracheal tube. This requires a reliable fit, may not be as secure as a tracheal tube and access to the airway is often limited and delayed during surgery. Occasionally a tracheostomy or submental intubation may be necessary if nasal intubation is contra-indicated and oral access is required.

Nasal fracture repair can cause significant haemorrhage. Nasal vasoconstrictors and nasal packing is used.

Orbital floor surgery usually accesses the orbital bones via the lower eyelid (transconjuctival) and retraction of the eye. The oculocardiac reflex resulting in bradycardia is common when retracting the eye. This reflex is reduced or abolished with an IV antimuscarinic agent.

Orbital floor surgery can lead to postoperative periorbital haematoma and risk of blindness. Coughing and laryngospasm on extubation must be avoided to decrease this risk. This can be minimized with use of remifentanil, or deep extubation and use of an LMA for awakening.

Upper face fractures

The upper face consists of the frontal bone, sphenoid, and upper half of the naso-orbital-ethmoidal complex.

Upper facial fractures can be accessed by the surgeon via facial incisions or via a coronal flap with an incision behind the hairline folding down the face to access the fracture. This minimizes scarring to the face.

These facial fractures may be associated with cerebrospinal fluid (CSF) leak, dural tears and risk of ascending infection. Nasal intubation may be contraindicated. If oral intubation will interfere with surgical access, a tracheostomy or submental intubation may be the best option.

Intraoperative hypotension is required to reduce blood loss. Remifentanil infusion usually provides a smooth and controlled reduction in blood pressure. These operations can take several hours so particular care is needed with patient pressure points, limiting fluids (unless catheterized), warming, and DVT prophylaxis.

Maxillofacial infection

Dental-related infection is common. Local spread of infection may involve the sublingual, buccal, parapharyngeal, submedial pterygoid, or submandibular spaces. Spread of infection along the fascial planes may lead to airway obstruction, mediastinitis, cavernous sinus thrombosis, and abscess rupture leading to infective soiling of the lungs. Haematogenous spread may cause systemic sepsis and endocarditis.

Patients may present with pain, swelling, trismus, and signs of developing airway obstruction; altered speech, drooling, dysphagia, stridor, and dyspnoea. Trismus may result from submasseteric inflammation and oedema commonly related to wisdom tooth infection. Unlike most maxillofacial trauma, trismus associated with infection is likely to remain post induction of anaesthesia. Parapharyngeal abscesses can progress rapidly to cause airway obstruction despite little external evidence of swelling. The inability to protrude the tongue is a good indicator of sublingual infection (the 'full' sublingual space disrupts the normal C-shape of the genioglossus muscle preventing tongue protrusion).

Ludwig's angina is a life-threatening sublingual cellulitis with parapharyngeal involvement into the neck and pretracheal tissues. This can develop rapidly into upper airway obstruction. The upper airway may be grossly distorted and a surgical airway also involves incising the infected tissue. This may be difficult and risks development of mediastinitis.

Dehydration may also be an issue due to swallowing difficulties.

Anaesthetic technique

A full airway assessment should predict difficulties with facemask ventilation, laryngoscopy, intubation, and emergency surgical airway access. Flexible nasendoscopy may be performed to assess the airway anatomy.

As for any difficult airway, the plan is made in conjunction with the team and may include IV induction with muscle relaxation, gaseous induction, elective transtracheal oxygenation, awake fibreoptic intubation or awake tracheostomy under LA in order to secure the airway.

Trismus may not improve post induction and forcing open the mouth can rupture the abscess. Awake fibreoptic intubation should be considered.

During laryngoscopy, the vocal cords and surrounding tissues must be carefully examined. A throat pack is used to absorb debris. Broad-spectrum antibiotics are administered to treat the infection and dexamethasone used to reduce oedema.

Postoperative management

If the vocal cords are swollen and displaced, a decision to leave the patient intubated may be made to avoid postoperative airway obstruction. Patients presenting with Ludwig's angina, parapharyngeal involvement or preoperative stridor may require prolonged intubation until infection and oedema resolves. This can be assessed with the presence of an air-leak around the ETT with cuff deflated and normalization of anatomy on nasendoscopy.

Orthognathic surgery

Orthognathic surgery is performed to correct dentofacial deformity, which has an impact on facial function as well as self-esteem. These operations involve surgical fracture of either, or both, the maxilla and mandible in order to reposition the jaw. A nasal tube is required to allow access to the oral cavity and allow the teeth to be placed on occlusion. Hypotensive anaesthesia is advantageous particularly during fracture of the maxilla to reduce blood loss. A smooth emergence to avoid coughing reduces the risk of postoperative haemorrhage.

Further reading

Chesshire NJ & Knight DJW (2001). The anaesthetic management of facial trauma and fractures. *CEPD Reviews*, 1(4):108–12.

Morosan N, Parbhoo A, & Curry N (2012). Anaesthesia and common oral and maxilla-facial emergencies. *CEACCP*, 3:1–6.

11.11 Dental anaesthesia

General anaesthesia dental procedures

All dental procedures requiring GA should now be performed within a hospital environment and are typically suitable for day surgery. Most patients requiring GA will be children or have a learning disability. Patients who have medical comorbidity which increases the risk of community dental procedures, e.g. haemophilia and liver disease may also be referred for hospital treatment. Many of these cases may be performed under LA.
Procedures include:

- Simple extractions
- Extractions of permanent molar teeth
- Complex reconstructive dentistry.

Considerations for dental general anaesthesia

Patient factors

Patients may be paediatric, have a learning disability, or high levels of anxiety. Paediatric patients will be susceptible to frequent upper respiratory tract infections, which increase the risk of laryngospasm. Patients with learning disabilities may have concurrent congenital medical concerns and communication and compliance may be an issue. Premedication may be necessary.

Surgical factors

Dental surgery involves a shared airway and there is a risk of airway obstruction from debris, bleeding, and dental packs. LA may be used concurrently and often contains adrenaline to reduce bleeding. Systemic absorption of adrenaline may occur.

Conduct of dental general anaesthesia

Premedication with oral midazolam may be considered for non-compliant patients. The induction may be inhalational or IV as appropriate for the patient.

The choice of airway is dictated by the planned surgery with both number and position of teeth being a consideration. A single extraction of a front tooth may be performed very rapidly and a nasopharyngeal airway may suffice. An LMA is appropriate for most procedures. Vigilance is required due to the risk of displacement in the shared airway. The dental surgeon will usually place a bite block between the opposite teeth to open the mouth, but extraction of mandibular teeth may cause downward pressure on the mandible resulting in airway obstruction. Counter pressure on the mandible can prevent this.

Extraction of wisdom teeth may be associated with increased difficulty of extraction. The associated bleeding and debris usually necessitates intubation. Short-acting muscle relaxants are preferable (or rocuronium and sugammadex to allow rapid reversal). Intubation on high doses of short-acting opiate, e.g. alfentanil is an alternative. A pharyngeal pack is required to prevent debris soiling the airway and must be recorded and removed at the end of the procedure as per NPSA guidelines.

Analgesia requirements are proportional to the number of teeth removed and the difficulty of the extractions. Paracetamol is sufficient for simple extractions. For more complicated extractions, diclofenac and dexamethasone may be added. Anticipated difficult procedures may also receive a LA block.

At the end of the procedure, the patient is extubated awake or the LMA is removed awake. The head down, left lateral position is preferable.

Dental sedation

Conscious sedation (see section 17.4) may be performed in registered dental practices by a fully trained anaesthetist. From the RCoA working party for safe sedation in adult practice, conscious sedation is defined as 'a technique in which the use of a drug or drugs produces a state of depression of the central nervous system enabling treatment to be carried out, but during which verbal contact with the patient is maintained throughout the period of sedation. The drugs and techniques used to provide conscious sedation should carry a margin of safety wide enough to render loss of consciousness unlikely'.

The working party encourages single drug sedation as combinations may be more prone to cause loss of consciousness. Midazolam is frequently used, sometimes in combination with opiates, and propofol TCI sedation may be used by experienced practitioners. Oximetry is a minimum requirement but ECG and NIBP monitoring may be required. Oxygen and resuscitation equipment must be available.

The history of dental chair general anaesthesia

In the past, patients were anaesthetized in the community with minimal monitoring (oximetry and sometimes ECG) and often no IV access. Gas induction with volatile anaesthesia and nitrous oxide was used and maintained via a nasal mask for longer cases. The sitting position was maintained throughout to provide easier access for the dentist and to help airway maintenance.

Many deaths occurred during the 1970s and 1980s due to poor monitoring, lack of skilled assistance, and resuscitation equipment. A working party in the early 1990s advised avoidance of GA where possible and the same standards of assistance, monitoring, and equipment for GA in the dental surgery as would be provided in hospital. Although surgeries were registered and inspected, there was poor compliance with these recommendations. Further high-profile deaths resulted in the General Dental Council and Royal College of Anaesthetists 1999 guidance. This stated that GA should only be used where LA will be insufficient to control pain, where age/emotional maturity will not allow treatment under LA, or where dental phobia may be induced or prolonged. This guidance also produced restrictions on who was providing anaesthesia. Finally, the Department of Health encouraged centralization of services and from 2002, GA could not be provided within a dental surgery in the UK.

Further reading

Cantlay K, Williamson S, & Hawkings J (2005). Anaesthesia for dentistry. *BJA CEPD Reviews*, 5(3):71–5. doi:10.1093/bjaceaccp/mki020.

Chapter 12

Day surgery

233

Day surgery

The strict definition of day surgery is when a patient is admitted and discharged on the same day as the surgical procedure. Increasingly, units offer 23h stay or other short stay arrangements which apply the principles of day surgery but should be considered as an inpatient admission. In 2000, the NHS Plan set a target for 75% of elective surgery to be performed as day surgery. A small 'basket' of procedures regularly performed in day surgery were used for audit and as performance markers. These procedures were mostly minor surgery lasting <1h. Over recent years day surgery has evolved. The increase in minimally invasive surgical techniques has made many more procedures suitable for day surgery. An increasing drive to reduce the length of stay and improve the quality of recovery with initiatives such as the Enhanced Recovery programme is now bringing some of the principles of day surgery care to the inpatient population.

Benefits of day surgery

There are several potential advantages to providing day surgical services (see Box 12.1).

Box 12.1 Potential benefits of day surgery

- Less risk of late cancellation—beds are not subject to pressure from emergency work
- High patient throughput per bed
- Reduced medical/nursing supervision per patient
- Reduced costs of care
- Reduced risks of hospital-acquired infection
- Less psychological upheaval for patients
- Increased patient involvement with care
- Increased patient satisfaction.

Facilities required for day surgery

Several models exit for provision of day surgical services:

Self-contained unit

A self-contained day surgery unit is the ideal. The unit should contain:

- Reception area with consulting rooms
- Pre-assessment area
- Preoperative preparation area (with changing rooms, lockers)
- Theatres
- Recovery area
- Postoperative ward and step-down area
- Administration office
- Car park and drop-off area.

This model is the most efficient for the day surgery pathway. Procedures are not influenced by emergency admissions or emergency theatre work. Patient transfer is rapid and reduced waiting times improve flow.

Day surgery ward using main theatres

A day surgery facility may provide preoperative and postoperative care whilst the surgical procedure and recovery is performed in main theatres. This is often the design in older hospitals where day surgery facilities have not been specially built for purpose. There is some reduction in efficiency with the increased patient journey to main theatres and this model increases the possibility of procedures being delayed by emergency use of theatres.

Day surgery admissions to inpatient wards

This is not a desirable model for providing efficient or high-quality day surgery care. Day surgery admissions are highly influenced by emergency surgical admissions so the risk of late cancellation is increased. Inpatients have increased nursing needs and the day surgery patient preparation and postoperative care suffers a reduction in quality as a consequence.

Paediatric facilities

Ideally, paediatric day surgery facilities will be separate from the adult service. The environment should reflect the special psychological needs of children and the extra space required for accompanying families. All facilities should conform to the standards of a general paediatric unit with specialized paediatric staff.

Delivering same sex accommodation

The NHS agenda to deliver same sex accommodation also applies to day surgery facilities. Only areas where the patients are fully clothed and first stage recovery are exempt.

Day surgery staffing

Clinical lead of day surgery

The clinical lead is often a consultant anaesthetist, ideally with management experience, who should represent day surgery at Board level. The clinical lead is responsible for the development of local policies, guidelines, and clinical governance.

Day surgery manager

The day surgery manager is often from a nursing background and is responsible for the day-to-day running and development of the service.

Nursing staff

Nursing staff are specially trained in day surgery care and may also perform preoperative assessment. Self-contained units encourage multiskilled staff with extended roles, and nurses may mix theatre and ward duties to ensure a flexible workforce.

In the UK, in preoperative assessment, requirements are for one nurse per 20 patients. In the day surgery ward areas, requirements are for one nurse per seven patients with one healthcare assistant also allocated.

Quality measures for day surgery

- Cancellations—may reflect poor patient selection
- DNA rates—may reflect poor administration
- Number of procedures performed—percentage of total surgery performed as day case
- Type of procedures performed
- Unexpected admissions
- Complication and infection rates
- Audit of pain/nausea and vomiting
- Patient satisfaction
- Re-admissions rates (<30 days post procedure).

BEAT: the British Association of Day Surgery (BADS) efficiency assessment tool

BADS provides a directory of procedures with examples of the percentage of cases performed as day case, 23h or <72h admission. This allows hospitals to compare their own practice with the national standards and identify areas where improvement is necessary.

Further reading

British Association of Day Surgery website: <http://www.daysurgeryuk.net>. RCoA *Bulletin*, Issue 69 (September 2011): <http://www.rcoa.ac.uk/system/files/CSQ-Bulletin69.pdf>

12.2 Guidelines for provision of day case surgery

Day surgery guidelines

The AAGBI and British Association of Day Surgery released updated guidelines for day surgery and short stay surgery in 2011. Local guidelines may vary depending on services provided within a hospital or in stand-alone units. The guidelines focus on appropriate patient selection, effective preoperative assessment, patient preparation, and protocol-driven, nurse-led discharge.

Patient selection for day surgery

A majority of patients will be appropriate for day surgery unless there is a valid reason that extra care during an overnight stay may be of benefit (Box 12.2). Local guidelines for inclusion and exclusion criteria should be made with multidisciplinary agreement. Social, medical, and surgical factors should all be considered.

Box 12.2 Criteria for day case surgery

Social criteria
- Patient understanding and consent for day surgery.
- Responsible escort available for journey home and 24h after general anaesthesia.
- Appropriate social circumstances, e.g. telephone and toilet facilities, proximity to hospital.

Medical criteria
- Fitness for procedure—this should be assessed on an individual patient basis for a particular procedure rather than using arbitrary limits related to age, ASA grade, or BMI.
- Obesity should not be a contraindication to day surgery. Most recovery problems associated with obesity occur in first-stage recovery and resolve early. Obese patients benefit from day surgery anaesthetic techniques and early mobilization.
- Stable chronic disease.

Surgical criteria
- Procedures with no significant risk of complications which require immediate medical attention, e.g. haemorrhage or cardiovascular instability.
- Procedures with controllable postoperative symptoms using oral medication and/or local anaesthetic techniques.
- Procedures where the patient can return to oral intake within a few hours.
- Procedures that allow the patient to mobilize within a few hours.

Although most day surgery procedures are elective, urgent procedures may be performed through day surgery, either by immediate transfer of the patient following assessment, or booking admission if the patient is safe to wait and can manage symptoms with oral medication. This can offer an efficient way of managing 'minor emergencies' such as incision and drainage of abscesses or ERPC which are often delayed by more major cases in the emergency theatre.

Paediatric day surgery facilities may offer care to full-term infants over the age of 1 month. Preterm infants should, however, be >60 weeks postconceptual age with no recent apnoeas, respiratory or cardiovascular disease, and no family history of sudden infant death syndrome or adverse social circumstances.

Preoperative preparation

Nurse-run, consultant-led, pre-assessment clinics should be used to assess day surgery patients. This service is ideally provided within the day surgery unit using the day surgery nursing staff. Patients may be seen on the same day that the procedure is booked by the surgical team or within a few weeks of the anticipated operation date. Any patients with more complex medical history should be seen early to allow time for a specialist opinion and optimization if required. The aim of preoperative preparation is to educate the patient about the day surgery pathway, impart procedure-specific information and details of postoperative care (both in verbal and written format where possible), and to identify any medical and social risk factors.

Recovery and discharge

First-stage recovery

This occurs in the theatre recovery and is the period until the time that the patient is fully awake with return of protective reflexes and has controlled levels of pain.

Second-stage recovery

The period on the day surgery postoperative ward from arrival from first-stage recovery until the patient satisfies the criteria for discharge. Early postoperative symptoms such as pain and nausea will be managed here as well as occasional emergencies such as haemorrhage.

Discharge

Day surgery discharges should be protocol driven and nurse led. Discharge planning commences in pre-assessment with identification of an escort and discharge plans for the patient. Local policies for agreed discharge criteria are followed and the day surgery staff receive competency-based training in the discharge process.

Several clinical discharge criteria are required to be met (see Box 12.3).

Box 12.3 Clinical discharge criteria (day surgery)
- Vital signs stable for 1h
- Orientated
- Adequate pain control
- Minimal nausea, vomiting, or dizziness
- Ability to mobilize and dress
- Tolerated oral intake
- Passed urine
- Minimal bleeding.

The information that the patient receives upon discharge should include:
- General post anaesthesia information, e.g. no driving.
- Procedure specific information, e.g. symptoms to expect, postoperative care.
- Follow-up appointments, e.g. wound care arrangements.
- Analgesia advice—the patient should be given an analgesic supply with written instructions.
- A contact number for seeking advice in the event of problems.
- Discharge summary for patient and GP.

The types of procedures typically considered suitable for day-case surgery are wide-ranging (see Box 12.4), and the boundaries are continually being extended (see Box 12.5).

Box 12.4 The NHS Plan 2000—'basket' of day surgery procedures

1. Orchidopexy
2. Circumcision
3. Inguinal hernia repair
4. Excision of breast lump
5. Anal fissure excision
6. Haemorrhoidectomy
7. Laparoscopic cholecystectomy
8. Varicose vein stripping
9. Transurethral resection bladder tumour
10. Dupuytren's contracture excision
11. Excision of ganglion
12. Carpel tunnel decompression
13. Arthroscopy
14. Bunion operation
15. Removal of metalwork
16. Cataract extraction
17. Squint surgery
18. Myringotomy
19. Tonsillectomy
20. Submucous resection
21. Reduction of nasal fracture
22. Correction of bat ears
23. Hysteroscopy
24. Laparoscopy
25. Termination of pregnancy

Reproduced from Basket (2000) NHS Plan © Crown Copyright 2000. http://www.nlg.nhs.uk/files/nationalplan.pdf

---

Box 12.5 The British Society of Day Surgery now has a 'Trolley' of procedures which also includes:

- Laparoscopic hernia repair
- Thoracoscopic sympathectomy
- Partial thyroidectomy
- Transcervical resection of endometrium
- Eyelid surgery
- Arthroscopic shoulder decompression
- Arthroscopic meniscectomy
- Wide local excision breast lesion with axillary clearance and many more…

Further reading

Association of Anaesthetists of Great Britain and Ireland; British Association of Day Surgery (2011). Day case and short stay surgery 2. *Anaesthesia*, 66:417–34.

12.3 Advances in day case anaesthesia

Anaesthesia for day surgery

The main aim of anaesthetic techniques for day surgery is to allow the rapid return of a normal conscious state with good analgesia and avoidance of nausea and vomiting. Longer-acting sedative drugs are avoided and judicious use of opiates reduces sedation and nausea. Pre-emptive simple analgesia and prophylactic non-steroidal analgesics, unless contraindicated, help to reduce opiate requirements but the increasing use of both regional and central neuraxial blockade may replace any opiate use. Prophylactic antiemetics should be routinely used in day case patients at risk of postoperative nausea and vomiting (see section 4.1).

Regional anaesthesia for day surgery

Local anaesthetic infiltration, field blocks (e.g. ilioinguinal blocks for hernia surgery), and peripheral nerve blocks may all be used for analgesia to avoid opiate use, or may be used to provide anaesthesia for day case procedures. The use of ultrasound has improved the safety of nerve blocks and also allows the identification of smaller nerves to allow more peripheral limb blocks to be performed successfully. This can provide analgesia whilst limiting motor blockade.

These techniques have allowed procedures such as shoulder surgery to be performed as day cases, whereas traditionally the postoperative opiate requirements may have necessitated inpatient stay. Regional techniques may also allow day case surgery in patients with severe medical comorbidity.

Patients may be discharged with residual sensory and/or motor block if they are given full instructions as to how to protect the limb e.g. arm sling, and have appropriate help and support at home. Written instructions should be provided to explain the expected duration of the block and who to contact with concerns. Prolonged motor block in the lower limb may obviously preclude mobilization and require longer stay.

Central neuraxial blockade for day surgery

The use of spinal anaesthesia in day surgery patients has increased the opportunity for day surgery procedures in patients with cardiac and respiratory disease as well as the obese. It has been shown to have low morbidity and high rates of patient satisfaction. Spinal anaesthesia avoids the risk of airway complications, nausea, and vomiting, and may not require first stage recovery. Patients can immediately resume oral intake, which may also make this a preferable technique in patients with diabetes.

Choice of spinal needle

Spinal anaesthesia is performed with a pencil-point needle of 25G diameter or smaller to reduce the risk of post-dural puncture headache.

Choice of local anaesthetic

Short-acting local anaesthetics are desirable but there is some concern with the occurrence of transient neurologic syndrome when using lidocaine intrathecally (10–40% incidence with a dose >40mg). Bupivacaine and ropivacaine are recommended by the manufacturers for intrathecal use. Intrathecal hyperbaric 2% prilocaine has also recently been licensed. As experience with this increases, it may offer an ideal short-acting, effective spinal block.

Dose of local anaesthetic

As the dose used is proportional to the duration of the block, the minimal dose to provide sufficient anaesthesia should be used. Unilateral positioning is used to control the spread of the block to the operative side. Small doses of fentanyl (e.g. 10mcg) will improve the quality of the block and are not associated with respiratory depression. Typical doses quoted are:

- 5mg heavy bupivacaine with 10mcg fentanyl made up to a volume of 3mL to provide anaesthesia for knee surgery.
- 7.5mg heavy bupivacaine and 25mcg fentanyl to provide anaesthesia for inguinal hernia surgery often in combination with ilioinguinal block.

Intraoperative management

Hypotension is rare with low-dose intrathecal local anaesthetic. If hypotension occurs it should be managed with vasopressors as opposed to large volumes of IV fluids which may cause bladder distension if there are difficulties voiding.

Supplementation of the block is possible using the following methods:

- Local anaesthetic infiltration
- Local anaesthetic field block, e.g. ilio-inguinal
- Administration of short-acting IV opioids.

Recovery and discharge

The recovery time is extended following spinal anaesthesia, being on average 3–5h. Prior to mobilization the patient must demonstrate the ability to straight leg raise against gravity or full power plantar flexion and return of proprioception in the big toe. Prior to discharge, the patient must also pass urine. Information about the complications of spinal anaesthesia, including post-dural puncture headache, should be provided and the patient should be followed up at 48–72h post procedure.

Diabetes and day surgery

Most 'stable' diabetics are suitable for day surgery. Good diabetic control is indicated by a glycosylated haemoglobin level <8% with no recent hypoglycaemic episodes or recent admissions with complications (see section 5.2). The patient must be familiar with home glucose monitoring, understand medication changes during disturbed glycaemic control, and be able to recognize and manage hypoglycaemia. The surgical procedure should be minor or intermediate, allow return to oral intake early (missing no more than one meal), and should be scheduled for first on the list, preferably in the morning.

A suggested scheme for the practical management of diabetic patients according to the timing and extent of surgery is provided (see Box 12.6).

If any diabetic patient has a blood glucose <5mmol/L, a dextrose infusion should be considered. Diabetic control suitable for discharge requires a blood glucose measurement within the range 5–13mmol/L. The patient must be tolerating oral intake and receive written information about the possibility of delayed hypoglycaemia or hyperglycaemia postoperatively. Patients should increase the frequency of home glucose monitoring for 24h post surgery. It is extremely important for patients with diabetes to have access to a 24h emergency contact.

Box 12.6	Guidelines for management of patients with diabetes in the day surgery unit

Minor surgery—morning list

Night before:	⅔ dose long-acting insulin if taken.
Morning:	Fasted from midnight, omit morning tablets or insulin with vigilance for hypoglycaemia.
Arrival:	If glucose 5–13mmol/L, proceed.
Post surgery:	Give late breakfast with normal medication or insulin.

Minor surgery—afternoon list

Day before:	Medication as normal.
Morning:	Light breakfast with tablets as normal or ½ normal insulin dose.
Arrival:	If glucose 5–13mmol/L, proceed.
Post surgery:	Give late lunch with any normal medication taken then. If insulin treated, give ¼ daily dose of short-acting insulin.

Intermediate surgery

Intermediate surgery may be possible in a tablet treated diabetic if performed in the morning. Insulin-treated diabetics may require insulin sliding scales. This is now possible in some day surgery units but requires increased medical supervision with specialist staff.

Morning:	Fasting from midnight and omit normal tablets.
Arrival:	Glucose 5–13mmol/L—proceed.
Post surgery:	Light snack following surgery. With lunch give ¼ dose of oral hypoglycaemic medication.

Further reading

Gupta A, Axelsson K, Thörn SE, *et al.* (2003). Low dose bupivacaine and fentanyl for spinal anesthesia during ambulatory inguinal herniorrhapy. *Acta Anes Scand*, 47:13–19.

Nair GS, Abrishami A, Lermitte J, *et al.* (2009). Systematic review of spinal anaesthesia using bupivacaine for ambulatory knee arthroscopy. *Br J Anaesth*, 102:307–15.

Chapter 13

Anaesthesia for general surgery (including transplantation)

13.1 Perioperative management of complex cases in general surgery

This section deals with some aspects of management in relation to various complex procedures in upper GI and hepato-pancreatico-biliary (HPB) surgery. More general aspects of complex perioperative care (including risk stratification, epidural analgesia, goal-directed therapy, and enhanced recovery programmes) are discussed in other sections.

Pancreatic resection

Most pancreatic resections are performed for malignant disease. The incidence of pancreatic cancer is increasing. Most patients present with unresectable tumours and have a median survival time of only 4–6 months. For patients with operable disease, pancreatic surgery is a major undertaking and carries with it a significant perioperative mortality and morbidity.

The potential for complications is high, due to a number of factors (Box 13.1):

- Technically highly complex procedure
- Frequently multiorgan resection
- Predominantly elderly patient population with significant comorbidity.

Box 13.1 Complications of pancreatic surgery

General
- Pneumonia
- Pulmonary embolism
- Myocardial infarction

Pancreas-specific
- Pancreatic or biliary leak/fistula
- Haemorrhage (e.g. from splenic artery pseudoaneurysm)
- Intra-abdominal abscess
- Delayed gastric emptying (TPN may be required post-op).

Some surgeons use octreotide (a somatostatin analogue) perioperatively to reduce pancreatic exocrine secretions, although the evidence remains limited that this reduces complications such as pancreatic leak.

The anaesthetic procedure requires large-bore IV access combined with invasive monitoring (arterial and central venous lines). Epidural analgesia is usually employed in an attempt to limit the physiological stress response and to provide good postoperative analgesia. The procedure is usually accompanied by major fluid shifts requiring high-volume fluid replacement. It frequently becomes necessary to begin a vasopressor infusion intraoperatively to combat a SIRS-like response. If the epidural is judged satisfactory and there is haemodynamic stability, the patient may be extubated in theatre, but a period of post-op IPPV is equally commonly employed.

Hepatic resection

The commonest indication for liver resection surgery is to treat metastases arising from colorectal cancer. Resections may also be performed for primary hepatocellular carcinomas, cholangiocarcinoma, or, less commonly, for benign tumours or cysts. A left or right hepatectomy may also be performed as the donor component of living-donor liver transplantation.

Surgical anatomy of the liver

The liver is a highly vascular organ and receives some 20% of the cardiac output—80% via the portal vein (formed behind the neck of the pancreas from the confluence of splenic and superior mesenteric veins) and 20% via the hepatic artery (a branch of the coeliac trunk). Blood drains into the IVC via right, middle, and left hepatic veins. Variations in this 'typical' arrangement are common.

The arrangement of the liver's blood supply and biliary drainage allows it to be functionally subdivided into eight segments: each segment has a separate portal and arterial supply and venous drainage. The functional divisions are invisible on the liver surface, but allow resection of segments without disruption to the vascular supply of adjacent parenchyma.

The liver has a remarkable capacity to regenerate. A residual volume of >25% is required to reduce the risk of early liver insufficiency. Aggressive preoperative chemotherapy may cause functional impairment of even apparently normal residual parenchyma. Selective portal vein embolization or ligation on the diseased side may be undertaken pre-operatively to increase the size of the eventual post-resection remnant. Occasionally, however, the hypertrophy results in a caval compression syndrome.

Conduct of anaesthesia—low CVP

The anaesthetic set-up will obviously require large-bore peripheral and/or central venous access together with standard central venous and arterial monitoring. Some practitioners monitor cardiac output or some other parameter such as stroke volume variation. Intraoperative blood gas analysis is essential, and usefully supplemented by point-of-care tests of coagulation.

Epidural analgesia is commonly employed, with careful monitoring of perioperative coagulation parameters.

It is important to maintain a relatively low CVP during the resection to reduce bleeding. Resection usually takes place using the CUSA (cavitron ultrasonic surgical aspirator), which disrupts the hepatic parenchyma, leaving vessels intact, allowing these to be clipped or sutured. The requirement for a low CVP often necessitates intraoperative use of a vasopressor (typically metaraminol boluses and/or a noradrenaline infusion) to maintain an adequate MAP.

Running a low CVP has several important consequences:

- Sudden blood loss will produce *severe* hypovolaemia.
- IVC compression from packs/retraction will cause significant impairment of venous return.
- A low CVP creates the potential for venous air embolism.

Pringle's manoeuvre

Occlusion of the hepatic artery and portal vein (Pringle's manoeuvre) will reduce blood loss during hepatic resections, but creates warm hepatic ischaemia. Most surgeons restrict an individual occlusion to a maximum of 15min duration, with 5min reperfusion before re-clamping. It becomes especially important to monitor electrolytes, glucose, and coagulation status during and after repeated Pringle manoeuvres. There is anecdotal evidence that N-acetylcysteine (NAC) infusions may have a protective effect in terms of limiting hepatic damage.

Postoperative considerations

The majority of patients can be woken at the end of surgery, especially if epidural analgesia has been employed. Careful monitoring of vital signs and hepatic function is important in the early postoperative period.

Oesophagectomy

Oesophageal cancer occurs predominantly in patients aged >50 years, and the incidence increases with age, with a marked male preponderance. Whilst the mortality from oesophagectomy has declined over the last decades, it remains in the region of 10%.

The surgery may be performed through open (transthoracic or transhiatal) or minimally invasive approaches. One-lung ventilation (OLV) is usually employed.

Anastomotic leak is the most frequent surgical complication, and postoperative pulmonary complications are the most common serious morbidity and an important predictor of mortality.

Thoracic epidural analgesia is associated with a reduced incidence of anastomotic leak. It is important to maintain perfusion pressure. Short-acting vasopressors may be safely used intraoperatively in the normovolaemic patient, but noradrenaline infusions may be associated with splanchnic hypoperfusion.

In terms of fluid therapy, a goal-directed approach (see section 13.10) should be employed. Excessive fluid administration may impair anastomotic healing and worsen acute lung injury. A protective ventilation strategy during OLV may reduce the incidence of pulmonary complications.

Carcinoid syndrome

Carcinoid tumours arise from enterochromaffin tissue, most commonly within the GI tract or lungs.

Carcinoid syndrome occurs in some 10% of patients—mainly those with gut-derived tumours—whereby vasoactive substances secreted by carcinoid tumours (most commonly arising from the appendix or small bowel) escape hepatic metabolism and exert systemic effects.

The syndrome is typically characterized by intermittent flushing, hypotension, diarrhoea, and/or bronchospasm, related to release of 5-hydroxytryptamine (5-HT) and other mediators.

Carcinoid heart disease is classically right-sided, with endocardial fibrosis affecting tricuspid and pulmonary valves.

In terms of anaesthesia, a thorough cardiovascular assessment is obviously crucial. In addition, a perioperative octreotide infusion (50mcg/h) reduces tumour hormonal activity and should be commenced at least 12h prior to surgery.

The objectives are to provide stable, controlled haemodynamics, often in the face of a difficult laparotomy. Epidural analgesia is frequently employed, with care to avoid excessive hypotension.

A period of high-dependency care is appropriate postoperatively, with ongoing IV then subcutaneous octreotide administration.

Splenectomy

Splenectomy may be performed as an elective procedure in patients with ITP and, in certain instances, in a variety of other haematological disorders (Box 13.2). In addition, the spleen is the most commonly injured organ in cases of abdominal trauma, often necessitating urgent splenectomy. There is a trend towards attempted splenic preservation through more conservative surgery or non-operative management in carefully selected cases of splenic trauma.

Patients with blood disorders who present for splenectomy may well be anaemic, thrombocytopenic, or have other coagulopathies. They may also bear the systemic consequences of previous chemotherapy or glucocorticoid treatment.

When considering platelet transfusion in a splenectomy patient who is thrombocytopenic, this should take place *after* ligation of the splenic vessels, to avoid sequestration in the spleen. Postoperatively, it is important to closely monitor the platelet count, since a rebound thrombocytosis may occur.

> **Box 13.2 Indications for splenectomy**
> - Immune thrombocytopenic purpura:
>   - If persistent thrombocytopenia despite high-dose glucocorticoid therapy.
> - Haemolytic anaemias:
>   - Hereditary spherocytosis (treatment of choice)
>   - Hereditary elliptocytosis (if symptomatic)
>   - Thalassaemias (splenectomy may reduce haemolysis, transfusion requirements and discomfort)
>   - Sickle cell disease (in a minority of patients with excessive red cell sequestration or splenomegaly)
>   - Autoimmune haemolytic anaemia (after failure of steroid treatment).
> - Hypersplenism in other disorders:
>   - Felty's syndrome, myelofibsosis, chronic leukaemias.
> - Trauma:
>   - Operative intervention if continuing blood loss or other injuries; a spleen-preserving strategy may be employed in selected cases.
> - As part of another surgical procedure:
>   - e.g. distal pancreatectomy.

In non-traumatic cases, splenectomy may be performed through an open or laparoscopic approach. Haematological issues usually preclude neuraxial blockade. It is, of course, essential to ensure adequate venous access and availability of blood products (and rapid infusion devices).

Complications of splenectomy include rebound thrombocytosis (aspirin therapy may be commenced if the platelet count exceeds $1000 \times 10^9/L$), left subphrenic abscess (especially in cases of trauma), and left lower lobe atelectasis.

Overwhelming post-splenectomy infection (OPSI) is a rare, but potentially, lethal complication. Most cases occur in the first few years after splenectomy. The relative risk is lowest in trauma, and higher in haematological disorders. The long-term risk in adults is approximately 1%. Patients are routinely vaccinated against encapsulated Gram-positive organisms (pneumococci, meningococci and *Haemophilus*), in addition to receiving antibiotic prophylaxis, but no strategy is uniformly protective.

Further reading

Mills GH (2011). Anaesthesia and the perioperative management of hepatic resection. *Trends Anaesth Crit Care*, 1:147-152.

Ng J-M (2011). Update on anesthetic management for esophagectomy. *Curr Opin Anaesthesiol*, 24(1):37–43.

Powell B, Mukhtar A, & Mills, GH (2011). Carcinoid: the disease and its implications for anaesthesia. *CEACCP*, 11(1):9–13.

13.2 Anaesthesia and malignant disease

Cancer is the second leading cause of death in the developed world, and >50% of cases occur at just four sites: bronchus, breast, colorectal, and prostate. The toxicity of chemotherapeutic drugs has obvious relevance for the anaesthetist, but there are wider issues—for example, an increasing realization that perioperative factors may impact upon the risk of tumour recurrence.

Systemic effects of malignant disease

Neurological
Pain is perhaps the commonest symptom, occurring in 75% of patients with advanced malignancy. Approximately 70% of patients also experience significant psychological distress or clinical depressive illness.

Nutritional and metabolic
Cancer cachexia, characterized by anorexia, weight loss, weakness, and impaired immunity affects some 50% of patients. Hypercalcaemia occurs in 10% of patients. This may be hormonal in origin (e.g. in bronchial carcinoma) or reflect bony destruction from metastatic disease (e.g. breast cancer or myeloma). Hyponatraemia may occur through a syndrome of inappropriate ADH secretion (SIADH), and is most commonly seen in small cell lung cancer.

Haematological
Neutropenia is common, either from the effects of chemotherapy or from bone marrow infiltration, and predisposes to infection. Anaemia tends to worsen as the malignant process progresses. Many patients are hypercoagulable, and indeed thrombotic phenomena may be the first sign of an occult malignancy.

Cardiovascular
Cardiac toxicity is an important and frequently challenging effect of chemotherapy, manifesting as cardiac failure or arrhythmias. Radiotherapy may also induce a cardiomyopathy. Provision of adequate vascular access is important in malignant disease for a variety of reasons (to administer chemotherapy or blood products, or to provide parenteral nutritional support). Central line (including portacath) insertion may be difficult if patients have had multiple previous lines or cannot tolerate lying flat.

Renal
Pre-renal failure may occur from hypoperfusion due to dehydration or cardiac failure: hypercalcaemia may contribute. Intrinsic renal impairment in malignant disease typically results from sepsis or nephrotoxic drugs. Advanced pelvic malignancy typically produces an obstructive uropathy and post-renal failure.

Local effects of malignant disease

Superior vena caval obstruction (SVCO) is typically seen in association with primary lung tumours, and may present acutely or more gradually with facial oedema, plethora, and headache. Associated tracheal compression (i.e. anterior mediastinal syndrome, AMS) may produce frank airways obstruction in addition to the features of SVCO and may be seen in lymphoma. The anaesthetic challenges in such cases are obvious, and rigid bronchoscopy may be required to secure the airway.

Spinal cord compression is a devastating complication of disseminated cancer. It is usually diagnosed late but heralded by pain: this should be the trigger for early imaging (usually MRI) and consideration of surgical decompression.

Effects of radiotherapy

Even with modern equipment, radiotherapy carries with it the risk of serious damage to adjacent tissues. Head and neck irradiation frequently results in long-term difficulties for the anaesthetist as regards airway management, and difficult intubation should be anticipated.

According to its location, radiotherapy may affect all organ systems:
- Acute radiation pneumonitis and chronic lung fibrosis
- Pericarditis ± effusion (often asymptomatic)
- Radiation nephropathy with hypertension and proteinuria (may respond to ACEI)
- Radiation hepatopathy: characterized by an early acute phase with hepatomegaly and deranged liver function tests, and a later chronic phase with progressive cirrhosis

Toxic effects of chemotherapy

Over 200 different agents are in current use in anticancer chemotherapy. For the purposes of classification, they fall into a relatively small number of categories (see Box 13.3).

Box 13.3 Major classes of chemotherapeutic agents
Alkylating agents Cyclophosphamide, melphalan, chlorambucil, busulphan, cisplatin.
Antimetabolites Methotrexate, 5-fluorouracil (5-FU), gemcitabine.
Natural products Vinca alkaloids (e.g. vincristine), epipodophylatoxins (e.g. etoposide), taxanes (e.g. paclitaxel, docetaxel).
Antibiotics Anthracyclines (e.g. doxorubicin), bleomycin.
Monoclonal antibodies Trastuzumab (Herceptin®), bevacizumab (Avastin®).

The toxic effects of chemotherapy are perhaps best considered on a system-by-system basis:

Cardiovascular
Cardiovascular complications of chemotherapy are rare, but potentially life threatening, and are a particular feature of the anthracyclines. The incidence is higher in the presence of pre-existing cardiac disease and if there has also been radiotherapy (e.g. in breast carcinoma). The effects include cardiac myocyte necrosis and fibrosis, resulting in cardiomyopathy, heart failure, and arrhythmias. 5-FU, cyclophosphamide, and taxanes are also well recognized to cause cardiac toxicity.

This is of particular significance since all these agents may be used in combination in the treatment of breast cancer, requiring close monitoring of cardiac function and limitation of total exposure. Women with Her-2 receptor positive disease may also receive Herceptin® (trastuzumab) which causes direct cardiotoxicity in about 5% of patients. The risk is markedly increased with concurrent anthracycline therapy.

Anthracycline toxicity may be immediate, early, or late—immediate forms (manifesting as tachycardia and mild reductions in stroke volume) are usually transient, but late manifestations represent irreversible cell death and carry a mortality of up to 30%. It is thus imperative that strict dose-limitation is applied to potentially curative anthracycline chemotherapy.

Respiratory

Many chemotherapy regimens may provoke secondary respiratory infections on account of immunosuppression, and some agents—in particular, gemcitabine—may cause a pneumonitis.

Of particular significance, however, is *bleomycin*, which is often used with curative intent to treat germ cell tumours and Hodgkin's disease. It may cause life-threatening pulmonary fibrosis. Pulmonary toxicity occurs in 6–10% of patients, and the incidence is higher in the presence of renal impairment or previous radiotherapy exposure. Oxygen therapy can both induce and exacerbate bleomycin lung injury. Oxygen concentrations should be kept to the minimum possible during and after anaesthesia in patients previously treated with bleomycin. There remains a lifelong risk of lung injury provoked by high FiO_2 after bleomycin exposure, and patients should be issued with an alert notice to this effect.

Management of bleomycin-induced lung injury includes discontinuation of the drug and administration of corticosteroids, although these have no proven benefit. If IPPV is required, the mortality approaches 100%.

Gastrointestinal

Mucositis is common in patients treated with either chemo- or radiotherapy, reflecting damage to the rapid-turnover cell population within mucous membranes.

Diarrhoea is frequently seen with antimetabolites and alkylating agents, and may even be life threatening. Infective causes must be sought out and treated.

Nausea and vomiting remain extremely common during chemotherapy. Different agents are stratified according to risk to plan appropriate preventive and treatment strategies.

Renal

Several classes of chemotherapeutic drugs are nephrotoxic, including the platinum-based agents: the effects are additive with concurrent dehydration or NSAID use.

Hepatic

Abnormal liver function tests are often seen patients with malignancy from a variety of causes including direct hepatotoxicity (e.g. 5-FU and methotrexate), veno-occlusive disease, infection or metastatic disease.

Neurological

Syndromes affecting both the peripheral and central nervous systems may occur directly or indirectly from chemotherapy, although there is a wide differential diagnosis such as metastatic disease (brain or spine) or a paraneoplastic syndrome. A common manifestation is peripheral neuropathy: autonomic neuropathies sometimes occur and may cause arrhythmias. Some agents, e.g. methotrexate, may produce an acute encephalopathy manifesting as confusion, seizures, or focal neurological deficits.

Haemopoietic

Bone marrow suppression and immunodeficiency are obviously extremely common side effects of most chemotherapy regimens. Granulocyte colony stimulating factor (G-CSF) is sometimes used to accelerate replenishment of white cell populations without the risks attached to leucocyte transfusions.

Metabolic

Tumour lysis syndrome is a potentially serious metabolic derangement, usually occurring shortly after the onset of chemotherapy,

typically in lymphomas and leukaemias. Manifestations include hyperuricaemia, hyperkalaemia, and uraemia, and it may progress to acute renal failure. Care should be taken *not* to routinely administer a corticosteroid (e.g. for prophylaxis against PONV) to a patient with untreated lymphoma.

Effect of anaesthetic technique on tumour outcome

There is increasing interest in the potential effect of anaesthesia on long-term patient outcome after cancer surgery.

The likelihood of tumour metastasis depends on the balance between a tumour's metastatic potential and the host defences. An intact cellular immune system—and, in particular, its natural killer (NK) and cytotoxic T-cell population—represents the critical host defence. Part of the stress response to surgery is a reduction in cell-mediated immunity.

The potential effects of drugs used in anaesthesia have been studied in both *in vitro* and animal models, and in some human studies:

* Both ketamine and volatile agents inhibit NK cell activity in rodents, whilst N_2O is well known to interfere with DNA and purine synthesis, and has been demonstrated to suppress neutrophil and mononuclear cell function. In a mouse model, N_2O exposure acts as a potent accelerator of liver and lung metastasis.

* Local anaesthetic agents have been reported in several *in vitro* models to have cytotoxic or antiproliferative (via EGF receptor inhibition) effects on tumour cells.

* Opioids (both perioperatively and in chronic therapy) have been shown to suppress cell-mediated and humoral immunity in both mouse and human studies.

* COX-2 inhibitors have shown antitumour and antiangiogenic activity in an animal model.

* Two major retrospective analyses have suggested that regional anaesthesia (epidural, spinal, or paravertebral) is associated with lower rates of tumour recurrence, and these findings are supported by animal studies. Prospective human trials are awaited. Several mechanisms have been postulated to explain the observed effects of neuraxial blockade, including attenuation of the immunosuppressive stress response and reduced opioid requirements.

* Perioperative allogeneic blood transfusion may be associated with an increased risk of tumour recurrence, through so-called transfusion-associated immunomodulation (TRIM). Laboratory and clinical evidence suggest reduced cellular immunity and cytokine production following blood transfusion, which may relate to the white cell component. Whether TRIM actually worsens cancer outcome (and whether leucocyte depletion reduces TRIM) remains to be elucidated.

Further reading

Allan N, Siller C, & Breen A (2012). Anaesthetic implications of chemotherapy. *CEACCP*, 12(2):52–6.

Arain MR & Buggy DJ (2007). Anaesthesia for cancer patients. *Curr Opin Anaesthesiol*, 20(3):247–53.

Carr C, Ng J, & Wigmore T (2008). The side effects of chemotherapeutic agents. *Curr Anaesth Crit Care*, 19(2):70–9.

Snyder GL & Greenberg S (2010). Effect of anaesthetic technique and other perioperative factors on cancer recurrence. *Br J Anaesth*, 105(2):106–15.

Organ donation and transplantation (ODT) has, undoubtedly, been one of the highlights amongst medical advances during the last 50 years. Arguably, it benefits not only recipients (whose lives may be changed immeasurably), but also donors and their relatives, for whom something positive can emerge out of tragedy in the case of deceased organ donation.

An adequate supply of organs is, of course, crucial to the success of a transplant programme, yet in the UK there is a 7:1 excess of potential renal transplant recipients over available donors (Fig 13.1).

In the UK, the lack of donors prompted the creation of an Organ Donation Taskforce in 2008, charged specifically with doubling rates of donation over 5 years. Donation rates have improved, but still fall short of the target.

Donation after brainstem death (DBD), both in the UK and other countries, has reached a plateau. One direct consequence of the taskforce initiative has been acceptance of the concept of donation after cardiac or circulatory death (DCD) to enlarge the donor pool. The UK has been at the forefront on this, where in 2009–2010, 35% of all donors were from a DCD source. Overall rates of deceased organ donation in the UK still fall well short, however, of those reported in mainland Europe and North America (Fig. 13.2).

The entire process of ODT raises important legal, moral, and ethical concerns. These span a range of issues, including the diagnosis of death, mechanisms of consent, and management of potential donors.

Diagnosis of death: an emerging consensus

There is an emerging consensus towards a unifying concept of human death. This states that all human death involves the irreversible loss of *two* essential capacities:

- The capacity to breathe
- The capacity for consciousness.

Both these capacities are functions of the brain, which, unlike any other organ, is both essential and irreplaceable.

Three sets of criteria can each be used to demonstrate irreversible loss of these capacities: somatic, circulatory, and neurological. The most appropriate set of criteria is determined in each case by the circumstances in which the doctor is called upon to make the diagnosis.

Somatic criteria

These can be assessed simply by external inspection of the corpse, and include signs such as massive cranial injury, hemicorporectomy, decomposition, or rigor mortis. Paramedics sometimes use such 'Recognition of Life Extinct' (ROLE) criteria in cases where death is so obvious that attempts at resuscitation should not be made.

Somatic criteria are largely impractical in cases of recent death.

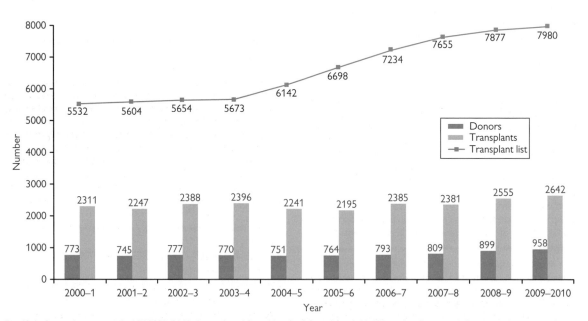

Fig. 13.1 Organ donation in the UK 2000–2010. Reproduced from Murphy PG, and Smith M, 'Towards a framework for organ donation in the UK', *British Journal of Anaesthesia*, 2012, 108, supplement 1, pp. i56–i67, figure 1, by permission of The Board of Management and Trustees of the British Journal of Anaesthesia and Oxford University Press. Data from NHS Blood and Transplant. 'Annual summary statistics on donation and transplantation in the UK'. Available from <http://www.uktransplant.org.uk/ukt/statistics/latest_statistics/latest_statistics.jsp> accessed 17 October 2011.

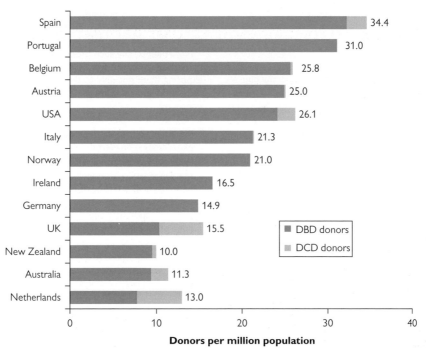

Fig. 13.2 International Rates of DBD and DCD (2009). Reproduced from Murphy PG, and Smith M, 'Towards a framework for organ donation in the UK', *British Journal of Anaesthesia*, 2012, 108, supplement 1, pp. i56–i67, figure 2, by permission of The Board of Management and Trustees of the British Journal of Anaesthesia and Oxford University Press. Data from Transplant Procurement Management. Available from <http://www.tpm.org> accessed 17 October 2011.

Circulatory criteria

These are based on the knowledge that irreversible structural anoxic brain damage occurs after the cerebral circulation ceases. They have long been used, both in hospital and community settings, as a basis for diagnosing death.

There are certain essential components for diagnosing death using circulatory criteria, including an agreement that further resuscitation will not be attempted, *and* a minimum period of observation following circulatory arrest.

The *observation period* is particularly important, and countries vary as to the safe minimum considered an acceptable standard for DCD: 2min in the USA and Australia, 5min in the UK and Canada, and 20min in Italy.

Successful transplantation after DCD requires a short warm ischaemic time (WIT), making the issue of the minimum acceptable observation period a crucial one. It has been argued that a period of 2–5min is too short—that neither the heart nor the brain can yet be considered irreversibly damaged, and that CPR might yet restore function—taken to its extreme, such an argument claims that in DCD donation, organs are being taken before death has occurred. The counter argument to this is fundamentally the additional criterion that no further attempts at CPR will be performed—otherwise many hours would be required to pass before it could be certain that cardiac and cerebral function had irreversibly ceased.

Neurological criteria

These allow for confirmation of death in cases of profound coma, when mechanical ventilation maintains cardiorespiratory activity. There is international acceptance of neurological criteria for determining death in this setting. Three essential components are employed:

1. An established aetiology, capable of causing structural brain damage (and therefore irreversible loss of the capacity for consciousness and the capacity to breathe).

2. Exclusion of reversible causes (e.g. hypothermia or metabolic disturbances).

3. Demonstration of profound coma, apnoea and absent brain-stem reflexes (fixed pupils—II and III; absent vestibulo-ocular reflex—III, IV, VI, and VIII; absent corneal reflex and absent response to supraorbital pressure—V and VII; absent gag reflex—IX and X)

Consent for organ donation: opt-out versus opt-in

Arguably, the process of donation would be straightforward (at least as far as the issue of consent is concerned) if unequivocal confirmation were readily available to relatives and clinicians that the patient had, during life, expressed the wish to become an organ donor—i.e. that the patient had signed the organ donor register (ODR) *and* discussed their position with relatives.

Currently, however, less than a third of actual donors in the UK appear on the ODR, and in only 50% of cases where consent to organ donation is obtained are the specific wishes of the individual known. Various explanations have been put forward for a relative reluctance to join the ODR:

• Feelings of disgust towards the whole process of organ procurement.

• A fear that registering on an ODR might hasten one's own death ('tempting fate').

• A concern that doctors might not try so hard to save one's life, so as to allow for organ donation to proceed.

• A fear that loss of the body's integrity might have serious repercussions for an afterlife.

It is also important to consider the reasons why families commonly refuse to consent to organ donation:

• Concern re: disfigurement of a loved one.

- Feeling that the patient has suffered enough.
- Uncertainty as to the patient's wishes.
- Disagreement amongst family members.
- Religious or cultural reasons.
- Inability to accept the death and/or lack of understanding of brainstem death.

Given these difficulties, alternative approaches have been proposed in respect of the issues relating to consent.

One suggestion is that the UK transplant authorities should more actively reach out to potential donors, perhaps through embracing modern technologies such as social networking, but is there an alternative approach to requiring formal consent?

It has been argued that consent to a procedure after death (i.e. where the individual, having signed the form during life, does not have to live with the consequences) is less robust—perhaps, in a sense, less crucial—than would be the rock-solid consent required for living donation. Taking this further, if a less rigid requirement for consent were applied, then approaches to potential donors or their relatives might be easier and more organs might become available.

The alternative position recommended by many is the so-called 'opt-out' approach of *presumed consent*. In essence, if there has been no actual and expressed objection on the part of the donor, then consent is implied—the views of the relatives may or may not be taken into account. In the harshest implementation of such an approach, donation would go ahead even in the face of relatives' disagreement.

An alternative proposal, currently being investigated, is that of *mandated choice*, where an individual is absolutely required to express his or her wish in one way or the other.

Such arguments sound compelling, but many perceive the current system of 'opt-in' as allowing for a positive decision taken without state interference, one that helps relatives (and donors) take something positive out of a tragedy, but one that remains an act very much as a gift from the individual—one given without the perception of bullying or the inference that loss of life means loss of control over one's body or that of a loved one.

Ethical issues in living donor transplantation

Living donor transplantation (LDT) has become the treatment of choice for end-stage renal failure. The transplant procedure can be performed at an optimal time, with much improved long-term graft survival. Additionally, fewer patients are therefore on the cadaveric waiting list, improving the chances of transplantation

for those with no potential live donor. Live donation has also been successfully performed for other organs, including liver, lung, bowel, and pancreas.

Nonetheless, any such procedure involves retrieving an organ or part of an organ from an otherwise healthy individual and exposing them not only to the risks of surgery, but also potentially to long-term complications. These concerns raise several questions:

- *How safe is the procedure?* This is of paramount concern—for live kidney donation, the mortality is 0.03%. Long-term life expectancy is unaltered.
- *What is the donor's motivation?* Several categories of motivation amongst live donors have been identified—a natural desire to help, a feeling of moral duty, the knowledge or belief that the other person would do the same for them, or an expectation that one's own life will improve (perhaps with improved health of a spouse). A minority of donors feel a sense of coercion, perhaps from other family members.
- *What are the donor's feelings about donation?* These are potentially complicated: donors often feel they are the recipient's only option (even if dialysis is an alternative). Interestingly, males tend to regard donation as a gift, females as their obligation.
- *What are the recipient's feelings?* There are often feelings of guilt, especially if there is a close relationship with the donor. This may lead to distress, most notably amongst adolescent recipients of parental grafts.

All potential donors go through a detailed work-up process and an independent assessor must be satisfied that the donor is competent, willing to donate, suitable to donate both medically and psychologically, and aware of the risks, benefits and alternatives.

Whilst many transplant centres previously disapproved of living donation between strangers, there are many examples of successful unrelated donations on an entirely altruistic basis. It has been proposed that the parties should at least remain anonymous until after the procedure has taken place.

Paired-exchange programmes allow for unrelated donation across pairs or even amongst a wider pool, when live-related donation is prevented through issues of tissue incompatibility.

Further reading

Papalois V & Mazaris E (2010). Ethical issues in living donor transplantation. In N Hakim, R Canelo & V Papalois (Eds) *Living Related Transplantation*, pp. 1–37. London: Imperial College Press.

Thompson JP, Murphy PG, & Bodenham AR (eds) (2012). Diagnosis of death and organ donation. *Br J Anaesth*, 108(Suppl 1):i1–i121.

13.4 Anaesthesia for renal transplant surgery

Renal transplantation is the preferred therapeutic option for the majority of patients with end-stage renal disease (ESRD). It confers a long-term survival advantage over lifelong haemodialysis or peritoneal dialysis, which are the only alternative treatments.

Careful preoperative assessment is required on account of significant comorbidities.

The transplant procedure itself requires a meticulous anaesthetic technique, especially in relation to haemodynamics and fluid/electrolyte balance.

The increasing use of living donors raises important additional concerns both for the safety of the donor and of the organ.

Preoperative assessment of patients with ESRD

Patients with ESRD frequently have multiple comorbidities, both related to the underlying aetiology of their renal disease, and due to the pathophysiological sequelae of chronic renal failure (see Table 13.1).

The commonest causes of ESRD are diabetic nephropathy and hypertension.

Table 13.1 Pathophysiological changes in ESRD	
Abnormality	Mechanism / Clinical manifestation
Anaemia	↓ rbc production (lack of erythropoietin + bone marrow fibrosis) and ↓ rbc survival
Platelet dysfunction	Normal plt count but reduced aggregation/factor III activity promoting bleeding diathesis
Systemic hypertension	Produces LVH / cardiomyopathy ± hypertensive crises (malignant hypertension)
Cardiac disease	Heart failure (from hypertension/uraemic cardiomyopathy / fluid overload); coronary artery disease (accelerated atherosclerosis); uraemic pericarditis; arrhythmias (from hyperkalaemia or hypocalcaemia)
Acid-base and electrolyte disturbances	Metabolic acidosis; ↑K^+ (arrhythmias); ↓Ca^{++} (arrhythmias, osteodystrophy); ↑Mg^{++} (hypotension, potentiation of muscle relaxants)
Endocrine disturbances	2^0 hyperparathyroidism; renal osteodystrophy; osteomalacia
Gastrointestinal abnormalities	Uraemic gastroenteritis; nausea and vomiting; peptic ulcer disease; GI bleeding
CNS disturbance	Behavioural changes; memory loss; neuromuscular irritability; myoclonus; convulsions; lethargy / coma (uraemic encephalopathy)
Dialysis-related problems	Hypovolaemia; disequilibrium syndrome (cerebral oedema); systemic anticoagulation; peritonitis

Cardiovascular assessment

Cardiovascular mortality in uraemic patients is 10–20 times higher than in the general population, and identification of *ischaemic heart disease* (IHD) is a key component of the preoperative work up. Cardiovascular assessment is dealt with in detail in section 1.1. There is a high prevalence of silent IHD in patients with ESRD, especially in those with diabetes. The resting ECG is often abnormal (LVH + strain etc.) and exercise ECG may be difficult to interpret, DSE is therefore frequently undertaken, proceeding to coronary angiography if there are signs of reversible ischaemia.

There is a higher prevalence of *cardiac failure* in patients on dialysis. Therapies such as β-blockers, ACEI, and ARA (see section 1.13) need to be optimized. LVEF frequently improves following renal transplantation.

Hypertension

Hypertension is extremely common in patients with ESRD. It predisposes to the development of LVH and ischaemia. A value of ≤140/90mmHg is typically set as the target BP in dialysis patients. ACEIs decrease mortality in congestive heart failure and may slow the progression of diabetic and other proteinuria-associated nephropathies. Both ACEIs and ARAs may reverse LVH and improve LV function independent of BP reduction (see section 1.13). It may not be necessary to defer surgery if BP remains high despite treatment in a patient who is otherwise fit for surgery (see section 1.15).

Diabetes

Diabetic nephropathy is the commonest cause of ESRD in the Western world, and diabetic patients have a higher mortality than patients with ESRD from other causes. Diabetes is an important risk factor for IHD. Optimal glycaemic control in the peri-transplant period is associated with a lower mortality.

Anaemia

Decreased production of erythropoietin contributes to anaemia in ESRD. Erythropoietin therapy improves cardiac status and reduces mortality, but may promote hypertension in dialysis patients; the aim should be for a *gradual* correction of anaemia towards a target Hb of 10–12g/dL.

Anaesthetic management of the transplant procedure

The overriding aims are to maintain stability in terms of fluid and electrolyte balance and haemodynamic status.

Immediate preoperative preparation

The results of the preoperative assessment should be reviewed. As a minimum, patients will require FBC, urea and electrolytes, cross-match, and ECG at the time of admission.

In respect of the serum potassium (K^+), the following guidelines may reasonably be followed:

- K^+ <5mmol/L: no problem.
- K^+ >6mmol/L: indication for preoperative dialysis.
- K^+ 5–6mmol/L: judge each case on its merits; many patients with ESRD run consistently high serum K^+ levels and tolerate them well. Dialysis may delay the transplant procedure and prolong the graft ischaemic time in cadaveric donation. Close liaison between anaesthetist, nephrologist and surgeon underpins successful management.

Monitoring and vascular access

Forearm and antecubital veins should be avoided in case they are required for future fistula formation. Measurement of CVP is widely considered to be essential, preferably via a newly-inserted RIJV line (subclavian access is relatively contraindicated since complications may again compromise a future fistula). An existing permacath *may* be used in exceptional cases, using a strict no-touch technique and taking care to aspirate the heparin lock.

Arterial lines are *not* routinely inserted unless there is serious concern about the patient's cardiac status.

There is increasing interest in the use of oesophageal Doppler monitoring to ensure the adequacy of fluid replacement during renal transplantation.

It is imperative to monitor neuromuscular blockade: premature contraction of the abdominal muscles may cause avulsion of the renal vascular pedicle and loss of the organ.

Venous gases should be monitored routinely, more frequently if there have been concerns, for example, about K^+ levels.

Conduct of anaesthesia

Induction agents

Propofol can safely be used for induction (and maintenance) of anaesthesia in patients with renal failure; thiopentone can also be used. These should be given judiciously, with availability of fluids and α-agonists to combat hypotension.

Inhalational agents

Sevoflurane is known to be degraded to compound-A by the CO_2 absorber within circle systems, an effect increased with low fresh gas flows. Although compound-A has been demonstrated to be nephrotoxic in rats, no harmful effects have been reported in patients with renal dysfunction. Whilst isoflurane and desflurane are safe, enflurane should be avoided because of fluoride ion accumulation.

Muscle relaxants

Suxamethonium should be used with caution. It is considered safe for RSI if the preoperative K^+ is <5.5mmol/L. Intubating doses typically elevate the serum K^+ by 0.5–0.7mmol/L. However, in the presence of neuropathy (e.g. uraemia, diabetes), or after repeated doses, the use of suxamethonium may trigger dangerous hyperkalaemia.

Non-depolarizing agents should be chosen whose excretion does not primarily depend on renal function. Atracurium is typically used (ester hydrolysis and Hofmann elimination), but its metabolite laudanosine is partially eliminated through the kidney.

Both vecuronium and rocuronium are mainly metabolized by the liver (although their metabolites are excreted in the urine). Whilst renal failure prolongs elimination half-life, studies have not consistently demonstrated prolonged durations of action of these agents in renal failure, even after several incremental doses.

Opioids

The action of morphine is prolonged in renal failure owing to accumulation of morphine-6-glucuronide, an active metabolite.

High- or repeated dose pethidine may cause accumulation of norpethidine, with a risk of seizures. Oxycodone is sometimes used as an alternative, but its excretion is also demonstrably impaired in ESRD.

Of the short-acting agents, there is no significant alteration of the pharmacokinetics of fentanyl, alfentanil, or remifentanil.

Intravenous fluid therapy

This is a cornerstone of management. Restoration (if necessary) and maintenance of intravascular volume is the single most important intraoperative measure to improve the likelihood of early graft function. Crystalloids are the solutions of first choice. Isotonic 0.9% saline was traditionally used but actually more frequently results in the need to treat hyperkalaemia or acidosis than is the case with balanced solutions such as Hartmann's. Alternatively, haemofiltration fluid (e.g. Monosol®) is used, both intraoperatively and especially postoperatively. Observation of the trend in CVP response guides therapy. Regular monitoring of K^+ is important, whatever fluid is employed.

Synthetic colloids are reserved for severe hypovolaemia where rapid volume expansion is required. There is little evidence in favour of one or other type of colloid. Debate continues as to whether HES solutions specifically impair renal function in renal transplant recipients. The most recent evidence suggests the dose should be limited to 15mL/kg/day and accompanied by sufficient volumes of crystalloid.

Intraoperative haemodynamics

Systemic hypotension may have serious consequences during renal transplantation, especially after graft reperfusion. It is imperative to ensure an adequate circulating volume: vasopressors should be used judiciously, and very much as 'second-line' therapy. Some controversy remains over whether long-term ACEI or ARA therapy should be continued immediately preoperatively.

Intraoperative hypertension may result from hypovolaemia or from excessive sympathoadrenal activity. With the possible exception of ACEIs and ARAs, long-term antihypertensive medication should be continued immediately preoperatively. It is obviously important to ensure adequate intraoperative analgesia and muscle relaxation. Hypertensive episodes may be treated with appropriate short-acting agents, e.g. labetalol.

Management at reperfusion

Diuretics (e.g. furosemide), osmotic agents (e.g. mannitol), and even dopamine may sometimes be administered around the time of reperfusion in an attempt to promote diuresis. There is, however, limited evidence to support any of these therapies (see Box 13.4).

Management of hyperkalaemia

The anaesthetist should be constantly alert to the possibility of

> **Box 13.4 Agents sometimes given at graft reperfusion**
>
> *Furosemide* reduces oxygen consumption in the loop of Henle, and is used frequently, both in ARF and during renal transplantation. There is no evidence, however, that it shortens ARF duration, reduces the need for dialysis or improves outcome. By altering the corticomedullary redistribution of blood flow, loop diuretics may actually be harmful.
>
> *Mannitol* is widely used in renal transplantation, acting as an initial volume expander. It also enhances release of vasodilatory prostaglandins in the kidney, and may act as a free radical scavenger. Over-zealous administration may actually result in renal failure: it should be used at most judiciously, and with accompanying hydration.
>
> There is no evidence that low-dose *dopamine* has any specific or clinically significant renal-protective effect. Its use may occasionally be justified to raise BP in the early postoperative period when there is a disparity between donor and recipient blood pressure.

hyperkalaemia, both intra- and postoperatively. As a general rule, K^+ >6mmol/L requires treatment: the options are set out in Box 13.5.

Postoperative management

Careful attention to fluid balance and haemodynamics must continue postoperatively, and a detailed handover between anaesthetist, surgeon, and nephrologist helps to facilitate this. The patient's analgesic requirements are usually met with an opioid-based PCA combined with regular paracetamol. A typical initial postoperative fluid regimen would be 100% replacement of the previous hour's urine output, commonly with Monosol®.

> **Box 13.5 Options for hyperkalaemia management**
>
> - IV insulin + dextrose (10–15IU Actrapid® in 50mL 50% dextrose).
> - Salbutamol (5–10mg nebulized or 250–500mcg slow IV).
> - Consider 50mL of 8.4% $NaHCO_3$ and/or 10mL of 10% calcium gluconate for serious hyperkalaemia, especially if ECG changes.

Anaesthesia for living-donor renal transplantation

Living-donor renal transplantation provides significant advantages to the recipient, including improved graft and patient survival, and a shorter waiting time to transplant. In respect of the donor, however, it exposes an otherwise healthy subject to the risks of major surgery.

The nephrectomy procedure is usually laparoscopic. Preoperative and generous intraoperative IV hydration are used to maintain renal perfusion, usually without CVP monitoring to reduce the risk of complications. Robust thromboprophylaxis is essential. Some centres employ postoperative epidural anaesthesia, whilst others use PCA fentanyl or morphine.

Further reading

Jankovic Z & Sri-Chandana S (2009). Anaesthesia for renal transplant: Recent developments and recommendations. *Curr Anaesth Crit Care* 19(4):247–53.

Sprung J, Kapural L, Bourke DL, *et al*. (2000). Anesthesia for kidney transplant surgery. *Anesthesiol Clin North America* 18(4):919–51.

13.5 Anaesthesia for liver transplantation

Introduction: indications for liver transplantation

Liver transplantation (LT) has evolved into a highly effective therapy for acute and end-stage chronic hepatic failure and it remains the sole definitive treatment for these conditions (Box 13.6). 1-year survival is now 90%. A successful liver transplant programme relies on a high degree of cooperation between multiple specialties, medicine, surgery, anaesthesia, critical care, haematology, nursing, etc.

Box 13.6 Primary indications for LT

Chronic liver disease
- Common:
  - Alcoholic liver disease
  - Hepatitis B or C cirrhosis
- Other:
  - Autoimmune hepatitis
  - Sclerosing cholangitis
  - Primary biliary cirrhosis.

Acute liver failure (ALF)
- Common:
  - Paracetamol overdose (UK)
  - Acute viral hepatitis (developing world)
- Other:
  - Acute seronegative hepatitis
  - ALF complicating pregnancy.

Preoperative considerations

The LT procedure represents a major challenge to all organ systems, and a comprehensive anaesthetic assessment is essential. Liver transplant candidates are becoming progressively older, and with greater comorbidities.

Cardiorespiratory disease

LT provokes a major haemodynamic stress, particularly after reperfusion. A fall in systemic arterial pressure coupled with a rise in pulmonary artery pressure, sometimes compounded by arrhythmias, may herald a period of profound instability, which will be exacerbated by pre-existing cardiovascular disease.

Coronary artery disease

It was previously thought that IHD was less prevalent in end-stage liver disease (ESLD) than in the general population (low LDL, lower systemic pressures, and high oestrogen levels), but evidence suggests that in fact the reverse is true. Patients may be relatively asymptomatic due to a poor exercise capacity in the setting of advanced chronic liver disease.

There are no specific guidelines in respect of how to identify IHD in LT patients. Most studies have, therefore, applied more general guidelines aimed at non-cardiac surgery (see sections 1.1–3) to the liver failure population. These comprise an assessment of functional capacity and cardiac risk factors ± non-invasive testing.

DSE has been widely advocated as the investigation of choice, but many patients with ESLD do not mount a satisfactory response to dobutamine, because of pre-existing vasodilatation ± β-blockade. The negative predictive value of DSE remains high in ESLD (i.e. a negative test predicts a very low risk of ischaemic complications) but the positive predictive value is low. There is growing interest in other methods of assessment, including CPET and CTCA. An abnormal non-invasive test should lead to consideration of angiography, which is relatively well tolerated provided coagulopathy is corrected. A transradial approach is sometimes used.

In those patients requiring revascularization, cardiac surgery pre-LT is certainly high risk. Percutaneous techniques are better tolerated, but drug-eluting stents are generally avoided.

Cardiomyopathy

Patients with cirrhosis typically have a high cardiac output, a diminished contractile responsiveness to stress, and impaired diastolic relaxation. The underlying mechanisms may involve abnormal calcium exchange and autonomic dysfunction. So-called cirrhotic cardiomyopathy may only become apparent postoperatively when normal vascular tone is restored, and may manifest as acute decompensated heart failure, particularly in patients with elevated right heart pressures preoperatively. A preoperative TTE is therefore performed routinely to assess LV, RV, and valvular function. LV dysfunction is not a contraindication to LT, but medical therapy for heart failure must be optimized (see section 1.13) and continued perioperatively.

Pulmonary heart disease

Two distinct pulmonary syndromes are associated with ESLD:

Hepatopulmonary syndrome (HPS): intrapulmonary shunting produces V/Q mismatch and hypoxia. PA pressures are typically normal and LT may be curative.

Portopulmonary hypertension (PPHTN): this is a form of pulmonary hypertension with progressive pulmonary vasoconstriction and remodelling causing raised PVR and typically late hypoxaemia. By definition, there is associated portal hypertension. If left untreated, LT often becomes contraindicated. Approximately 5–10 % of potential LT candidates have moderate-to-severe PPHTN (mean PAP 35–50mmHg) with a mortality of up to 50% after LT. A preoperative PAP of >50mmHg is associated with an even higher mortality, although some series have reported better outcomes.

An accurate diagnosis of PPHTN is crucial in pre-transplant assessment; there are many other causes for raised PAP on ECHO, e.g. LV dysfunction or volume overload, and many patients with high RV pressures on ECHO are subsequently found to have normal PAP. Raised PAP and/or RV dysfunction on ECHO should prompt right heart catheterization to measure PAP, PVR, and PCWP. Moderate-to-severe PPHTN requires referral to a physician for a possible trial of pulmonary vasodilator therapy, after which the right heart catheter should be repeated. Intraoperative protective strategies for patients with raised PA pressures include use of TOE to monitor RV function, availability of inhaled nitric oxide, and a consideration of venovenous bypass or a 'piggy-back' technique to minimize RV overload at reperfusion.

Coagulopathy

The value of standard laboratory tests (e.g. INR) in the assessment of a LT patient's coagulation profile is increasingly challenged. Changes in the coagulation profile in liver disease are a reflection of the complex interplay that exists between pro-coagulant and anticoagulant forces. It is important to reflect on normal liver function:

- Synthesis of all coagulation factors (except von Willebrand's factor).
- Synthesis of antithrombotic factors (proteins C and S, antithrombin III).
- Synthesis of fibrinolytic agents (e.g. plasminogen).
- Clearance of activated coagulation factors.

It is unsurprising, therefore, that liver failure brings with it exceedingly complex changes in the normal delicate balance of haemostasis. An INR measurement is only taking account of a small part of the overall haemostatic picture, and using it to guide important treatment decisions (e.g. giving FFP) is likely to be misguided.

Renal impairment

Impairment of renal function is a common complication in ESLD, and is associated with an increased risk of perioperative complications. In its most severe form it manifests as the hepatorenal syndrome (see section 4.8). The postulated trigger is splanchnic vasodilatation, and therapy with volume expansion and vasopressors (e.g. terlipressin) may improve outcome. The syndrome may not always be reversed by successful liver transplantation.

Management of the transplant procedure

The transplant procedure is generally described in three stages:
- Stage I: dissection
- Stage II: anhepatic phase
- Stage III: reperfusion.

During stage I, the 'old' liver is mobilized in preparation for removal: this stage may be complicated by steady or even massive haemorrhage from venous collaterals.

During stage II, cross-clamping of the IVC and portal vein reduces venous return by 40–50%. This may be ameliorated to some extent by judicious volume and vasopressor therapy, and in some instances, by an extra-corporeal veno-venous bypass (VVB) circuit between femoral and internal jugular veins. VVB is, however, associated with potentially fatal complications, and most centres use it selectively at most. An increasingly preferred alternative is a "piggyback" technique in which the IVC is side-clamped (rather than cross-clamped) to preserve some flow, usually with an additional porto-caval shunt.

Reperfusion at the onset of stage III usually brings with it haemodynamic instability as accumulated potassium and vasoactive metabolites enter the systemic and pulmonary circulations. A successful piggyback technique mitigates against this to some extent.

Vascular access and haemodynamic monitoring

As an absolute minimum, the LT procedure requires direct arterial BP monitoring and a CVP line. There is a good argument for a femoral arterial line, which may be more representative in the face of hypotension and/or vasoconstrictors.

Detailed information is required intraoperatively in respect of preload and cardiac function, and a PAC was traditionally used (Fig. 13.3). Increasingly, there has been a move towards relatively less invasive monitoring, and TOE is frequently used. Some centres also monitor femoral venous pressure. Other techniques of cardiac output monitoring (e.g. pulse contour analysis and oesophageal Doppler monitoring) have been investigated.

In acute liver failure, ICP and/or jugular venous bulb S_vO_2 monitoring may be employed. Large-bore venous access is obviously a pre-requisite, and a rapid infusor central venous line is usually inserted to allow for massive transfusion.

Fluid management

This is a subject of continuing debate, but a policy of relative fluid restriction during stages I and II may limit bleeding from venous collaterals, and lessen the risk of acute RV overload upon

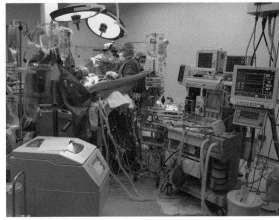

Fig. 13.3 Photo of liver transplant theatre set-up. Note cell salvage, rapid infuser, PAC trace, and continuous cardiac output monitoring.

declamping at the onset of stage III. This approach usually means a greater reliance on vasopressors, and potentially a greater renal morbidity.

A rapid infusion device and intraoperative red cell salvage (see section 16.7) are usually employed.

Management of coagulopathy

Each stage of the LT procedure brings its own typical spectrum of changes in respect of coagulation:
- Stage I: the primary issue is usually surgical bleeding, and ongoing fluid resuscitation depletes clotting factors and platelets.
- Stage II: platelets and clotting factors continue to decline, and tissue thromboplastin accumulates.
- Stage III: reperfusion may be attended by a severe coagulopathy which has multiple causes including fibrinolysis, an endogenous heparin effect, hypothermia, hypocalcaemia, haemodilution, etc. Occasionally, a patient may become hypercoagulable at this time.

Arbitrary and/or over-administration of blood products are neither beneficial nor supported by evidence. It may result in volume overload and even a hypercoagulable state with the risk of hepatic artery thrombosis and potential graft loss.

TEG® is used successfully in many centres to guide therapy in terms of coagulation factors and antifibrinolytics. In terms of the latter, the use of aprotinin is now restricted (due to a potential excess of cardiovascular events)—tranexamic acid is more widely used.

Monitoring of potassium

Cardiac arrest occurring at the time of reperfusion is an ever-present concern, and real efforts must be made to control hyperkalaemia during stages I and II, especially if there has been a large red cell transfusion requirement.

Postoperative management

Advances in surgical and anaesthetic techniques have led to an increase in early extubation and fast-tracking in selected patients.

Further reading

Hannaman MJ & Hevesi ZG (2011). Anesthesia care for liver transplantation. *Transplant Rev*, 25(1):36–43.

Ozier Y & Klinck J (2008). Anesthetic management of hepatic transplantation. *Curr Opin Anesthesiol*, 21(3):391.

Raval Z, Harinstein ME, Skaro AI, et al. (2011). Cardiovascular risk assessment of the liver transplant candidate. *J Am Coll Cardiol*, 58(3):223–31.

13.6 Management of the transplant recipient for non-transplant surgery

A greater number of patients survive long term following organ transplantation. They may present either for elective treatment or require unplanned emergency interventions.

General considerations

It is, of course, a priority to involve the patient's transplant team at an early stage, and to obtain details of the transplantation procedure and the current immunosuppression regimen. Preoperative graft function should be evaluated, and the presence of rejection confirmed or refuted. The function of other organs may have been compromised by illness or immunosuppression.

Exclude rejection

Three categories of rejection are described: hyperacute, acute, and chronic. These are distinguished by time and mode of onset, and by the pattern of immune cell involvement.

Rejection may be suggested by functional deterioration of the transplanted organ. It may be accompanied by constitutional symptoms, including fevers, chills, and fatigue, accompanied by leucocytosis. Definitive diagnosis requires tissue biopsy. Organ-specific symptoms are as follows:

- Heart: dyspnoea, decreased exercise tolerance, angina.
- Lung: dyspnoea and hypoxaemia. Chronic rejection may manifest as *bronchiolitis obliterans*, presenting with dyspnoea and dry cough, typically 8–12 months post transplantation.
- Liver: jaundice, change in colour of urine or stool, pruritus, weight gain, raised AST, bilirubin, PT, decreased albumin.
- Kidney: azotemia, proteinuria, hypertension, weight gain, oedema.
- Pancreas: epigastric tenderness, glucose intolerance, raised amylase or lipase.
- Intestine: diarrhoea, blood in stool, nausea, vomiting, and abdominal pain.

If rejection is suspected, elective surgery should be postponed, and the transplant team contacted.

Concerns related to immunosuppression

Immunosuppressive drugs reduce both the incidence and severity of rejection episodes and are key to successful transplantation (Box 13.7).

A common approach is so-called 'triple therapy', typically comprising a steroid (prednisolone), an antimetabolite (azathioprine or mycophenolate mofetil), and a calcineurin inhibitor (ciclosporin).

As time progresses after transplantation, doses are typically reduced, agent's eliminated, or new agents added. Immunosuppressant drugs should be continued up to the time of surgery. If the route of administration requires changing perioperatively, the transplant team should be informed.

Infection-related considerations

Infection is an ever-present possibility in the context of immunosuppression. All interventions should be performed with strict asepsis, and efforts should be made to avoid nasotracheal or nasogastric interventions that might cause bacteraemia. In addition to a general risk of infection, there is a specific risk of opportunistic infections (including CMV, *Pneumocystis* pneumonia, fungal infections and EBV infection). Epstein–Barr virus (EBV) infection may lead to post-transplant lymphoproliferative disease.

Box 13.7 Important classes of immunosuppressant drugs

Corticosteroids
- Interfere with antigen presentation by disrupting IL-1 metabolism.

  Side effects include adrenal suppression, susceptibility to infection, impaired wound healing, salt and water retention, glucose intolerance, hypertension, electrolyte abnormalities, peptic ulceration, osteoporosis, myopathy, and psychological disturbances.

Calcineurin inhibitors (ciclosporin, tacrolimus)
- Calcineurin induces IL-2 transcription (mRNA). Inhibitors bind to immunophilins (intracellular proteins), leading to suppression of T cell function; they also inhibit other lymphokines.

  Side effects include renal impairment (exacerbated by NSAIDs); neurotoxicity; diabetogenesis, and hyperlipidaemia.

- Ciclosporin also causes hepatotoxicity, electrolyte disturbance, gingival hypertrophy and possible lymphoproliferative disease.

- Tacrolimus is associated with cardiomyopathy (also nausea, vomiting, flushing, hyperkalaemia, psychological disturbances, headache, and tremor).

Antimetabolites (azathioprine, mycophenolate mofetil)
- Azathioprine causes competitive inhibition of DNA synthesis: it is a prodrug broken down to mercaptopurine, a purine analogue. It prevents lymphocyte clonal expansion, down-regulating the immune response; but also causes non-specific marrow suppression especially thrombocytopaenia.
- Mycophenolate mofetil (MMF) is a newer agent and more selective. It, too, is a prodrug, broken down to mycophenolic acid. It inhibits the pathway for guanosine nucleotide synthesis via inosine monophosphate dehydrogenase, and prevents lymphocytic proliferation.

  Side effects include diarrhoea, nausea, vomiting, leucopenia, and opportunistic infections. Long-term therapy predisposes to lymphoma and other forms of lymphoproliferative disease.

Monoclonal antibodies
- OKT3 is targeted against CD3 lymphocytes.
- Basiliximab reacts against the Il-2 receptor of T cells.

Many transplant patients receive long-term prophylaxis (e.g. with co-trimoxazole or antifungals).

The presence of active infection requires elective procedures to be postponed.

Organ-specific considerations

Heart transplantation

- Interrupted autonomic innervations means that increases in cardiac output are met with increases in stroke volume, not heart rate.
- Cardiac preload optimization is important; anaesthesia-induced vasodilatation should be treated promptly since the patient cannot raise a compensatory tachycardia.
- The transplanted heart is paced by the *donor* atrium. Heart block (SA node dysfunction or AV block) may necessitate permanent pacing.

- Atrial arrhythmias are common (up to 50% of patients).
- Neurally-mediated cardiac reflexes are absent (e.g. baroreceptor responses to cardiac sinus massage or Valsalva manoeuvre).
- The heart responds to endogenous catecholamines and direct-acting drugs but not indirect agents.
- Accelerated coronary atherosclerosis occurs in 10–20% of patients at 1 year and up to 50% at 5 years.
- Relevant investigations include ECG (note presence of double P wave), echocardiography, stress echo, and cardiac catheterization.

Lung transplantation
- There is decreased mucociliary clearance. After double-lung transplant (DLT) carinal innervation is ablated (preserved after single-lung transplant). The result is an increased risk of silent aspiration, retention of secretions, and infection.
- Respiratory rate, and rhythm, airway tone, and function are unaffected. Improvements in respiratory function occur soon after transplantation:
  - After 1 week: FEV_1 normalizes.
  - After 1 month: arterial pCO_2 normalizes (and the ventilatory response to CO_2).
  - After 12–18 months: only mildly restrictive pulmonary function tests after DLT. Single-lung transplant recipients continue to have impaired pulmonary function tests because of the presence of the native lung.
- Relevant investigations include gases, CXR, and lung function tests.
- Care during intubation is required to avoid trauma to anastomosis.
- Disruption of lymphatic drainage and vascular permeability after transplantation makes it important to avoid excessive perioperative fluid administration as this may lead to acute pulmonary oedema.

Renal transplantation
- The original pathology (e.g. hypertension or diabetes) frequently persists and requiring ongoing treatment since there remains the potential of subsequent renal injury to the transplanted organ.
- Use of NSAIDs is contraindicated.
- Morphine may accumulate depending on the degree of renal impairment.
- Transient hypovolaemia and/or hypotension may result in exaggerated renal injury in renal transplant recipients.
- A gradual reduction of graft function is to be expected over the years following transplantation (optimal donors give better results than marginal donors).

Liver transplantation
- Patients awaiting transplantation pose a greater challenge than those already transplanted.
- Those on a waiting list usually have advanced cirrhosis, but there is a spectrum from minimal functional impairment to ESLD (hyper/hypocoagulablity, thrombocytopaenia, portal hypertension, ascites, pleural effusions, hyponatraemia, renal impairment, etc.).
- Avoid NSAIDs but paracetamol is usually safe.
- During the period following liver transplantation:
  - Procoagulant factors normalize by day 2; diminished fibrinolytic activity by day 7; anticoagulant activity normal by day 7–14.

- By week 2 after transplant, synthetic function is essentially normal.
- During the first 3 months, the bilirubin level will improve but aminotransferase enzymes and ALP may remain elevated.
- Encephalopathy, pulmonary hypertension, hepatorenal and hepatopulmonary syndrome resolve over weeks to months.
- Patients presenting for surgery following recovery from liver transplantation are generally in good health.
- Beware recurrence of primary pathologies: recurrence of viral hepatitis (especially hepatitis C); primary biliary cirrhosis, autoimmune hepatitis; alcoholic liver disease.
- LFTs and drug disposition are unlikely to be significantly altered until late disease (15% or less hepatocyte function).
- A persistently raised bilirubin and ALP may suggest biliary obstruction; a raised AST is the most sensitive early indicator of rejection.

Pancreas transplantation
- Control of blood glucose concentrations occurs immediately following reperfusion of the transplanted organ.
- Patients may require additional insulin due to the stress of surgery and steroid administration.
- A major problem following transplantation is the risk of surgical complications: intra-abdominal infection and abscess, vascular graft thrombosis, anastomotic leaks.

Intestinal transplantation
- Bowel motility returns by day 7–15, but gastric emptying may take longer to return.
- Absorption of dietary sugars occurs when motility returns, fat malabsorption may persist for a time.
- Clinicians should be vigilant for dehydration, chronic diarrhoea, and malnutrition. Diarrhoea and dehydration are common: due to a short native or transplant colon, fat malabsorption, rejection, or infection. Preoperative electrolytes should always be measured.
- Graft-vs-host disease (GVHD) may occur in post-transplant patients—migration of lymphocytes between graft and host. Unexplained haemolysis, pancytopaenia, pneumonitis, GI changes (diarrhoea, ulceration of oral mucosa), altered mental state, and skin rash should arouse suspicion of GVHD.
- Immunosuppression may be problematic due to an abundance of lymphatic tissue.
- Rejection episodes are frequent, leading to bacterial translocation and sepsis.

Further reading

Blasco LM, Parameshwar J, & Vuylsteke A (2009). Anaesthesia for noncardiac surgery in the heart transplant recipient. *Curr Opin Anaesthesiol*, 22(1):109–13. doi:10.1097/ACO.0b013e32831c83e0.

Keegan MT & Plevak DJ (2004). The transplant recipient for nontransplant surgery. *Anesthesiol Clin North Am*, 22(4):827–61. doi:10.1016/j.atc.2004.05.006.

Kostopanagiotou G, Smyrniotis V, Arkadopoulos N, *et al.* (1999). Anesthetic and perioperative management of adult transplant recipients in nontransplant surgery. *Anesthes Analg*, 89(3):613–22.

13.7 Anaesthetic implications of transurethral resection syndrome

TUR syndrome is an infrequent yet potentially fatal condition that results from excessive absorption of irrigation fluid (usually hypo-osmolar 1.5% glycine in the UK) via open prostatic or venous sinuses (but is also well described after TURs of the bladder and transcervical resections of the endometrium). It results in hypervolemia, hyponatraemia, and/or hyperglycinaemia. Clinically this can manifest as an encephalopathy together with cardiac and/or respiratory failure (Box 13.8). Milder forms may go unrecognized, especially in the elderly population.

Box 13.8 Features of the TUR syndrome

Cardiovascular system
- Initial rise in systolic pressure and wide pulse pressure.
- Eventual hypotension as system pushed along the Frank–Starling curve into cardiac failure.
- Bradycardia.
- Respiratory distress due to pulmonary oedema.
- ECG changes: nodal rhythms, ST changes, U waves, wide QRS.

Central nervous system
- Drop in GCS score with confusion, restlessness, disorientation, and cerebral oedema.
- Nausea and vomiting due to hyponatraemia and cerebral oedema.
- Visual disturbances including transient blindness—due to glycine toxicity.
- Pupillary dilatation with sluggish reflexes.
- Convulsions and coma.

Miscellaneous
- Abdominal pain.

Mild to moderate TUR syndrome occurs in 1–8% of resections and the overall mortality is 0.2–0.8%. Severe TUR syndrome, however, carries a mortality of up to 25%. The signs and symptoms sometimes present as early as 20min after resection starts but may begin as late as 24h postoperatively. General anaesthesia masks the CNS manifestations, and the dominant features are unexpected hypertension, arrhythmias or bradycardias, and eventual hypotension and pulmonary oedema.

Irrigation fluid

The ideal irrigation fluid should be isotonic, non-haemolytic, non-toxic, non-conductive (particularly for high-frequency diathermy current), easy to sterilize, and cheap.

Unfortunately 0.9% saline and Hartmann's solution conduct electricity. Excessive absorption of normal saline can also give rise to a hyperchloraemic acidosis.

Glycine is almost ideal as it is electrically neutral, has good optical properties, and is non-allergenic and non-haemolytic. However it is hypo-osmolar (188msom/L).

Irrigation fluid is absorbed at a rate of 10–30mL/min. Various factors increase the rate of absorption—see Box 13.9.

Box 13.9 Factors that increase rates of irrigation fluid absorption

- Large numbers of open venous sinuses: implied by amount of blood loss and size of prostate (>60–100g increased risk).
- Inexperienced surgeon.
- Prolonged surgery (>1h).
- Reduced peripheral/systemic venous pressure: hypovolaemia or vasodilatation.
- Hydrostatic pressure of irrigation fluid: >60cmH$_2$O. This drops each time surgeon drains the bladder.
- Capsular or bladder perforation: this may occur in 10% of TUR cases. The irrigating fluid pressure only needs to exceed the intra-abdominal pressure of 0.5kPa (and not the venous pressure of 1.5kPa) to be absorbed.

Pathophysiology

Cardiac failure

At a mean rate of 20mL/min, 1L of hypo-osmolar irrigation fluid can be absorbed. This not only can lead to a drop in serum sodium concentration of between 5–8mmol/L, but also increases cardiac preload, whilst systolic and diastolic pressures rise. This may cause a reflex bradycardia. Eventually cardiac contractility falls. In addition there is dilution of serum proteins and a fall in oncotic pressure. These changes favour movement of fluid from the vascular to the interstitial compartment, with the risk of pulmonary and cerebral oedema as well as accumulation in the peri-prostatic and retroperitoneal spaces. The eventual low cardiac output state is therefore a function of fluid egress (causing a relative hypovolaemia) *and* low contractility: this is exacerbated by, and can be mistaken for, the sympathetic block of subarachnoid anaesthesia.

Hyponatraemia and water intoxication

Several mechanisms are thought to play a role in the hyponatraemia found in these patients:
- Initially a dilutional effect predominates.
- Secondly, there are losses of sodium within the stream of irrigation fluid that gets drained out and into the fluid that accumulates in the retro-peritoneal and peri-prostatic spaces.
- Finally, large amounts of glycine are thought to stimulate supranormal release of atrial natriuretic peptide that promotes a natriuresis

Sodium is essential for normal membrane excitability particularly in the heart and brain. Moderate falls in plasma sodium have only a minimal effect, as predicted by the Nernst equation. It seems that *hypo-osmolality* is more important, and that hyponatraemia without hypo-osmolality rarely causes CNS disturbances.

Acute hypo-osmolality rapidly leads to free water absorption in the brain parenchyma leading to cerebral oedema and raised intracranial pressure.

Symptoms and signs invariably occur when plasma sodium falls below 120mmol/L. Signs include depressed myocardial contractility, hypotension, bradycardias, wide QRS complexes, and prolonged action of neuromuscular blocking agents. Once [Na$^+$] falls below 100mmol/L, ventricular tachycardia, fibrillation, cardiac arrest, seizures, and coma can occur.

Glycine toxicity

Glycine is a major inhibitory neurotransmitter in the brain and acts on chloride channels in a similar way to GABA. It has a redistribution half-life of 6min but a terminal half-life that is dose dependent and varies from 45min to several hours. *In vitro*, glycine has been shown to cause oedema of cardiac myocytes, and >1% solutions have been associated with depressed myocardial contractility and ischaemic changes on ECG up to 24h post procedure, especially if the procedure exceeded 1h.

N-methyl D-aspartate (NMDA) activity is enhanced by glycine and this may play a role in associated seizure and encephalopathy activity. It follows that magnesium, which blocks the NMDA channel and has membrane-stabilizing effects, may be useful in this setting. Although formal trials are lacking, it should at least be considered, with the caveat that any muscle weakness may worsen transiently.

Separate troublesome effects of glycine are retinal toxicity and hyper-ammonaemia. The livers and kidneys metabolize glycine by oxidative deamination to glyoxylic acid and ammonia. Ammonia in turn depresses endogenous dopamine and noradrenaline release and may exacerbate encephalopathy. Signs of glycine toxicity include nausea, vomiting, apnoeic spells, transient blindness, weakness, oliguria and anuria. These usually occur 1h after surgery and may progress to coma and death if not treated.

Prevention of TUR syndrome and precautions

The key in the treatment of TUR syndrome lies in prevention, and in *early* recognition of signs and symptoms (Box 13.10).

> **Box 13.10 Prevention of TUR syndrome**
>
> - Consider regional anaesthesia: less blood loss, less pulmonary oedema, early recognition of CNS symptoms, recognition of capsular and bladder perforations (shoulder and periumbilical pain assuming block to T10).
> - Limit resection time to <60min.
> - Limit hydrostatic pressure of irrigation fluid to <60cmH$_2$O.
> - Experienced surgeon.
> - Good and frequent communication between patient (if awake), anaesthetist, and surgeon.
> - Measure irrigation fluid absorption.
> - Consider normal saline as irrigation fluid and use bipolar diathermy.
> - Consider alternative surgical techniques like vaporization (laser/ultrasound) that possibly cause less bleeding and no need for diathermy so normal saline can be used as irrigation fluid.
> - Identify high-risk patients: pre-existing hyponatraemia, pulmonary oedema or large prostate.

Measuring fluid absorption

This is important, and various methods are described. Perhaps the easiest method is to record the difference between the infused volume and the drained volume. However this is confounded by urine production, spillage, and bleeding. Another method uses increases in body weight as a surrogate marker of fluid absorption but this requires a bed with a weighing scale incorporated. Some centres add 1% ethanol to the irrigation fluid and breath-analyse the patient frequently throughout the procedure: a positive breath test implies significant fluid absorption. Sustained increases in CVP can also be used, but this is fairly insensitive to slow rates of fluid absorption.

Treatment of TUR syndrome

See Box 13.11.

> **Box 13.11 Treatment of TUR syndrome**
>
> *Immediate*
> - Stop surgery.
> - Stop IV fluids.
> - Coagulate bleeding points.
>
> *Supportive*
> - 100% oxygen.
> - Intubate and ventilate if necessary.
> - Adrenergic drugs/atropine/calcium for bradycardia and hypotension.
> - Benzodiazepines for seizures.
> - Consider IV magnesium.
> - Active warming if hypothermic.
> - Invasive monitoring: admit to HDU or ITU.
>
> *Specific therapy*
> - Measure plasma Na$^+$ osmolality and blood gases.
> - Diuretic therapy to treat initial pulmonary oedema: options are furosemide (may worsen hyponatraemia) or mannitol.
> - Hypertonic saline (3%) if [Na$^+$] <120mmol/L or if symptoms are severe. Correct no faster than 1–2mmol/h. Maximum rise should not exceed 12mmol in 24h. Stop once [Na$^+$] >125mmol/L and symptomatic improvement.

Calculating the dose of 3% hypertonic saline

Correction of serum sodium needs to be no more than 1–2mmol/h to avoid the development of central pontine myelinolysis. Possible calculations to estimate treatment regimen include:
- Method 1: 1.2–2.4mL/kg/h.
- Method 2: 2 × (0.6 × weight or TBW) = number of mL of 3% saline over 1h.

Hypertonic saline must only be used with great caution, and specialist advice should be sought.

Other potential problems in TUR surgery

It is important to understand the other serious complications that can occur during and after TUR surgery, especially that of the prostate. These patients are frequently frail with multiple comorbidities, poor cardiac and respiratory reserve, and sluggish autonomic reflexes. As a result they are less tolerant of hypo- and hypervolaemia, hypothermia, and anaemia.
- Haemorrhage: typical losses are 500mL but difficult to quantify.
- Fibrinolysis: from urokinase released from prostatic tissue.
- Myocardial ischaemia in up to 25% of patients. MI in 1–3%.
- Hypothermia: exacerbated by sympathetic blockade. Patients should receive active warming including warmed irrigation fluids.
- Bladder/urethral/capsular perforations.
- Bladder spasm/penile erection/clot retention.
- Postoperative cognitive impairment/delirium (separate to TUR syndrome).

Further reading

Gravenstein D (1997). Transurethral resection of the prostate (TURP) syndrome: a review of the pathophysiology and management. *Anesth Analg*, 84(2):438–46.

O'Donnell AM & Foo ITH (2009). Anaesthesia for transurethral resection of the prostate. *CEACCP*, 9(3):92–6. doi:10.1093/bjaceaccp/mkp012.

13.8 Anaesthesia for bariatric surgery

Introduction

The so-called global obesity epidemic continues to increase. Some 25–30% of adults in the UK and USA are clinically obese (BMI ≥30) and about 4% are morbidly obese (BMI ≥40). The implications both for the individual and for society are considerable. Obesity is associated with significant health risks, especially in terms of cardiovascular morbidity and mortality. The estimated financial costs to healthcare systems related to obesity are huge ($100 billion annually in the USA). The success of bariatric surgery compared to non-surgical treatments for obesity led to it being approved in the UK by NICE, subject to various criteria being met (see Box 13.12).

Box 13.12 NICE criteria for bariatric surgery

Criteria for surgery
- BMI >40 kg/m^2 or 35–40 with significant comorbidity that could be improved with weight loss.
- All appropriate non-surgical measures have been tried but have failed to achieve or maintain adequate, clinically beneficial weight loss for 6 months (surgery can be first line if BMI is >50kg/m^2).
- The person has received, or will receive, intensive management in a specialist weight loss service.
- The person is fit for anaesthesia and surgery.
- The person commits to the need for long-term follow-up. NICE guidelines on Obesity CG43.

Contraindications
- Inflammatory diseases of the GI tract.
- Upper GI bleeding.
- Portal hypertension.
- Liver cirrhosis.
- Chronic pancreatitis.
- Weight >180kg: may make laparoscopic approach difficult (relative contraindication).

Criteria for surgery: National Institute for Health and Clinical Excellence (2006) Adapted from 'CG 43 Obesity: guidance on the prevention, identification, assessment and management of overweight and obesity in adults and children'. London: NICE. Available from http://guidance.nice.org.uk/CG43. Reproduced with permission.
Contraindications: Reproduced from Sabharwal, A., and Christelis, N., 'Anaesthesia for bariatric surgery', *Continuing Education in Anaesthesia, Critical Care and Pain*, 2010, 10, 4, pp. 99–103, by permission of Oxford University Press.

Types of surgery and benefits

Bariatric procedures reduce caloric intake by altering the anatomy of the GI tract. Operations are classified as either *restrictive* or *malabsorptive*.

Evidence suggests there is an increase in life span following surgery and that surgery yields savings in overall healthcare expenditure.

Restrictive procedures

These are designed to limit nutrient intake by creating a small gastric reservoir, with a narrow outlet to delay emptying, thus augmenting feelings of satiety.

The most commonly performed restrictive procedures are the *gastric band* and the *vertical sleeve gastrectomy*. The gastric band is placed around the proximal stomach to create a small gastric pouch. In common with other procedures, it is usually performed laparoscopically. The band has a collar that can be inflated or deflated with saline. Inflation constricts the band at the proximal stomach reducing the rate at which food empties.

Procedure-specific complications include erosion or migration of the band, erosive oesophagitis, upwards herniation of the stomach inside the band, and disconnection of the subcutaneous reservoir. Continuing patient motivation and careful follow-up are required for the procedure to be successful.

The sleeve gastrectomy permanently reduces the stomach to about 15% of its original size, and may be a more attractive option for higher BMI patients if a gastric bypass is not considered suitable.

Malabsorptive procedures

Malabsorptive procedures bypass varying portions of the upper gastrointestinal tract to reduce absorption. The commonest is the *Roux-en-Y gastric bypass*, which includes a restrictive component. The gastric pouch (15–30mL) is anastomosed to a segment of proximal jejunum thereby bypassing most of the stomach, and the duodenum. It is considered to be the most effective long-term procedure for very obese patients, but complications are more frequent, and potentially more serious.

Some surgeons perform an initial sleeve gastrectomy, proceeding to a Roux-en-Y bypass as a second procedure, after initial weight loss, which facilitates surgery and reduces perioperative risk.

Complications of Roux-en-Y bypass include anastomotic leak, gastric pouch outlet obstruction, and jejunostomy obstruction in addition to the predictable complications of major surgery in obese patients.

In 10% of patients dumping syndrome can occur following the ingestion of a high-sugar liquid meal. The release of vasoactive neurotransmitters and fluid shifts causes splanchnic vasodilation coupled with a relative hypovolaemia. This can lead to diarrhoea and abdominal cramps. Symptoms can normally be alleviated with dietary modification.

Benefits of surgery

Prospective data confirm the success of bariatric surgery in promoting weight loss, which averages 25% at 2 years. A consistent finding is also that, in up to 70% of cases, many of the complications of obesity will resolve, namely diabetes, dyslipidaemia, and OSA. Evidence suggests there is an increase in life span following surgery and that surgery yields savings in overall healthcare expenditure.

Patient assessment

Perhaps a majority of 'routine' patients presenting for bariatric surgery will present no additional challenges other than their actual obesity. As the BMI increases, however, so does the risk of certain important comorbidities (see Box 13.13).

Box 13.13 Important comorbidities in morbid obesity

Cardiovascular
- Systemic hypertension
- Ischaemic heart disease
- Heart failure
- Arrhythmias
- Obesity cardiomyopathy.

Respiratory
- OSA
- Obesity hypoventilation syndrome
- Pulmonary hypertension
- Cor pulmonale.

Others
- Diabetes mellitus/metabolic syndrome.

In respect of preoperative assessment, a consensus has emerged that, for the majority of patients, a protracted period of investigations is unnecessary. The general principles of risk assessment as described in Chapter 1 still apply. Specifically, the preoperative evaluation before bariatric surgery should focus on:

- Detecting sleep-disordered breathing syndromes, namely OSA and obbesity hypoventilation syndrome (OHS).
- Identifying potential airway management and/or vascular access difficulties.
- Patient education about the perioperative management plan and anticipated goals (e.g. preoperative smoking cessation and early postoperative mobilization)

Sleep-disordered breathing syndromes

Obesity is a major causative factor for both OSA and OHS (Pickwickian) syndrome. Some 70% of bariatric patients may have OSA, but data are lacking that routine preoperative sleep studies are either cost-effective or that they improve outcome. Thus sleep study (polysomnography) referrals should be individualized, based on clinical assessment and/or validated questionnaire tools (see section 11.2).

There is evidence that effective CPAP administration in severely affected patients produces benefits across a range of parameters, including improvements in both systemic and pulmonary hypertension, ventilatory drive, and LV function. Thus patients already receiving CPAP should be advised to adhere strictly to their prescribed regimen during the period leading up to surgery. It is not certain for how long newly treated patients would require CPAP in order to achieve significant improvements in physical status and perioperative risk.

Preoperative airway assessment

Litigation data confirm that obesity to be a frequent factor amongst claims related to airway management during anaesthesia, most especially at extubation. A thorough preoperative assessment of the airway is essential.

The vast majority of patients presenting for bariatric procedures do not present intubation difficulties, provided sensible precautions are taken in terms of positioning and equipment. Difficult mask ventilation is perhaps more common. Predicting likely difficulty remains something of an art: a Mallampati score >3 is predictive of difficult intubation, whilst BMI, neck circumference, and a history of OSA are not.

Most practitioners would agree that anaesthesia for bariatric surgery becomes significantly more hazardous if patients are smokers. It should be incumbent upon any bariatric programme to stress to all patients the importance of not smoking, ideally for a period of 8 weeks prior to surgery.

Conduct of anaesthesia and postoperative care

Airway management

Optimal positioning throughout the periods of pre-oxygenation, mask ventilation and laryngoscopy is essential. Patients should be placed in the 25–30° reversed Trendelenburg position. The usual approach will be proper pre-oxygenation, followed by IV induction and immediate administration of a neuromuscular blocking agent. This will assist subsequent attempts at mask ventilation and permit earlier intubation.

Airway difficulties occur more frequently during *extubation*, and this requires just as much planning. The patient should again be sitting up (before anaesthesia is reversed). Anecdotally, the advent of sugammadex has been welcomed in respect of this patient group, who should be extubated when fully awake and reversed from neuromuscular block. It is important *not* to perform manoeuvres (turning the patient, suctioning etc.) during the phase of emergence, since this is likely to promote coughing and desaturation.

Other aspects

There are no data suggesting different outcomes whether anaesthesia is maintained with volatile agents or a TIVA technique. If volatiles are used, it is sensible to use an agent with low blood solubility (such as desflurane) to facilitate faster emergence and return of airway reflexes.

Pharmacokinetics in obese patients are complicated, both in the case of opioids and muscle relaxants, doses should be according to ideal, rather than actual, body weight.

Careful positioning is essential to avoid slippage or pressure-related-injuries (even rhabdomyolysis), and a dedicated bariatric table plus associated equipment is mandatory.

Robust thromboprophylaxis is a cornerstone of perioperative care and should usually comprise TED stockings, calf compression devices, LMWH, and early mobilization.

A multimodal analgesic technique is appropriate, usually including LA wound infiltration, paracetamol and NSAIDs, and opioids as required.

The required postoperative care environment will be decided based upon the patient's pre-existing condition, the nature and duration of surgery, and on local practices and facilities. Encouraging early mobilization is particularly important. There is no evidence that postoperative CPAP increases the incidence of surgical complications such as anastomotic disruption.

Anaesthesia for patients after previous bariatric surgery

There is evidence that the presence of a gastric band may cause oesophageal dysmotility, perhaps more commonly if there was a previous history of gastro-oesophageal reflux.

There is no evidence that deflating the band prior to anaesthesia reduces the risk of aspiration. Whether or not rapid sequence induction is required is open to debate, but adequate preoperative fasting followed by induction in a reverse Trendelenburg position with smooth intubation are obviously important.

The use of LMAs may be inadvisable in this patient group.

Patients who have had malabsorptive procedures are also at increased risk of regurgitation and aspiration, probably on account of altered oesophago-gastric peristalsis.

Further reading

DeMaria EJ (2007). Bariatric surgery for morbid obesity. *NEJM*, 356(21):2176–83. doi:10.1056/NEJMct067019.

NICE (2006). *CG43: Obesity*. <www.nice.org.uk/guidance/CG043>.

Sabharwal A & Christelis N (2010). Anaesthesia for bariatric surgery. *CEACCP*, 10(4):99–103.

Schumann R (2011). Anaesthesia for bariatric surgery. *Best Pract Res Clin Anaesthesiol*, 25(1):83–93. doi:10.1016/j.bpa.2010.12.006.Society for Obesity and Bariatric Anaesthesia website: <http://www.soba.org.uk>.

13.9 Enhanced recovery

The concept of enhanced recovery after surgery (ERAS) is relevant across all surgical subspecialties. It was pioneered by Kehlet in the early 1990s, and has been most commonly applied in the setting of major abdominal surgery (e.g. colonic resection). It is, however, also pertinent to other disciplines such as orthopaedics and cardiac surgery.

The essential tenet is that a *combination* of measures including optimal pain relief, minimally invasive surgical techniques, early postoperative enteral feeding, and early mobilization act together to improve postoperative outcome. The concept challenges the view that a stress response to surgery is inevitable—or, at least, maintains that it may be reduced by appropriate surgical, anaesthetic, nutritional, and supportive techniques.

An Enhanced Recovery Partnership Programme has been established in the UK by the Department of Health in partnership with other bodies in order to accelerate and support implementation of ERAS across centres and across specialties.

The emphasis is on a multidisciplinary approach that combines numerous elements (Fig. 13.4).

Pre-assessment

Preoperative assessment allows for estimation of risk (see section 1.1) and affords an opportunity to optimize patients with comorbidities prior to surgery. It will also ideally allow individual members of the multidisciplinary team to communicate with the patient with respect to the likely postoperative course and to set out goals in terms of mobilization and discharge.

Preoperative fasting and bowel preparation

Avoidance of preoperative dehydration may reduce postoperative pain and nausea, and clear fluids taken up until 2h before surgery do not increase the risk of aspiration.

Clear carbohydrate-rich fluid loading reduces postoperative insulin resistance. It is suggested this may reduce muscle catabolism and render patients more able to benefit from early postoperative nutrition. A suggested regimen is 800mL of a 12.6% solution of complex carbohydrate the evening before surgery, and a further 400mL 2–3h pre-op.

Bowel preparation (e.g. with oral sodium phosphate) was traditionally considered necessary before all colorectal resections, but is unpleasant for the patient and may result in significant fluid and electrolyte deficiencies, particularly in the elderly. It is now considered to be of no benefit in routine colonic surgery, and may even increase the risk of anastomotic leak.

Premedication

It is suggested that, where possible, patients should not routinely receive preoperative anxiolytic medication since this increases postoperative sedation. There may be a role for α_2-agonists, such as clonidine, which are opioid-sparing.

Thromboprophylaxis

Thromboprophylaxis is, of course, a fundamental consideration in all surgical procedures (see section 1.20). Graduated compression stockings should be routine, and are usefully combined intraoperatively with intermittent pneumatic calf compression devices. Kehlet et al. suggest that the latter should be avoided postoperatively since they may hinder early mobilization.

LMWH is now standard chemoprophylaxis and can safely be timed around epidural insertion and removal. Epidurals per se may also reduce thromboembolic complications.

Antibiotic prophylaxis

Single-dose antimicrobial prophylaxis is considered as effective as multidose regimens (albeit with a repeat dose intraoperatively in the case of prolonged procedures). Prophylaxis should be administered *before* skin incision, and, in colorectal surgery, should be active against both aerobic and anaerobic bacteria (e.g. co-amoxiclav or a cefuroxime/metronidazole combination).

Anaesthetic technique and postoperative analgesia

The anaesthetic technique should be geared towards rapid recovery, and a multimodal, opioid-sparing technique using short-acting agents is considered preferable. Some authors favour TIVA in respect of an association with speedy recovery and a reduced incidence of PONV.

Epidural analgesia is associated with improved postoperative analgesia, swifter ambulation, a reduced incidence of postoperative pulmonary complications, and a reduced duration of ileus after colorectal surgery (see section 26.5).

Spinal anaesthesia may confer similar advantages in selected patients.

Epidurals require careful maintenance postoperatively, particularly after the patient begins to sit up when the block height may recede.

Some authors have reported opioid-sparing effects with less invasive techniques such as transversus abdominis plane (TAP) blocks and rectus sheath catheters.

Paracetamol should be given routinely throughout the postoperative course. In the absence of contraindications, NSAIDs may be added to the analgesic regimen, particularly once the epidural has been discontinued.

Other agents, such as gabapentin, clonidine, ketamine, and magnesium may usefully contribute.

Surgical technique

Minimally invasive surgical techniques are encouraged since they are generally associated with a shorter length of hospital stay and reduced postoperative pain. In terms of laparotomy, the consensus is that incisions should be kept to a minimum length, but whether transverse or vertical midline incisions are preferable remains a point of contention.

Nasogastric intubation
Nasogastric tubes were previously routinely left in place for several days after major abdominal surgery. Evidence now suggests that they may predispose to pulmonary aspiration and prolonged ileus, and that, if inserted, they should be removed at the end of the procedure. Obviously, some upper GI procedures (e.g. pancreatoduodenectomy) will require a period of postoperative nasogastric decompression.

The enhanced recovery pathway

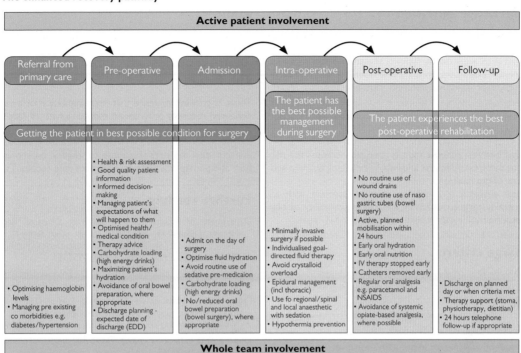

Fig. 13.4 Enhanced recovery pathway. Reproduced from Department of Health, 'Delivering enhanced recovery: Helping patients to get better sooner after surgery', 2010, http://webarchive.nationalarchives.gov.uk/20130107105354/http://www.dh.gov.uk/en/Publicationsandstatistics/Publications/PublicationsPolicyAndGuidance/DH_115155 and reused under the terms of the Open Government Licence (OGL) http://www.nationalarchives.gov.uk/doc/open-government-licence/open-government-licence.htm.

Maintenance of normothermia

Hypothermia is associated with an increased stress response, increased oxygen consumption, more blood loss, and a higher incidence of postoperative wound infection. Temperature measurement both pre- and intraoperatively is now considered mandatory for all but the shortest procedures, coupled with provision of adequate warming devices such as warming mattresses and upper body forced-air blowers.

Perioperative fluid management

Preoperative aspects—avoidance of bowel preparation, access to clear fluids until 2h pre-op, and carbohydrate loading—have already been discussed.

In terms of intra- and postoperative fluid therapy, a balance clearly has to be struck between over-restriction of fluid, which may diminish effective circulating volume and cause hypoperfusion, and fluid overload, which may in itself impair tissue oxygenation.

Kehlet proposed a simple strategy for avoidance of fluid overload: 'Clearly, the best way to limit postoperative intravenous fluid administration is to take the drip down'.

There is obviously considerable variation in fluid requirements according to preoperative volume status and the nature of the surgery. Goal-directed fluid therapy, tailored to the patient's individual needs, would therefore seem to be the optimal approach, guided by ODM or some other non-invasive estimate of stroke volume (see section 13.10).

Abdominal drains and urinary catheters

Meta-analyses suggest that drains do not reduce leak rates or other complications after routine colonic anastomoses. Kehlet and colleagues consider that abdominal drains significantly impede early and appropriate mobilization, and counsel against their routine use.

Urinary catheters are similarly suggested to be a hindrance to mobilization, and it is recommended they only remain during the period of epidural analgesia.

Postoperative nausea and vomiting

A multimodal approach is recommended to reduce the incidence of PONV, which otherwise causes patient distress and delays resumption of normal feeding. Strategies include avoidance of dehydration, a balanced analgesic technique to reduce opioid use, avoidance of nitrous oxide (± volatile agents), and routine use of antiemetic agents including corticosteroids.

Promotion of gut motility

A prolonged postoperative ileus delays recovery. Several aspects of ERAS aim to minimize postoperative gut dysfunction, including epidural analgesia, minimal opioid use, avoidance of fluid overload, early oral intake, and early mobilization.

Postoperative nutrition

There is no clear advantage in keeping patients fasting after elective GI resection, particularly if other measures to avoid prolonged ileus are in place. Patients should be encouraged to recommence oral intake within a few hours of surgery. Early feeding reduces all-cause infection risk and hospital length of stay.

Early mobilization

Prolonged bed rest reduces muscle strength, increases the risk of venous thromboembolism, and impairs both lung function and the return of gut function.

Effective analgesia is, of course essential, together with an appropriate nursing environment and ready availability of key staff—especially physiotherapists—who can set daily goals.

Discharge criteria

The discharge process should begin at the preadmission session, when goals can be set and any special needs identified. Essential discharge criteria include:

- Good pain control on oral analgesics.
- Stable oral intake of food and fluids.
- Independently mobile (or at pre-admission level).

Audit

Regular feedback and audit of outcomes is inherent to the success of an ERAS programme.

The future

There is growing evidence that implementation of a successful enhanced recovery programme reduces length of stay. Further studies need to address potentially wider benefits in terms of long-term survival. There is evidence that anaesthetic technique impacts upon the stress response to surgery, on immune function, and perhaps on tumour recurrence (see section 13.2).

Further reading

Department of Health (2011). *Delivering Enhanced Recovery – Helping patients to get better sooner after surgery*. <http://www.dh.gov.uk/en/Publicationsandstatistics/Publications/PublicationsPolicyAndGuidance/DH_115155>.

Fawcett WJ, Mythen MG, & Scott MJP (2012). Enhanced recovery: more than just reducing length of stay? *Br J Anaesth*, 109(5):671–4.

Fearon KC, Ljungqvist O, von Meyenfeldt M, *et al.* (2005). Enhanced recovery after surgery: A consensus review of clinical care for patients undergoing colonic resection. *Clin Nutr*, 24(3):466–77.

Kitching AJ & O'Neill SS (2009). Fast-track surgery and anaesthesia. *CEACCP*, 9(2):39–43.

13.10 Goal-directed therapy and perioperative optimization

Patients undergoing major surgery (e.g. elective and emergency colorectal resections, open aortic surgery, and upper GI resections) are at risk of major complications, including death (see section 1.1).

The stress response to surgery entails a substantial increase in oxygen consumption (Vo_2), from about 110mL/min/m^2 to 170mL/min/m^2. This is normally met by an increase in cardiac output and by increased tissue oxygen extraction.

From the work of Shoemaker and others (originally in critical care and subsequently in the perioperative setting), it has been postulated that patients with limited physiological (cardiovascular or respiratory) reserve cannot easily repay their 'oxygen debt', and will be at greater risk of complications. In turn, it is suggested that strategies to increase perioperative oxygen delivery (Do_2) might bear fruit in terms of improved outcome.

Increasing Do_2 involves optimization of fluid balance (goal-directed therapy, GDT), with or without further manipulation of haemodynamics using inotropes or vasoactive agents. Flow-based monitors are used to guide such interventions. Numerous studies have been conducted over the last 30 years, some of which have demonstrated improvements in morbidity and, in some cases, mortality. The strategy remains controversial but high profile. NICE now recommends use of ODM to guide GDT in major colorectal surgery.

Oxygen debt and Shoemaker's hypothesis

Oxygen is the required substrate for aerobic metabolism within mitochondria. Since there is no storage reservoir of oxygen, a constant supply is required which must match any changing metabolic needs to avoid tissue hypoxia.

At rest and in health, Do_2 comfortably exceeds global oxygen consumption (Vo_2). With moderate reductions in Do_2, tissue oxygen extraction (Vo_2:Do_2 ratio) will increase to maintain aerobic metabolism. Below a critical Do_2, Vo_2 becomes supply-dependent, and anaerobic metabolism will occur (Fig 13.5).

Global oxygen delivery (Do_2) is described by the equation:

$$Do_2 \text{ (mL/min)} = \text{cardiac output (L/min)} \times \text{arterial oxygen content (CaO}_2)$$

Expanding:

$$Do_2 = CO \times [(1.39 \times Hb \times SaO_2) + (0.003 \times PaO_2)]$$

In health, Do_2 is augmented by increasing cardiac output and tissue oxygen extraction. If disease prevents this, then tissue dysoxia in the face of increased metabolic demands may result in cellular and organ dysfunction.

The presence of an oxygen debt can be demonstrated in both postoperative and critically ill patients. Shoemaker and others observed that the magnitude and duration of oxygen deficit after major surgery was greatest in non-survivors, and least in those who survived without complications (Fig. 13.6).

Shoemaker hypothesized that increasing oxygen delivery in high-risk patients to match physiological values they had observed in survivors might improve outcome for subsequent patients. Thus emerged the concept of a 'supranormal' target in respect of oxygen delivery.

From the equation for Do_2, assuming that Hb and SaO$_2$ are optimized, it is the *cardiac output* that is most readily manipulated in order to increase Do_2. This is achieved using fluids and inotropes to improve blood flow.

Goal-directed therapy in practice

There is certainly evidence that different fluid regimens affect outcome after major surgery. There remains much contention, however, over what goals should be set, and which monitoring techniques should be used in seeking to achieve them.

It should be realized that the term 'optimization' does not necessarily mean seeking to achieve pre-defined, supranormal goals

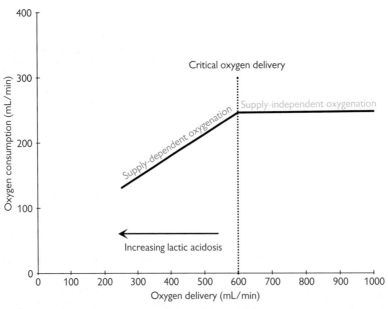

Fig. 13.5 Oxygen delivery and consumption.

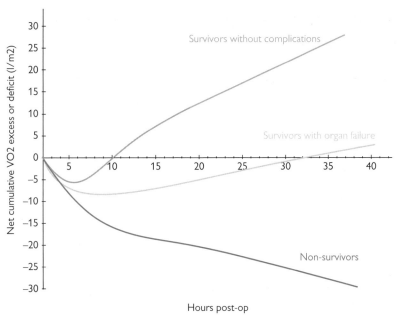

Fig. 13.6 Oxygen debt and postoperative survival. Reproduced from Shoemaker W et al., 'Tissue oxygen debt as a determinant of lethal and nonlethal postoperative organ failure', *Critical Care Medicine*, 16, 11, figure 2, p. 1119, Copyright Society of Critical Care Medicine and Wolters Kluwer 1988, with permission.

as per Shoemaker's original work, but rather, tailoring therapy to the best-achievable haemodynamics (guided by monitoring) in the individual patient.

Several studies have demonstrated reductions in morbidity and/or mortality resulting from interventions with fluid therapy alone or in combination with inotropes. Other studies have demonstrated no difference or even worse outcomes from goal-directed fluid therapy.

In addition, and, on the face of it, perhaps paradoxically, there has been simultaneous work emphasizing the dangers of over-hydration, and suggesting that fluid *restriction* may improve outcome in surgical patients.

How can these different schools of thought be reconciled? It has been suggested that the relationship between a patient's volume status and clinical outcome approximates to a J-shaped or U-shaped curve (Fig. 13.7). In essence, volumes

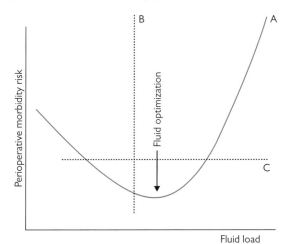

Fig. 13.7 Schematic relationship between fluid status and outcome. Reproduced from Bellamy MC, 'Wet, dry or something else?', *British Journal of Anaesthesia*, 2006, 97, 6, pp. 755–757, by permission of The Board of Management and Trustees of the British Journal of Anaesthesia and Oxford University Press. doi:10.1093/bja/ael290.

of fluid administered may vary greatly for the same observed perioperative risk.

Which goals to target and which monitor?
It is fair to say that the concept of GDT is, in itself, not a new one. Every day in anaesthesia, medicine, and critical care, clinicians aim to achieve or maintain particular parameters, whether arterial pressure, oxygen tension, or haemoglobin concentration.

If one accepts the tenet of avoiding an oxygen debt as an important factor in improving survival (Fig. 13.6), then it would seem logical that therapeutic goals should reflect *oxygen flux* – i.e. that standard parameters of heart rate, blood pressure, or CVP might be insufficient, and that oxygen delivery (Do_2) or at least, cardiac output, should be targeted *and* monitored.

Most of the earlier work in GDT involved use of the PAC, but this is undeniably invasive with at least the potential for serious complications.

More recent studies have employed monitoring techniques that are perceived as less invasive. Use of the ODM has been a major focus of research interest and, more recently, the technique has been embraced by NICE, although not without controversy. NICE recommends that the ODM should be used during major or high-risk surgery, citing a reduced incidence of complications and shorter length of stay compared to using conventional techniques (even if the latter includes invasive monitoring). It also suggests an average cost saving of over £1000 per patient. The advice has been criticized on several counts, including its reliance on a small number of clinical trials in heterogeneous patient populations. Additionally, the manufacturer's recommendations in respect of treatment algorithms for interventions based on readings from the ODM have changed since most of the studies were conducted. The new guidance places greater emphasis on maximizing stroke volume (Fig. 13.8).

One compelling argument is that no monitor should be allowed to supersede in importance over the therapy it seeks to direct, i.e. it is the *intervention* (fluid, oxygen, etc.) that is important, not the monitoring device itself.

What fluid should be used?
Arguably, there has been greater emphasis on monitoring devices in GDT than on which actual fluid(s) to prescribe. In the

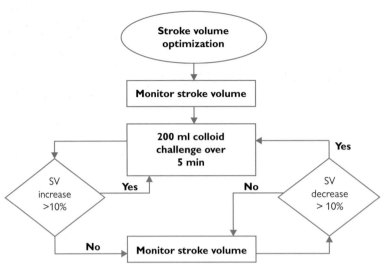

Fig. 13.8 ODM treatment algorithm. Reproduced from Challand C, et al. 'Randomized controlled trial of intraoperative goal-directed fluid therapy in aerobically fit and unfit patients having major colorectal surgery', *British Journal of Anaesthesia*, 2012, 108, 1, pp. 53–62, by permission of The Board of Management and Trustees of the British Journal of Anaesthesia and Oxford University Press. doi:10.1093/bja/aer273.

ODM-guided studies, a wide variety of fluids have been used. Does the type of fluid matter?

In critical illness, concern has been expressed regarding possible accumulation of high-molecular-weight starches and a possible excess of AKI. Conversely, crystalloids are regarded as being required in larger volumes to produce an equivalent response, leading to large positive fluid balances and oedema (e.g. of bowel anastomoses).

Currently, despite the push for ODM-guided fluid optimization in the UK, there remains a need to investigate more closely the effects of different fluids. Additionally, when treatment takes place in the context of an enhanced recovery (ER) programme (see section 13.9), it is important to evaluate the effects of separate components of ER (e.g. monitoring devices and fluids against aggressive physiotherapy in expediting patient discharge).

Use of inotropes

Some studies of GDT have reported improved outcomes using inotropes or vasodilators in addition to fluids to achieve augmented Do_2. Dobutamine and dopexamine have been most widely studied. The latter is a dopamine analogue with actions at β-adrenoceptors and at peripheral dopamine receptors. It is a positive inotrope and peripheral vasodilator, but is also perceived to improve splanchnic perfusion. This may reduce intestinal translocation of bacterial products or endotoxin. In patients with higher cardiac risk, excessive beta stimulation may be harmful, and these drugs should be used with caution.

Further reading

Bellamy MC (2006). Wet, dry or something else? *Br J Anaesth*, 97(6):755–7. doi:10.1093/bja/ael290.

Challand C, Struthers R, Sneyd JR, *et al.* (2012). Randomized controlled trial of intraoperative goal-directed fluid therapy in aerobically fit and unfit patients having major colorectal surgery. *Br J Anaesth*, 108(1):53–62. doi:10.1093/bja/aer273.

Doherty M & Buggy DJ (2012). Intraoperative fluids: how much is too much? *Br J Anaesth*, 109(1):69–79. doi:10.1093/bja/aes171.

Ghosh S, Arthur B, & Klein AA (2011). NICE guidance on CardioQ(TM) oesophageal Doppler monitoring. *Anaesthesia*, 66(12):1081–3. doi:10.1111/j.1365-2044.2011.06967.x.

Lees N, Hamilton M, & Rhodes A (2009). Clinical review: Goal-directed therapy in high risk surgical patients. *Crit Care*, 13(5):231. doi:10.1186/cc8039

Morris C & Rogerson D (2011). What is the optimal type of fluid to be used for peri-operative fluid optimisation directed by oesophageal Doppler monitoring? *Anaesthesia*, 66(9):819–827. doi:10.1111/j.1365-2044.2011.06775.x.

Chapter 14

Cardiac anaesthesia

269

Cardiothoracic anaesthesia remains an area of specialist practice, but the underlying principles are applicable to any patient with cardiac disease undergoing non-cardiac surgery. With an ageing population, the number of such patients is likely to rise in the future.

Assessment

In addition to standard questioning, preoperative assessment of the cardiac surgical patient must focus on the presence, severity, and distribution of coronary artery disease, valvular heart disease, evaluation of myocardial function, and other factors directly relating to the surgical procedure(s) to be performed. Close assessment of renal and respiratory function is usually also warranted in this group of patients who often have a history of smoking, diabetes, or hypertension, and frequently all three!

Many patients will be receiving antiplatelet or other anticoagulant therapies. In some elective cases, these can be discontinued in a timely manner, but often, patients present as emergencies requiring urgent intervention.

The practical conduct of cardiac anaesthesia is likely to be similar for most patients (Box 14.1), with a degree of fine tuning depending upon the severity of the specific pathologies involved.

Monitoring

Cardiac surgery poses potentially unique physiological changes in patients whose cardiac reserve is limited in terms of valvular or myocardial performance and/or coronary perfusion.

Manipulation of the mediastinum, great vessels, and heart may in itself cause major alterations in preload, afterload, and intrinsic cardiac function. Patients thus require more extensive and usually more invasive monitoring than other groups.

ECG

A five-lead system is used to allow all standard and augmented limb leads to be monitored, together with a single chest lead (usually in the V5 position). Three leads will usually be on continuous display (one looking at each of the three coronary artery territories, e.g. II, V, and aVL) but full seven-lead analysis can usually be shown on the monitoring if needed.

Arterial blood pressure

Invasive blood pressure monitoring is mandatory and usually inserted pre-induction. The radial artery is typically used: left-sided lines can rarely give falsely low readings due to subclavian artery compression from sternal retraction.

Central venous access

Usually inserted post induction and mostly used for multi-port venous access rather than for intraoperative assessment of cardiac filling pressures.

Temperature

The majority of cardiac patients are cooled to a greater or lesser extent depending upon the procedure. This is primarily to provide cerebral protection in the face of potentially reduced or compromised circulation. Multiple sites can be used—rectal, urinary, naso-oesophageal, or tympanic.

Urine output

The bladder is routinely catheterized and hourly urine output monitored.

Pulmonary artery catheter

With the advent of other, less-invasive systems of cardiac output monitoring and the increasing role of TOE in cardiac surgery, the use of the PAC has declined. However, it remains useful in patients with pulmonary hypertension, right heart failure, and in more specific circumstances (e.g. cardiac or pulmonary transplantation).

Transoesophageal echocardiography

There has been a huge expansion in the use of TOE in the operating room over the last decade. Although not always specifically indicated, it has become almost routine in most cardiac surgical procedures (see section 1.8).

Cerebral monitoring

Processed, simplified EEG monitoring (e.g. BIS®) and near infra-red spectroscopy (NIRS) are increasingly being used in cardiac anaesthesia to assess anaesthetic depth and cerebral perfusion respectively. Their effects on outcome have not yet been fully evaluated.

Laboratory tests

Formal laboratory testing is often not practicable during cardiac anaesthesia because of the inevitable time delays. Point-of-care (POC) testing for blood gas analysis including haemoglobin and electrolyte measurement, and activated clotting time (ACT) to assess anticoagulation are mandatory. Other POC testing modalities include thromboelastography (TEG®) and platelet function analysis (PFA) either using modified TEG® or other technologies (see section 10.2).

Box 14.1 Course of typical cardiac procedure
• Controlled induction
• Sternotomy ± conduit preparation
• Heparinization
• Cannulation of aorta/venous drainage
• Cardiopulmonary bypass (CPB)
• Rewarming
• Wean from CPB
• Reversal of heparin
• Decannulation
• Closure of wounds and transfer to ICU.

Conduct of anaesthesia

The overriding aims at *induction* are to minimize two important cardiovascular insults:
• The fall in SVR often seen with hypnotic agents
• The increased sympathetic drive caused by direct laryngoscopy.

The drop in SVR reduces diastolic blood pressure, and in turn, coronary perfusion to the left ventricle.

High-dose opioids

The most commonly used technique involves administration of moderate-to-high doses of opioids (e.g. fentanyl 5–10mcg/kg) coupled with smaller doses of hypnotic and a muscle relaxant. This provides excellent protection from the stress of laryngoscopy whilst giving adequate anaesthetic depth and relative cardiovascular stability.

Remifentanil is seen by many as an ideal drug for cardiac surgery because of its unique pharmacokinetics and its potential use postoperatively for sedation on the ITU. However, its cost and, perhaps more importantly, the tendency for bradycardia, have limited its use.

Induction agents

The choice is largely down to individual preference: any agent may be used in small doses. In cases of critical aortic or left main stem stenosis, etomidate is sometimes preferred.

Neuromuscular blockade

Historically *pancuronium* was the muscle relaxant of choice because of its long duration and slight vagolytic action. Sternotomy itself does not mandate full paralysis, although few would advocate no neuromuscular block. Indeed because of the induced hypothermia during CPB patients can shiver if not adequately paralysed. However, with the trend towards early extubation, even in non-fast-track patients, there is increasing use of medium duration muscle relaxants (especially *rocuronium*). The histamine release seen with *atracurium* makes this agent potentially less haemodynamically stable.

Maintenance

There is increasing evidence that the use of volatile agents for maintenance of anaesthesia has beneficial effects in terms of myocardial protection, not unlike those of ischaemic preconditioning. The effects are much more marked when used in the pre-CPB period (i.e. prior to the ischaemic insult). Volatiles can be added to the oxygenator of the CPB system and thus can be provided throughout the period of surgery - reliance on opiates or TIVA for anaesthesia during CPB is unnecessary. However, many anaesthetists also run propofol infusions during bypass as this allows the establishment of the infusion prior to the post-CPB period when there is greater potential for haemodynamic instability and provides a smooth transfer to the postoperative care environment.

Blood pressure control

Post-induction control of systemic pressure usually requires a combination of vasoconstrictors (usually α-agonists) and vasodilators (usually nitrates, although α-antagonists and directly-acting drugs such as hydralazine may also be required). Blood pressure swings may occur at several stages relatively early in the procedure. Following laryngoscopy, the next most stressful stage is sternotomy. Supplemental doses or boluses of opiate are usually required at this stage. There often follows a period of low stimulation during conduit harvesting when the systemic pressure often drifts downwards. Following this, manipulation of the aorta in preparation for aortic cannulation can lead to a baroreceptor response and hypertension (just at the time that the surgeon needs the pressure low for cannulation!)

Anticoagulation

CPB mandates full anticoagulation. This is usually achieved with heparin 300–500IU per kg given at the request of the operating surgeon (usually at the end of internal mammary artery harvesting during CABG) and targeted to an ACT of 400–500sec or 3–4 x baseline. (Use of cardiotomy suction and insertion of aortic and venous lines is usually permitted when the ACT reaches 300sec.) The ACT is a reliable measure of heparin effect before during the early stages of CPB, although during longer pump runs and post weaning it becomes less reliable because of variable activation of the clotting cascade (see also section 14.3).

Set-up for CPB

The surgeon performs all line insertions for the set-up of CPB, but there are a number of critical stages of which the anaesthetist must be aware. The first stage, usually aortic cannulation, requires the ACT to be >300sec and the surgeons will usually request that the systolic pressure is <100mmHg as this helps to reduce the chance of iatrogenic aortic dissection. Venous cannulation can also be problematic as manipulation of the atria often leads to dysrhythmias, especially atrial fibrillation. This may lead to severe compromise in some patients and may require cardioversion or sometimes even rapid institution of bypass.

Cardiopulmonary bypass

CPB as we recognize it today has advanced dramatically since its inception in the 1950s. It has allowed the development of cardiac surgery from a limited number of short, risky procedures to the modern-day world of complex revascularization, valve replacements and repair, artificial hearts and cardiac and lung transplantation. In essence, it enables surgeons to operate on a still, bloodless field whilst still maintaining organ perfusion. Advances in monitoring, pump technology, oxygenators, and circuits have led to safer surgery with morbidity and mortality of <5% for the majority of routine cases, and cardiopulmonary bypass is not directly implicated in the majority of these. Problems and complications, whilst rare, can however be rapidly fatal and swift recognition and management is required.

Knowledge of the basic structure and layout of cardiopulmonary bypass circuits is useful for all those involved in cardiac anaesthesia (see Fig. 14.1).

At the onset of CPB deoxygenated blood drains by gravity from the right heart via a wide-bore tube into the venous reservoir. Here it may mix with blood from a variety of cardiotomy suckers, vents or other drains that usually operate via separate pumps. This mixed blood is then pumped out of the reservoir through the oxygenator (usually combined with the heat exchange mechanism). These hollow-fibre systems have relatively high intrinsic resistance and so the blood has to be pumped through. Modern membrane oxygenators cause a much reduced inflammatory response compared to the old bubble oxygenators possibly because of the reduced exposure of the blood to a blood-gas interface, and are extremely efficient at gas exchange. Temperature control is usually via a separate device that controls the temperature of the counter-current fluid in the oxygenator (see section 14.2). Oxygenated blood leaves the oxygenator and returns via an arterial line filter into the aortic cannula (which is placed distally to the aortic cross clamp).

Integral to the circuit (but omitted from the diagram for clarity) are a number of other devices to help the perfusionist: there are assorted line pressure monitors; mixed venous blood saturation monitors and sometimes real-time in-line blood gas analysis devices; various emergency bypass routes should a particular component need urgent replacement; mechanisms for manual control of the rotary pumps (something not easily available with centrifugal pumps); sampling ports and ports for additional blood and fluid administration if required.

Administration of cardioplegia, when used, involves a separate mixing system which blends the cardioplegia solution with blood taken from the arterial line. This is then cooled (or occasionally warmed) and administered into the aortic root, directly into the coronary artery ostia or in a retrograde manner via the coronary sinus depending on the surgical requirements.

Establishment of CPB

The onset of CPB provides a unique set of circumstances with a fairly standard physiological response. Bypass commences with the opening of the venous pipe(s) allowing passive flow to the pump reservoir. If venous flow is inadequate the bypass reservoir will not fill properly—which can lead to potential air entrainment.

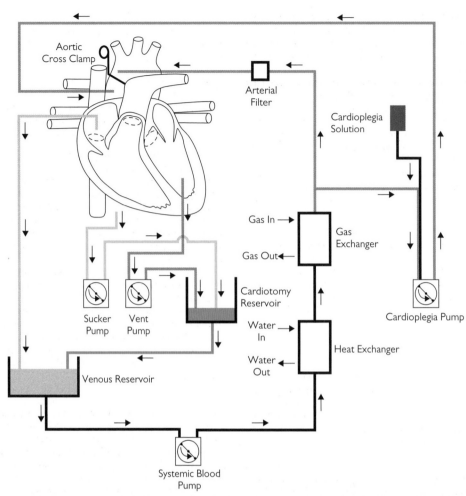

Fig. 14.1 A typical cardiopulmonary bypass circuit. Reproduced from Machin and Allsager, 'Principles of cardiopulmonary bypass', *Continuing Education in Anaesthesia, Critical Care and Pain*, 2006, 6, 5, figure 1, p. 177, by permission of The Board of Management and Trustees of the British Journal of Anaesthesia and Oxford University Press.

Poor venous flow can be due to air locks, poor placement, kinks, or forgotten clamps.

As the venous flow increases, the perfusionist will gradually increase the aortic return to the patient aiming for a target flow of 2.2–2.5L/min/m². Once this flow rate has been achieved, CPB is fully established and ventilation of the lungs can cease; the lungs are usually disconnected to improve the surgical field. The heart should be completely emptied by full CPB, although this may not be achieved until the aortic cross clamp is applied in cases of significant aortic regurgitation or other shunts.

Control of mean arterial pressure (MAP)
Even with the use of pulsatile flow during CPB, the pulse pressure is usually low and hence MAP is a more accurate variable to monitor. Systemic blood pressure invariably will fall following the onset of CPB. This initial fall is primarily due to vasoplegia which itself results from decreased blood viscosity and haematocrit caused by haemodilution from the pump prime. It is usually short-lived. Mean arterial pressure is maintained at an appropriate level for the patient mainly via the use of vasoconstrictors as required, although temporary reductions in MAP for surgical needs are more rapidly provided by alteration of the pump flow. More prolonged vasoplegia because of profound and prolonged inflammatory response to CPB is less common than in the past because of advances in CPB circuit technology and techniques; however, it does still occasionally occur and can extend in to the postoperative period.

Hypothermia
Most centres will use moderate hypothermia during bypass—typically 32–34°C but can be lower. This has the effect of reducing systemic and cerebral oxygen requirements and therefore increasing the tolerance of lower bypass flows and MAP. Deep hypothermic circulatory arrest (DHCA) is still sometimes used for complex aortic work and some congenital cardiac surgery. The temperatures employed for this are of the range of 18–22°C (see section 14.2).

Myocardial preservation techniques
Whilst systemic hypothermia causes cerebral protection, the myocardium is usually excluded from the CPB circuit and so must be protected via different strategies. Broadly speaking there are two techniques: cardioplegic arrest and cross-clamp-fibrillation. Cardioplegia is essentially a solution containing potassium, magnesium, and procaine; the absolute amounts vary depending on which particular type is used. It is used to arrest the heart in diastole and provides excellent operative conditions. Cardioplegia can be used to facilitate all types of cardiac surgery. The solution

is usually administered antegrade via the aortic root with a cross-clamp distal to it or under direct vision into the coronary ostia. If there is concern about coronary artery patency then cardioplegia can be also administered retrograde via the coronary sinus.

Cross-clamp-fibrillation is perhaps a more advanced technique that uses intermittent cross clamping of the aorta and subsequent fibrillation of the heart (either spontaneously on cross-clamping or by use of a direct current fibrillator device). The duration of fibrillation that can safely be tolerated is around 10–15min and thus this technique is only really suitable for the 'bottom ends' of coronary artery surgery (i.e. veno- or arterio-arterial anastomoses to the coronary arteries) or other very quick procedures. The cross-clamp is released at the end of the ischaemic period and the heart can then be defibrillated and sinus rhythm restored.

General points
Throughout bypass, the perfusionist has prime control over the running of the CPB, but this must be done in close liaison with the surgeon and the anaesthetist. The ACT, blood gases, haemoglobin or haematocrit, acid–base balance, electrolytes, and blood sugar should be monitored at least every half an hour. Fluid management to maintain pump volume is usually done in conjunction with the anaesthetist and may require red cell transfusion and colloids as appropriate.

Weaning from bypass

Before bypass is discontinued the patient's physiology and cardiopulmonary status should be in as good a position as possible to resume the normal role of provision of oxygen delivery to the body and most anaesthetists and cardiac surgeons will have a mental checklist which they will run through before making the decision to wean from bypass (see Box 14.2).

Box 14.2 Criteria for weaning from CPB

- Normothermia (36–37°C).
- Electrolytes and acid–base balance normalized.
- Haemoglobin adequate.
- De-airing of cardiac chambers and grafts.
- Lung ventilation established.
- Aortic cross-clamp removed.
- Heart rate and rhythm compatible with weaning (epicardial pacing may be required).
- Consideration of need for positive inotrope/other mechanical support if necessary.

Temperature
The patient's temperature should be normalized as hypothermia causes coagulopathy, arrhythmias and an increased afterload (as well as potentially increasing oxygen consumption on the ICU).

Blood gas analysis
Electrolytes and an adequate haematocrit should be maintained throughout bypass. Similarly, during bypass the patient should not be allowed to develop an uncontrolled acidosis, and the use of bicarbonate is still required sometimes.

Lungs
Re-expansion and resumption of ventilation of the lungs must occur and this is often done as part of the process of de-airing of the cardiac chambers (assisted by TOE).

Removal of cross-clamp
The aortic cross-clamp must be removed and with this the restoration of normal coronary artery flow (or indeed flow down the new grafts) will occur.

Heart rate and rhythm
The heart may return spontaneously to normal sinus rhythm upon reperfusion. Epicardial pacing may be required in some patients before weaning from bypass, especially following prolonged bypass or if preexisting conduction deficits were present.

Ventricular and circulatory support
The role and use of inotropes or mechanical devices to facilitate weaning from CPB is long established and a detailed description is not appropriate here. The exact thought process and decision as to which drugs or devices may be required will depend on individual patient requirements, personal preference of anaesthetists and surgeons, institutional practice and availability of expertise (e.g. mechanical ventricular assist devices are only available in a few centres in the UK).

All positive inotropes have been used to facilitate weaning and none has been shown to have superior outcomes over any other. Mechanical support is usually a second-line intervention, often after standard weaning practices have been unsuccessful.

Usually consideration of whether or not inotropes may or may not be required is made in light of several factors, including preoperative ventricular performance (both left and right ventricles), operative procedure, and presence of co-morbidities such as pulmonary hypertension.

Weaning process
Once the criteria discussed in the previous paragraphs have been duly considered, then a decision is made (usually by the surgeon) to come off bypass. The venous drain is progressively clamped by the perfusionist and as the heart fills the patient's cardiac output returns. Once venous drainage is fully occluded the venous pipe is removed and any remaining blood in the CPB reservoir can be slowly returned via the aortic cannula to the patient, titrated against blood pressure or other parameters of filling as necessary. Once the patient has been successfully separated from the bypass circuit, then the aortic line is removed. Reversal of the heparin usually with protamine (3–5mg/kg or 1mg per 100IU of heparin) should be administered, again at the surgeon's request. The exact timing will depend on many factors. (See section 14.3 for further details of dosing and administration.)

Following successful weaning from CPB and decannulation, there follows a period of surgical haemostasis, anterior chest drain insertion, and chest closure. During this time, rechecking of the ACT and blood gases following resumption of normal physiological status occurs; further assessment of any coagulopathy and administration of blood products and stabilization of the haemodynamics should also take place prior to transfer to the postoperative care environment.

Postoperative period

The complexity of open cardiac surgery invariably requires a period of postoperative care on an ITU. Even with straightforward and uneventful surgery, there is often a degree of rebound hypothermia, there are residual effects from any opioids used, there is always the potential for bleeding, and most patients require some degree of fluid resuscitation and some degree of lung recruitment all of which require a period of postoperative ventilation and stabilization prior to waking. The duration of this postoperative ventilation is widely variable but most cardiac surgical patients without complications should be awake and extubated within 2–6h of returning to the ICU.

Some patients, for example, those who are undergoing minimally invasive surgical procedures, or those who have relatively little comorbidity, may be suitable for more rapid waking and may well be extubated at the end of surgery in theatre. However, these patients often still require critical care facilities and so many of the advantages of so-called 'fast-tracking' are lost, as it does not necessarily improve throughput of the ICU.

Further reading

Machin D & Allsager C (2006). Principles of cardiolpulmonary bypass. *CEACCP*, 6(5):176–81.

Morgan E, Mikhail M, & Murray M (2002). *Clinical Anaesthesiology* (3rd edn, pp. 435–60). New York: McGraw-Hill Publishing.

Woods S & Gray S (2009): Cardiopulmonary bypass *Anaesth Intens Care Med*, 10(9):416–20.

14.2 Methods of cooling and rewarming during cardiac surgery and complications

Principles

Historically, cooling in order to achieve cardiac arrest was performed by surface cooling or immersion. This provided both a bloodless field as well as cerebral protection. With the advent of CPB, the need for circulatory arrest almost disappeared, and more moderate levels of hypothermia were found to be equally neuroprotective without the problems associated with extensive cooling.

Cooling during cardiac surgery is used primarily to reduce the cerebral metabolic rate of oxygen ($CMRO_2$) and thus protect the brain from ischaemic or hypoxic injury during CPB. Even with the use of moderate hypothermia, however, there is an increased incidence of temperature-related complications.

In respect of induced hypothermia, temperatures fall into three ranges (see Box 14.3).

Box 14.3 Induced hypothermia: temperature ranges
• Mild: 32–36°C
• Moderate: 28–32°C
• Deep: 15–28°C

Deep hypothermia is usually only used in conjunction with circulatory arrest.

It should be remembered that although cardioplegia is administered at around 4°C, the cooling associated with CPB is *not* for myocardial protection.

The degree to which the patient is cooled depends to some extent on the individual surgeon and the procedure that is being performed. Most coronary surgery will only require mild hypothermia, whilst valvular surgery will usually require mild to moderate cooling. Deep hypothermic circulatory arrest (DHCA) is usually only required for complex aortic or complex congenital surgical procedures.

Methods of cooling/rewarming

Cardiopulmonary bypass

The use of heat exchangers as part of the CPB circuit is the primary cooling method used in cardiac surgery. In modern systems these are integrated into the oxygenators using hollow-fibre technology allowing multi-lumen passage of blood in one direction and fresh gas and water in the opposite (counter-current) direction (not unlike the arrangement of fluid flow in diafiltration systems). These are, therefore, quite high resistance circuits and require the main bypass pump to be placed upstream (see section 14.1).

The blood in the circuit is therefore exposed to a large surface area membrane in continuity with high counter-current water flow that allows for active cooling and rewarming. The temperature of the water itself is controlled through a completely separate machine and is set by the perfusionist. In this way, core temperature can be decreased by approximately 0.5–1°C per minute depending on the temperature differential in the heat exchanger (normally set at 8–10°C difference). The process is reversed for rewarming.

Fluid warmers

The use of IV fluid warming is dependent on flow and as such is not used as a primary means of warming during cardiac surgery. However, it can be used following cessation of CPB to mitigate cooling effect of fluids, especially blood products and may help prevent rebound hypothermia. There is some evidence that their use in the postoperative setting may help speed up full rewarming (i.e. reduction of the core-peripheral gradient) and thus speed up the time to extubation.

Forced air warmers

These are widely available and often used as an adjunct to rewarming on CPB, as well as for continued warming in the post-operative period. They are not, however, particularly efficient at increasing body temperature, although their use does cut down convective loss and so helps to maintain body temperature even when normal homeostasis is lost. Using them in conditions of ischaemia or circulatory arrest can be associated with thermal injury to the tissues, and they must be used with caution.

Heated operating mattress

As with forced air warming, electrically heated mattresses placed on operating tables underneath the patient can be used to help rewarming or help maintain normothermia pre- and post- bypass. They tend to be relatively expensive but are more efficient than forced air warming since they prevent conductive loss.

Ice packs

Ice packs can be placed in highly vascular areas like the groin or axilla to help achieve cooling. They are also commonly placed around the head for circulatory arrest to maximize cerebral cooling. The ice can cause frostbite if placed directly onto skin and is usually wrapped in plastic bags. Alternatively, a commercially available head cooling system may be employed.

Deep hypothermic circulatory arrest

This rather unique set of physiological circumstances is employed to allow complex procedures to take place without any conventional systemic circulation. It is mostly used for complex aortic procedures, especially those involving the head and neck vessels, including arch dissections and aneurysms, as well as complex congenital surgery. It has also been used for complex cerebral aneurysm work and some major renal cell tumours. The processes used are similar to standard moderate hypothermic techniques, albeit with a few modifications:

- Cooling to 18–20°C takes longer to achieve. Although this clearly adds to the overall time of the procedure, the slower and more extensively the brain is cooled, the better the neuroprotection seems to be.

- The time period for which the circulation can be safely stopped is not fully established, although the incidence of significant neurological injury increases once 30min of circulatory arrest have elapsed.

- The perfusionist can run into problems with overload of the CPB system as the venous return (i.e. passive flow to the pump) is caused by gravity. The venous reservoir can overfill necessitating sometimes rather urgent removal of volume.

- Rewarming takes longer, but there is evidence to show that rapid rewarming (and indeed hyperthermia following DHCA) may in fact increase cerebral perfusion, which in the adult population may increase embolic load and thereby worsen neurological outcomes (see pH-stat vs α-stat discussed later).
- Some form of cerebral circulatory monitoring is often employed (e.g. NIRS). If there are significant alterations in these readings, they can often be offset by using selective antegrade perfusion of one or both carotids (assuming an intact circle of Willis) or sometimes retrograde perfusion via the jugular veins.
- Complications associated with hypothermia seem to be much more severe following DHCA.

Cooling following cardiac arrest

Cooling patients to 32–34°C for 12–24h following return of spontaneous circulation (ROSC) after out-of-hospital cardiac arrest has been shown in at least two major studies to improve outcome (both neurological and mortality) following VF arrests (see section 5.7). The scope of this practice has recently been extended to all post-cardiac arrest cases from outside hospital (and in some cases those from within hospitals). The sooner cooling is begun following ROSC the better this outcome seems to be. The techniques available for this include all those mentioned above, but there are also intravascular cooling devices and specifically designed cooling devices now commercially available to assist in this process. The complications of this cooling for 24h seem to be less marked, perhaps because they can be acted on at a more leisurely pace especially during the rewarming period (which itself occurs over several hours).

Complications of hypothermia

Physiological
Although many of the changes associated with hypothermia are concerning, in practice the majority are not severe, except following DHCA. Nonetheless, coagulopathy, thrombocytopenia, arrhythmias, shivering in the post-operative period and altered glycaemic control can all prove problematic.

Blood and circulation
- Vasoconstriction
- Increase blood viscosity
- Coagulopathy and platelet dysfunction
- Left shift of oxy-haemoglobin curve with reduced oxygen delivery.

Metabolism
- Metabolic acidosis
- Impaired glucose metabolism
- Decrease drug metabolism
- Electrolyte imbalance: particularly hypokalaemia.

Cerebral
- Vasoconstriction
- Reduced cerebral oxygen consumption.

Renal
- Reduced GFR
- Impaired Na^+, H_2O, and glucose reabsorption.

Gastrointestinal
- Gastric dilatation and ileus
- Submucosal erosions and haemorrhage.

Cardiac
- Bradycardia
- Arrhythmias
- Impaired contractility.

Physical

Altered gas absorption—pH-stat vs α-stat
- As temperature decreases so the solubility of gases increases. This is most notable with CO_2.
- Measurement of CO_2 and pH at low temperature thus needs some care.
- 'pH-stat' measurement often requires the addition of CO_2 to the oxygenator to maintain a pH at 7.4. The pH is measured at the actual patient temperature and leads to relative hypercarbia. CBF is controlled by pCO_2 and this therefore tends to lead to an increase in CBF. The increase in CBF may lead to better cerebral cooling (i.e. more of the brain is more effectively cooled) but there is the risk of increasing the microemboli load.
- 'α-stat' measurement measures the pH at 37 °C, without the addition of CO_2. This may normalize or reduce cerebral blood flow but therefore sometimes leads to reduced efficiency of cerebral cooling.
- In adult practice, most centres will use α-stat management as the majority of post-operative neurological injury is probably caused by macro and microemboli.
- In the paediatric population (especially neonates) the effects of hypoperfusion seem to dominate in terms of neurological outcome and so pH-stat is still often used.
- Some centres advocate the use of pH-stat whilst cooling (improved efficiency of cerebral cooling) and α-stat during rewarming in an effort to limit the extent of emboli.

Gas embolization
- Gas solubility in blood increases with cooling (discussed earlier).
- Rapid rewarming may lead to gas bubble formation and embolization with the risk of end-arteriolar ischaemia.
- The systemic effects of this may manifest as regional wall motion abnormalities, cerebral microvascular injury, gut ischaemia and renal injury, although it may be difficult to prove this as the causative event in the face of multiple potential aetiological factors.
- Rewarming speed is limited to allow gases to equilibrate and prevent bubble formation.

Further reading

Barnard M & Martin B (2010). *Cardiac Anaesthesia* (pp. 280–6). Oxford: Oxford University Press.

14.3 Coagulation management during cardiac surgery

Thrombogenesis during cardiac surgery

The primary indication for anticoagulation during cardiac surgery is to prevent clot formation within the CPB circuit and conduits.

Anticoagulation may also be required for other extra-corporeal circuits, including intra-aortic balloon pumps, renal support, ECMO, and ventricular assist devices. Despite advances in CPB circuit technology (reduced complement activation and heparin-bonded lines), exposure of blood to the artificial surface is one of the most potent activators of complement and thrombin, rendering anticoagulation mandatory.

Multiple factors related to the CPB circuit affect the intrinsic coagulation system. These include the degree of haemodilution from the bypass prime, duration of the bypass run, reinfusion of cardiotomy-suction blood (which is highly activated because of the degree of exposure to tissue factor) and the degree of hypothermia (especially when circulatory arrest is used).

Preoperative anticoagulation

Many cardiothoracic patients are already anticoagulated preoperatively for existing medical conditions such as atrial fibrillation or existing prosthetic valves.

Increasingly, many patients with acute coronary syndromes are presenting for urgent surgery having had dual anti-platelet therapy (usually aspirin and clopidogrel) and who may also have received the glycoprotein IIb/IIIa antagonist abciximab (ReoPro®). The latter can be of particular concern as its effects are difficult to measure and can persist for 7–10 days.

Elective patients who are anticoagulated are bridged in a conventional manner using UFH or high-dose LMWH. Increasingly some less invasive cardiology and electrophysiology procedures are being performed without stopping anticoagulation. The availability of prothrombin complex concentrates (PCC) (Beriplex® or Octaplex®) means that if significant bleeding or other complications ensue, then anticoagulation can rapidly be reversed.

Available drugs

Heparin

The most commonly used anticoagulant, heparin, is a mucopolysaccharide extracted from bovine lung or porcine intestinal mucosa. It works by increasing the efficacy of antithrombin III. Anti-thrombin III itself works by binding to and inactivating thrombin, effectively arresting the coagulation cascade within the common pathway. However, as heparin concentrations increase there is a progressive inhibition of factors IXa, XIa, and XIIa. The main advantage of heparin over other available anticoagulants is its titratability, ease of monitoring and ease of reversal if required.

As a naturally occurring substance, heparin is occasionally implicated in true allergic reactions, and can cause thrombocytopenia.

Direct thrombin inhibitors

Drugs such as hirudin (derived from *Hirudo medicinalis*, or the medical leech) and its derivatives lepirudin (recombinant hirudin) and bivalirudin all directly inhibit thrombin. They do not affect platelet function and have been shown to be safe in heparin-induced thrombocytopaenia (HIT). They have a relatively short half-life and need to be given by infusion. Whilst the effect may be short-lived, the effects cannot easily be reversed

(as with heparin) and they require time to allow the effects to wear off at a time when usually all efforts are being made to stop bleeding. Therefore, although they have a role in patients unable to tolerate heparin, they are not widely used outside these groups.

Prostacyclin (PGI₂)

This is a naturally occurring substance that can be administered as an infusion to inhibit platelet aggregation. Its main use in cardiac surgery is in the critical care unit in circumstances when heparin is contraindicated, for example, following HIT, or because of its other potentially beneficial effects such as those on the pulmonary vascular bed.

Monitoring coagulation during cardiac surgery

During cardiac surgery, and when using other extra-corporeal circuits and balloon pumps on the critical care unit, rapid and often repeated assessment of anticoagulation is required. Formal, conventional laboratory tests of anticoagulation such as activated partial thromboplastin time (aPTT) can of course be used and remain the gold-standard for assessment of heparin effect. However, point-of-care tests are usually preferred in the cardiac surgical setting because of the rapidly changing nature of the processes, both physical (CPB) and physiological.

Activated clotting time (ACT)

The ACT remains the most commonly used test of heparin effect in this field, but its use is now largely confined to the cardiac theatre and interventional radiology suite. Measured in seconds, it is similar to a whole blood clotting time but uses kaolin, celite or another activator as an accelerant to yield meaningful information more rapidly. Originally this required the addition of whole blood to a test tube containing the activator and some mechanical assessment of clot formation to be made. Several systems now exist, but the more modern devices require less than 1mL of blood to perform the assay and results are given within 5min (often using accelerated automated algorithms to give results more rapidly than the actual answer would otherwise appear). Most systems work by detecting the presence of fibrin within the sample. The normal range is 90–140sec (depending on which device is used) with an ACT >300sec required for aortic cannulation and usually >400–500sec before the start of bypass.

The ACT is not without its limitations. It becomes a less reliable marker of heparin effect in the post-bypass period (as a result of hypothermia, factor deficiency, haemodilution and altered platelet numbers and activity). It is also unreliable in the presence of the serine protease inhibitor aprotinin (Trasylol® Bayer HealthCare) because this drug artificially prolongs the celite-based assays.

Other tests, such as direct heparin assays (Hepcon® Hemostasis Management System) or measuring factor Xa levels are gaining support, but are not widely available in the UK.

Thromboelastography (TEG®)

The principle of TEG® relies on the viscoelastic properties of a developing blood clot and produces characteristic patterns that vary depending on different aspects of clot formation. TEG® gives an assessment of speed of onset of coagulation (R-time), adequacy of clot (maximum amplitude, MA) and fibrinolysis. TEG® can yield both quantitative and qualitative assessments of clot function within 15–20min and helps establish whether there is deficiency of platelets, fibrinogen, or clotting factors.

The presence of heparin during CPB means that the TEG® needs to be performed using heparinase that destroys any heparin that may be present. This allows assessment of the underlying coagulation at any stage during the bypass run (especially if prolonged) and during re-warming, which in itself means that blood products can be ordered prior to weaning in a more targeted manner than in the past.

TEG® has been shown to be more reliable at predicting bleeding in postoperative cardiac patients (compared to APTT or PT), possibly because it uses whole blood (i.e. including the platelet surface) as would occur *in vivo*. Its main limitation is the lack of effect seen with aspirin and clopidogrel or other antiplatelet agents, although additional, more complex assays overcome this. For further more detailed discussion of the use of TEG® see section 10.2.

Reversal

Protamine
Protamine is a protein derived from salmon and other fish sperm, although human forms also occur in nature. It is now produced commercially using a recombinant process.

It works by binding to heparin, directly forming an inactive complex that is finally cleared by the reticulo-endothelial system.

It is administered as a slow IV bolus in a dose of at least 1mg per 100IU of heparin used. Further, additional doses may be required to return the ACT to baseline as heparin can be sequestered in the peripheral circulation and there may be a variable degree of endogenous heparin release from mast cells as part of the inflammatory response.

Allergic reactions can cause histamine release and associated hypotension, although these are possibly less common with the recombinant forms. Protamine can also cause pulmonary hypertension (PHT), and care must be used in patients with pre-existing RV dysfunction or PHT. Protamine is a component of some insulin preparations and these patients are at increased risk of allergic reactions.

Before administering protamine it is usual to inform the perfusionist, who will usually turn off and remove pump suckers at this stage; the venous line will usually have already been removed.

Other methods of reversal
Most other anticoagulants have no specific or targeted reversal agent. If they require reversal in an emergency situation, then increasingly, factor concentrates are being used for this purpose.

Other drugs

Antifibrinolytics
Drugs that reduce blood loss following cardiac surgery have been widely adopted into practice. The serine protease inhibitor Aprotinin (Trasylol®) and lysine analogues such as tranexamic acid (Cyclokapron®) or ε-aminocaproic acid (EACA, Amicar®) are the most widely studied products.

Aprotinin has fallen from favour in recent years over concerns about increased mortality and morbidity (myocardial infarction, stroke, and renal failure) although it may be seeing a return in the near future. Tranexamic acid is widely used in the UK, without seemingly attracting adverse outcomes but with perhaps less efficacy. EACA is not available in the UK but is used in North America.

Although associated with reduced measured blood loss postoperatively, these drugs do not seem to reduce re-exploration rates.

Desmopressin (DDAVP)
Desmopressin has been used in patients with acquired and inherited von Willebrand's disease, platelet disorders and mild haemophilia A. It has also been used to some extent in patients on antiplatelet therapy. It works by causing release of von Willebrand factor (vWF) from platelets, which enhances platelet adhesion and an increase in factor VII activity. Its widespread use in cardiac surgery is limited by its limited efficacy outside of these groups.

Recombinant factors
Recombinant factor VII (rFVII, NovoSeven®, Novo Nordisk, Denmark) and other recombinant factors have all been trialled in cardiac surgery. Although most demonstrate efficacy at reducing blood loss, there are concerns over thrombotic complications, especially in the arterial tree.

Complications of anticoagulation

Bleeding
The most obvious complication of use of anticoagulants in the cardiac setting is perioperative blood loss. Cardiac surgery uses approximately 6% of packed red cells (PRCs) in the UK whilst accounting for <1% of all surgical procedures performed. However, the success of multimodal approaches to reduce allogeneic blood use in this population means that the majority of these patients will receive only one or two units of PRCs, with only the minority requiring major transfusions of PRCs and other products.

Heparin-induced thrombocytopenia (HIT)
A reduced platelet count associated with cardiac surgery is not uncommon; however it rarely falls below $70–90 \times 10^9/L$ in the absence of a pathological consumptive process. HIT is an auto-immune condition that can be life-threatening. Heparin binds to platelet factor 4 (PF4) and antibodies are formed to this complex. It usually occurs within 5–10 days of exposure, and leads to thrombocytopenia and paradoxical thrombus formation. Further transfusion of platelets can make the process worse. Treatment is by stopping the heparin, use of an alternate anticoagulant if required (see 'Available drugs'), and general haematological supportive care. The diagnosis is confirmed by ELISA for antibodies to the heparin-PF4 complexes, but the diagnosis should be made primarily on clinical grounds in discussion with a haematologist and treated as HIT if there is a high degree of suspicion.

Further reading

Lesserson, L & Enriquez, L (2011). Coagulation monitoring. In JA Kaplan, DL Reich, & SN Konstadt (eds), *Kaplan's Cardiac Anaesthesia* (6th edn, p 496–519). New York: Elsevier.

14.4 Bypass-related issues in cardiac surgery

Medical and anaesthesia-related issues

Anaemia and acidosis

The main cause of anaemia during CPB is haemodilution. The decision to transfuse is usually based on the haematocrit, the volume requirements of the perfusionist, evidence of worsening acidosis, a rising lactate, or a combination of these. It is rarely necessary if the Hb is >8g/dL whilst on CPB. Other causes of low haemoglobin include blood loss (especially occult loss) and haemolysis. The latter is less common with modern bypass systems but increases with increasing bypass time and may be implied when there is haematuria.

Metabolic acidosis during CPB is multifactorial but usually results from global changes in perfusion, compounded by development of anaemia, alterations in temperature and prolonged bypass duration. However, other causes should be borne in mind, especially if there is little response to standard corrective measures. These include hepatic and renal failure, or gastrointestinal or limb ischaemia (often embolic). The latter situations are often detected late, as they may not manifest until after the CPB run has finished.

Awareness

Historically, the incidence of awareness during cardiac surgery was considered to be higher than in a general surgical population.

The use of TIVA with propofol at 20mg–150mg/h (in addition to high-dose opioids) was the only way to try to avoid this. With the addition of a volatile agent (normally isoflurane in the UK) to the bypass gases the incidence of awareness has fallen further (vent gases from the oxygenator can be connected to the anaesthetic gas monitoring, although correlation with end-tidal values has not been established). The increased availability of processed EEG monitoring (BIS ®/Entropy®) has allowed more accurate control and assessment of depth of anaesthesia during CPB.

Coagulation issues

Failure of heparinization

An absolute inability to anticoagulate a patient is rare, but a degree of heparin resistance is often seen in the cardiac surgical population because of recent heparin exposure and thus a relative lack of antithrombin III. This may paradoxically require administration of FFP prior to heparinization to replenish the levels. In elective cases, there is time to rectify the problem, but the situation can be more problematic in the emergent situation.

Coagulopathy

The CPB prime is about 1.5–2.0L in volume and consists of a variable amount of crystalloid and/or colloid, sometimes with a small amount of mannitol and usually 5000–10 000 units of heparin. The onset of CPB leads to rapid haemodilution of the circulating volume. In paediatrics and occasionally in adult practice the pump may be also primed with blood. Activation of platelets and clotting factor consumption still occurs despite systemic heparinization and is worsened by the duration of bypass and extreme hypothermia. In part this is due to complement activation by exposure of the blood to non-physiological surfaces of the bypass tubing. Heparin-bonded circuits are available but they are expensive and there is little clinical evidence to support their use. Monitoring of coagulation remains the mainstay of care with replacement of blood products with FFP, platelets and cryoprecipitate when needed (see section 10.2 for further details).

Platelet dysfunction

Platelet dysfunction may result from mechanical stresses caused by roller pumps during CPB. Centrifugal pumps have less effect, as do the newer generations of roller pump, but prolonged bypass times often lead to deteriorating platelet activity. This may compound any preoperative antiplatelet therapy that may have been given.

Clots within CPB circuit

These are, fortunately, rare. They can usually be detected by the appearance of clots in the reservoir but are also suggested by high arterial line pressures if there is clot in the distal circuit or filter. Should clotting occur during coronary artery bypass grafting (i.e. closed heart surgery) then cardiac massage can be performed which may allow a replacement circuit to be connected. If, however, the left-sided cardiac chambers are open, then there is no ability to support the systemic circulation easily and the outcome may be extremely poor. Manual support of the circulation via internal massage or if possible short-term weaning from CPB is essential whilst the CPB pump or component is changed. Re-heparinization may also be beneficial. Changing pumps or parts of the circuitry is complex, high risk, and involves at least two or three perfusionists: it is not undertaken lightly.

Haemodynamic instability

The onset of CPB is usually associated with a profound drop in SVR as the peripheral vasodilatation occurs in response to a bolus of low oxygen-carrying fluid. This may require use of vasoconstrictors by the perfusionist and is usually short-lived. In a small number of cases this vasodilatation may persist. This is due to the activation of complement and other components of the inflammatory cascade and can be severe and persistent in some patients. Advances in circuit technology and the use of membrane oxygenators have reduced the incidence and severity of this and other manifestations of a severe inflammatory response (e.g. CPB-associated ARDS or 'pump lung'). However, persistent hypotension or haemodynamic problems might relate to anaphylactic reactions to drugs or fluids within the prime or any recently administered drugs and should be considered in such circumstances.

Unexplained volume loss during CPB can be due to several factors. Profound vasoplegia can cause an apparent volume loss, but the temporal relationship with the onset of CPB and the speed of onset is usually a clue to the true cause. Retroperitoneal bleeding (especially if femoral cannulation has been used), aortic dissection, volume loss into one or other thoracic cavity or blood loss from vein harvesting sites which are subsequently re-draped and covered should all be considered. Rarely there are small, unnoticed leaks from parts of the bypass circuits or connectors.

Neurological injury

Apart from death, major neurological injury is perhaps the most feared complication of cardiac surgery and has received a lot of interest in recent years. As the incidence of type 1 injury (major, focal neurological deficits) has stabilized so interest has focused on type 2 injury, the rather ill-defined neurocognitive decline that is seen in some patients. Both are usually related to embolic phenomena of either particulate matter or possibly small gaseous emboli. Microemboli (defined as those <200 microns) are not filtered out by in-line filters and can be caused by small gas bubbles, platelet fragments or clumps, cholesterol particles or other fragments of atheroma which may become dislodged from the aorta during cannulation and other manipulations. Despite advances in technology which may help detect these phenomena (such as NIRS, transcranial Doppler sonography, and even BIS®), currently there is little that can be done to prevent such events occurring other than good surgical technique or perhaps off-pump CABG.

Intracranial haemorrhage is extremely rare, but often catastrophic in the face of anticoagulation or coagulopathy.

Patients with known carotid artery stenosis are potentially more susceptible to type 1 injury, and may well require combined carotid endarterectomy and cardiac surgery. If they do not fulfil the criteria for carotid artery surgery then it is important to maintain the perfusion pressure at normal levels for the patient.

Finally, it should be remembered that the majority of major type 1 events occur in the postoperative period and are often the result of the combination of ongoing inflammatory response, coagulation and platelet dysfunction and unstable atheromatous plaques.

Renal injury

Renal injury following cardiac surgery is multifactorial. The role of perfusion pressure and flow on renal function is well known and mean arterial pressure during bypass should be maintained as close to normal as is feasible. Significant haemolysis and haemoglobinuria or myoglobinuria may exacerbate renal injury as well as worsening any hyperkalaemia.

Surgical/technical problems

Aortic dissection

Limited dissection can occur during aortic cannulation or rarely can be due to the 'jet' striking the posterior aortic wall. It can extend up in to the carotids or subclavian arteries or distally around the arch to the descending aorta. Attempts to establish full bypass, especially if the cannula is within the false lumen can be catastrophic and the key to avoiding this is early detection of the dissection.

Other than visual recognition of a dissection by the surgeon, factors that may suggest its occurrence include high line pressures, loss of radial artery pulsation or pressure and identification by TOE (extending false lumen). Limited anterior dissections can often be controlled and repaired, however more extensive damage may require extensive reconstruction.

Carotid/subclavian artery occlusion

Incorrect placement of the cannula can lead to obstruction or malperfusion of the arch arteries, especially if the cannula is placed distally in the ascending aorta. Signs include unilateral facial blanching, unilateral decline in NIRS scores or other neuromonitoring, conjunctival oedema or low radial artery pressure.

Venous return failure and air locks

Maintenance of the volume return to the venous reservoir is essential for the proper functioning of CPB. Failure to achieve this runs the risk of gas entrainment into the arterial side of the circuit and the development of an air lock or the risk of massive gaseous embolus. Most CPB systems will have level monitors on the venous reservoir. Assuming that volume loss is not a problem, then there are a number of possible causes.

Surgical manipulation of the heart is the commonest cause for reduction in venous return. If the surgeon is deliberately altering the position of the heart or temporarily occluding the venous line to size CABGs, then he should inform the perfusionist prior to doing so.

When establishing or weaning from bicaval bypass then it is common to use a single cannula for some of the time. Poor drainage via a single venous cannula is not uncommon and full bypass may not be established until proper venous drainage is achieved.

Air locks on the venous side are not uncommon, but are often not highly problematic. Air can be entrained from loose purse strings around the cannula or because the right side of the heart is open either deliberately or inadvertently.

Once the surgeon has been informed and the problem identified, simple solutions such as adjustment of the cannula may be all that is required. If this repeatedly fails to address the issue then use of bicaval venous drainage may be considered.

Massive systemic air embolism

This is a rare but usually catastrophic event. The majority of causes relate to problems within the CBP circuit. Air entrainment from the venous reservoir, loss of pump control, erroneous connections, and non-airtight connections leading to air entrainment elsewhere have all been implicated in the past. Occasionally it may occur when the heart starts to eject before de-airing has been performed but after removal of the aortic cross clamp or because of paradoxical embolization across a septal defect.

The occurrence of significant systemic gas embolism is an acute emergency (see Box 14.4).

Critical ischaemia will occur wherever air is injected into the arterial circulation and can also produce an 'airlock' where even if perfusion is re-established the ischaemia may persist.

Box 14.4 Suggested action plan for massive gas embolism

- Stop bypass.
- Trendelenburg position—allows air to pass up against gravity and out of the cranial circulation.
- If related to air within the arterial circuit then remove the aortic cannula and flush through circuit.
- Connect arterial line to venous cannula (in SVC) and flush at 1–2L/min to reverse cerebral flow and hopefully push air out of carotids into the aorta.
- Intermittently compress carotids to purge vertebral arteries.
- Technique can be repeated with IVC if whole body embolism suspected.
- Vasoconstrict to raise SVR and hopefully increase perfusion pressure to drive bubbles across the vascular bed.
- Consider neuroprotection post-op—cooling, prolonged sedation.

Further reading

Jameel S, Colah S, & Klein AA (2010). Recent advances in cardiopulmonary bypass techniques. *CEACCP*, 10(1):20–3. doi:10.1093/bjaceaccp/mkp042.

14.5 Off-pump cardiac surgery

The original studies of CABGs in animals were performed on the beating heart. With the advent of CPB in the 1950s and the ability to perform multivessel grafting in relative safety, surgery on the beating heart fell out of fashion. True open-heart surgery, of course, still mandates a bloodless, motionless operative field.

As the safety and efficacy of coronary artery surgery improved, and attention began to focus on the negative aspects of CPB as previously described, there has been a recurrence of interest over the last two decades in so-called 'off-pump' surgery for coronary artery bypass grafting (OPCAB).

Initially, the uptake of *multivessel* bypass grafting performed on a beating heart was seen only in certain centres, performed by enthusiasts for the technique. In the early 2000s, concern over long-term graft patency rates, possibly reflecting slightly alterations in distal anastomotic techniques, has meant that the numbers of these individuals has slowly declined, although there are still some centres where up to 50–70% of bypass grafts (including redo coronary artery surgery) are performed off-pump.

There has been concern over the completeness of revascularization in some cases, as grafting an unfavourable target vessel in the presence of haemodynamic compromise may persuade the surgeon to stop grafting the vessel rather than convert to an on-pump procedure. Patient selection may also play a role and some will actively seek out a surgeon performing OPCAB.

Surgical issues

Both cross-clamp-fibrillation *and* OPCAB techniques are considered relatively advanced techniques for coronary artery revascularization, mostly because of the time constraints these techniques place on the distal anastomosis. Although most cardiac surgeons will perform single left internal mammary artery (LIMA) to left anterior descending artery (LAD) grafts off-pump, multivessel grafting is technically more challenging and not undertaken by all.

Haemodynamic issues
With off-pump surgery there is the added difficulty of maintaining adequate systemic cardiac output during grafting. Depending on the vessels to be grafted, the heart may need to be rotated, and both atria and especially the right ventricle can be compressed reducing both systemic and pulmonary venous return. Tissue stabilization devices (e.g. Medtronic Octopus®) and heart stabilization devices (e.g. Medtronic Starfish® and Urchin®) are available to help position the heart such that haemodynamic change is minimized and the target vessels can be approached in a controlled manner. These devices in themselves have been shown to cause regional wall motion abnormalities which may further compound the problem, although these are all mechanical in nature and usually resolve when the heart is returned to a more anatomical position.

Grafting sequence
If multivessel grafting is undertaken, the sequence in which the grafts are performed is usually different from an on-pump technique. The reason for this is that flow to the IMA arises from the subclavian vessels and so occurs whilst an aortic cross clamp is in place. Therefore, opening of the IMA graft will restore myocardial blood flow to the LAD (or other grafted vessel) irrespective of whether CPB is used or not. Hence, the IMA target vessel (almost invariably the LAD or branch thereof) is usually grafted last in on-pump surgery using cardioplegia but is often grafted first with off-pump techniques as it restores coronary artery

flow to about 50% of the LV before potentially compromising manipulation and positioning take place.

Vein grafts are often done in any order, but with sequential distal and proximal anastomoses. Whilst this reduces the ischaemic time, it requires repeated side-clamping of the aorta to perform the 'top end' anastomosis, as with the cross-clamp-fibrillation technique.

Bleeding
Although there is obviously no need for aortic or venous cannulation, many of the sites of iatrogenic bleeding following cardiac surgery are not related to these alone. Mammary harvest sites, side branches of conduits, distal and proximal anastomotic sites as well as sternal wires are all frequently implicated in post-cardiac surgical bleeding and it has been shown that although overall measured chest tube loss in off-pump surgery may be reduced, re-exploration rates are similar. Heparin is still required in all cases although many will only use 'half-dose' regimen unless the case is at particularly high risk of emergent conversion to an on-pump case.

Perfusion
Most surgeons will require a perfusionist to be on stand-by, usually with the pump primed. Overall surgical time might be slightly shorter than that for on-pump surgery, but with little overall economic savings in terms of theatre time and costs.

Benefits
It is thought that the benefits of OPCAB where they exist are seen particularly in the elderly or those with poor ventricular function. Many of these patients have multiple complex comorbidities and the reduction in morbidity is primarily due to the avoidance of the CPB. However, these are already a higher-risk group of patients and thus comparisons are harder to draw. Much more detailed sub-group studies are required before there will be a definitive answer about the true risks and benefits of OPCAB from a surgical perspective.

Anaesthetic concerns

The anaesthetic approach for OPCAB is as for any cardiac surgical case. Many OPCAB cases are done for single vessel grafting and as such are often targeted as fast-track cases. Thus temperature control during the whole operation, judicial administration of opiates or use of ultra-short-acting drugs, including muscle relaxants is required. In other respects, the basic approach, induction, monitoring etc. are the same as for all cardiac cases (see section 14.1).

Control of haemodynamics
This is sometimes much more challenging during off-pump surgery, mostly as a direct result of surgical manipulation of the heart. Fluid management is very much in control of the anaesthetist and as intraoperative echocardiography images are of extremely variable benefit, many advocate the use of real-time cardiac output monitoring to guide fluid replacement. Most patients will require volume loading of 500–1000mL as a minimum (with blood and blood products as required). Use of vasoconstrictors to maintain the MAP during grafting of the circumflex and posterior descending artery (PDA) territories is often unpredictable as the position of the heart can lead to obstructed flow in the right side with pooling of drugs injected into it. The use of inotrope infusions may be of benefit as long as they are commenced prior to surgical positioning, but may run into the same problems if

the abnormal position is maintained for too long. In most cases a degree of tolerance of mild hypotension (as long as it is not prolonged), cautious volume loading and use of vasoconstrictors allows surgery to proceed without too much compromise.

If there are signs of persistent and unresolving hypotension, new regional wall motion abnormalities on TOE, new ECG changes or other signs of ongoing ischaemia then conversion to an on-pump operation may be required.

Once the heart is repositioned after performing the distal anastomosis, the surgeon will usually immediately wish to do the 'top end'. At this stage the patient's own homeostatic mechanisms are trying to restore normal haemodynamics and this along with potentially pooled vasopressors often causes a moderate overshoot of the blood pressure at a time when the surgeon wants the systolic below 100mmHg in order to safely side-clamp the aorta. Forward planning is the key here, and small boluses of GTN (50mcg) can avoid delays or the need for an impatient surgeon to temporarily clamp the IVC. It is rare to need other vasodilators to overcome this.

Arrhythmias

These may be more common intraoperatively and haemodynamic instability as a result of new or fast atrial fibrillation or ventricular arrhythmias will require aggressive treatment including internal cardioversion or conversion to CPB. The loss of the atrial component of left-ventricular filling can be particularly destabilizing in these patients during circumflex and PDA grafting. Postoperatively, however, the incidence of atrial fibrillation is possibly reduced.

Electrolyte imbalance

Hypokalaemia and hypomagnesaemia will require correction by the anaesthetist rather than relying on the perfusionist. This may be a contributing factor to the increased incidence of arrhythmia.

Ventilation

Ventilation is obviously maintained throughout. However, the surgeons will often request a reduction in tidal volume or reduction in PEEP during grafting as the lungs can cause mediastinal movement or encroach on the operative field. This is not a problem for a short while but can cause atelectasis if prolonged which may delay post-operative weaning, extubation and recovery. Recruitment manoeuvres undertaken around the time of sternal closure may be beneficial, although care should be taken with hyper-expanding the lungs if the LIMA has been used.

Neurological injury

One of the presumed advantages of OPCAB is a reduction in neurological damage following cardiac surgery. This has not been borne out in clinical trials and there has been much speculation as to why this should be. Although the embolic load is almost certainly reduced in terms of microemboli, macroemboli still occur because of repeated partial side-clamping of the aorta to perform proximal anastomoses which can lead to plaque disruption and instability. Displacement of the heart to perform the distal anastomoses often increases CVP and although MAP may be maintained the cerebral perfusion pressure may fall below normal autoregulatory levels thereby causing a hypoperfusion injury. This remains a key area of research interest. Aortic non-touch techniques, including bilateral IMA harvest and 'Y-grafting' may be beneficial, but are not without their own difficulties and limitations.

Renal injury

This is an area where there is some evidence of benefit of OPCAB over on-pump surgery. However, the complex aetiology of acute renal failure (ARF) following cardiac surgery means that this is hard to prove in individual cases but patients with chronic renal failure or those at high risk of ARF may benefit from off-pump techniques.

Inflammatory response and coagulopathy

A large number of studies have tried to prove a reduction in the inflammatory response using OPCAB. The assumption that use of CPB causes a worsened inflammatory response compared with OPCAB has not been confirmed by these trials (although depending on the markers used there is usually a trend towards a reduced level of systematic inflammatory response in OPCAB). This is probably a reflection of the strength of the inflammatory response to cardiac surgery per se and not just that of CPB. Coagulopathy equally tends to be less severe, but as mentioned earlier the bleeding risk is not significantly reduced.

Postoperative course

There are little firm data in heterogeneous groups of patients to support OPCAB as reducing length of stay, significant morbidity, such as post-op respiratory tract infections, or mortality. Subgroup analysis shows inconsistent benefit in some groups.

Further reading

Alston RP (2012). Anaesthesia for off-pump coronary artery bypass grafting surgery. *Anaesth Intens Care Med*, 13:510–12. doi:10.1016/j.mpaic.2012.08.006.

Hett DA (2006). Anaesthesia for off-pump coronary artery surgery. *CEACCP*, 6(2), 60–62. doi:10.1093/bjaceaccp/mkl005.

14.6 Postoperative complications after cardiac surgery

The postoperative course of cardiac surgical patients remains one of the most potentially complex of all high-risk surgical patients. With advances in surgical and anaesthetic techniques, many patients now require shorter postoperative ventilation, which potentially means a reduced stay in ICU. Nevertheless, most patients will spend 24–48h in some form of critical care unit. During this time patients are closely monitored for respiratory, neurological, renal and circulatory dysfunction and may need support for some or all of these systems.

Haemodynamic issues

Bleeding and coagulopathy

Postoperative bleeding is extremely common after cardiac surgery, with approximately 50–60% of patients receiving allogeneic blood transfusions. Most patients can lose volumes of the order of 200–500mL without this being considered abnormal (although the rate at which the loss occurs must clearly be taken into account). It can be due either to surgical causes, coagulopathy or a combination of both. As a general rule, acute rapid severe loss is likely to be surgical in nature whilst ongoing slower ooze is more suggestive of coagulopathy. Severe coagulopathy will result in bleeding from all wound and puncture sites.

Risk factors
In many cases of bleeding after cardiac surgery, more than one risk factor will be present (see Box 14.5).

> **Box 14.5 Risk factors for bleeding after cardiac surgery**
>
> - Preoperative antiplatelet or anticoagulant therapy (e.g. aspirin, clopidogrel, warfarin, heparin, GP IIb/IIIa inhibitors)
> - Surgical factors (including redo surgery and long bypass times)
> - Abnormal temperature (persistent hypothermia, or use of deep hypothermic circulatory arrest)
> - Other haematological abnormalities (including massive transfusion, and pre-existing coagulopathies—e.g. haemophilia)
> - Metabolic derangement (reduced ionized calcium, uraemia, hepatic failure).

Signs
The commonest sign of bleeding is persistent chest drain loss. Other signs include falling haemoglobin concentration (although many patients will have a varying degree of haemodilution from both the bypass prime and postoperative fluid challenges), haemodynamic instability (often not severe unless tamponade is suspected) or more subtle signs such as unexplained oliguria, poor ventilation or oxygenation (due to blood loss into the thoracic cavity).

Management
The management of postoperative bleeding requires close liaison between the surgeon and anaesthetist or intensivist.

Early echocardiography may be required if tamponade is suspected, but can also be useful in terms of fluid management and optimization of cardiac function. Transoesophageal echo is now usually preferred in these circumstances as TTE often results in poor image quality in ventilated patients with anterior chest drains.

Correction of any coagulopathy is essential. This should ideally be guided by near-patient testing. Reliance on conventional laboratory testing is often unreliable or time-limited in the presence of ongoing bleeding, especially when empirical treatment of a presumed coagulopathy is often used. See section 14.3 for further details.

General supportive measures should also be undertaken: all efforts should be made to correct any hypothermia (including warming of blood and fluid); excess hypertension should be controlled and correction of ionized calcium may also be required.

Apparent complete cessation of bleeding from one or other chest drain should always be treated with caution as it may imply occlusion of the drain by clot. In this circumstance the risk of tamponade will increase if there is concealed persistent bleeding.

Re-exploration
The decision to re-explore the chest for bleeding is rarely straightforward, except in the case of actual or impending cardiac tamponade. The rate, total volume of loss and evidence of systemic compromise (e.g. rising lactate secondary to anaemia) must all be taken into account. Re-exploration rates will vary depending on many factors but in general are around 4–8%. Those patients who require re-exploration have higher rates of complications (including significant sternal wound infections and wound breakdown), and as a consequence prolonged ICU and hospital stays.

Hypertension

Postoperative hypertension has a variety of causes (Box 14.6) and although it can usually be controlled with nitrates or other vasodilators, this may not always be the best course. Identification of the cause should be sought first and appropriate therapy commenced. Untreated hypertension leads to increased myocardial work, high pressure along grafts and suture lines, and an increased the risk of postoperative bleeding.

> **Box 14.6 Causes of postoperative hypertension after cardiac surgery**
>
> - Inadequate sedation or analgesia, especially around the time of extubation (awareness is now much less common with the use of short-acting NMBAs).
> - Persistent hypothermia (with a subsequent increase in SVR).
> - Sympathetic vasoconstriction or left ventricular hypertrophy.
> - Intracranial pathology (haemorrhage or infarct) should be considered in all cases.
> - Rarely, malfunctioning infusion pumps or inadvertent boluses may cause fluctuant hypertension.
> - Technical issues such as transducer malposition should always be ruled out.

Treatment should ideally focus on addressing the cause and only then should generic pharmacotherapy be started although this is very much an oversimplification. Common first-line agents include IV nitrates or β-blockade.

Hypotension

The potential causes of hypotension are multiple (see Box 14.7) but whilst several are potentially life threatening and need rapid attention, most are less frequently encountered—other than hypovolaemia and non-life-threatening arrhythmias.

> **Box 14.7 Causes of postoperative hypotension after cardiac surgery**
>
> - *Cardiac*—myocardial infarction, kinking of bypass graft(s), poor myocardial protection, left or right ventricular dysfunction, valvular failure (native or artificial), arrhythmia, tamponade
> - *Circulatory*—systemic inflammatory response or ongoing vasoplegia, true hypovolaemia, massive bleeding, sepsis
> - *Respiratory*—tension pneumothorax
> - *Pharmacological*—excess sedatives or nitrates; inadvertent cessation of inotropes
> - *Technical*—transducer misplacement or incorrect calibration.

Often, in the postoperative setting, the cause is apparent or suggested (e.g. ongoing chest drain losses causing hypovolaemia). Treatment involves the establishment and treatment of likely or obvious causes. In the absence of any such signs or if response to simple fluid challenges does not correct the hypotension, then early echocardiography should be performed to assess left ventricular function, volume status and to exclude early tamponade. Cardiac output monitoring is also frequently used in the post-operative setting to optimize filling and cardiac output, although the specific type of device will vary from centre to centre.

Perioperative cardiac tamponade

Cardiac tamponade is the accumulation of fluid (or clot) within the potential space between the visceral and parietal pericardia. In the acute setting, the pericardium is relatively non-distensible and any fluid within it will compress usually one or more of the lower pressure chambers of the heart (atria or right ventricle) leading to inadequate filling during diastole, causing low cardiac output and eventually cardiac arrest.

Even though the pericardium is opened during surgery, small volume isolated collections or thrombus formation within chest drains means that the blood often does not escape from the confines of the pericardium postoperatively and thus can still cause pathology.

Tamponade is more common after valve surgery than bypass grafting, and more common with mechanical valves because of the requirement for anticoagulation, albeit often delayed in this circumstance. The classical triad described by Beck of muffled heart sounds, raised CVP and low blood pressure is a poorly diagnostic and late sign. Early detection relies on a combination of high suspicion and early echocardiography.

Warning signs

- Resistant or worsening oliguria
- Rising lactate despite adequate fluid resuscitation
- Low blood pressure resistant to supportive measures
- Tachycardia
- Raised CVP showing marked, sustained rise with a fluid challenge.

Management

- Immediately summon the surgeon, the chest may need to be opened imminently on ICU.
- TOE/TTE—TOE is usually preferred as TTE may not identify posterior collections well.
- Correct any coagulopathy.
- If there is high suspicion of tamponade then ensure adequate sedation and paralysis; inform the blood bank and request products; inform the theatre team.

Ultimately, the treatment of actual or suspected tamponade in the postoperative setting is by re-exploration and relief of the tamponade. Occasionally this may necessitate opening the chest on the ITU, which has many incumbent problems. Any haemodynamic compromise frequently resolves immediately on re-opening of the sternum. This may be seen even if there have been no absolute diagnostic echocardiographic features prior to re-exploration suggesting that tamponade was imminent.

There is no role in the perioperative setting for attempted percutaneous pericardial drainage.

Low cardiac output

Despite optimum myocardial preservation during cardiopulmonary bypass, myocardial performance can be significantly impaired during the early postoperative period. This is sometimes a result of reperfusion injury but often reflects a degree of myocardial oedema or worsening of preoperative function as a result of the effects of intraoperative ischaemia or cardioplegia. Clearly the degree to which individual patients are affected will vary, with some requiring little more than fluid optimization whereas other may require prolonged inotropic or mechanical support.

Signs

Important signs of low cardiac output are:

- Oliguria
- Hypotension, reduced capillary refill time, and cool peripheries
- Metabolic acidosis and raised lactate
- Hypoxia resulting from pulmonary congestion.

Aetiology

Causes of low cardiac output are multiple but should be considered systematically:

- Low preload: due to hypovolaemia, cardiac tamponade
- Decreased contractility: due to myocardial stunning or hibernation, pre-existing poor LV function, graft kinking or incomplete revascularization
- Arrhythmias
- Increased afterload: due to vasoconstriction, LV outflow tract obstruction
- Diastolic dysfunction
- Right ventricular compromise.

Management

Treatment will obviously depend on the aetiology but should follow basic supportive principles.

- Adequate volume resuscitation (although hypervolaemia may cause over-distention of the cardiac chambers potentially causing tension on atrial suture line or stretching of grafts).
- Early echocardiography to assess left-ventricular preload, regional wall motion abnormalities or valvular lesions.
- Inotropes or vasopressors should be used as indicated.
- Prompt treatment of arrhythmias.
- Correction of electrolyte abnormalities and low haemoglobin.
- Consider mechanical support (IABP or VAD if available) if necessary.

Arrhythmias

The incidence of tachy- and bradyarrhythmias following cardiac surgery is relatively high, although these are mostly relatively benign and of supraventricular origin. Ventricular arrhythmias are less common (although more common than in a general surgical population) and treatment of these should follow current resuscitation guidelines.

Approximately 25% of patients will develop atrial fibrillation post-operatively and although often self-terminating or resolving when electrolyte abnormalities are corrected, a large number of these will require cardioversion (pharmacological or electrical). A significant percentage of this later group will be prescribed amiodarone, for a period of weeks following surgery although this is usually only until they are reviewed in the postoperative surgical outpatients.

Bradycardia is similarly common, especially immediately post bypass or after valve surgery. This is usually easily corrected by use of surgically placed epicardial pacing wires, and is often a short term problem, although many valve patients will ultimately require permanent pacemakers (see section 14.7).

Many tachyarrhythmias resolve with correction of underlying fluid deficits, electrolyte imbalance, or removal of mechanical irritants such as chest drains. All persistent arrhythmias or those causing significant haemodynamic compromise should be treated following national or local guidelines and the exact therapies used will depend on the degree of compromise experienced by the patient and individual clinician preferences.

Complications in other organ systems

Respiratory complications

The majority of cardiac patients are at high risk of developing pulmonary complications postoperatively. Pre-existing lung disease, smoking history, prolonged bypass and poor analgesia can all increase this risk significantly. Mild complications may occur in up to 50% of patients, whereas those requiring complicated prolonged ventilation are much less common, affecting between 5% and 8% of patients.

Atelectasis, infection, consolidation, and acute lung injury

The commonest complication in most patients is basal atelectasis following sternotomy and bypass. In some this will progress to infection and consolidation, and can occur in the very early stages postoperatively.

Pulmonary oedema either as a consequence of left ventricular failure or as a result of an acute lung injury (ALI) is less frequent but should be considered in patients with poor LV function. The incidence of ALI following cardiac surgery has declined in recent years with improvements in CPB technology, but still occurs (and indeed can occur in off-pump surgery) because of the exaggerated systemic inflammatory response seen in some patients following cardiac surgery.

Effusions

Pleural effusions (which are often caused by blood in the immediate postoperative setting) are usually later developments but should be considered in all post-cardiac surgical patients as they are relatively common, especially in those requiring prolonged ITU management. Significant effusions should be drained.

Management of respiratory complications

The management of respiratory failure ranges from simple antibiotic therapy (usually IV in the first instance) to non-invasive ventilation or CPAP through to the fully-invasive protective ventilation strategies used in ARDS. Many of this latter group will require tracheostomy and prolonged weaning.

All cardiac patients require a certain amount of respiratory physiotherapy and the importance of this should not be underestimated.

Renal dysfunction

A significant proportion of the cardiac surgical population will develop a degree of acute renal impairment in the postoperative period. The majority will resolve without the need for haemofiltration or dialysis but about 5% of an unselected cardiac ITU population will require renal replacement therapy and this has a disproportionate impact on cardiac ITU facilities.

The causes are usually multifactorial, but pre-existing chronic renal impairment, low cardiac output states, prolonged bypass, and hypovolaemia will all predispose to ARF. Direct nephrotoxins are an unusual aetiological factor unless the patients have been referred following recent ischaemic episodes requiring angiography and hence exposure to intravenous contrast.

Oliguria in the early postoperative period is usually as a result of relative hypovolaemia, a low cardiac output state, hypotension or a combination of these. Initial efforts should therefore be directed towards optimizing these factors. However, patients will often require large amounts of fluid in the early postoperative phase and excessive volume-loading of an often struggling heart may lead to worsening failure (and indeed can cause atrial stretch and tensioning of suture lines). Early use of diuretics either as intermittent boluses or as infusions may help to avoid this.

Neurological complications

Other than death, perhaps the most feared consequence of cardiac surgery is a major stroke. Neurological complications have been of concern since the very earliest days of cardiac surgery. They can be divided into type I (focal) lesions and type II lesions (more diffuse and often non-specific).

Types of injury

The incidence of type I injury is around 1–2% for CABG surgery but rises to about 5% for open heart surgery (especially on left-sided structures). Factors which increase the risk of stroke are: age >70 years, diabetes, previous strokes, prolonged bypass, recent MI, and peripheral vascular disease. Outcomes are very variable but they tend to be somewhat more favourable than if they had occurred in isolation.

Other focal lesions which are often overlooked include peripheral nerve injuries (especially the saphenous nerve from vein harvesting (3%), and brachial plexus injuries from sternal retraction (<1% although much more common in thoracic surgery). Ophthalmic injury may present with visual field defects and this is often very subtle. However, if formal testing of visual fields is conducted, then the incidence of defects may be as high as 25% in some studies, although the impact on the individual patient is usually low.

More diffuse neurological injury (type II) resulting in neurocognitive change is much more common. However, trying to quantify the true incidence is difficult as the changes are often subtle and are often only revealed using complex psychological testing. However, figures of the order of 35–80 % have been reported in several studies.

Aetiology of neurological injury

The aetiology of most neurological injury in the adult population is almost invariably embolic, whether it is particulate (atheromatous plaque rupture, platelet clumps, cholesterol fragments—especially implicated in ophthalmic injury) or gaseous (which is to some extent implicated in much of the neurocognitive change). The incidence of intracranial haemorrhage perioperatively is extremely low but, because of the use of anticoagulants for bypass, this tends to have very poor outcomes. Hypoperfusion injury from low-flow states is more common in the paediatric setting (where atheromatous disease is not a problem) and when deep-hypothermic circulatory arrest has been used.

Historically CPB was implicated in many strokes. It was hoped that off-pump coronary surgery would reduce the incidence of neurological injury, but the majority of surgeons still require to perform repeated side-clamping of the aorta in order to complete the top-end anastomoses. This may cause plaque rupture within the aorta, with mural thrombosis and embolization. Advances in CPB technology, the use of membrane oxygenators and the lower thrombogenicity of the circuits, means that the intraoperative risks are probably lower. However, a significant number of strokes occur postoperatively and the general inflammatory response that occurs may in itself be partly to blame.

Patients with symptomatic carotid artery disease which would warrant carotid endarterectomy may also require cardiac surgical procedures. In this circumstance it is often sensible to perform a combined procedure although the evidence for this is limited and conflicting.

Wound infections and breakdown

Surgical wound infections (particularly those related to the sternal wound) are a significant complication in cardiac surgery. The majority are superficial and require only antibiotic therapy (intravenous or oral as appropriate).

Deep sternal wound infections with osteomyelitis, sternal breakdown, and instability are uncommon (<1% of patients undergoing sternotomy) but significantly increase hospital stay, costs, and mortality. These patients often require extensive and repeated debridement, vacuum dressings and the most severe infections will require plastic surgical reconstruction either using pectoralis major or omental flaps.

Further reading

Change DCH & Bainbridge D (2008). Postoperative Cardiac Recovery and Outcomes. In JA Kaplan (ed), *Essentials of Cardiac Anaesthesia* (pp. 519–65). New York: Saunders.

14.7 Cardiac pacing

In principle, all pacing systems consist of some form of generator and a mechanism to deliver the current to the heart. These can either be completely internalized as permanent pacemakers (see section 1.10) or various components may remain outside the patient depending on the circumstance.

Current has to flow between two points in order to stimulate the heart. Older implanted systems used the box as one electrode and delivered the current along a unipolar lead to the heart; the current would then return to the box over a much larger area. This required higher currents than are now used and these devices were also more susceptible to interference. With the advent of bipolar leads (where the two electrodes are both placed distally on the pacing lead) the currents required are much lower and these systems are less susceptible to interference. Modern permanent leads are also shielded to help prevent electrical interference.

Temporary pacing systems are usually small battery operated devices. Epicardial pacing (generally used in the cardiac surgical setting) usually requires two separate wires placed in close proximity on the atrium or ventricle, and the potentials needed are similar to those for bipolar leads. Most temporary generators can use transvenous or epicardial wires as indicated.

In simple terms, a pacemaker can do one of two things: it can sense an intrinsic myocardial current ('sensing') or it can generate one ('pacing'). The different modes that are available with even the simplest temporary devices rely on these very basic principles.

The specific chambers that are paced will depend on the individual patient requirements, although almost invariably the ventricles are the primary chamber requiring pacing with the atria being secondary. Exactly how and when each chamber is paced (or not) depends upon the settings of the generator (see 'Pacing modes').

Indications for pacing procedures

There are multiple reasons why patients require pacing (see Box 14.8). It is now rare in the non-cardiac or non-emergency setting for patients to require temporary pacing purely to facilitate surgery. If a patient has a symptomatic bradyarrhythmia or symptomatic heart block then they probably require permanent pacing. Patients undergoing emergency surgery with symptomatic disease that would warrant pacing should be discussed with a cardiologist (ideally an electrophysiology specialist) but with the wide availability of transcutaneous pacing, the need for urgent temporary transvenous pacing is now rare.

Box 14.8 Indications for pacing

- Acute MI with asystole or symptomatic bradycardia or block
- Heart block: Mobitz II, third-degree, or trifascicular block
- Sinus node disease
- Facilitation of weaning from CPB
- Prevention of supraventricular tachyarrhythmias
- Hypertrophic obstructive cardiomyopathy
- Cardiac resynchronization therapy.

Cardiac resynchronization therapy (CRT) and biventricular pacing

CRT is often used as an essentially palliative procedure for end-stage heart failure. It should be noted that the biventricular pacing often used in CRT (when both right and left ventricles are paced) is different to dual-chamber pacing (which implies atrioventricular pacing). Biventricular pacing is usually combined with atrial pacing and therefore requires three leads: right atrial, right ventricular and left ventricular (the latter usually placed in the great cardiac vein via the coronary sinus) which can be seen on the CXR. These devices often have defibrillation modes also (see later).

Current delivery

There are several ways of delivering pacing current to a heart.

Transcutaneous external electrodes

External pads are placed across the chest, in a similar position to that for external cardioversion or defibrillation. Although very easy in concept, this technique is only used as an emergency bridging therapy as it has limited efficacy and is uncomfortable due to the higher currents required (50–90mA). Sedation may be required.

Transvenous pacing

Transvenous pacing is the mainstay of emergency pacing outside of a cardiac surgical setting. Wires are usually balloon-tipped and are inserted through an introducer sheath usually in the right internal jugular vein (although any venous access can be used) ideally using fluoroscopy. The tip should sit in the right ventricular apex but can be used wherever electrical capture is reliably achieved. They are not actively fixed to the endocardium (unlike permanent leads) and are thus susceptible to movement. They are normally bipolar.

Epicardial pacing

Surgically placed wires are the commonest form of pacing seen on a cardiac surgical ITU. The majority are required simply in order to facilitate weaning from CPB, although with some interventions, e.g. aortic valve replacement, the incidence of postoperative bradycardia and heart block is higher and wires are often placed prophylactically.

Two wires (one live, one neutral) are placed into the myocardium of the ventricle (usually the right) or tacked on to the right atrium (or indeed both atrium and ventricle). These are then externalized through the anterior chest or abdominal wall and connected to the external pacing generator. When they are no longer required they can simply be pulled out. However, these have a limited duration of use (7–10 days) before they start to become unreliable in terms of function and also become increasingly difficult to remove. Risks of removal always include atrial or ventricular myocardial damage leading to potential concealed bleeding, tamponade or sudden collapse. Postoperative decisions about the need for permanent pacing, commencement of formal anticoagulation if required and exact timing of temporary wire removal often require some careful thought.

Permanent pacing systems

Pacing wires are normally inserted via the left brachial or cephalic veins under X-ray guidance to rest in the right atrial appendage (atrial pacing), right ventricle (ventricular pacing) or coronary sinus (left ventricular pacing). The generator is implanted usually subcutaneously in the left subclavian region. The procedure is usually done under local anaesthesia with sedation. Modern permanent systems are highly sophisticated programmable devices and can include rate-responsive variable pacing, antitachycardia modes and defibrillation functions. They should be checked regularly and will need alteration before surgery due to the effects of diathermy and shivering (see 'Pacing modes').

Pacing modes

The functionality of pacemakers is described by a standardized NASPE (North American Society of Pacing and Electrophysiology) and BPEG (British Pacing and Electrophysiology Group) pacemaker code (see Table 1.6, section 1.10).

The intention is to try to get the paced heart to function as closely to normal sinus rhythm as possible. If the AV node is intact and the primary reason for pacing is to increase the rate (e.g. for weaning purposes) then a simple atrial mode may be all that is required (at least in the perioperative setting). More complex modes will be required depending on the pathophysiology.

Rate response functions are only really used in implantable devices and increase the heart rate in response to exercise by detecting changes in thoracic impedance and blood temperature. Rate modulated is the commonest mode although others exist.

The anti-tachycardia modes (fifth letter) are rarely used but can pace (P), shock (S) or both (Dual (D)).

The different modes available may be best understood by discussing some of the more commonly used modes and their indications. It should be remembered that many of the modes described are now available with temporary pacemakers as well as permanent systems.

VOO/AOO/DOO

These modes are the most simple available and also the most dangerous. There is no sensing and the pacemaker will pace the relevant chambers asynchronously. Although useful in the emergency situation, the risks of inappropriate ventricular pacing and the potential for R-on-T pacing leading to tachyarrhythmias or ventricular fibrillation are clear and these modes should only be used for short periods of time with immediate availability of defibrillation. These are sometimes used before and during chest closure when diathermy may cause interference with the sensing functions.

AAI

Here the atrium is paced and sensed via a single atrial lead (or two epicardial leads). Sensing an atrial beat leads to the inhibition of pacing. There will then follow a period when the device will wait for another beat to be sensed; if one is not sensed then the device will pace the atrium. This is most commonly used in PPMs for sick sinus syndrome or to facilitate weaning from bypass.

VVI

This is analogous to AAI except that it applies to the ventricle. It is commonly used when there is a low ventricular rate with an unreliable atrial component e.g. in atrial fibrillation. It is also commonly used as the initial mode to facilitate weaning from bypass. Ventricular sensing is enabled to prevent pacing on top of a normal complex, which can potentially cause an R-on-T response.

DDD

This is probably the commonest pacing mode used in permanent systems and is also widely used postoperatively. It obviously requires both atrial and ventricular leads. Sensing of a beat in either the atrial or ventricular leads will cause inhibition of the paced beat. If no ventricular response is sensed following an atrial beat, then the device will pace the ventricle.

Atrial or ventricular pacing?

The specific reasons why pacing of one chamber may be preferred over another will obviously vary with the individual. Much will depend on the presence of an intact atrio-ventricular node and the ability of either chamber to generate spontaneous beats (i.e. either atrial or ventricular complexes).

Sometimes, the reasons are more related to manipulation of the patient's physiology. Cardiac output is a function of heart rate and depending on the underlying electrical activity (e.g. slow AF) it may only be necessary to pace the ventricle in order to increase the rate and thus the cardiac output. Patients with diastolic dysfunction (e.g. those with left-ventricular hypertrophy secondary to aortic stenosis or hypertension) may well be initially weaned from CPB using ventricular pacing alone, but because these ventricles rely much more on the atrial component to achieve an optimum preload cardiac output in this case may be significantly improved by adding in atrial pacing.

These decisions are obviously tailored to the individual patient, and in the context of cardiac surgery, following discussion between the surgeon and anaesthetist.

In general it is preferable to pace the atria only and rely on intrinsic AVN conduction and ventricular response than to rely on complete reliance on pacing control. This is often actually what occurs with DDD pacing modes.

Sensitivity and pacing thresholds

The understanding of thresholds is important when trying to establish why a patient may or may not be appropriately pacing.

Pacing threshold

The pacing threshold is the current or voltage at which the relevant chamber achieves capture. This is usually of the order of about 1–2mV for a ventricle. The actual voltage used to pace the chamber is usually double the threshold to ensure capture. Pacing thresholds should be checked once or twice daily with temporary systems. Increasing pacing thresholds may be a sign of lead damage, lead displacement or fibrosis at the point of attachment.

Appropriate attempted pacing by a device may result in no myocardial depolarization if there is failure to capture which may relate to the pacing threshold being too low.

Sensitivity

If the device senses a voltage greater than the set sensitivity for that chamber, this is interpreted an intrinsic cardiac beat. Thus, the higher this voltage is set, the lower the sensitivity of the device. It is unusual to have to alter the sensitivity with most temporary devices.

However, an over sensing system may misinterpret a signal as an intrinsic beat and so fail to pace (even with good capture); an under sensing system may pace inappropriately potentially causing R-on-T events.

14.8 Principles of intra-aortic balloon counterpulsation and other assist devices

Intra-aortic balloon pump counter-pulsation

Intra-aortic balloon pump (IABP) counter-pulsation is the most widely used circulatory assist device for critically ill patients with cardiac failure. In addition to its use in cardiac surgery patients (typically to allow separation from CPB), it is increasingly being used on cardiac critical care units in patients following acute coronary syndromes or in patients with post-infarct ventricular septal defects or other complications awaiting surgical intervention (see Boxes 14.9 and 14.10). The device is usually inserted percutaneously via the femoral artery and is available in a range of sizes suitable for both adult and paediatric patients.

Principles

The balloon lies in the descending aorta distal to the left subclavian artery and proximal to but not occluding the renal arteries. It is inflated with helium (which allows easier rapid inflation of the balloon and possibly causes fewer embolic problems should the balloon leak or rupture) and is synchronized to inflate and deflate either with the ECG or arterial pressure waveform (sensed at the distal end of the catheter). The IABP deflates immediately prior to systole (actually during the phase of isovolumetric contraction) and inflates during diastole.

In essence, the device increases cardiac output without increasing myocardial oxygen demand.

The reduction in afterload in pre-systole facilitates ejection from the left ventricle (increasing cardiac output) thereby reducing left ventricular work.

Inflation during diastole increases the MAP and thereby coronary artery perfusion thus improving myocardial oxygen delivery.

Systolic blood pressure is usually increased, but sometimes falls. MAP is, however, augmented, and this is most important in terms of coronary perfusion.

Box 14.9 Indications for IABP insertion

- Weaning from CPB
- Cardiogenic shock (typically post MI)
- Post-infarct VSD or acute mitral regurgitation
- During or after failed angioplasty
- Refractory or unstable angina
- Cardiomyopathy
- Bridge to ventricular assist device placement or other intervention.

Insertion and placement

A device of appropriate size is chosen for the patient and the insertion distance estimated from the 3rd rib to the groin. Ideally the catheter should be inserted under fluoroscopic guidance, but in the perioperative or critical care situation, correct placement can be confirmed via TOE and subsequent CXR.

The catheter is inserted aseptically into the femoral artery using a Seldinger technique. Once placement is confirmed the patient will usually receive systemic heparinization to reduce the risk of thromboembolism.

Box 14.10 Contraindications to IABP placement

Absolute
- Severe aortic regurgitation
- Untreated aortic dissection
- End-stage cardiac disease with no prospect of recovery.

Relative
- Uncontrolled sepsis
- Abdominal aortic aneurysm (or aortic stent)
- Tachyarrhythmias
- Severe peripheral vascular disease.

Settings

The catheter is connected to a console that controls the delivery of fixed volumes of helium (20–50mL) to inflate the balloon within the aorta. The catheter has distal sampling ports that act as pressure transducers. The pump is synchronized either to the arterial pressure waveform or to the ECG.

The balloon is timed to inflate after the aortic valve closes (corresponding to the dicrotic notch on the arterial waveform or the peak of the T-wave) and deflate immediately before the aortic valve opens (corresponding to the point just before the upstroke on the arterial waveform or at the peak of the R-wave on the ECG). The augmentation ratio is typically 1:1 although lower ratios (1:2 or 1:3) can be used to assess underlying cardiac function when weaning is being considered.

The typical changes in the arterial waveform are illustrated in Fig. 14.2.

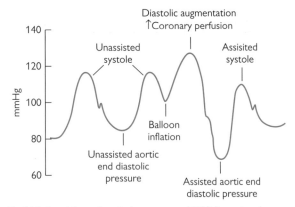

Fig. 14.2 Arterial waveform in the presence of IABP. Reproduced from Punit Ramrakha and Jonathan Hill, *Oxford Handbook of Cardiology*, Second edition, 2012, Figure 18.10, page 823, with permission from Oxford University Press.

A number of potentially important complications are associated with IABP insertion (see Box 14.11).

(see Box 14.11)

> ### Box 14.11 Complications of IABP insertion
>
> - Limb ischaemia
> - Thromboembolism
> - Malposition causing renal or cerebral ischaemia
> - Balloon entrapment
> - Balloon rupture and ensuing gas embolism
> - Infection
> - Haemolysis and thrombocytopenia
> - Compartment syndrome
> - Vascular injury—aneurysm, haematoma and bleeding
> - Aortic dissection.

Ventricular assist devices

Ventricular assist devices (VADs) have existed in some form for several decades. Their role has hitherto largely been limited to the management of cardiac failure in highly specialist cardiac centres (usually transplant centres), owing to their cost and complexity (Box 14.12).

> ### Box 14.12 Ventricular assist devices: indications and complications
>
> *Indications*
>
> - As a bridge to *transplantation*—usually for end-stage cardiomyopathy
> - As a bridge to *recovery*—e.g. following myocarditis or failure to wean from CPB
> - As a *destination therapy*—i.e. permanent systems where transplant is not an option (rare in the UK).
>
> *Complications*
>
> - Sepsis
> - Pump failure—mechanical/electrical failure, cannula displacement
> - Multiorgan failure
> - Thromboembolism—CVA and distal vascular ischaemia
> - Bleeding—from anastomotic sites or following anticoagulation
> - Insufficient pump output causing hypotension and syncope.

With newer technology and increased ease of use, there was hope that VAD applications might become more widespread. However, the numbers of patients for whom these devices are demonstrably truly beneficial remains relatively small. Many patients require protracted ITU and in-patient stays.

The devices may be extracorporeal or largely implanted internally. Amongst external devices, the pump unit is *ex-vivo* (e.g. the Thoratec HeartMate® XVE) and is similar to a miniature form of bypass system; indeed some systems use modified CPB pumps for this purpose. With internal devices, the pump is implanted in the body with tunnelled leads to the controller and power supply outside the body (e.g. the Jarvik 2000®).

Devices can deliver pulsatile or non-pulsatile flow depending on the system. Newer units allow ambulation and a degree of return to normal life albeit often with considerable limitations. Most devices can be used to support the left ventricle, right ventricle or both, and many newer units do not require formal systemic anticoagulation.

Further reading

Barnard M & Martin B (2010). Ventricular assist devices. In *Cardiac Anaesthesia* (pp. 287–96). Oxford: Oxford University Press.

Krishna M & Zacharowski K (2009). Principles of intra-aortic balloon pump counterpulsation. *CEACCP*, 9(1):24–8.

14.9 The adult patient with congenital heart disease and implications for anaesthesia

Over the last few decades survival into advanced adulthood with the more complex and serious forms of congenital heart disease (CHD) has increased and there will soon be more adults alive with CHD than children. The consequence of this is that the non-specialist anaesthetist is likely to be exposed to this complex spectrum of patients. They may present at a local hospital for emergency or elective surgery (including on the labour ward), or as a result of admission to a general intensive care unit. There are also those patients who may present *de novo* in adulthood with previously undiagnosed disease.

It is important that all general anaesthetists have a basic understanding of congenital cardiac disease, the implications these conditions have for the patient undergoing general anaesthesia and, perhaps most importantly, when the risks are such that discussion or referral to a specialist unit may be more appropriate.

General approach

A multidisciplinary team including experts in CHD should make decisions about whether and where an individual 'GUCH' patient should undergo non-cardiac surgery. Specialist anaesthetic input should inform the process where necessary. In the urgent situation this may not be possible but efforts should be made to discuss the case with regional centres.

Broadly, there are a number of steps to consider:

- Establishing the structural lesion(s) present and whether or not these have been corrected in any way.
- Functional assessment both on a global scale and specifically looking at the heart and the pulmonary and systemic circulations.
- Urgency and complexity of the illness/surgical procedure to be performed and the proximity and feasibility of timely transfer to the nearest specialist centre.
- Consideration of the effects of anaesthesia on the individual's circulation (especially the effects of positive pressure ventilation and reduction in systemic afterload).
- Availability of high dependency care postoperatively.

Classification

As discussed in section 1.19, CHD encompasses a wide range of potential pathologies. Most classification systems are based on anatomical definitions.

Patients who have undergone surgery often still have some form of residual functional deficit (even if there is anatomical correction of their condition). A working classification of CHD is presented in Table 14.1.

Table 14.1 A working classification of CHD from the GUCH perspective		
Simple	Intermediate	Complex
Corrected or isolated ASD Corrected or small VSD Corrected patent ductus (PDA) Mild or isolated mitral, aortic or pulmonary valve disease	Coarctation Tetralogy of Fallot Ebstein's anomaly Moderate-to-severe pulmonary valve disease Uncorrected PDA or ASD Abnormal pulmonary venous drainage Right or left ventricular outflow tract obstruction (VOTO)	Presence of cyanosis Eisenmenger's syndrome Single ventricle Mitral/pulmonary/ tricuspid atresia Fontan circulation Transposition of great vessels/truncus arteriosus

Assessment

A thorough history and examination should be undertaken. Patients with CHD will often have extensive records and advanced investigations including left and right heart catheter studies, ECHO studies, or other imaging. If these are not readily available or there is no recent correspondence from tertiary centres, then the minimum investigation required preoperatively should be a transthoracic echo to establish the underlying structural and functional status (ideally performed by someone with expertise in congenital cardiac disease). It may be beneficial in the perioperative setting to draw a diagram of the anatomy and flow directions. Beyond this, there are some key interlinked factors that can have a significant impact and must be considered.

Cyanosis

The presence of cyanosis is sometimes used to help classify CHD. Its impact on function is significant; these patients have more comorbidities and have higher perioperative risk. Cyanosis is the result of right-to-left shunting or mixing of systemic and pulmonary venous blood in a single common chamber. Estimation of the pulmonary to systemic flow ratio is important in trying to determine the severity of the shunt.

The long-term consequences of chronic cyanosis are significant and can further reduce peripheral oxygen delivery:

- Polycythaemia (raised haematocrit and hyperviscosity)
- Neurocognitive change and impaired neurological function
- Renal impairment
- Paradoxical embolus and brain abscess
- Gallstones as a result of increased haemoglobin turnover.

Factors that can affect the severity of the cyanosis include alterations in pulmonary blood flow and PVR, low systemic arterial pressure and SVR, hypercapnia, acidosis, and raised lactate (see sections 1.18 and 2.6).

Pulmonary circulation

Many patients with CHD have a degree of pulmonary hypertension (PHT) often as a result of increased flow through the pulmonary artery. This is usually longstanding and frequently irreversible (even if the primary lesion is corrected). The consequence of this is that there is usually a variable amount of right ventricular (RV) dilatation, RV failure, and tricuspid regurgitation.

Increases in pulmonary artery pressure (PAP) may cause left-to-right shunts to reverse (the Eisenmenger circulation) or pre-existing right-to-left shunts to worsen. Such changes cause cyanosis to develop or worsen.

Complex variations in pulmonary blood flow, including Blalock–Taussig shunts, variants of the Fontan circulation, or right ventricular outflow tract obstruction (RVOTO) are potentially affected by increases in PVR. This has significant implications for anaesthesia and positive pressure ventilation.

Ventricular function

Quantification of both LV and RV function is vital in these patients. RV failure is more common. The right ventricle does not normally hypertrophy in the face of increased afterload; instead it tends to dilate leading to failure and tricuspid regurgitation.

It is also important to consider which morphological (left or right) ventricle is supporting the pulmonary and systemic circulations or indeed whether there is only a single ventricle supporting both. These patients are rare but complex and should preferably be referred to regional centres.

Comorbidities

Other comorbidities that may be present include:

Arrhythmias

Patients with CHD are more likely to develop arrhythmias (especially atrial, although there are associations with Wolff–Parkinson–White syndrome (Ebstein's anomaly)). Heart block and bradyarrhythmias may also exist.

Respiratory

The effects on PAP predominate, but CHD patients have increased respiratory problems including reduced compliance (often associated with kyphoscoliosis), mass effects from enlarged cardiac chambers compressing lung lobes, phrenic nerve injury, and haemoptysis.

Haematological changes

Other than changes in haematocrit, many patients have a degree of coagulopathy including vWF abnormalities, and many require anticoagulation.

Acquired cardiac disease

The increasing chronological age of grown-up patients with CHD means it is important to assess for the presence of acquired cardiac disease, notably ischaemic heart disease.

Neurological

Central neurological damage may occur as a result of paradoxical emboli causing cerebral infarcts or abscesses. Scarring from these events may also cause seizures. There are often associated psychosocial and developmental limitations as a result of the disease itself or because of associated disease or syndromes (for example, in Down's syndrome).

Intrathoracic nerve injuries may also exist including the vagus, phrenic and recurrent laryngeal nerves, often as a result of previous surgery.

Postoperative care

In general, most patients with CHD are likely to need a period of time in a high dependency unit following surgery. The duration of stay may be protracted with an increased chance of multisystem failure. It is probably shrewd to discuss all cases with CHD requiring time on a non-specialist unit with local centres of expertise (ideally before surgery if at all possible).

Specific syndromes and their implications for anaesthesia

Most patients with 'simple' CHD that has been corrected can probably be treated as normal or as for any other adult with underlying valvular disease (considering relevant factors such as anticoagulation and functional capacity).

Patients with more complex disease are probably best managed in centres with advanced experience in dealing with adults with CHD. However, in the urgent or emergency situation it often falls to a non-expert to cope.

General principles

- Strict asepsis with all invasive procedures (because of the much greater risk of endocarditis in patients with CHD).
- Meticulous attention to removing air bubbles from all venous lines (because of the potential for residual ASDs, VSDs, or other right-to-left shunts).
- Consider placement of external defibrillator pads pre-induction (especially if known to be pro-arrhythmic or systemically unwell).

- Cautious and slow IV induction (as circulation times are often prolonged).
- Close attention to electrolytes and use of short central venous catheters (and caution with the wires during insertion) because of the risk of provoking arrhythmias.
- Careful control of $PaCO_2$ and consideration of the effects of positive pressure ventilation on the pulmonary circulation.
- Careful balance of systemic and pulmonary circulations if shunting is present.
- Intra-operative TOE may be of benefit if feasible.
- Good analgesia is vital. Even in cyanotic patients the ventilatory response to hypercarbia is preserved.

Atrial septal defects

Adult patients may present *de novo* with previously undiagnosed ASDs. The majority (70%) are secundum defects with a defect in the fossa ovalis and usually left-to-right shunting (Note: a patent foramen ovale (PFO) is a failure of the atrial flap to endothelialize following closure at birth and is not a true deficit in the fossa ovalis. It is rarely associated with any shunt and is probably very common—it is a coincidental finding in 25% of postmortem examinations). Sinus venosus defects involve the superior part of the inter-atrial septum and are often associated with anomalous pulmonary venous drainage. Primum defects are uncommon and often associated with atrioventricular canal (endocardial cushion) defects. This latter condition is more prevalent in Down's syndrome.

Patients become more symptomatic with increasing age (and the associated decrease in left ventricular compliance), on exertion or in conditions that cause the left atrial pressure to rise. Older individuals with previously undiagnosed ASDs may present with established PHT. The majority of secundum defects can now be closed percutaneously with specific closure devices (although this may not lead to resolution of the PHT).

In uncomplicated cases, the main concern for the anaesthetist is avoidance of increased PVR and paradoxical embolus.

Ebstein's anomaly

This abnormality of the tricuspid valve (TV) is frequently associated with a PFO or secundum ASD. There is dyplasia of the TV (usually the septal leaflet) with displacement of the valve towards the RV apex. There is a tendency for the right atrium (RA) to be extremely large with a relatively small RV. The increase in RA pressure may cause cyanosis as a result of right-to-left shunting across the ASD. Many of these patients (some 25–30%) develop supraventricular tachyarrhythmias. This is a particular concern as these patients have a higher incidence of aberrant Wolff–Parkinson–White pathways. They also have a higher incidence of conduction defects so may present with bradycardias or varying degrees of heart block.

Clearly the increased risk of supraventricular and potential rapid ventricular response is the key consideration for non-specialists. Care with Seldinger wires and central venous catheters, and the prompt and aggressive treatment of any tachyarrhythmias (including direct current cardioversion) is vital as even SVTs are poorly tolerated.

Ventricular septal defects

Uncorrected isolated VSDs in adults are uncommon. The majority will be small although the potential for increased PAP exists and larger shunts will usually present in adulthood with Eisenmenger's syndrome. Non-Eisenmenger patients are considerably more stable. (Patients who develop a VSD following acute myocardial infarction are significantly more complex and have a much poorer prognosis.)

The anaesthetic implications are similar to those for an ASD, although paradoxical embolus is much less common. Patients with VSDs are at much increased risk of endocarditis compared with other CHD.

Patent ductus arteriosus

As with other conditions that cause increases in pulmonary flow, the long term issues with PDA in adults is pulmonary hypertension and volume overload of the heart.

Unrepaired these patients have a high mortality with about 33% dying by the age of 40 and two-thirds by the age of 60. As with VSDs, they are at significantly increased risk of endocarditis even compared with other forms of CHD. Many lesions can be closed percutaneously.

Eisenmenger's syndrome

Eisenmenger's syndrome or circulation is the potential end point of many of the previous conditions with an uncorrected, large left-to-right shunt causing increased pulmonary arterial flow. With time the increased flow causes irreversible changes in the pulmonary vasculature such that the PVR is so high that flow across the shunt lesion reverses. Cyanosis develops dependent on the degree of shunt. The syndrome can be precipitated by acute increases in PVR as a result of intercurrent infection, pulmonary embolus or even as a result of increased airway pressures in patients undergoing positive pressure ventilation; this may return to normal with restitution of the non-pathological state.

Prolonged survival with Eisenmenger's is possible, even from childhood, but patients are at risk of sudden cardiac death and overall mortality increases with the duration of the syndrome. These patients display many of the side effects of chronic cyanosis.

Anaesthesia is extremely high risk in this population. Any reduction in the SVR usually worsens both the shunt and cyanosis. The PVR is usually considered fixed and has no response to pulmonary vasodilators. Factors that increase the PVR should be avoided. These include hypothermia, hypoxia, hypercarbia, acidosis, and hypovolaemia. The effect of α-agonists on the pulmonary vasculature may worsen the PVR; however, the effect exerted by these agents on the SVR is greater, and reduces the shunt: this outweighs the negative impact on the PVR.

Generally, unless the surgical condition can be managed with local anaesthesia alone (with the incumbent risks of anticoagulation which is almost universal in these patients) then these patients are best managed in centres of expertise.

Transposition of the great arteries (TGA)

TGA is the abnormal connection of the great arteries to the ventricles: the pulmonary artery arises from the anatomical left ventricle (which receives oxygenated blood from the pulmonary veins via the left atrium); the aorta (including the coronary arteries) arises from the right ventricle and receives deoxygenated blood from the venae cavae via the right atrium. There may be other abnormalities including VSDs or abnormalities of the coronary arteries.

Congenitally corrected TGA is a variant where the flow of deoxygenated and oxygenated blood is normal in terms of great vessel outflow, but there is discordance with the anatomical right and left ventricles: the pulmonary circulation is supported by a morphological left ventricle and the systemic circulation is supported by a morphological right ventricle.

Adults who present with TGA will almost certainly have had surgery in childhood, unless congenitally corrected. The exact nature of the surgery will depend on their age and thus the era in which they were born. Atrial switch procedures (Mustard and Senning) were the standard until the mid-1980s. These procedures involved atrial baffles to redirect flow appropriately; however, the systemic circulation remains supported by a morphological right ventricle which tends to lead to heart failure. Later complications include baffle leaks (leading to cyanosis) and

there is also an increased incidence of arrhythmia and sudden death. Patients who underwent atrial switch procedures are now uncommon and should be managed in specialized centres.

In recent years, the arterial switch has taken over. The great arteries are transected and joined to their anatomically appropriate ventricles along with reimplantation of the coronary arteries. This procedure has better outcomes (90% survival at 10 years) than the atrial switch although truly long-term figures are not yet established.

Those individuals with congenital corrected TGA or who have had an uncomplicated arterial switch (in the absence of coexistent CHD) may be treated as normal; this should be assessed on a case-by-case basis. Those with other lesions or degeneration of the primary repair are usually complicated and should be referred to specialist centres.

Tetralogy of Fallot

This is the commonest form of cyanotic heart disease seen in adults. It consists of RV outflow tract obstruction (usually subvalvular), subsequent RV hypertrophy (which develops in utero), a large VSD with the aorta overriding the VSD such that flow across the VSD can often be bi-directional causing cyanosis if there is a reduction in SVR.

The majority of adults will have had some form of surgery, usually to close the VSD and to relieve the pulmonary outflow tract obstruction. They may require on-going revision of leaks and correction of pulmonary regurgitation.

Implications for the non-specialist include the risk of arrhythmias (often ventricular), pulmonary regurgitation and recurrent RV outflow tract obstruction and RV failure. As with other complex CHD, these individuals are usually best managed by specialist centres.

The single ventricle and the Fontan circulation

Single-ventricle patients are rare. The dominant ventricle may be morphologically left or right but usually has inflow from both atria, either because of atresia of one or other atrioventricular valves or because of the so-called double-inlet ventricle where both atrioventricular valves have the majority of their connection to one ventricle. This leads to mixing of pulmonary and systemic blood potentially causing cyanosis, the severity of which varies depending on the degree of pulmonary outflow tract obstruction.

The Fontan circulation is the culmination of a number of ways of palliating patients with a single ventricle. The modern Fontan comprises a total cavopulmonary connection (TCPC) where the superior and inferior venae cavae are connected to the right pulmonary artery either directly or via conduits, although other variants may still present. Thus, there is maintenance of 'normal' circulation but with entirely *passive* flow on the right side. This leads to a unique physiology and set of problems for the anaesthetist. As with other CHD many patients are now surviving to adulthood and are presenting for non-cardiac surgery.

Patients with Fontan physiology are at particular risk of thrombosis (especially atrial), supraventricular arrhythmias, and various protein-losing states, which have a poor long-term prognosis. The 'failing Fontan' (i.e. those with limited exercise tolerance) are a particularly worrying group of patients.

Anaesthesia in these patients is extremely complex and is usually best performed in expert centres. A number of principles require consideration:

- Maintenance of preload.
- Avoidance of hypercarbia, acidosis, and hypoxia.
- Avoidance of changes in PVR.
- Use of spontaneous ventilation is attractive; however, this may lead to hypercarbia. If positive pressure ventilation is used PEEP (<5cmH$_2$O) may help to preserve the functional

residual capacity (reducing PVR) without significant effects on cardiac output or right-sided flow.

- Regional anaesthesia and neuraxial techniques may be beneficial if feasible.
- High incidence of arrhythmias which should be aggressively managed.

Pregnancy and congenital heart disease

Pregnant women with CHD may be particularly complex, especially around the time of delivery. Specific risks include:

- Recurrent miscarriages.
- Worsening heart failure (often as a result of the cardiovascular changes associated with pregnancy).
- Issues surrounding use of anticoagulants and thrombotic states.
- Risk of endocarditis.
- The extra stresses of labour and delivery.

Those at particular risk include women with Eisenmenger's syndrome (or any cyanotic state), pulmonary hypertension, LV outflow tract obstruction and impaired ventricular function. Many of those who would present too high a risk are counselled against pregnancy.

Some patients only come to the attention of the anaesthetist late in pregnancy (i.e. in the 3rd trimester or towards the time of delivery) by which time many of the high-risk changes in physiology have occurred. As such, those who have tolerated these are probably low risk and may deliver normally.

Operative delivery is not usually required solely for maternal cardiac indications. Epidural analgesia is often beneficial, especially in the early stages of labour. The effects of increased intrathoracic pressure during the second stage of labour may have detrimental effects on the pulmonary blood flow in certain patients and may require closer observation in this group (e.g. those with PHT). Blood loss and auto-transfusion around the third stage of labour or during operative delivery may precipitate cardiovascular collapse or heart failure. Also the use of oxytocin may precipitate a pulmonary hypertensive crisis or significant increases in SVR causing right or left ventricular failure.

Management of these potentially complex patients should involve obstetricians, cardiologists, and anaesthetists with sub-speciality interests in these patients. See section 24.3.

Further reading

Ashley E, Barnard M, & Cordery. (2005). Adult congenital heart disease and management on the ICU. *Care Crit Ill*, 21(3):83–6.

Diller G-P & Gatzoulis MA (2007). Pulmonary vascular disease in adults with congenital heart disease. *Circulation*, 115(8):1039–50. doi:10.1161/CIRCULATIONAHA.105.592386.

Nanda S, Nelson-Piercy C, & Mackillop L (2012). Cardiac disease in pregnancy. *Clin Med*, 12(6):553–60.

Russell IA, Rouine-Rapp K., Stratmann G, *et al.* (2006). Congenital heart disease in the adult: a review with internet-accessible transesophageal echocardiographic images. *Anesthes Analg*, 102(3):694–723. doi:10.1213/01.ane.0000197871.30775.2a.

Chapter 15

Thoracic anaesthesia

297

15.1 Preoperative assessment in thoracic surgery

Advances in anaesthetic management, diagnostic and surgical techniques, and perioperative care have expanded the envelope of patients with lung cancer now considered to be 'operable'.

The term 'resectability' is determined by the anatomical stage of the tumour, whereas 'operability' is dependent on the extent of the procedure and the physiological status of the patient.

Assessment of lung function

Evaluation of lung function remains the most important aspect of preoperative assessment. It establishes the risk of operative mortality and impact of lung resection on quality of life, especially in relation to acceptable post-resection dyspnoea.

Dynamic lung volumes
The most valid test for post-thoracotomy respiratory complications is the predicted postoperative forced expiratory volume in 1sec (ppo FEV$_1$), which is calculated as:

$$\text{ppo FEV}_1 = \text{Pre-op FEV}_1 \times \% \text{ remaining lung}$$

The right upper and middle lobes combined are approximately equivalent to each of the other three lobes with the right lung 10% larger than the left lung. Some consideration needs to be made about the preoperative contribution of the lobes to be resected, as many are often functionally inactive and so do not contribute to the pre-op FEV$_1$. Once established, the ppo FEV$_1$ can be used to risk stratify patients as follows:

- Low risk = >40% ppo FEV$_1$
- Moderate risk = 30–40% ppo FEV$_1$
- High risk = <30% ppo FEV$_1$.

Transfer factor (TL$_{CO}$)
Carbon monoxide transfer factor (TL$_{CO}$) is the most useful test for the gas exchange of lung and it correlates with the total functional surface area of alveolar–capillary interface. The 2010 British Thoracic Society guidelines recommend measurement of lung TL$_{CO}$ in all patients regardless of spirometric values. An analogous ppo TL$_{CO}$ can be estimated:

- Low risk = >40% ppo TL$_{CO}$
- Moderate to high risk = <40% ppoTL$_{CO}$.

Split lung function tests
Other techniques have been used to predict postoperative lung function including spirometry, quantitative ventilation and perfusion scintigraphy (V/Q scanning). Ventilation scintigraphy or perfusion scintigraphy should be considered in any patient who has ppo FEV$_1$ <40% to help predict postoperative lung function particularly in pneumonectomy patients and for postoperative care planning.

CT or MRI
Quantitative CT scanning has been reported to be simpler and more accurate in the prediction of postoperative FEV$_1$ in patients undergoing pulmonary resection. Dynamic perfusion MRI currently has the best reported test performance compared with quantitative CT and perfusion SPECT and may be at least as accurate as quantitative CT. It is not currently widely used, although almost all patients presenting for lung resection will have had CT assessment of their tumour for staging.

Exercise testing
Formal assessment of cardiopulmonary interaction may include:

Stair climbing
This is a traditional, simple, and still extremely useful test in ambulatory patients. Ability to climb two or more flights is associated with decreased mortality and correlates well with CPET.

6-minute walk test
The 6MWT is a useful measure of functional capacity targeted at people with moderate to severe lung disease. The objective of this test is to see how far a patient can walk in 6min. Good performance on the 6MWT has been associated with improved surgical outcomes as well as predictors of morbidity and mortality in patients with COPD and pulmonary hypertension. The 6MWT does not determine peak oxygen uptake, the cause of dyspnoea on exertion, or evaluate the causes or mechanism of exercise limitation. The information provided by a 6MWT should be used to complement CPET.

Shuttle walk test
This is determined as the total distance covered by walking between two cones 10m apart at a pace that is progressively increased. Its advantage is that it shows better correlation with peak oxygen uptake than the 6MWT. Disadvantages include less widespread use and more potential for cardiovascular problems. The British Thoracic Society recommends the shuttle walk test as functional assessment in patients with moderate to high risk of postoperative dyspnoea using a distance walked of above 400m as a cut off for good function.

Cardiopulmonary exercise testing (see section 1.2)
Formal CPET, usually involving cycling against a progressively increasing resistance, allows calculation of the maximum oxygen consumption (Vo$_2$ max) and the anaerobic threshold (AT). It is becoming increasingly available. The Vo$_2$ max is the most valid predictor of post thoracotomy outcome:

- Low risk = >20mL/kg/min
- Moderate risk = 15–20mL/kg/min
- High risk = <15mL/kg/min.

Postoperative quality of life/dyspnoea
Lung cancer surgery is associated with a greater impact on quality of life scores compared with other chronic diseases or cancers, and this may persist for >5 years. Pneumonectomy is associated with a poorer quality of life for a longer duration compared with lobectomy.

Quality of life after surgery may be more related to cardiopulmonary fitness, and pulmonary function assessment alone is a poor predictor of patients' perceptions of physical disruptions in day-to-day activities. As discrepancies may exist between, on the one hand, patients' perceptions about their residual physical and emotional status, and on the other, objective functional measures, lung function tests and exercise tests cannot be taken as sole surrogates for quality of life evaluation. A quality of life instrument should always be used. A risk assessment algorithm for postoperative dyspnoea is shown in Fig. 15.1.

Other aspects of risk

Cardiovascular morbidity
This is discussed in detail in sections 1.1–1.5 and the same principles should be applied in thoracic surgical patients as in patients undergoing other major non-cardiac surgery.

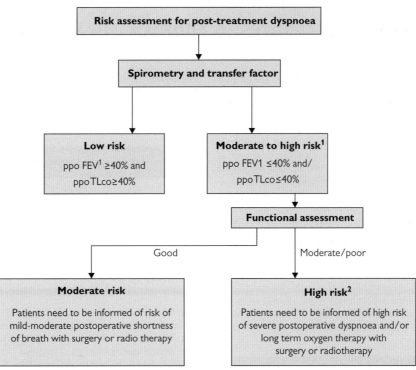

Fig. 15.1 Risk assessment algorithm for postoperative dyspnoea. Reproduced from *Thorax*, E Lim et al., 'Guidelines on the radical management of patients with lung cancer', 65, Suppl 3, copyright 2010, with permission from BMJ Publishing Group Ltd and the British Thoracic Society.

All thoracic surgery constitutes 'high-risk' surgery for the purposes of risk stratification according to the revised cardiac risk index.

Age
In patients >80 years, the rate of respiratory complications (40%) is double that expected in a younger population and the rate of cardiac complication (40%), particularly arrhythmias, is nearly threefold. The mortality from pneumonectomy (22% in patients >70 years), particularly right pneumonectomy, is excessive.

Renal dysfunction
Renal dysfunction after pulmonary resection surgery is associated with a high incidence of mortality. The factors associated with high risk of renal impairment are given in Box 15.1.

Smoking
Smoking should be discontinued for at least 6–8 weeks before surgery to decrease secretions and to reduce pulmonary complications. Both gaseous and particulate phases of cigarette smoke can deplete glutathione and vitamin C and may promote oxidative injury to tissues. Unfortunately, many patients will not quit smoking for as little as 24h. Even this has theoretical beneficial effects on the oxygen carrying capacity of haemoglobin; acute inhalation of cigarette smoke releases carbon monoxide, which increases carboxyhaemoglobin levels, nitric oxide, and nitrogen dioxide which can lead to formation of methaemoglobin.

Box 15.1 Factors associated with increased risk of post-thoracotomy renal impairment

- Previous history of renal impairment
- Current diuretic therapy
- Pneumonectomy
- Postoperative infection
- Blood loss requiring transfusion.

Chronic obstructive pulmonary disease
COPD frequently coexists with surgical pathology of the chest. The severity of COPD is graded according to spirometry data (see Table 15.1).

Table 15.1 Severity of COPD according to FEV_1 and FVC

Severity	Post-bronchodilator FEV_1 : :FVC	% predicted FEV_1
At risk	> 0.7	≥ 80
Mild	≤ 0.7	≥ 80
Moderate	≤ 0.7	50–80
Severe	≤ 0.7	30–50
Very severe	≤ 0.7	< 30

Reproduced from the *Global Strategy for the Diagnosis, Management and Prevention of COPD, 2013*, copyright Global initiative for chronic Obstructive Lung Disease (GOLD), with permission.

Preoperative interventions in patients with COPD aimed at correcting hypoxemia, relieving bronchospasm, mobilizing and reducing secretions, and treating infections may decrease the incidence of postoperative pulmonary complications.

Cor pulmonale occurs in 40% of adult COPD patients with FEV_1 <1L and in 70% with FEV_1 <0.6L. Patients for pneumonectomy with ppo FEV_1 <40% should have transthoracic echocardiography to assess right heart function. Elevated right heart and PAP places such patients in a very high-risk group.

Further reading
Lim E, Baldwin D, Beckles M, *et al.* (2010). Guidelines on the radical management of patients with lung cancer. *Thorax*, 65(Suppl 3):iii1–ii27. doi:10.1136/thx.2010.145938.

15.2 Common procedures in thoracic surgery

The emphasis of thoracic surgery underwent a major change during the second half of the 20th century. Previously, the majority of surgery related to the treatment of tuberculosis and its complications, whereas now most work relates to the diagnosis and treatment of lung cancer and other intrathoracic tumours.

In broad terms, thoracic surgery encompasses surgery on the *lungs* (either as an open procedure via thoracotomy or as video-assisted thoracoscopic surgery (VATS)), and surgery of the *mediastinum and main airways*, or of *other intrathoracic structures* (oesophagus, sympathetic chain).

Rigid bronchoscopy as a diagnostic and therapeutic measure has become less common with the advent of flexible fibreoptic bronchoscopy, but presents itself as a specific anaesthetic challenge.

Thoracotomy

The management of the patient presenting for formal anterolateral thoracotomy remains one of the more challenging cases for an anaesthetist. Common indications for thoracotomy are listed in Box 15.2.

Box 15.2 Major indications for thoracotomy

- Lung resection (including lobectomy, pneumonectomy, diagnostic tissue sampling)
- Drainage and decortication of empyema
- Repair of bronchopleural fistula
- Oesophagectomy and other surgery of the oesophagus
- Radical treatment for recurrent pneumothorax (including resection of bullous disease)
- Lung volume reduction surgery (LVRS)
- Single lung transplantation
- Traumatic lung or diaphragmatic injury
- Occasionally for access to the heart or to the pericardium
- Anterior approach to the thoracic spine for scoliosis surgery
- Open thoracic sympathectomy
- Resection of hydatid cysts.

Some of these procedures will be undertaken by non-thoracic surgeons and may indeed occur in non-thoracic surgical centres. Posterior thoracotomies are still occasionally undertaken if the anatomical location of the lesion is suitable for this approach. In general, however, the surgical access is not as good and the procedure is rarely performed.

The anaesthetic management of all patients undergoing thoracotomy is often very similar, although the specific needs for invasive monitoring and the immediate postoperative destination of these patients is more dependent on the procedure than on the anaesthesia per se.

Important anaesthetic concerns obviously arise in the context of one-lung ventilation (OLV):

Assessment of difficult endobronchial intubation or lung isolation

The most useful predictor of difficult endobronchial intubation is the CXR. Distal airway problems not detected by plain CXR film may be seen on chest CT scans. Formal airway assessment is often unhelpful in predicting difficult endobronchial intubation.

Prediction of hypoxia risk during one-lung ventilation

It is sometimes possible to identify patients who are most at risk for desaturation during OLV for thoracic surgery. The factors that correlate with desaturation during OLV are listed in Box 15.3.

The practicalities of OLV are described in detail in section 15.3.

Box 15.3 Factors that correlate with an increased risk of desaturation during OLV

- High percentage of ventilation (V) or perfusion (Q) to the operative lung on preoperative V/Q scan.
- Poor PaO_2 during two-lung ventilation, particularly in lateral position intraoperatively.
- Right sided surgery.

Video-assisted thoracoscopic surgery

Minimally invasive surgery has gained rapidly in popularity over the last two decades. The ability to perform intrathoracic procedures using minimally invasive techniques has clear advantages over those requiring open thoracotomy.

Many procedures can be performed using single- or two-port techniques, although often one of these incisions may be extended to a mini-thoracotomy without having huge impact on postoperative complications.

In common with other forms of minimally invasive surgery, the applications are ever increasing, and more complex procedures, including lobectomies, are now being performed using VATS techniques (Box 15.4). The potential advantages (decreased wound size, a lesser physiological insult, reduced analgesia requirements, reduced complication rates and a shorter hospital stay) are perhaps offset slightly by the increased duration of the procedure although this is often only marginal.

Some thoracoscopic procedures are performed by non-thoracic surgeons (e.g. thoracoscopic sympathectomy, which is traditionally the province of the vascular surgeon).

Box 15.4 Typical procedures amenable to VATS technique

- Diagnostic wedge resections of lung or other tissue (including lymph node sampling for biopsy)
- Drainage of pleural effusions and pleurodesis
- Abrasion pleurodesis for recurrent pneumothorax
- Bullectomy
- Adhesiolysis
- Simple drainage and decortication of early empyema
- Thoracoscopic sympathectomy (sometimes bilateral)
- Lobectomy in selected patients
- Pericardial window formation
- Minimally invasive mitral valve surgery (MIMS).

Some VATS procedures may ultimately require formal thoracotomy and this has to be taken into consideration when assessing the patient and also when planning immediate postoperative discharge location. Whilst a critical care facility would not routinely be required for the majority of VATS procedures, the patient's comorbidities, the extent of the surgery, and the possible need for conversion to an open procedure should all be taken into account when scheduling these cases.

Surgery on the mediastinum

Surgery on the anterior mediastinum is performed for a variety of different reasons, some of them complex and unusual. Again, as a result of the different structures present, some mediastinal surgery is performed by non-thoracic surgeons.

The commonest intervention is *mediastinoscopy*, usually performed to derive a tissue diagnosis on anterior mediastinal masses, including lymph nodes. It is possibly the least invasive of all thoracic surgical procedures but also potentially the most dangerous. The proximity of the aortic arch to the masses and nodes being sampled should never be underestimated and there should always be the facility to convert to an immediate sternotomy should the great vessels be damaged or if there is uncontrollable haemorrhage.

Open resection of mediastinal tumours, including some retrosternal thyroid masses, thymic tumours, thymectomy for myasthenia gravis, and other, often congenital lesions, requires a formal median sternotomy. In general, these patients have fewer of the comorbidities seen in cardiac surgical patients, and although immediate postoperative care should probably be in a critical care facility, the duration of the ICU stay and complication rates are much lower than for patients undergoing cardiac surgery.

Procedures on the lower trachea and carina are often very complex, and may require input form thoracic surgeons, ENT specialists, and sometimes chest physicians. Open approaches to these structures usually require thoracotomy or median sternotomy and may require cardiopulmonary bypass. They are uncommon and each case should be discussed at a multidisciplinary team meeting to agree on the surgical plan, anaesthetic plan, and postoperative care process.

The posterior mediastinum contains the oesophagus and descending aorta. Oesophageal surgery including resection and reconstruction is usually performed via anterolateral thoracotomy either alone or in combination with cervical or midline laparotomy incisions. OLV and good postoperative analgesia are cornerstones of management (see section 13.1).

Descending thoracic aortic surgery is commonly performed by vascular surgeons in regional centres, or increasingly by interventional radiologists in combination with vascular and cardiac surgeons. Such procedures are complex and require a multidisciplinary team approach.

Bronchoscopy and associated procedures

With the advent of fibreoptic bronchoscopy, rigid bronchoscopy is now less commonly performed, at least for diagnostic procedures. A number of indications remain, however, and bring with them specific requirements for anaesthesia.

Most commonly, rigid bronchoscopy is performed prior to lung resection to assess the position of the tumour, especially if the tumour is close to the main bronchi. It is sometimes used to perform trans-tracheal biopsies of mass lesions in the mediastinum.

Therapeutic rigid bronchoscopy is performed for retrieval of foreign bodies, and for formal lavage and treatment of retained secretions (especially with distal airway collapse or consolidation).

Therapeutic bronchoscopy for laser treatment of tracheal or endobronchial tumours (that are often not suitable for surgical intervention for a variety of reasons) is becoming increasingly used, albeit often for palliative reasons. These cases often involve thoracic surgeons, ENT surgeons, and/or chest physicians working together. They carry a risk of major airway haemorrhage, pneumomediastinum, and pneumothorax and are usually performed in super-specialist centres.

Rigid bronchoscopic techniques are associated with all the difficulties of the shared airway and (usually) the inability to provide inhalational anaesthesia and positive pressure ventilation. When coupled with laser therapy to tumours, then the additional risks of laser surgery are superimposed (see sections 11.9 and 15.4).

15.3 One-lung ventilation in thoracic surgery

Intentional collapse of the lung on the operative side facilitates most thoracic procedures but complicates anaesthetic management (see Box 15.5 for indications). The collapsed lung continues to be perfused whilst no longer ventilated, and the patient develops a right-to-left intrapulmonary shunt.

Box 15.5 Indications for one-lung ventilation

- Patient related:
  - To confine infection to one lung
  - To confine bleeding to one lung
  - To separate ventilation to each lung
- Bronchopleural fistula:
  - Tracheobronchial disruption
  - Large lung cyst or bulla
- Severe hypoxemia due to unilateral lung disease
- Procedure related:
  - Repair of thoracic aortic aneurysm
  - Lung resection
- Pneumonectomy:
  - Lobectomy
  - Segmental resection
- Thoracoscopy:
  - Oesophageal surgery
  - Single-lung transplantation
  - Anterior approach to the thoracic spine
- Bronchoalveolar lavage.

Techniques for one-lung ventilation

Three techniques can be employed:
- Placement of a double-lumen tube (DLT).
- Use of a single-lumen endotracheal tube in conjunction with a bronchial blocker.
- Use of a single-lumen bronchial tube.

Double-lumen tubes

The advantages of DLTs are relative ease of placement, the ability to ventilate either or both of lungs, and the ability to suction either lung.

Various types of DLTs are available but they share the following characteristics:
- A longer bronchial lumen that enters the right or main left bronchus, and a shorter tracheal lumen that remains in the trachea.
- A preformed curve to allow preferential entry into one or other bronchus.
- Both bronchial and tracheal cuffs.

Ventilation can be delivered to only one lung by clamping either the bronchial or tracheal lumen with both cuffs inflated; opening the port on the appropriate connector allows the ipsilateral lung to collapse. As the bronchial anatomy varies between two sides, tubes are designed specifically for either right or left bronchus. Different types of DLT are compared in Table 15.2.

The most commonly used double lumen tubes are of the Robert–Shaw type. The single-use polyvinyl chloride DLTs currently in common usage have incorporated high-volume/low-pressure tracheal and bronchial cuffs, and follow in principle the original Robert–Shaw design. They are available in sizes 35, 37, 39, and 41Fr. It is important to choose a size appropriate to the patient to lessen the chance of iatrogenic airway injury. Useful guidelines in adults are as follows:
- Males: <170cm use 39Fr; >170cm use 41Fr.
- Females: <160cm use 35Fr; >160cm use 37Fr.

Table 15.2 Different types of double-lumen tube

Name	Carinal hook	Shape of lumen	Bronchus inflated
Carlens	Present	Oval	Left
White	Present	Oval	Right
Robert–Shaw	Absent	D-shaped	Left or right

Placement of DLTs

After laryngoscopy, the DLT is passed with distal curvature concave anteriorly and is rotated 90° (toward the side of bronchus to be intubated) after the tip enters the larynx. It is advanced until resistance is felt; the average depth at insertion, from the teeth for a left DLT is 29cm in an adult and varies ±1cm for each 10cm of patient height above/below 170cm. Correct tube placement should be established using the protocol given in Box 15.6, and confirmed with flexible fibreoptic bronchoscopy.

Box 15.6 Protocol for checking placement of a left-sided DLT

1. Inflate the tracheal cuff.
2. Check for bilateral breath sounds. Unilateral breath sounds indicate that the tube is too far down.
3. Inflate the bronchial cuff (1–2mL).
4. Clamp the tracheal lumen.
5. Check for unilateral left-sided breath sounds:
   - Persistence of right-sided breath sounds indicates that the bronchial opening is still in trachea (tube needs to be advanced).
   - Unilateral right-sided breath sounds indicate incorrect entry of the tube in the right bronchus.
   - Absence of breath sounds over the right lung and left upper lobe indicates tube is too far down the left bronchus (tube needs to be pulled back).
6. Unclamp the tracheal lumen and clamp the bronchial lumen.

Check for unilateral right-sided breath sounds. Absence or decreased breath sounds indicates that the tube is not far enough down and the bronchial cuff is occluding the distal trachea.

When the bronchoscope is advanced into the tracheal lumen, the carina should be visible and the bronchial tip of the tube should be seen entering the left bronchus; additionally, the top of the bronchial cuff (coloured blue) should be visible but should not extend above the carina. If the bronchial cuff of a left-side DLT is not visible, it may be low enough to obstruct the orifice of the left lower lobe; the tube should be withdrawn until the bronchial cuff is visible. The bronchial cuff should ideally be inflated only to a point at which the audible leak from the open tracheal lumen disappears while ventilating only through the bronchial lumen. Tube position should be reconfirmed after repositioning for surgery.

Malpositioning of DLTs

This is usually indicated by poor lung compliance and low exhaled tidal volume.

Problems with left-sided DLTs are usually related to one of the following possibilities:

- If the tube is too deep, the bronchial cuff can obstruct the left upper or the left lower lobe orifice. In some patients the bronchial lumen may be within the left upper or left lower lobe bronchus but the tracheal opening remains above the carina; this situation is suggested by the collapse of one of the left lobes when the bronchial lumen is clamped. Worse, if the surgical procedure is in the right thorax, when the tracheal lumen is clamped, only the left upper or left lower lobe will be ventilated; hypoxia usually develops rapidly.

- When the tube is not advanced far enough, the bronchial cuff can occlude the right main bronchus.

- The tube may enter the wrong bronchus—the fibreoptic bronchoscope can be used to reposition it to the correct side.

Problems with right-sided DLTs arise because the orifice of the right upper lobe is close (1.0–2.5cm) to the carina. It is very easy to occlude the right upper lobe orifice with the bronchial tube cuff and, hence, the preference for using left-sided DLTs.

Complications of DLTs

- Hypoxaemia due to tube misplacement or occlusion.
- Traumatic laryngitis.
- Tracheobronchial rupture resulting from over-inflation of bronchial cuff.
- Inadvertent suturing of tube to bronchus during surgery.

Bronchial blockers

Bronchial blockers are inflatable devices that are passed alongside or through a single-lumen tube to selectively occlude a bronchial orifice.

Advantages

In patients with a recognized and/or unrecognized difficult airway, placement of a DLT with direct laryngoscopy can be extremely difficult and at times, impossible. This includes patients with cervical spine injuries and/or pathology. In this situation, placement of a single-lumen ETT is easier and often necessary, requiring the need for a bronchial blocker for subsequent lung isolation.

Placing a DLT in patients with distorted tracheobronchial anatomy is often difficult and at times, contraindicated. Use of a bronchial blocker, in this situation, is more often successful and safe.

Often, intubated patients present for surgery requiring OLV including trauma patients and patients from the emergency department and ICU. Also, the particular surgery or intraoperative events (i.e. massive fluid infusion) will require postoperative ventilation. Use of a bronchial blocker negates the need to change the ETT in these situations, therefore avoiding the possibility of losing the airway altogether. Furthermore, some of these patients may not tolerate periods of apnoea. Some bronchial blockers can be placed during continuous ventilation.

Bronchial blockers can provide selective blockade of a specific lobe. This is particularly useful in the patient with an isolated air leak, haemorrhage, or infection in one lobe, thereby allowing ventilation of more lung units. Finally, bronchial blockers are useful in patients who have had a prior pneumonectomy and now present for a selective lobectomy.

Limitations

Collapse of the desired lung is often slow because of the small size of channel within the blocker. Bronchial blockers are more easily dislodged during patient positioning and surgical manipulation of the lung. Bronchial blockers present the potential risk of perforating a bronchus or lung parenchyma causing a pneumothorax.

Single-lumen bronchial tubes

Single-lumen bronchial tubes are less often used now. They have tracheal and bronchial cuffs. In a right-sided single-lumen tube, inflating the bronchial cuff isolates and ventilated the right lung. When the bronchial cuff is deflated and the tracheal cuff is inflated, both lungs can be ventilated. A much larger slit in the bronchial cuff (compared with right-sided DLTs) results in a high success rate of ventilating the right upper lobe. The left-sided single-lumen tube should be positioned with the help of a bronchoscope.

Management of one-lung ventilation

The greatest risk of OLV is hypoxemia. Fortunately, blood flow to the non-ventilated lung is decreased by *hypoxic pulmonary vasoconstriction* (HPV). The stimulus for HPV is primarily the alveolar oxygen tension (PAO_2), which stimulates precapillary vasoconstriction redistributing pulmonary blood flow away from hypoxemic lung regions via a pathway involving NO and/or cyclo-oxygenase synthesis inhibition. Factors known to inhibit HPV and thus worsen the right-to-left shunting include:

- Very high or very low pulmonary artery pressures
- Hypocapnia.
- High or low mixed venous PO_2.
- Vasodilators such as nitroglycerin, nitroprusside, β-adrenergic agonists (including dobutamine and salbutamol), and calcium channel blockers.
- Pulmonary infection.
- Inhalation anaesthetics.

Factors that decrease blood flow to the ventilated lung can be equally detrimental; they counteract the effect of HPV by indirectly increasing blood flow to the collapsed lung. These are:

- High mean airway pressures in the ventilated lung due to high PEEP, hyperventilation, or high peak inspiratory pressures.
- Low FiO_2, which produces hypoxic pulmonary vasoconstriction in the ventilated lung.
- Vasoconstrictors that may have a greater effect on normoxic vessels than hypoxic ones.
- Intrinsic PEEP that develops due to inadequate expiratory times.

Ventilation during one-lung anaesthesia

It is possible to improve gas exchange by altering the ventilatory variables (Box 15.7) such as:

- *Tidal volume:* should be adjusted to keep the peak airway pressure <35cmH$_2$O and the plateau airway pressure <25cmH$_2$O. A reasonable starting point for OLV is 4–6mL/kg. The ventilatory rate may be increased to maintain the same minute ventilation.

- *Positive end-expiratory pressure:* most patients do not increase PaO$_2$ with added PEEP during OLV. Patients with either normal or supranormal (restrictive lung disease) lung elastic recoil will benefit from low levels (5cmH$_2$O) of PEEP during OLV.

- *Volume control versus pressure control:* pressure control useful in patients with severe obstructive disease to limit airway pressure. It is also helpful in patients at risk of acute lung injury (pneumonectomies, lung transplantation).

- *FiO$_2$:* the FiO$_2$ should be increased at the start of OLV to 100% and then can be decreased as tolerated over the next 30min.

Box 15.7 Techniques to improve oxygenation during OLV

- First-line therapy is to increase the FiO_2, which is an option in essentially all patients (except those who received bleomycin that potentiates pulmonary oxygen toxicity).
- *CPAP* (5–10cm H_2O) with oxygen to the non-ventilated lung is the most useful ventilation manipulation: most effective when there is partial re-expansion of the lung, which unfortunately can interfere with surgery.
- *PEEP* (5–10cm H_2O) to the ventilated lung will improve oxygenation in patients with normal lung mechanics and those with increased elastic recoil due to restrictive lung diseases.
- Periodic inflation of the collapsed lung with oxygen.
- Early ligation or clamping of the ipsilateral pulmonary artery during pneumonectomy.
- *Alternative ventilation methods:* several alternative methods of OLV, all of which involve partial ventilation of the non-ventilated lung, have been described and improve oxygenation during OLV. These techniques are useful in patients who are particularly at risk for desaturation, such as those with previous pulmonary resections of the contralateral lung:
  - Selective lobar collapse of only the operative lobe in the open hemi thorax by placement of a blocker in the appropriate lobar bronchus of the ipsilateral operative lung.
  - Differential lung ventilation by partially occluding the lumen of the DLT to the operative lung.
  - Intermittent reinflation of the non-ventilated lung by regular re-expansion of the operative lung via an attached CPAP circuit.
  - Two-lung high-frequency positive-pressure ventilation (HFPPV).
  - Conventional OLV of the non-operative lung and high-frequency jet ventilation of the operative lung.

With the advent of fibreoptic bronchoscopy, coupled with high-resolution CT and MRI scanning, the necessity for *rigid* bronchoscopy, both diagnostic and perioperative, has declined. However, it is still often used to check tumours located proximally in the tracheobronchial tree to assess their location and resectability immediately prior to surgery.

It is also increasingly used for therapeutic laser surgery or endobronchial stent placement for otherwise unresectable tumours.

The ability to perform increasingly complex procedures in thoracic medicine (such as flexible endobronchial ultrasound (EBUS)-guided biopsies) has led to an increasing requirement for the provision of general anaesthesia even for relatively simple flexible bronchoscopic work.

There are other scenarios in which rigid bronchoscopy is used, particularly in ENT surgery (see Chapter 11).

Fibreoptic bronchoscopy

Local anaesthesia for fibreoptic bronchoscopy (and indeed awake fibreoptic intubation) is covered in Chapter 11, and should be familiar to all anaesthetists.

General anaesthesia for fibreoptic bronchoscopy and related procedures is relatively straightforward assuming there are no specific airway concerns. Endotracheal intubation and use of an adapted catheter mount allows continued closed-circuit anaesthesia whilst still performing the bronchoscopy.

The technique should also permit therapeutic bronchoscopy on patients in intensive care without too much loss of PEEP and risk of desaturation. On occasion, however, the bronchoscope may sub-totally occlude the ETT and hence interfere with ventilation, so close observation of tidal volumes and arterial oxygen saturation is needed.

Rigid bronchoscopy

Anaesthesia

Rigid bronchoscopy mandates general anaesthesia. In the past, deep inhalational anaesthesia with spontaneous ventilation was often described as a technique for rigid bronchoscopy (especially for retrieval of inhaled foreign bodies where there was concern that positive pressure ventilation might propel the foreign body further into the lung).

In practice this is difficult to achieve and may in fact make the surgical procedure more difficult because of tracheal and laryngeal stimulation leading to coughing and subsequent lung movement, which is almost unavoidable using this technique.

The current standard is probably to use a total intravenous anaesthetic (TIVA) technique and the combination of propofol and remifentanil is well suited to this; it allows deep anaesthesia whilst allowing the rapid return of normal protective airway reflexes, irrespective of the duration of the procedure performed. Whether this is done using target-controlled infusions (TCI), standard infusion devices or even by manual injection of the drugs depends on individual preference and available technology. If the duration of TIVA is likely to be very short (e.g. rigid bronchoscopy immediately prior to lobar resection or pneumonectomy) then manual injection of propofol with more conventional opiate use works well as these patients are usually fully paralysed and will probably revert to an inhalational technique after the bronchoscopy has been performed (usually via a double-lumen endobronchial tube). For longer procedures

then some form of infusion is usually required. The usual caveats apply relating to depth of anaesthesia monitoring and reliability of IV access so as to avoid the potential for awareness.

Neuromuscular blockade

Muscle relaxants are invariably required, if only to facilitate the initial placement of the bronchoscope. Thereafter, a combination of propofol and remifentanil is usually enough to suppress the laryngeal reflexes sufficient for the duration of the procedure. However, a balance must be struck to allow for the potential cardiovascular side effects of this combination. Some practitioners advocate the use of topical local anaesthesia (e.g. laryngojet 4%) to aid this.

The use of sugammadex to rapidly reverse even the most profound neuromuscular block from rocuronium or vecuronium now allows provision of optimal surgical conditions, even for very short diagnostic procedures without necessitating the use of deep anaesthesia to obtund laryngeal reflexes.

Emergence from anaesthesia

Once the surgical procedure is completed there is the question of how to maintain the airway and anaesthesia whilst the patient is allowed to awaken. If not performed by the surgeon on removal of the bronchoscope, then oropharyngeal suction should be performed (some advocate doing this under direct vision). The infusions should be stopped at an appropriate time for them to wear off by the end of the procedure and reversal of the neuromuscular block administered if appropriate (a situation rendered much easier by sugammadex). If rapid reversal and awakening is likely then use of a simple oropharyngeal or nasopharyngeal airway and standard face-mask support may be all that is required until the return of spontaneous ventilation. If a more prolonged recovery is predicted, then most would advocate the use of a laryngeal mask airway which allows smoother emergence, and if necessary continued maintenance of anaesthesia using a volatile agent.

Recovery is usually rapid and the procedures are not particularly painful postoperatively. Most patients experience some degree of haemoptysis following bronchoscopy and should be warned that this is to be expected.

Ventilation

Intermittent positive pressure ventilation

Conventional ventilation can be used for bronchoscopy. Ventilating bronchoscopes, such as those made by Storz have standard 15mm attachments that allow connection of normal anaesthetic circuits. However, this often means using intermittent apnoea to allow the surgeon access to the airways. In the interests of surgical expediency and also for the provision of continuous ventilation it is usually more convenient to use an open-ended bronchoscope, which requires some form of jet ventilation. This may not always be acceptable, for example, in small children when barotrauma may be of more concern, or in other circumstances where the use of high-pressure gas may potentially worsen the situation, for example, with bronchopleural fistulae.

Jet ventilation

In most circumstances where procedures are of short duration, then the use of some form of manual, low-frequency jet ventilation using either a Sanders injector or Manujet III (VBM, Germany) will suffice.

Jet ventilation works by using high-pressure (4 Bar) oxygen that is delivered to the bronchoscope via a side attachment (see Fig. 15.2). Air is entrained from the open end via a Venturi effect

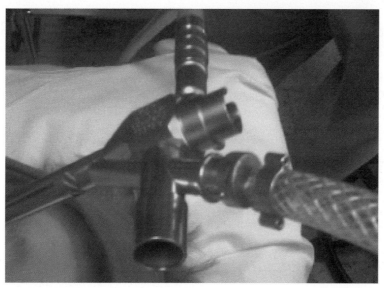

Fig. 15.2 Typical equipment for jet ventilation.

diluting the FiO_2 to about 0.8–0.9. Rates of 10–12 breaths per minute are usually adequate to maintain oxygenation, although it should be remembered that it is often difficult or impractical to monitor inspired and expired gases (notably CO_2) and the risk of hypercarbia must be borne in mind.

Intermittent side-stream assessment can be performed (but this requires suspending ventilation); transcutaneous CO_2 devices are available, but these are not widely used. Repeated blood gas sampling can also be used, but this usually requires an arterial line, which is unlikely to be placed for a straightforward diagnostic procedure.

Barotrauma is not normally a problem if an open-ended bronchoscope is used, since expiration occurs as normal via the open end, thus limiting any global pressure build up. However, it is possible that air-trapping can occur distal to any obstruction especially when foreign bodies are involved, but also if a tumour exerts a ball-valve effect within the lumen of a bronchus. One must, therefore, be constantly alert to this possibility, including the development of pneumothoraces, which are likely to tension.

Further reading

Evans E, Biro P, & Bedforth N (2007). Jet ventilation. *CEACCP*, 7(1):2–5. doi:10.1093/bjaceaccp/mkl061.

15.5 Postoperative care of thoracic surgical patients

Respiratory care

The incidence of serious respiratory complications following thoracic surgery is around 5–10% for patients without underlying lung disease. It is significantly higher in patients with significant pre-existing diffuse lung disease (up to 90% in some series).

Certain aspects of management may influence the frequency and severity of postoperative respiratory complications:

Perioperative fluids and ventilation
Measures that have been demonstrated to reduce postoperative respiratory complications include:
- Relative fluid restriction (13–20mL/kg/24h)
- Limited tidal volume and airway pressure ventilation.

These are discussed in section 15.3.

Responding to changes in oxygen requirements
Thoracic patients tend to have higher initial oxygen requirements that usually reflect residual collapse or atelectasis. Subsequent increases in oxygen requirements may be a sign of deteriorating lung function either because of infection or pulmonary oedema, both of which need early and aggressive therapy. Often the initial persistent collapse will resolve with the establishment of suction on drains.

Management of sputum retention
This is often a problem, especially in patients who have had extensive lung resections and may have had pre-existing borderline pulmonary function. Humidification of inspired gases, physiotherapy, and sometimes the insertion of a mini-tracheostomy is required.

General measures
Postoperatively, the importance of *adequate analgesia* and the ability to take proper vital capacity breaths when required is probably the most important component of respiratory care. Early mobilization and physiotherapy are possibly equally important but are unlikely to be achieved without adequate analgesia.

Other modalities of respiratory support (including non-invasive ventilation and CPAP) are valuable, especially following pneumonectomy when the avoidance of frank post-operative respiratory failure is crucial. Patients who require re-intubation post pneumonectomy have an especially high mortality.

Cardiac care

Arrhythmias
The most common arrhythmia is atrial fibrillation, which occurs in up to 40% of cases, higher in post-pneumonectomy patients. The aetiology is often complex but around 30% of these are as a result of sepsis and may be an early indicator of this. Management of arrhythmias should follow standard protocols (see section 1.9).

Myocardial ischaemia
The incidence of myocardial ischaemia in the thoracic surgical cohort is higher than in the general surgical population (some 3–5%), and is associated with a high mortality (40–70%). Patients known to have coronary artery disease are obviously at greater risk, and these patients need careful preoperative assessment and probably require invasive monitoring intra- and postoperatively.

Haemodynamic instability
The possibility of occult blood loss should always be considered in even a marginally unstable postoperative patient. The thoracic cavity can hold a large volume of blood, especially if the drains are malpositioned, kinked, or occluded (e.g. by clot). Mediastinal shift occurring after lung resection may in itself cause instability.

Over-administration of crystalloids may worsen lung injury. Limited resuscitation of the hypotensive patient with colloids is appropriate, but most centres have a low threshold for starting vasopressors or inotropes early rather than exposing patients to large volume loads.

Pain management

Thoracotomy incisions are notoriously painful and require multimodal pain management to achieve analgesia adequate enough to allow good ventilation of the operative lung.

Regional analgesia

Thoracic epidural analgesia
This probably remains the gold standard for pain relief, although epidural use has declined in some institutions owing to concerns about potential risks and the emergence of other techniques perceived as less invasive.

Paravertebral block (PVB)
PVB can be performed either preoperatively by the anaesthetist or under direct vision by the surgeon (ideally with a continuous infusion postoperatively). When combined with PCA, it provides similar analgesia without the excess morbidity or mortality.

Complications from PVB are unusual, the most significant being pneumothorax, which is clearly perhaps less significant in the presence of a chest drain.

Infiltration/intercostal blockade
If regional techniques are not feasible (usually because of intraoperative conversion or localized infection) then a good alternative is to use multilevel intercostal nerve blockade either by the surgeon under direct vision or by the anaesthetist, in combination with PCA.

After VATS procedures, local wound infiltration is usually performed.

Opioid analgesia
Patients undergoing VATS operations will have varying analgesic requirements depending on the procedure and the individual patient. Many patients undergoing biopsies or other simple procedures may only require small amounts of IV opioids in recovery and can be maintained on oral opioids until the drains are removed at which time the pain usually rapidly diminishes.

By contrast, patients undergoing pleurodesis (especially using talc or abrasion) often have high analgesic requirements during the first 24–48h, necessitating large doses of IV opioids or PCA. Pain management is restricted by surgical concerns over NSAID use and the potential for these drugs to reduce the efficacy of the pleurodesis itself (although NSAIDs are often contraindicated in many thoracic patients anyway). Many patients with malignant disease will already be receiving opioids, and small doses of ketamine or α_2-agonists may play a useful adjunctive role.

Some institutions use spinal opioids for thoracic surgery (mostly with preservative-free morphine), usually in combination with a PCA or even PVB. The technique is gaining in popularity, although some concerns remain in respect of possible delayed respiratory depression.

Chest drain management

All thoracic surgical procedures, except perhaps pneumonectomy, mandate the placement of wide-bore intercostal drain(s) postoperatively. Mostly these are for drainage of *air*, allowing the operative lung to re-expand. The use of additional drains for *fluid* (including empyema drainage, pleural effusions, and blood) will vary depending on the specific circumstances.

Most chest drains are placed anterolaterally, just below the thoracotomy incision or through one of the VATS port incisions. As a general rule, anterior drains are directed apically and are intended to drain air, whilst basal drains are placed behind and are intended to drain blood or other fluids. In complex situations, this may vary. True anterior drains (in the 2nd intercostal space, mid-clavicular line) are usually reserved for loculated or complex apical pneumothoraces. These are more commonly performed in critically ill patients with ARDS or those with complex bullous disease. They are not routinely used following surgery, and carry a much greater risk of vascular damage (internal thoracic artery, subclavian vessels).

Underwater seals

Most drains are attached to underwater seals. The simplest arrangement is a wide-diameter bottle with the chest drain connection inserted some 2–3cm into the fluid. The volume of water in the bottle above the distal end of the drain connection should be greater than the total volume of the tubing connecting the two. This is usually provides low resistance to allow efflux of air from the thoracic cavity but prevents entrainment of air back into the pleural cavity, even when a deep inspiratory effort is made (with intrapleural pressure reaching some $-60cmH_2O$ to $-80cmH_2O$) so long as the drain is well below the level of the patient's chest. The addition of suction ensures this.

Multiple bottle systems are cumbersome and complex and are not widely used.

Suction

A low degree of suction (−2kPa to −4kPa) is applied to the drain bottle(s) in most cases. This allows better re-expansion of the lung and also encourages drainage of air and fluid. The systems need to be low-negative pressure but high-displacement vacuums so that they can cope with all but the most severe air leaks.

The exceptions are when there is a severe persistent air leak or bronchopleural fistula (BPF) or following pneumonectomy. Severe air leaks and BPF are perpetuated by suction, although the risk of recurrent uncontrolled pneumothorax needs to be weighed against this. Most persistent air-leaks improve with the resumption of negative pressure ventilation and the aim should be to achieve this as soon as possible.

Post-pneumonectomy

The use of chest drains post-pneumonectomy is not normally recommended unless there is significant concern over the risk of ongoing bleeding. The air cavity in the resected hemithorax gradually fills with fluid over a period of days to weeks. Any air is slowly reabsorbed. However, if there is an imbalance between the rate of production of fluid and the rate of air re-absorption, the residual air can slowly tension or the excess fluid can cause mechanical compression both causing mediastinal shift and haemodynamic instability. This needs to be monitored radiographically in the early postoperative phase. Some advocate balanced pleural drainage which may require intermittent clamping of a drain or alternatively the injection or aspiration of air.

In cases where a drain *is* used post pneumonectomy, using suction carries a risk of negative intrathoracic pressure and mediastinal shift *towards* the operative side and should be avoided.

Removal of drains

Drains should be removed when they are no longer draining significant air or fluid (usually after a period of at least 12–24h). They are often taken off suction or clamped for a period of time prior to removal. In order to reduce the risk of pneumothorax during the removal process, they should be removed either during *expiration* if spontaneously breathing (i.e. when the transpleural pressure is greatest) or if undergoing positive pressure ventilation then during *inspiration*. A CXR should always be performed post-removal.

Bronchopleural fistula

A BPF is a potentially serious complication. Although BPF can occur following lobectomy, it is more common following pneumonectomy and is defined simply as a persistent air leak following resection with a connection between the bronchial stump and the lung cavity.

The incidence is low (1–2% following pneumonectomy) but there is an associated high morbidity and mortality. The main concern stems from the risk of infected pleural fluid contaminating the non-resected lung. In the case where a pneumonectomy patient requires early reventilation because of respiratory failure, the risk of development of a BPF is greatly increased.

Patients tend to present 3–10 days postoperatively with increasing respiratory distress, increasing oxygen requirements, and may be overtly septic. The presence of an air–fluid level on CXR is usually diagnostic.

Most patients will require urgent re-exploration and closure of the defect. The contralateral lung needs rapid isolation to protect it from further contamination. This is usually performed with some sort of rapid sequence induction and placement of a DLT, ideally without any positive pressure ventilation prior to isolation (although this is often difficult to achieve in reality). This needs to occur with simultaneous cardiovascular resuscitation as required.

Further reading

Raiten JM & Blank RS (2011). Anesthetic management of post-thoracotomy complications. In P Slinger (ed) *Principles and Practice of Anesthesia for Thoracic Surgery* (pp. 601–8). New York: Springer.

15.6 Management of pneumothorax

A pneumothorax is a collection of air within the pleural space. There are three mechanisms by which this can occur:

- Communication between alveolar spaces and pleura
- Communication between atmosphere and pleural space
- Presence of gas-forming organisms within the pleural space.

It is an important diagnosis, and a common clinical problem. All anaesthetists should have an understanding of the diagnosis, management, and anaesthetic implications of pneumothorax. Pneumothoraces resulting from formal thoracic surgical procedures mandate drainage postoperatively and are discussed in section 15.5.

Classification

From a clinical perspective, pneumothoraces are classified as spontaneous, traumatic, or iatrogenic (see Box 15.8).

Box 15.8 Classification of pneumothorax

- Spontaneous:
  - Primary: no apparent underlying lung disease
  - Secondary: clinically apparent underlying lung disease (COPD, cystic fibrosis, etc.)
- Traumatic:
  - Blunt or penetrating chest trauma
- Iatrogenic:
  - Secondary to medical interventions (pleural biopsy, CVC line, pleural aspiration, barotrauma, etc.)

Primary spontaneous pneumothorax (PSP)
PSP typically occurs in young, tall, thin individuals. It is more common in men than women, and smoking is a risk factor. The classical presentation is with sudden, ipsilateral chest pain. Dyspnoea is generally mild. The classical signs of reduced or absent breath sounds and vocal fremitus, and hyper-resonance to percussion, depend on the size of the pneumothorax. Tension pneumothorax (presenting with rapidly evolving cardiorespiratory collapse) is extremely rare in PSP.

For a spontaneous pneumothorax to occur, there must have been a communication between the alveolar spaces and the pleura. The most commonly accepted explanation is spontaneous rupture of a subpleural bleb. Up to 90% of patients are found to have small, usually apical, blebs or bullae on CT or at thoracoscopy, especially those with recurrent episodes.

Recurrent episodes occur in up to around 50% of patients, especially in those who continue to smoke.

The standard imaging modality for diagnosing PSP is an erect CXR, taken during inspiration. CT scanning is reserved for complex cases.

The size of a pneumothorax has previously been suggested as a way to assess its severity and hence to guide intervention. However, size may not correlate well with symptoms (especially in SSP) and is often underestimated on a plain radiograph. A 2cm pneumothorax at the hilar level on the plain film approximates to a 50% pneumothorax by volume.

A wide variety of management options are available for management of PSP:

- Observation
- Simple aspiration
- Catheter drainage
- Chest tube placement (± medical pleurodesis)
- VATS procedure (with bullectomy/pleurectomy/pleurodesis).

A patient who presents with a first episode of a small apical pneumothorax can usually safely be observed, or even discharged and followed up as an outpatient.

In the presence of symptoms, evacuation of air is required, usually by simple manual aspiration rather than formal intercostal drainage.

After a second episode, consideration may be given to attempting recurrence prevention. Increasingly, the trend is towards a VATS procedure.

Secondary spontaneous pneumothorax (SSP)
These occur in the presence of underlying lung disease. They are associated with greater morbidity and mortality as the physiological consequences of the pneumothorax are usually much more significant, and treatment must be undertaken urgently. Tuberculosis is now less common as the underlying cause, and COPD now predominates (see Box 15.9). Depending on the underlying cause, the peak incidence of SSP occurs later in life than that of PSP.

Box 15.9 Some typical causes of secondary pneumothorax

- Airway disease:
  - COPD
  - Acute severe asthma
  - Cystic fibrosis
- Infection:
  - Tuberculosis
  - *Pneumocystis carinii* pneumonia
- Connective tissue disease:
  - Marfan's syndrome
  - Ehlers–Danlos syndrome
- Malignant disease:
  - Lung cancer.

In the presence of emphysematous bullae, CXR diagnosis of pneumothorax may be difficult. CT confirmation may be required.

These patients should usually be admitted and given supplemental oxygen as appropriate to their underlying condition. Needle aspiration is generally less successful in this group (although may be attempted if 1–2cm) and most of these patients require at least small-bore intercostal drain placement. They should be referred to a chest physician and those with a persistent air leak (defined as persistent bubbling for >48h) should be discussed with a thoracic surgeon for consideration of formal pleurodesis.

Traumatic pneumothorax
Pneumothorax may occur after both penetrating and blunt chest trauma. If positive pressure ventilation is required, then chest tube placement is mandatory. The drain should usually be of large bore (28–36 French), especially if there is an associated haemothorax.

Iatrogenic pneumothorax
The commonest causes of pneumothorax associated with medical interventions are:

- Transthoracic needle aspiration of pleural effusion
- Subclavian approach to CVC insertion
- Thoracocentesis
- Transbronchial lung biopsy
- Pleural biopsy
- Positive pressure ventilation.

Other causes relevant to anaesthesia and surgery relate to similar invasive procedures (attempted internal jugular cannulation and all forms of brachial plexus blockade), in addition to PVB, tracheostomy formation, jet ventilation, and other causes of barotrauma, including laparoscopic procedures.

Pneumothoraces resulting from positive pressure ventilation in critically ill patients are particularly dangerous: the positive pressure may cause a persistent leak, and they have a tendency to tension. Patients with acute lung injury may have recurrent episodes requiring multiple drains; the resulting pleural adhesions may cause loculated gas collections.

Ultrasound can be very effective for the diagnosis of pneumothorax, although in the presence of surgical emphysema, its efficacy is significantly reduced.

CT scanning remains probably the gold standard imaging modality for detection and assessment of pneumothoraces. This is especially true in loculated disease, mal-placed chest drains, or in the presence of surgical emphysema. However, obvious concerns about radiation dose and the practicalities of transferring critically ill patients to and from the CT scanner limit its overall use.

Patients in the ITU requiring ventilation for any reason who develop a pneumothorax should always undergo formal drain insertion because of the risk of tension.

Anaesthesia and pneumothorax

Surgical treatment of pneumothorax will be undertaken within thoracic centres. Most patients will already have drain(s) *in situ*. They are, however, at risk of developing contralateral pneumothoraces and it is important to be vigilant for any unexplained change in airway pressure or oxygenation during the procedure, especially during periods of single-lung ventilation.

Anaesthesia per se may increase the risk of pneumothorax. This mostly stems from the use of positive pressure ventilation and other iatrogenic causes. Other concerns include the use of nitrous oxide (which will tend to worsen any pneumothorax and may increase the risk of tension).

The safe timing of anaesthesia for unrelated surgery following PSP or SSP is not well established. If there has been some form of definitive treatment (pleurodesis or pleurectomy) then the risk of recurrence is low and surgery can probably proceed safely from 7–14 days. Anaesthesia following conservatively treated PSP is harder to gauge and a timescale similar to that advised in relation to flying (6–8 weeks) is perhaps more appropriate. In these cases, it would seem sensible to avoid nitrous oxide and to employ low-pressure ventilator settings, or allow spontaneous ventilation.

Tension pneumothorax

The diagnosis of tension pneumothorax (TPT) requires a high degree of suspicion and constitutes a medical emergency. Certain patients are at particular risk (see Box 15.10).

> **Box 15.10 Clinical situations with increased risk of tension pneumothorax**
>
> - ITU patients receiving ventilation (IPPV or non-invasive)
> - Multiple and/or chest trauma
> - Obstructive lung disease and acute severe asthma
> - Recent CPR
> - Presence of a clamped, blocked, or malpositioned chest drain
> - Miscellaneous causes (e.g. hyperbaric oxygen therapy).

In the awake patient, intrapleural pressure is negative throughout the ventilatory cycle ($-3cmH_2O$ to $-8cmH_2O$). In a ventilated patient, inspiratory pressures are typically $20cmH_2O$ or higher, followed by either physiological expiratory pressures or PEEP of $\geq 5cmH_2O$. TPT is sometimes defined as when IPP is positive throughout the respiratory cycle. In the awake patient, IPP must be subatmospheric during part of the respiratory cycle for the pneumothorax to continue to develop, hence the definition of an 'expiratory TPT'. A maximal expiratory effort in an awake patient can achieve an IPP of $-80cmH_2O$, which is able to overcome the increasing IPP as TPTdevelops.

In awake patients, from case reports, the dominant presenting features of TPT are chest pain and respiratory distress, with tachycardia and ipsilateral reduced air entry. Other 'typical' signs occur less consistently. In a ventilated patient, TPT presents with reduced saturations and haemodynamic compromise.

The diagnosis of a *tension* pneumothorax is commonly held to be a *clinical* one, hence the adage 'the CXR that should never have been taken...', although case reports have described the occasional value of a CXR to confirm the diagnosis in stable patients with equivocal signs, or in unstable ventilated patients without other signs.

The classical treatment of TPT is anterior needle decompression followed by tube thoracostomy. Needle decompression is sometimes controversial—it is arguably over-used almost as an investigative tool in the pre-hospital setting, and may fail, causing diagnostic confusion.

Further reading

Leigh-Smith S (2005). Tension pneumothorax--time for a re-think? *Emerg Med J*, 22(1):8–16. doi:10.1136/emj.2003.010421.

Noppen M & De Keukeleire T (2008). Pneumothorax. *Respiration*, 76(2):121–7. doi:10.1159/000135932.

Paramasivam E & Bodenham A (2008). Air leaks, pneumothorax, and chest drains. *CEACCP*, 8(6):204–9. doi:10.1093/bjaceaccp/mkn038.

Sahn SA & Heffner JE (2000). Spontaneous pneumothorax. *NEJM*, 342(12):868–74. doi:10.1056/NEJM200003233421207.

Chapter 16

Vascular anaesthesia

313

16.1 Resuscitation and management of ruptured aortic aneurysm

Incidence and mortality

Abdominal aortic aneurysm (AAA) is common with a prevalence of 2–5% in males over the age of 60 in the UK. Ruptured abdominal aortic aneurysm (RAAA) is responsible for approximately 1 in 200 deaths. The condition carries a high mortality with surgical mortality of 32–70%; however, many patients die before reaching hospital. In one study, 42% of patients with ruptured aneurysms died before hospital (often within 1h of the onset of symptoms).

Mortality is closely linked to the degree of preoperative hypotension and other related factors such as massive blood transfusion and cardiac arrest. Survival depends not only on the severity of rupture, but also the ability of the patient to compensate physiologically. This is linked to the premorbid state of the patient.

Also implicated in increasing mortality are:

- Increasing age
- Female gender
- Low intraoperative urine output
- Delays in diagnosis
- Prolonged surgery
- Inadequate surgical experience.

The site of rupture is important; 88% of cases rupture into the retroperitoneal space where the haemorrhage may be contained. In 12% there is rupture into the peritoneal cavity and occasionally into the inferior vena cava (aortocaval) or the duodenum (aorto-enteric), all of which are associated with even higher mortality.

Anaesthetic issues

The aim of anaesthesia is to facilitate definitive surgical management as rapidly as possible but there are some important considerations in the initial management (Box 16.1).

Box 16.1 Important initial considerations in RAAA
• Elderly patient • Comorbidities • Shock • Haemorrhage/resuscitation • Monitoring • Transferring patient (CT scan/hospital) • Trying to avoid delays to surgery.

Pre-clamp resuscitation

There are two opposing views on the optimum management of resuscitation. One view is that fluid resuscitation should be avoided as restoration of the BP may cause further haemorrhage leading to dilutional coagulopathy, massive blood transfusion, and technical surgical difficulties. The other is that fluid resuscitation should be started immediately since the longer the period of shock the greater the risk of developing cardiac complications and multisystem organ failure.

The main argument *for* preoperative fluid resuscitation is that the SBP at presentation is the single most important factor influencing survival of RAAA. Those patients presenting with a SBP of <90mmHg have a mortality rate of >60% in most series. Improving the circulating blood volume, and hence BP, might therefore improve outcome.

Some retrospective studies of RAAA have shown that the incidence of multisystem complications correlates with the duration of shock, and with an increased interval from diagnosis to surgery.

In the absence of definitive evidence it seems sensible to suggest that severe hypotension (systolic <70mmHg) is permissible, for a short period, if surgery is imminent. If delay is likely, for example the patient is to be transferred to another hospital for surgery, more aggressive resuscitation would be appropriate with consideration being given to the early use of blood and blood products.

Diagnosis of RAAA

Preoperative CT scanning when RAAA is suspected could cause delay and may be difficult in the unstable patient. However it improves diagnosis and may be useful for planning surgery, particularly if endovascular aneurysm repair (EVAR) is being considered.

Clinical diagnosis requires the classic triad of:

1. Back pain
2. Hypotension
3. Pulsatile abdominal mass.

In one recent review, only 26% of patients presented with all three of these factors.

CT is helpful in haemodynamically stable patients. Many of these patients with suspected ruptured aneurysms do not actually have them. In two recent studies of normotensive patients with known or suspected AAA and abdominal pain only 28% (18 of 65) and 63% (30 of 48) actually had a ruptured aneurysm.

RAAAs may be misdiagnosed as other diseases. In a recent review of 152 ruptured aneurysms, 30% were initially misdiagnosed, leading to significant delays in treatment. Misdiagnosis was more common in patients with no palpable pulsatile abdominal mass.

These patients were initially diagnosed as:

- Urolithiasis
- Diverticulitis
- GI haemorrhage
- Myocardial infarction
- Back pain
- Traumatic injury
- Sepsis.

The correct diagnosis was almost always made entirely on the basis of CT findings.

Anaesthetic management

Priorities in management include:
- Insertion of large-bore peripheral IV cannulae
- Blood cross-matching
- Rapid diagnosis
- Mobilization of theatre staff prior to immediate transfer.

Theatre management priorities include:

- Preparation of drugs
- Setting up of invasive and non-invasive monitoring equipment
- Provision for rapid infusion with fluid warming
- Warming blanket
- Infusion pumps
- Cell saver.

The abdomen should be prepared and draped with the patient awake and the surgeon scrubbed. It is advisable to have at least two experienced anaesthetists present and an anaesthetic assistant. In general, one anaesthetist should be responsible for continued resuscitation whilst the other concentrates on induction and maintenance of anaesthesia.

Invasive monitoring is best instituted following cross-clamping, when the patient is more haemodynamically stable.

Objectives of anaesthetic management include:

- Ongoing assessment of haemodynamic status
- Establishment of monitoring in the time available before surgery
- Maintenance of intravascular volume
- Treatment of coagulopathy
- Maintenance of optimal cardiac output and tissue oxygenation
- Control of haemodynamic changes due to aortic clamping and unclamping
- Postoperative ITU

Monitoring

All patients should have ECG, pulse oximeter, and non-invasive blood pressure (NIBP) monitoring. In severely shocked patients, NIBP and pulse oximeter may be unreliable. Direct intra-arterial monitoring is therefore essential for detection of beat to beat changes in BP and for arterial blood gas measurement, but surgery should *not* be delayed in order to insert an arterial line. An ECG may be the only monitor available prior to aortic cross-clamping in the moribund patient.

Additional monitoring requirements:

- Arterial blood gases
- Biochemistry
- Haemoglobin
- Lactate
- A coagulation screen and platelet count is recommended every 30min and deficiencies vigorously corrected.
- Core and peripheral temperature should be monitored and hypothermia avoided.
- A urinary catheter should be inserted prior to surgery.

Induction of anaesthesia

The haemodynamic status on reaching theatre is variable, but under-resuscitation is likely. Induction of anaesthesia may be followed by a catastrophic fall in BP when sympathoadrenal stimulation is obtunded and the tamponading effect of the abdominal muscles is lost.

Induction should therefore be followed by immediate aortic cross-clamping so that filling pressures are rapidly restored.

There is no evidence that the choice of induction agent alters survival in patients with haemorrhagic shock. Haemodynamically stable techniques are preferable to avoid life-threatening cardiovascular collapse and the use of propofol or thiopentone as an induction agent is probably best avoided. Etomidate provides very cardiostable anaesthesia, but there are unproven concerns about the effects of adrenocortical suppression in these patients. Many advocate the use of a technique based on high-dose opiates.

Endovascular aneurysm repair for RAAA

EVAR is increasingly being used for the emergency treatment of RAAA. It was first performed (successfully) at the Cleveland Clinic in 1994 and is now performed at many centres with good results.

Comparative efficacy of EVAR and open repair for RAAA is controversial as current evidence is subject to selection bias. The results of randomized control trials currently underway are awaited.

Anaesthetic issues

Guide wire placement can easily be done under LA. Some centres have used LA successfully for the entire procedure. Endoluminal balloon inflation, in cases of cardiovascular collapse, can also be done under LA and this may improve stability and allow the induction of GA.

Some authors advocate aggressive hypotension (50–70mmHg), for short periods, because of the increased chance of abdominal compartment syndrome (see section 4.6) in EVAR for RAAA, and the morbidity and mortality associated with this. Abdominal compartment syndrome causes hypotension, oliguria, and ventilatory failure. Intravesical pressure monitoring can be used to detect raised intra-abdominal pressure and laparotomy with haematoma evacuation may be required.

Further reading

Leonard A & Thompson J (2008). Anaesthesia for ruptured abdominal aortic aneurysm. *CEACCP*, 8(1):11–15.

16.2 Endovascular aneurysm repair

Patients are usually offered aneurysm surgery once the anteroposterior (AP) diameter of the aneurysm reaches approximately 5.5cm. After this, the annual risk of rupture exceeds the average risk of death following open repair. Once aortic aneurysms reach this size they expand exponentially, markedly increasing the annual risk of rupture. The 30-day mortality associated with RAAA is up to 80%. Of those that reach hospital alive and undergo emergency surgery, 40% will die within 30 days regardless.

Therapy is aimed at preventing rupture. Elective surgery prevents rupture and may be performed as an open operation or as an endovascular procedure. Open repair carries significant morbidity and mortality. The mortality in the UK for elective open infrarenal AAA repair is 6.2–7.5%. The 30-day mortality with EVAR ranges from:

- 1.7% in patients deemed fit for open repair
- 9% in those deemed unfit for open repair.

Evidence to support the use of EVAR

EVAR is a rapidly evolving technology, and with a relative lack of large randomized trials, the evidence is not clear-cut (see Box 16.2 for potential advantages). The largest randomized control trial performed (EVAR 1) studied 1082 patients who were anatomically suitable for EVAR and fit for open repair. Patients were randomized to either EVAR or open surgery. The study showed:

- Reduced perioperative mortality in EVAR group (2.3% vs 6% during hospital stay).
- After 4 years all-cause mortality was similar in the two groups (28%).
- Reduction in aneurysm-related death in EVAR group (4% vs 7%).
- Postoperative graft-related complications were higher in EVAR (41% vs 9%)
- After 12 months there was no difference in health-related quality of life.
- Costs actually higher in EVAR (£13 257 vs £9946).

Box 16.2 Potential advantages of EVAR
- Lower mortality
- Shorter hospital stay
- Less expensive
- Better quality of life
- Can be performed under local, regional, or general anaesthesia
- Suitable for patients with serious comorbidity.

EVAR technique

EVAR involves the use of a stent-graft to exclude aneurysms of the abdominal aorta. A stent-graft is a self-expandable stent, with an outer or inner fabric lining of Dacron® or polytetrafluoroethylene (PTFE) similar to the graft used for open aneurysm repair. The stent-graft is positioned between normal artery proximal to the aneurysm and normal artery distal to the aneurysm. Blood flows from normal artery through the stent-graft and back into normal artery. The outward radial force of the stent causes a seal preventing the flow of blood outside the stent-graft and into the aneurysmal sac. This proximal sealing zone is the non-aneurysmal infrarenal aortic neck. Almost all AAAs extend to the aortic bifurcation or beyond, so the distal sealing zone is both common iliac arteries (for purely aortic aneurysms), and the external iliac arteries for aorto-iliac aneurysms.

The stent-grafts are usually introduced through the common femoral arteries. Most surgeons will perform a surgical cut-down onto the vessels due to the size of the sheaths. If the femoral arteries are too small, the iliac artery may be exposed and a Dacron conduit anastomosed to this vessel to introduce the stent-graft. This requires an abdominal incision. Once the common femoral arteries are exposed, a J-wire is introduced through an arterial puncture needle. The stent-graft is introduced over the wire and positioned so that the junction between covered and uncovered stent is just below the lowermost renal orifice. A digital subtraction angiogram is obtained to confirm correct positioning of the stent-graft in relation to the renal orifices. Under GA the anaesthetist will be asked to stop respiration for digital subtraction angiography. The stent graft is deployed.

Anaesthesia for EVAR

Environment
Ideally there should be a dedicated theatre for EVAR equipped to the same standard as a vascular theatre with imaging of sufficient quality to perform complex EVAR. In reality these cases may be performed in the radiology department, which will cause logistical difficulties with:

- Equipment availability
- Drug availability
- Blood gas/ROTEM®/TEG® monitoring
- Storage of blood/blood products
- Help in an emergency
- Recovery/ITU.

It is essential that the facilities used are adequate for conversion to open repair in an emergency. The same standards apply to personnel. Imaging equipment in operating theatres often provides poorer quality images. This is acceptable for most cases but exceptions are:

- Obese patients
- Complex fenestrated devices.

Technique
Although conversion rates to open repair are low (<2%) the anaesthetist needs to be prepared for both this and massive haemorrhage. The bare minimum of general management should include the use of two large-bore IV cannulae, invasive arterial monitoring, a urinary catheter, and immediate access to a rapid infusion device. Additional monitoring is not routinely required though may be indicated in individual cases.

Patients are cross-matched as for open repair. The use of forced air warming devices and IV fluid warmers is strongly recommended, the duration of the procedure can exceed 3h and large volumes of fluid may need to be administered. Anaesthetic technique used may be:

- GA
- Regional
- LA.

For routine infrarenal EVAR, use of combined spinal epidural (CSE)/epidural is recommended, but GA should be considered for the following reasons:

- Use of heparin or antiplatelet therapy
- Anticipated prolonged surgery
- Likely sedation requirement/poor compliance
- Axillary approaches.

There is some evidence that regional or local anaesthesia may reduce postoperative complications. The EUROSTAR database looked at 5557 patients who had undergone EVAR across Europe. The registry suggests that 30% of EVARs are performed using local or regional anaesthetic techniques. They concluded that cardiac complications were significantly reduced in those patients who had local or regional anaesthesia. Duration of stay in ITU and length of overall hospital stay were also reduced.

However, those who are able to tolerate EVAR under LA are generally a highly selected group:

- With more favourable arterial access
- Undergoing no additional procedures
- Less likely to be overweight.

Other studies have concluded that the risk profile of the patient appears to be more important than the influence of any given anaesthetic technique. The ACC/AHA do not advocate any specific mode of anaesthesia for patients with cardiac disease. EVAR under regional or LA is feasible and effective, but there is no definitive evidence that they are superior to GA. The choice of anaesthesia should be tailored to the individual case.

Postoperatively, close surveillance is essential. In the UK most are cared for in a level 2 HDU.

Complications of EVAR

See Box 16.3.

Box 16.3 Complications of EVAR

- Deployment problems
- Stent-graft limb thrombosis
- Endoleak:
  - Type 1: failure of stent graft to seal
  - Type 2: back bleeding from lumbar vessels
  - Type 3: dislocation of the limbs from main body or tear in fabric
  - Type 4: porosity or endodistension
- Graft migration
- Rupture of Iliac artery
- Haemorrhage
- Embolization—distal, renal, gut
- Graft infection
- Conversion to open repair
- Paralysis, secondary to spinal cord ischaemia
- Cardiac complications
- Contrast-induced nephropathy
- Postimplantation syndrome.

Contrast-induced nephropathy

Contrast-induced nephropathy (CIN) is a potential complication following EVAR and has been defined as an absolute increase in serum creatinine of 44mmol/L or a relative increase of 25% from baseline, provided other causes of renal dysfunction are excluded (see section 3.5).

Clinical risk factors for CIN include:

- Chronic renal impairment
- Diabetes mellitus
- Perioperative dehydration
- Volume of contrast used
- Advanced age
- Perioperative use of other nephrotoxic drugs (including those who have been given contrast within the last 10 days).

Strategies to reduce CIN include:

- Generous perioperative IV fluid administration.
- Minimal use of contrast.
- Increased interval between contrast CT angiography and EVAR.
- Less complex procedures considered in those with significant renal impairment.
- Intravenous rehydration prior to the radiological procedure is probably beneficial.

There has been interest in the use of prophylactic antioxidants to prevent CIN, e.g. N-acetylcysteine and some meta-analyses have suggested a benefit, but individual studies looking specifically at its use in EVAR have not demonstrated this effect.

Paralysis

Due to the anatomy of the blood supply to the spinal cord, EVAR may result in cord ischaemia and paralysis. The risks are increased by a longer or more proximal stent. The incidence for infrarenal EVAR is quoted as about 1 in 400.

A CSF drain may be used to reduce the effects of cord ischaemia. This is not routinely done for infrarenal EVAR but may be considered for more proximal stents.

Blood loss

Average blood loss is about 400mL, but there is wide variation with longer procedures resulting in a higher loss. Haemorrhage will usually be concealed and only become apparent when the patient displays signs of hypovolaemia and shock.

Postimplantation syndrome

This is common and usually benign. Clinical characteristics include:

- Pyrexia
- Leucocytosis
- Elevated inflammatory markers.

Clinically it appears similar to sepsis, but without the presence of infection. Exclusion of larger aneurysms may cause significant fibrinolysis secondary to thrombus within the aneurysm sac leading to a state of coagulopathy. The majority of cases of postimplantation syndrome are self-limiting and usually settle within 2 weeks of surgery.

Further reading

Nataraj V & Mortimer AJ (2004). EVAR. *CEACCP*, 4(3):91–4.

The UK EVAR Trial Investigators (2010). Endovascular versus open repair of AAA. *NEJM*, 362:1863–71.

Aortic cross-clamping

Aortic cross-clamping causes profound physiological and pathological changes that affect every organ system. Occluding the blood flow in the aorta will cause end-organ ischaemia which may result in permanent damage with a corresponding increase in patient morbidity and mortality. When the clamp is removed the metabolites which have built up during the period of anaerobic metabolism are released into the general circulation causing another sequence of physiological and pathological disturbance.

The effects will depend on certain variables:

- The site of the clamp
- The length of time it is applied
- The patient's physiological reserve
- Whether the surgery is elective or emergency.

Cardiac effects

The level of the clamp is a key consideration; the more proximal the clamp, the more profound the effect on the patient. A suprarenal clamp has a much more significant effect than an infrarenal one.

Cardiac output = stroke volume × heart rate

Cardiac output = blood pressure/systemic vascular resistance

Once the aortic cross-clamp is applied, a sudden increase in system vascular resistance (SVR) occurs. This causes an increase in the workload of the heart, which can be demonstrated on transoesophageal echocardiography. So when the cross-clamp is applied either the blood pressure will rise or the heart will fail.

Infrarenal clamps may cause minimal changes but studies have shown supracoeliac clamps may be associated with:

- Mean arterial pressure increases up to 50%
- Filling pressures increase by 40%
- Ejection fraction is reduced by 40%.

Myocardial regional wall motion abnormalities were demonstrated in 33% of the study patients with a suprarenal clamp and >90% of those patients with a supracoeliac aortic cross-clamp. These changes occur even in those patients with normal preoperative myocardial perfusion scans.

The heart must maintain a cardiac output in the face of increased resistance to forward flow. It achieves this by:

- An increased preload from the central veins. This increases the stretch on the myocardial fibres and, according to Frank–Starling's Law, results in increased contractility.
- Increased sympathetic stimulation. This increases the heart rate and contractility, which maintains cardiac output.
- Help from the anaesthetist.

Therapeutic aims

Reduce afterload (decrease SVR) with vasodilatation:

- Anaesthetic agents
- Regional anaesthesia (epidural)
- GTN
- Sodium nitroprusside.

Increase contractility using inotropes:

- Adrenaline
- Dobutamine.

Increased contractility requires increased oxygen consumption. This is achieved in two ways:

1. Coronary vessels autoregulate and dilate to allow greater flow through those areas of myocardium with higher metabolic demand.
2. The flow of blood is redistributed from the epicardium to the subendocardium. This allows the heart to improve its inotropic state resulting in reduced LVESV whilst maintaining intraventricular pressures.

Role of the venous system

On cross-clamping the distal arterial blood supply is reduced. This reduces the return of blood to the venous system. As the venous system empties, the compliance of the vessels decreases according to Laplace's law and this encourages the veins to collapse and expel blood towards the major central veins. This is seen clinically with increased central venous pressure (CVP) and pulmonary capillary wedge pressure (PCWP). During infrarenal clamping, the majority of the redistributed blood may pool in the more compliant splanchnic system. This reduces the effective change in preload. The splanchnic system alone is thought to represent 70% of the redistributed blood and explains why the blood pressure changes can be modest in infrarenal cross clamping. Net effect depends on factors such as:

- Sympathetic tone
- Type of anaesthetic technique
- Vasopressor agents.

All these will cause arterial changes, but may also redistribute venous blood and affect preload.

Renal effects

The kidneys demand a relatively constant perfusion pressure, which is regulated by the afferent arterioles and humoral factors. Renal vessels can be severely affected by aortic cross-clamping whether it is supra or infrarenal.

Suprarenal cross-clamping can reduce renal blood flow by up to 95%. This can result in acute tubular necrosis (ATN) with a proportion of patients requiring renal replacement therapy which is associated with higher mortality.

Risk factors:

- Length of cross clamping
- Pre-existing renal impairment
- Age
- Diabetes.

Infrarenal clamping changes the distribution of the blood within the kidney with a decrease in cortical perfusion. This can cause reduced glomerular filtration rate (GFR) and lower urine output. GFR has been shown to decrease in 67% of patients after infrarenal aortic surgery whilst renal plasma flow decreased in 48% of patients. This reduction is maintained at 6 months postoperatively.

Spinal cord ischaemia

Within the spinal cord the blood supply is dictated by the difference between mean aortic pressure or anterior spinal artery pressure and CSF pressure or venous pressure, whichever is greater:

$$\text{Perfusion pressure} = \text{MAP} - \text{CSF pressure}$$

With the application of the cross-clamp, the anterior spinal artery pressure drops and venous engorgement occurs, reducing the effective perfusion pressure and increasing the risk of ischaemia. The spinal cord is dependent upon collateral supply for perfusion. The most distal supply is the artery of Adamkiewicz, which supplies the distal cord. Its anatomy is variable and it may originate from the distal thoracic to the infrarenal aorta. Both hypoxia and reperfusion injury have a part to play in the pathogenesis of neurological impairment and paraplegia. This is thought to be due to free radical production locally. The introduction of free radical scavengers has been shown to reduce the incidence of paraplegia in animal studies.

Paraplegia due to aortic cross-clamping is associated with many factors:

- The level of the cross clamp
- Duration of clamping
- Age
- Urgency of the operation
- Episodes of hypotension
- Aortic dissection.

Neurological damage secondary to aortic cross-clamping can be in the order of 40%, and only half will have any neurological recovery. Clearly the risks are less with infrarenal aortic clamping, however the figures quoted remain from 0.25–1%.

Techniques used to prevent neurological damage include:

- Surgical techniques
- Maintaining adequate blood pressure
- CSF drainage
- Cooling techniques
- Ischaemic preconditioning
- Free radical scavengers.

The viscera

Visceral ischaemia through reduced or altered blood flow can occur secondary to a number of causes. The mesenteric vessels are commonly affected by the aortic clamp resulting in vessel ligation or temporary occlusion. This can have serious consequences with a mortality of up to 50%. The bowel can be affected whether the aortic clamp is supra- or infrarenal. The most common site for clinical ischaemia is the descending colon, supplied by the inferior mesenteric artery. Blood flow to the gut can be altered by patient factors such as:

- Hypovolaemia
- Cardiac arrhythmias and reduced cardiac output

as well as operative factors such as:

- Emboli
- Thrombosis.

The incidence of visceral ischaemia varies from 1–10%.

Coagulation

Coagulation and haemorrhage continues to play an important part in morbidity and mortality associated with aortic surgery. Cross-clamping and the resulting ischaemia can lead to coagulopathy due to coagulation factor consumption and activation of fibrinolytic pathways.

Systemic effects of reperfusion

Cross-clamping results in anaerobic metabolism or even ischaemia/necrosis. This results in the build-up of metabolic waste products (Box 16.4).

Box 16.4 Products of anaerobic metabolism
• H^+
• ADP
• K^+
• Adenosine
• Hypoxanthine
• Xanthine oxidase
• Purines.

Upon clamp release these are washed into the systemic circulation and cause:

- Vasodilatation (decreased SVR)
- Cardiac dysfunction (decreased contractility, decreased cardiac output).

The combination of hypotension and cardiac dysfunction can cause profound hypotension and even cardiac arrest.

Risk factors for significant reperfusion syndrome include:

- Level of clamp
- Duration of clamping
- Hypovolaemia
- Comorbidity
- Emergency surgery
- Age.

Lung complications are common after aortic surgery. Some pulmonary morbidity is attributed to inflammatory mediators following cross-clamp release. This causes increased pulmonary vascular resistance (PVR), pulmonary hypertension, and increased pulmonary vascular permeability. These can lead to pulmonary oedema and acute lung injury and result in prolonged ventilation.

The increase in pulmonary capillary leak is a result of the release of humoral factors, such as thromboxane, released by ischaemic endothelial cells. Thromboxane induces neutrophils which results in platelet activation and the release of oxygen free radicals and elastase. Within the lungs these cause increased vascular permeability. Other mediators of the pulmonary capillaries include the renin–angiotensin system and complement. When activated during aortic surgery this raises levels of C3a and C5a, which are potent mediators of smooth muscle contraction and can also affect capillary permeability.

Further reading

Gelman S (1995). The pathophysiology of aortic cross clamping and unclamping. *Anesthesiology*, 82(4):1026–57.

Webb ST & Allen JSD (2008). Perioperative renal protection. *CEACCP*, 8(5):176–80.

16.4 Management of elective carotid surgery

Carotid endarterectomy (CEA)

CEA is a procedure to remove atheromatous plaque at or around the carotid bifurcation with the aim to prevent stroke. Large multicentre trials since the 1990s have established the current role of CEA in stroke prevention.

Stroke is the third most common cause of mortality in the Western world, with about 120 000 cases/year in the UK. Approximately one-third of patients die, one-third recover, and one-third suffer long-term disability. Costs for long-term care exceed £1 billion per year.

Carotid stenosis is implicated in about one-fifth of strokes. Currently 5000 CEAs are carried out in the UK each year, about half of which are performed under LA.

Indications for surgery

Large randomized control trials (European Carotid Surgery Trial 1991, North American Symptomatic Carotid Endarterectomy Trial 1991) have shown that CEA can reduce the risk of stroke in certain groups of patients. Symptomatic patients with 50–69% stenosis had marginal benefit and those with >70% (without near occlusion, or occlusion) had considerable benefit, providing surgical morbidity was <6%.

Current evidence suggests that patients with asymptomatic stenosis should be treated with best medical therapy.

Preoperative considerations

Patients for CEA have vascular disease and are likely to have the pattern of cardiovascular and smoking-related risk factors and comorbidity common to these patients.

Patients may already have suffered a stroke and need a detailed neurological assessment. If surgery under LA is planned, then their ability to communicate during surgery is a key consideration. Psychological and emotional issues are also important. A small number of patients absolutely refuse surgery under LA. All patients need appropriate explanation of what to expect in the anaesthetic room/operating theatre.

Antiplatelet therapy

Nearly all patients will have received antiplatelet therapy. Evidence suggests that a single dose of 75mg of clopidogrel the night before surgery, in addition to regular aspirin, reduces the incidence of postoperative embolic events.

Investigations

All patients should have routine blood tests and an ECG. Further investigations should be performed as indicated on an individual basis, according to the ACC/AHA guidelines. Control of hypertension, and other cardiorespiratory disorders, should be optimized.

The effectiveness of CEA in preventing stroke is closely related to the timing of surgery. Surgery should be performed within 2 weeks of symptoms and ideally within 48h. It is essential that anaesthetic assessment of the patient does not cause unnecessary delay.

Local anaesthesia

IV access, both 20G and 16G, is established in the contralateral arm, one with multiple port 'octopus' connectors incorporating non-return valves.

An arterial line is sited, under LA, preferably in the contralateral arm. Cardiovascular instability can be a major problem during surgery and a well-functioning arterial line is essential. Ideally a site accessible without interrupting surgery is recommended.

LA options

- Superficial cervical plexus block (see Box 16.5)
- Deep cervical plexus block (see Box 16.6)
- Combined cervical plexus blocks
- Cervical epidural
- Local infiltration.

Cervical plexus blocks are most commonly performed. The deep cervical plexus block may be performed via an interscalene approach under ultrasound control. It is, however, associated with a high incidence of serious complications. Superficial cervical plexus block with high volume of LA may offer comparable analgesia. A combination of lidocaine and bupivacaine is effective.

Box 16.5 Superficial cervical plexus block

- Patient supine, head turned to opposite side.
- Midpoint of posterior border of sternocleidomastoid.
- 22G needle immediately behind muscle perpendicular to skin.
- Insert until encounter the 'pop' of the cervical fascia.
- 15mL LA will form a 'sausage' along the posterior muscle border.

Box 16.6 Deep cervical plexus block

- Palpate the transverse processes of C3 along a line between the mastoid process and C6 transverse process.
- Needle perpendicular to skin is directed toward transverse process until contact at 1–2cm and then withdrawn 1–2mm.
- 10mL LA injected as single injection after aspiration.
- Some advocate three separate injections at C2, C3, and C4 using 4mL at each point.
- [NB: Risk of subarachnoid, epidural, and intravenous injection. Deep cervical plexus block causes phrenic nerve and recurrent laryngeal nerve block].

Surgical issues will impact on the effectiveness of the block. High lesions requiring vigorous retraction or high dissection can be difficult to adequately block. There is some crossover innervation from the contralateral cervical plexus which can be abolished by subcutaneous midline LA infiltration. The carotid artery itself is difficult to block and may be exquisitely sensitive to manipulation. Many surgeons will inject LA through the carotid sheath under direct vision in order to overcome this problem. Remifentanil infusions may also be helpful, but sedation is undesirable.

Perioperative considerations

- The patient is positioned to be as comfortable as possible and theatre temperature made suitable.
- A transparent drape should be used on the head and neck to minimize claustrophobia.
- Supplementary oxygen should be administered, either with a cut away mask or nasal sponge.
- Patients are not routinely catheterized or given IV fluids, unless there is a specific indication.

The anaesthetist must talk to the patient throughout the procedure in order to reassure and to check cerebral function. Sedation, if used, should be kept to a minimum to allow ongoing assessment. Changes in cerebral function may be subtle and regular checks of verbal and motor skills should be made both before and after internal carotid artery cross-clamping.

Cardiovascular instability can be a particular problem during CEA with rapid and profound hypertension or hypotension. Infusions of vasopressors and vasodilators should be available for immediate administration. Blood pressure should remain at (or above) normal values throughout, in order to maintain cerebral perfusion pressure. Systolic hypertension >180mmHg should be avoided, although most perioperative strokes are probably attributable to thromobembolism.

Heparin 3000–5000IU is administered prior to clamping.

General anaesthesia

Patients undergoing CEA under GA should have invasive blood pressure measurements established prior to induction to maximize cardiovascular stability. A reinforced tube is used and eye protection important. It is not necessary to infiltrate LA or perform a block.

The cardiovascular considerations are the same regardless of anaesthetic technique. SBP should be kept at, or above, the normal value of the patient whilst avoiding systolic hypertension. Long-acting opiates should be avoided to allow postoperative neurological assessment.

Extubation is performed while deeply anaesthetized. The patient should remain in the operating theatre with the surgeon present until neurological function can be assessed.

Postoperative management

- Regular neurological observations in recovery.
- All patients are anticoagulated.
- GTN or labetalol infusions are used to keep the systolic pressure at 120–180mmHg.
- Hypotension should be managed with a fluid bolus or may require vasopressors following review.

Oral analgesia is usually sufficient for postoperative pain relief. Patients may complain of headache and nausea.

Overnight HDU care is usual, but most patients are discharged from hospital after 2 days.

Severe postoperative complications are rare. These include bleeding, which may compromise the airway and be life threatening, stroke, and cerebral hyperperfusion syndrome.

Cerebral hyperperfusion syndrome

Case series report an incidence of up to 3%. Risk factors include reduced cerebrovascular reserve, second side operation, and prolonged postoperative hypertension. It usually presents in the early postoperative period but has been described up to 2 weeks postoperatively.

The syndrome is characterized by:
- Ipsilateral headache
- Hypertension
- Seizures
- Focal neurological defects.

This emergency requires treatment directed at controlling blood pressure to prevent cerebral oedema and haemorrhage.

General versus local anaesthesia

There has been much debate over the relative merits of LA or GA for CEA. A large scale randomized trial (GALA trial) showed no definite benefit of either technique over the other. Primary outcomes were stroke, MI, and mortality at 30 days.

Advantages/disadvantages of GA

If the patient has a GA then effective neurological monitoring cannot be carried out. Several techniques have been investigated to give surrogate measures of cerebral perfusion under GA. These include:
- Transcranial Doppler, measuring middle cerebral artery velocity
- Distal stump pressure measurement
- Cerebral oxygen consumption
- Somatosensory evoked potentials
- EEG interpretation.

None of these techniques have been found to be specific or sensitive enough. Therefore a shunt may be inserted during carotid cross-clamp to ensure adequate cerebral perfusion. The shunt runs from the proximal stump to the distal internal carotid artery (ICA). The insertion of the shunt is not without risk and may result in intimal damage, emboli, or thrombosis increasing the risk of postoperative stroke.

Some surgeons place a shunt in all patients having GA whereas others feel that no patients should have a shunt (on the grounds that only a small number of patients show signs of neurological impairment when the carotid is clamped). A policy of shunting those at high risk of developing ischaemia during clamping would seem ideal, but in practice it is difficult to select these patients.

The advantages of GA are airway control, maintenance of normocapnia/normoxia for CBF optimization, and reduction in cerebral metabolism which may be neuroprotective in the event of ischaemia. Many patients prefer this technique.

Advantages/disadvantages of LA

CEA performed under LA enables accurate, immediate assessment of neurological status. In the event of neurological changes on cross clamping the ICA a shunt can be inserted. This prevents unnecessary shunt insertion. The other complications of GA are avoided and LA may be associated with a shorter hospital stay.

Disadvantages include the complications of the regional block and poor access to the airway if GA conversion is required. Sedation may negate the benefits of LA.

Further reading

Ladak N & Thompson J (2012). General or local anaesthesia for carotid endarterectomy? *CEACCP*, 12(2):92–6.

Rerkasem K & Rothwell PM (2008). Local versus general anaesthesia for carotid endarterectomy. *Cochrane Database Syst Rev*, 4:CD000126.

16.5 Anaesthesia for sympathectomy

Thoracic sympathectomy

Thoracic sympathectomy is most commonly performed for idiopathic hyperhidrosis. It may also be performed to manage chronic regional pain syndromes, cardiac ischaemia, and long QT syndrome. Originally, the thoracic sympathetic chain was accessed via an open surgical approach. This high morbidity surgery is now avoided with the use of thoracoscopic procedures.

Anatomy

The sympathetic nervous system is derived from the spinal cord between T1 and L2. Fibres pass via an anterior root into the corresponding spinal nerve. They then synapse either in the paravertebral sympathetic chain or at a distant ganglion. The sympathetic fibres for skin and vessels re-emerge from the cord with skeletal fibres.

The sympathetic chains extend between the skull base and coccyx and are positioned 2–3cm lateral to the vertebral column. They descend behind the carotid sheath, passing over the heads of the upper ribs in the thorax and enter the abdomen. The paravertebral sympathetic chains continue into the pelvis and merge together at the level of the coccyx.

Thoracoscopic sympathectomy

The Society of Thoracic Surgeons Task Force recently reviewed the current literature and reached a consensus that primary hyperhidrosis of the palms, plantars, axillae, or face is best treated with endoscopic thoracic sympathectomy. Interruption of the sympathetic chain is best achieved by clipping, which gives the possibility of reversing the sympathectomy. Their recommendations for level of interruption are as follows:

- Top of the 3rd rib for craniofacial hyperhidrosis.
- Top of 3rd/4th rib for palmar only hyperhidrosis.
- Top of the 4th and 5th rib for palmar and axillary, axillary alone and palmar, axillary, and plantar hyperhidrosis.

Surgical complications are uncommon but include:

- Pneumothorax (4%)
- Horner's syndrome (0.5%)
- Haemothorax/chylothorax (0.5%).

Recurrence occurs in about 4% of cases and compensatory hyperhidrosis may occur in 50% patients.

Anaesthesia for sympathectomy

Preoperative considerations

The majority of patients undergoing endoscopic thoracic sympathectomy are young with minimal comorbidities. Rarely, this is also a surgical option for refractory angina, digital ischaemia, or prolonged QT syndrome. There is a small risk of conversion to thoracotomy and significant blood loss.

Intraoperative considerations

Standard monitoring is adequate; any invasive monitoring will be dictated by comorbidities. Due to the risk of major blood loss, large-bore IV access is necessary.

The choice of airway is discussed in Table 16.1. This is highly influenced by the surgical technique and exposure, and must be discussed with the surgeon. Traditionally, the choice is between endobronchial and endotracheal intubation.

Endobronchial ventilation via DLT results in:

- Loss of hypoxic vasoconstriction.
- Increased shunt during one-lung ventilation.
- Higher incidence of hypoxia.
- Residual atelectasis adds to hypoxia.

Whereas with endotracheal ventilation via single-lumen tube:

- The lung on the operated side is still ventilated.
- Partial collapse occurs due to the endoscopic CO_2 insufflation and lung retraction.
- Lower incidence of hypoxia.
- These conditions also apply to a patient self-ventilating with an LMA.

Due to the easier anaesthetic technique and reduced incidence of hypoxia, the endotracheal ventilation method is gaining in popularity. If this technique is chosen, the anaesthetist needs to pay careful attention to the rate and pressure of CO_2 insufflation. It is recommended that inflation pressures should be a maximum of 10mmHg. Higher pressures may be associated with a significant decrease in cardiac index. Signs of tension pneumothorax must be treated immediately with the release of CO_2 and re-inflation of the operative side.

The patient is positioned supine with 20–30° head-up tilt. The arm on the operative side is abducted by 90° to enable surgical access (for two thoracoscopic ports in the anterior axillary line). The patient will be draped to enable conversion to thoracotomy should it be necessary.

If a bilateral procedure is planned then both arms will need to be abducted in a crucifix position. The right side may be technically difficult due to the close proximity of the hemiazygous vein to the right sympathetic chain. Bilateral procedures are also more challenging for the anaesthetist. Profound hypoxia may occur when the second lung is collapsed due to residual atelectasis adding to shunt in the ventilated lung.

At the end of the procedure, the lung is re-inflated under direct vision and intrapleural LA administered as part of the multimodal analgesia required.

Postoperative considerations

There is no benefit from routine use of intrapleural drains, as the incidence of pneumothorax is low and those requiring drainage even lower. Most centres still routinely perform a CXR to exclude pneumothorax. A period of clinical observation in recovery is important to check for immediate complications.

Standard postoperative analgesia is required. Patients often complain of retrosternal or upper back pain, which is believed to be associated with pleural stretching, related to the capnothorax.

Table 16.1 Airway techniques for thoracoscopic sympathectomy

Anaesthetic technique	Advantages	Disadvantages
Double- lumen endobronchial tube (DLT)	Provides excellent surgical exposure with or without CO_2 insufflation, lung deflated before incision thereby decreasing risk of lung damage	Increased risk of iatrogenic laryngeal and tracheal trauma and hypoxia due to incorrect tube placement
Single-lumen endotracheal tube	Familiar, easier technique	Requires CO_2 insufflation and lung retraction to allow surgical access which increases the risk of lung damage and tension pneumothorax
Single-lumen endotracheal tube with a bronchial blocker	Familiar technique for securing the airway, as with DLT can provide excellent surgical exposure	Bronchial blocker requires a level of expertise to secure lung isolation. Lung deflation is longer than with DLT
LMA either spontaneous ventilation or positive pressure ventilation	A supraglottic airway that avoids iatrogenic trauma to the vocal cords and trachea	Will require CO_2 insufflation and relatively high ventilation pressure, which will increase the risk of gastric insufflation. If emergency conversion to thoracotomy is required then intubation will be required
Regional anaesthetic, both high thoracic epidural and multiple level intercostal nerve blocks have been described	Avoids airway intervention	Requires level of expertise and patient co-operation. As with an LMA if an emergency conversion to thoracotomy is required the patient will need intubation.

Further reading

Brock H, Rieger R, Gabriel C, *et al.* (2000). Haemodynamic changes during thoracoscopic surgery. The effects of one-lung ventilation compared with carbon dioxide insufflation. *Anaesthesia*, 55:10–16.

Cerfolio RJ, De Campos JR, Bryant AS, *et al.* (2011). The Society of Thoracic Surgeons expert consensus for the surgical treatment of hyperhydrosis. *Ann Thorac Surg*, 91(5):1642–8.

Rodríguez PM, Freixinet JL, Hussein M, *et al.* (2008). Side effects, complications and outcome of thoracocscopic sympathectomy for palmar and axillary hyperhydrosis in 406 patients. *Eur J Cardiothorac Surg*, 34(3):514–9.

Prevalence and health burden

More than a quarter of the adult population of the UK smoke (27% of men, 25% of women). Tobacco is the single greatest cause of preventable death worldwide. The WHO estimated that tobacco caused 4.9 million deaths in 2007 (approximately 1 in 10 adults). Smoking kills about 106 000 people each year in the UK.

Smoking causes a multitude of serious and potentially fatal diseases including cardiovascular disease, respiratory disease, malignancies, and reproductive problems.

The 'British Doctors Study' led by Richard Doll was a longitudinal study of 40 701 medical specialists from 1951–2001. In 1956 they demonstrated a statistical link between smoking and lung cancer. In follow-up reports they showed that >50% of persistent smokers die of a smoking-related disease.

Passive smoking is also known to be associated with health risks. After Scotland banned smoking in public places in 2006, there was a 17% reduction in hospital admissions for acute coronary syndrome; 67% of the decrease occurred in non-smokers.

Health problems associated with smoking

Many serious and potentially fatal diseases are caused by smoking (Table 16.2). Smoking also increases the incidence of more minor complaints such as respiratory tract infection.

Table 16.2 Diseases and conditions associated with smoking	
System	Condition
Cardiovascular	Hypertension Coronary artery disease Peripheral vascular disease Aneurysmal disease Cerebrovascular disease
Respiratory	COPD Lung cancer
Malignancies	Lung Oral, nasal, laryngeal Oesophageal, gastric, pancreatic Bladder, kidney, cervical Myeloid leukaemia
Reproductive	Infertility and erectile dysfunction Preterm delivery Stillbirth Low birth weight
Miscellaneous	Osteoporosis Peptic ulcer disease Sudden infant death syndrome

Cardiovascular disease

Coronary artery disease (CAD) is the leading cause of death in the UK and smoking is a major factor in its development. Smokers are 2–4 times more likely to develop CAD compared with non-smokers.

Also, smoking doubles an individual's risk for stroke and increases by more than 10 times the risk of developing peripheral vascular disease. Smoking exerts these effects by the prominent role it has in the aetiology of atherosclerosis.

Respiratory disease

Smoking is the most important cause of chronic obstructive pulmonary disease (COPD). Smoking is associated with a tenfold increased risk of death caused by COPD, with 90% of all COPD deaths occurring in smokers. The adverse respiratory effects of smoking are caused by inducing persistent airway inflammation, which causes a direct imbalance in oxidant/antioxidant capacity and increases proteolytic enzyme release. However, some of these effects are reversible. Stopping smoking will slow the average rate of decline in FEV_1 from 50–70mL per year to 30mL per year (the equivalent rate in non-smokers).

Malignancies

Smoking causes 30% of all cancer deaths and >80% of lung cancer deaths. Bronchial carcinoma is the most common fatal malignancy in the developed world and accounts for >50% of all cancer-related deaths. The risk of dying from lung cancer is more than 22 times higher among male smokers and about 12 times higher among female smokers compared with those who have never smoked.

Reproductive system

There is an increased rate of both male and female infertility amongst smokers. Smoking is associated with a number of pregnancy-related complications, including ectopic pregnancy, placental abruption, and preterm delivery. It increases the risk of stillbirth, death of the neonate within the first week of life, and the risk of sudden infant death syndrome. In addition, smoking is associated with some congenital defects such as cleft palate.

Mechanisms of disease development

Atherosclerosis

The chemicals (Box 16.7) present in inhaled tobacco smoke are absorbed into the circulation. Nicotine stimulates the release of catecholamines, whilst other products (perhaps including nicotine) injure the arterial endothelium and promote atherogenesis. Free radicals and aromatic compounds diminish the endothelial synthesis of nitric oxide. This results in impaired endothelium-dependent relaxation of arteries and is the earliest clinical sign of endothelial dysfunction.

Box 16.7 Some of the chemicals found in tobacco smoke
• Acetaldehyde • Acrolein • Acrylamide • Ammonia • Benzanthracene • Benzapyrene • Benzene • Carbon monoxide • Cresols • Hydrogen cyanide • Nitrogen oxides • Nitrosoanatabine • Nitrosonornicotine • Phenol • Toluene.

Smoking-induced changes at the endothelial surface result in upregulation of leucocyte adhesion molecules. The increased oxidation of low-density lipoprotein (LDL) in smokers has synergistic effects to promote monocyte adhesion and monocyte migration into the subintimal space. Continued stimulation of intimal cells by oxidized LDL leads to the development of atherosclerosis.

Smoking also potentiates thrombosis at the dysfunctional endothelium by increasing the concentration of plasma fibrinogen and altering the activity of platelets.

COPD pathogenesis

COPD is characterized by chronic inflammation throughout the airways, parenchyma, and pulmonary vasculature. Macrophages, T lymphocytes, and neutrophils are increased in various parts of the lung. Activated inflammatory cells release a variety of mediators including leukotriene B4, interleukin-8, tumour necrosis factor-α, and others capable of damaging lung structures or sustaining neutrophilic inflammation. Two other processes that may be important in the pathogenesis of COPD are an increase in proteinases relative to antiproteinases in the lung, and oxidative stress. Inflammation of the lungs is caused by exposure to inhaled noxious particles and gases. Cigarette smoke can induce inflammation and directly damage the lungs.

Cancers

There are over 5000 identified chemicals and more than 60 known carcinogens in cigarette smoke. The carcinogenicity of cigarette smoke can also be enhanced by the presence of tumour promoters and co-carcinogens. The reaction of carcinogens with DNA can cause mutations and, if unrepaired, can lead to the activation of oncogenes or the deactivation of tumour suppressors.

Epigenetic changes may also occur from exposure to tobacco carcinogens, leading to a change in gene expression.

Perioperative effects of smoking

Smoking not only causes disease, it also impacts on the treatment of that disease. Smokers suffer increased morbidity and mortality after vascular, cardiac bypass, and colorectal surgery. Smokers have a higher rate of unplanned admission to high dependency areas after surgery.

Smokers undergoing surgery have to contend with the associated comorbidity as well as a decrease in their oxygen carrying ability, caused by chronic exposure to carbon monoxide. This results in decreased oxygen availability to tissues at a time when the endocrine and hormonal responses to surgical stress cause an increased tissue demand for oxygen.

Smokers may develop polycythaemia as a result of chronic hypoxaemia. This, together with increased plasma fibrinogen and platelet activation, results in hypercoagulability and an increased risk of arterial thrombosis.

Smokers are at higher risk of life-threatening postoperative respiratory and cardiac complications following surgery.

Stopping smoking carries clear benefit in the perioperative period. Stopping days or weeks before surgery will allow the clearance of carbon monoxide and improvements in upper airway reactivity, while stopping for a few months may lead to a reduction in postoperative complications.

16.7 Principles of blood conservation and red cell salvage

Introduction

Despite increased knowledge of the hazards of allogeneic blood, perioperative transfusion is a common event in the UK, with surgical patients receiving approximately 40% of all donated blood. However, blood conservation techniques and use of autologous cell-salvaged blood can prevent the need for allogeneic blood in some patients.

Rationale for avoiding allogeneic blood transfusion:
- Risk of transfusion-related adverse event
- Limited availability of blood stock
- Financial cost of blood products
- Adverse effects of stored blood (reduced clotting factors, reduced oxygen carrying capacity)
- Worse clinical outcomes for some surgical patients (cardiac surgery, colorectal metastatic disease)
- Religious beliefs of some patients.

Preoperative management

Bleeding risk assessment
Planning blood conservation surgery must start with a preoperative patient risk evaluation. This identifies factors that are associated with an increased likelihood of requiring perioperative blood products such as:
- Advanced age
- Decreased preoperative red cell volume (small body size or preoperative anaemia or both)
- Complex surgery (especially re-do operations).

It is also important to identify patients who do not wish to receive blood or blood products due to religious reasons (e.g. Jehovah's Witnesses) and to document their specific requests.

Measures to increase red cell volume (RCV)
Of the risk factors already noted, the one that can be most easily manipulated preoperatively is decreased RCV.

$$RCV = \text{fraction of red cells} \times \text{blood volume}$$

RCV is an index of the red cell reserve that is likely to be depleted by operative intervention. It can be increased preoperatively in anaemic patients by use of iron supplements and erythropoietin.

Autologous blood donation
The patient's own blood may be removed 3–4 weeks prior to surgery and stored for future autologous donation. During this time the patient may be given iron supplements and erythropoietin to replenish RCV. However, pre-deposit programmes are expensive and still carry the risks associated with transfusion of stored blood and incorrect patient identification.

Impaired coagulation and antiplatelet drugs
Patients on anticoagulant therapy must be identified and managed according to their indication for treatment. In some cases it may be possible to discontinue drugs perioperatively, but others will require bridging therapy with short-acting agents.

Patients who are taking antiplatelet medications must be assessed on an individual basis. The risk of stopping medication must be weighed up against the risk of bleeding after considering coexisting risk factors for blood loss.

Bleeding diatheses should be identified and treated, e.g. desmopressin to reduce the bleeding time in patients with known von Willebrand disease or mild haemophilia A.

Intraoperative management

Acute normovolaemic haemodilution
This method of preoperative RCV conservation involves the venesection of one or two units of the patient's own blood prior to the start of the surgery. The patient is then given IV solutions to restore normovolaemia. Blood lost in theatre, will be of a lower haematocrit, (hence less RCV lost) and there is autologous blood available for transfusion after haemostasis has been achieved.

Antifibrinolytics
Antifibrinolytic drugs such as tranexamic acid may be used during surgery to prevent or reduce further bleeding where fibrinolysis is implicated. The use of these drugs may be guided by viscoelastic tests such as thromboelastography.

Topical haemostatic agents
Topical haemostatic adhesive materials can be applied to localized sites of bleeding by the surgeons:

Resorbable haemostatic gauzes such as Surgicel® provide a scaffold for clot formation and provide wound compression as they swell due to blood accumulation and coagulation.

Fibrin sealants are usually two-component systems in which a solution of concentrated fibrinogen and factor XIII are combined with a solution of thrombin and calcium to rapidly form a fibrin clot. Antifibrinolytics are added to some preparations to prevent clot lysis. These agents cannot be used in conjunction with intraoperative cell salvage.

Surgical techniques and equipment/devices
Techniques such as laparoscopic surgery, spinal anaesthesia, hypotensive anaesthesia, and devices such as tourniquets, electrocautery, laser, harmonic scalpel, etc. may be used to limit the amount of blood loss during surgery.

Intraoperative cell salvage (ICS)
ICS is indicated for patients with:
- Large blood loss anticipated (>1000mL or >20% blood volume).
- Low preoperative haemoglobin or increased risk of bleeding.
- Multiple antibodies or rare blood types.
- Objections to receiving allogeneic blood.

The blood is collected from the operative site, washed of any contaminants, and the red blood cells returned to the patient (Fig. 16.1).

A team approach, headed by an ICS lead clinician (often an anaesthetist, responsible for staff training and awareness) is required for effective utilization of autologous blood recovery techniques (Box 16.8).

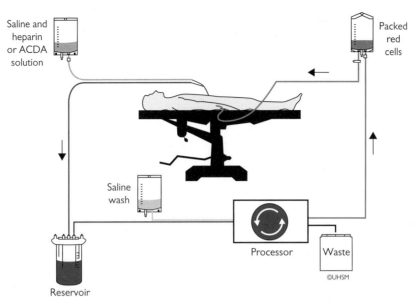

Fig. 16.1 Diagram of cell salvage circuit. Reproduced with permission from University Hospital of South Manchester NHS Foundation Trust Department of Medical Illustration.

Box 16.8 Technique of blood collection for ICS

- Theatre staff and surgeons should have prior warning of cases where ICS is likely to be used so appropriate suction systems can be set up.
- Large-bore suction tip (minimum 4mm Yankauer sucker) should be used.
- Low vacuum pressure suction should be used to avoid red cell haemolysis.
- To avoid air aspiration, blood should be suctioned from pools rather than surface skimming.
- Specialized double-lumen suction tubing (allowing addition of anticoagulant before it is returned to the ICS collection reservoir) must be used.
- Blood collection must be discontinued if the surgical field is contaminated with substances that are not licensed for IV use, e.g.:
  - Iodine
  - Topical antibiotics not licensed for IV use
  - Topical haemostatic agents
  - Orthopaedic cement.

Special considerations for ICS

There are a number of specific circumstances where the use of ICS is not recommended because potentially blood has been contaminated with bacteria, amniotic fluid, or malignant cells. In these cases, clinicians must take into account latest evidence and consider the risks and benefits of individual patients.

Bowel contamination

The manufacturers recommend that ICS devices are not used in surgery where there has been contamination by bowel content unless there is catastrophic haemorrhage.

Obstetrics

Use of ICS in obstetrics has been limited until recently by concerns of the risk of amniotic fluid embolism due to reinfusion of blood that may contain fetal contaminates. This theoretical risk may be minimized by the use of a leucocyte depletion filter with the ICS blood giving set.

Malignancy

The use of ICS in surgical patients with known malignancy is contraindicated due to the potential risk of spreading metastatic disease by reinfusion of malignant cells. There are, however, many reports of ICS being used in cancer surgery without evidence of recurrence.

Postoperative management

Postoperative cell salvage

In some patients, where postoperative loss is expected to be 500–1000mL (e.g. orthopaedic patients undergoing knee arthroplasty), blood can be collected in wound drains. This is then either filtered within the drain collection system and returned to the patient, or removed and washed before reinfusion. This is an inexpensive method of blood conservation, but it must be subject to appropriate collection (within 6h or as recommended by the manufacturer) and adequate documentation to ensure safe transfusion practice.

Diet

Although some patients may be placed on iron supplements after major joint replacement surgery, current studies show that these do not hasten return to normal RCV if adequate tissue stores are present. The emphasis should, therefore, be on maintaining optimal nutritional status throughout a perioperative pathway.

Jehovah's Witnesses

There is wide variation in acceptable transfusion practice within the Jehovah's Witness population. Some patients will accept blood component products or recombinant factors and others will not even accept autologous blood. It is crucial to establish and document the exact wishes of the individual prior to surgery.

Further reading

Bowley DM, Barker P, Boffard KD (2006). Intraoperative blood salvage in penetrating abdominal trauma. *World J Surg*, 30:1074–80.

Sullivan I, Faulds J, & Ralph C (2008). Contamination of salvaged maternal blood by amniotic fluid and fetal red cells during Caesarean section. *Br J Anaesth*, 101(2):225–9.

Neider AM, Manoharan M, Yang Y, *et al*. (2007). Intraoperative cell salvage during radical cystectomy does not affect long term survival. *Urology*, 69:881–4.

Chapter 17

Anaesthesia in the non-theatre environment

329

17.1 Anaesthesia in the non-theatre environment

Introduction

A remote site is defined by the Royal College of Anaesthetists as 'any location where an anaesthetist is required to provide anaesthesia or sedation away from the main theatre suite and where it cannot be guaranteed that help will be available'. This environment presents unique challenges as the demand for anaesthetic services outside the operating theatre increases (see Box 17.1).

Major surgical procedures are increasingly being replaced with interventional radiological procedures, as well as the need for anaesthetic services elsewhere. These areas are often geographically remote, creating relative isolation for the anaesthetist.

Each area also provides unique challenges depending on the nature of the procedure being undertaken. In addition, cases are often performed as emergencies or in critically ill patients.

Box 17.1 Common out-of-theatre locations

- Radiology department: CT, MRI, interventional procedures
- Psychiatric unit for ECT
- Coronary care unit for cardioversion
- Cardiac catheter laboratory for unstable patients undergoing revascularization
- Emergency department
- Endoscopy unit for sedation and anaesthesia for complex procedures
- Radiotherapy unit for planning and treatment.

Risks of remote site anaesthesia

The majority of the risks are associated with unfamiliarity and inadequate planning. These can be minimized by careful preprocedure preparation and good communication. The risks can be divided as follows:

Environment

The site is often isolated horizontally (e.g. corridors, locked doors, roads) or vertically (e.g. stairs and lifts). In addition, it may be hostile in terms of lack of light, unfavourable temperature, and equipment. There may be environmental hazards to staff such as radiation exposure, magnetic fields, and lack of scavenging, which may pose particular risks to pregnant patients. Doors may be locked or only opened using key cards or codes precluding easy movement around the department.

Equipment

There may be unfamiliarity with, or lack of availability of equipment or drugs. Equipment may differ to that found in the main anaesthetic suite and there may be a lack of specialized or complex equipment. Monitoring lines and ventilator tubing may need to be long and kept free of any machinery, and moveable equipment arms increase the risk of dislodgement of lines or airways. Many tables on which radiological procedures are undertaken do not tip.

Assistance

The trained anaesthetic assistant may also not be familiar with the environment and may not be able to gain access to equipment or drugs, especially in an emergency. Local staff may not understand the requirements and risks of anaesthesia. Also, assistance from other anaesthetists may not be readily available.

Patient

Patients are often complex or emergency patients that may be critically ill. In addition, procedures may be undertaken in children or in patients with learning difficulties.

Procedure

This may require a lengthy anaesthetic with varying degrees of stimulation to the patient. The patient may not be easily accessible in the event of an emergency and they may need to be monitored from a distance.

Preoperative preparation

Thorough preoperative assessment of the patient is vital to the same standard as a patient undergoing surgery. Understanding of the underlying pathology is essential and there should be careful examination and documentation of any deficits. Baseline cardiovascular, respiratory, and renal reserve should be evaluated. If contrast is to be used, previous reactions should be noted and iodine and shellfish allergies may predispose to a future reaction.

There should be guidelines and protocols in place to dictate standards that should be adhered to. Wherever possible, remote site anaesthesia should be supervised by an experienced consultant.

All anaesthetists should be familiarized with the area prior to undertaking the procedure and the location of all equipment, including resuscitation equipment, should be known. Where possible, anaesthetic equipment should be of the same standard as that in the main theatre suite and adequate training should be provided.

Good and timely communication is vital with all the personnel involved in the procedure. It is essential that the particular requirements of the procedure are known and that the nature of the procedure is discussed prior to it starting. It has been shown repeatedly that good communication and planning is critical to averting problems. Plans should be in place to manage patient transfer if required.

If there is any concern about the safety of a procedure being undertaken at a remote site, particularly in patients with complex medical disorders, e.g. ECT or endoscopy, then consideration should be made to conducting it in the main theatre suite.

Conduct of anaesthesia

The anaesthetic technique should be carefully chosen taking into account the patient factors, the nature of the procedure, and the particular requirements of the site. There is little data to support any specific technique, but this should be one with which the anaesthetist is most familiar. Factors to consider include the need for patient immobility, maintenance of physiological stability, manipulation of regional and systemic blood flow, managing anticoagulation, and the treatment of sudden complications during the procedure.

Attention to detail is vital and consideration of securing the airway with an endotracheal tube should be made in situations where immediate access to the patient would be difficult. However, this should be balanced with the need to minimize haemodynamic stress and allow smooth emergence from anaesthesia.

Patient positioning is important with meticulous attention paid to padding pressure areas. Secure IV access should be available that will allow drug and fluid infusion from a safe distance.

Often, radiological equipment needs to be deliberately cooled and so provision should be made to monitor the patient's core temperature and actively warm the patient and fluid infusions.

Mandatory monitoring should be as for any anaesthetic, as per the AAGBI guidelines. This should include a pulse oximeter, non-invasive BP cuffs, ECG, end-tidal gas monitoring, and capnography. Where muscle relaxants are used, a peripheral nerve stimulator is recommended. For complex procedures, particularly those that are intracranial or endovascular, an arterial line can facilitate monitoring and blood sampling. There should be a low threshold for bladder catheterization.

The anaesthetist should ensure that an adequate supply of oxygen is available. In cases of emergency, there should be immediate access to resuscitation equipment and it should be possible to summon a resuscitation team in a timely fashion. A full range of emergency drugs should be immediately available.

Contrast reactions are becoming rarer with the introduction of non-ionic agents although fatal reactions still occur with 1:10 000 exposures. Anaesthetists should be vigilant to the signs of allergic reactions, particularly in cases of previous reaction. Contrast nephropathy is more common and is the third most common cause of hospital acquired renal failure. To minimize this, fluid management should be aimed at maintaining normovolaemia and N-acetylcysteine and bicarbonate infusion pre- and post-procedure have both been shown to reduce the incidence.

A fully trained and experienced anaesthetic assistant, who is familiar with the remote site, should be available at all times and a team safety briefing should be undertaken.

Record keeping and documentation should be undertaken to the same standard as in the main theatre suite.

Postoperative care

If patients are to be recovered in the remote site then they should receive care to the same standard as that delivered in the main recovery area. The anaesthetist should remain with the patient until they are stable and able to be transferred to a ward or other area.

Specific requirements

Anaesthesia for MRI and ECT are discussed in sections 17.2 and 17.3 respectively.

Procedures in the radiology department

Patients requiring anaesthesia in the radiology department generally require either investigation or interventional procedures. The frequency of these is increasing, as is their complexity. Patients may be critically ill or have life-threatening conditions.

All staff working in the radiology department should be aware of the potential exposure to ionizing radiation and this should be kept to a minimum by the use of appropriate screens, lead aprons, and thyroid shields. Radiation exposure follows the inverse square law, that is, the exposure drops proportional to the square of the distance from the source. Therefore, the anaesthetist should remain as distant as is safely possible.

Interventional radiology procedures are becoming more common as they replace the need for surgery. These can be undertaken electively but can also involve treating unstable bleeding patients. Examples of these include ruptured abdominal aortic aneurysm, massive GI haemorrhage, or obstetric haemorrhage. Specific drugs and agents may be required including those needed to manipulate coagulation, intracranial pressure, and arterial blood flow.

Interventional neuroradiology has undergone significant advances over the past few years and procedures such as endovascular treatment of aneurysms and embolization of arterio-venous malformations becoming well established. In the case of coiling of aneurysms, general anaesthesia is preferred to minimize the risk of perforation through physiological stability and lack of patient movement.

Anaesthesia for radiotherapy

General anaesthesia for radiotherapy may be required for adults and children to alleviate pain and help with patient positioning. Monitoring is particularly remote and access very limited during treatment.

There are also particular risks of adverse effects of high concentrations of oxygen in the presence of some chemotherapy agents. The anaesthetic technique may need to be adjusted.

Anaesthesia for endoscopy

General anaesthesia in the endoscopy unit is unusual but may be required for high-risk patients with massive GI bleeds. However, it is more common that these patients are treated in the operating theatre.

Sedation techniques are more common in this area, although anaesthetists are not often involved.

Anaesthesia in the cardiac catheter lab

The increasing scope of interventions in the catheter lab has resulted in a greater need for anaesthetic input ranging from general anaesthesia for transcatheter aortic valve implantation (TAVI) to percutaneous coronary intervention (PCI) in patient in cardiogenic shock. The challenges relate to this being a high-risk patient population undergoing procedures with potentially life-threatening complications.

Performing angiography or PCI in patients in cardiogenic shock requires a skilled anaesthetist, especially given the acute nature of the situation. Patients often require endotracheal intubation and positive pressure ventilation that will help to offload a failing left ventricle. If the patient has suffered an out-of-hospital cardiac arrest, they may need to be cooled.

There are a number of potential complications including contrast reactions and hypothermia. Special care must be taken during patient positioning as optimal images are gained with the patient's arms above their head. Therefore, the brachial plexus is at risk of being damaged.

Further reading

Metzner J & Domino KB (2010). Risks of anesthesia or sedation outside the operating room: the role of the anesthesia care provider. *Curr Opin Anaesthesiol*, 23:523–31.

The Royal College of Anaesthetists (2013). Guidance on the provision of anaesthetic care in the non-theatre environment 2013. In *Guidelines for the Provision of Anaesthetic Services*. London: The Royal College of Anaesthetists. <http://www.rcoa.ac.uk/node/12211>.

17.2 Anaesthesia and safety for magnetic resonance imaging

Introduction

Since the first anaesthetics in magnetic resonance (MR) units were described in the 1980s, the number of hospitals acquiring MR units, and the scope for their use, has increased. The systems are becoming more powerful and interventional procedures have become possible. This increases the need for anaesthetic support and the provision for safe anaesthesia or sedation presents unique challenges due to the continuous presence of a strong magnetic field and restricted access to the patient.

Patients are often challenging: those requiring anaesthesia or sedation include children, adults with learning disorders or severe claustrophobia, and those who are unable to lie still or flat during the scan. Patients can also be critically ill.

Hazards of MR units

Magnetic field

The majority of the hazards relate to the fact that MRI depends on a constant strong magnetic field that is generated by superconductors which are cooled by liquid helium to 4.2°K. Most scanners operate between 0.1 to 2.0 Tesla (1T=10 000 Gauss). The strength of the field falls off exponentially as the distance from the magnet increases and Gauss lines are used to determine safe operating zones.

The risks of long-term exposure to electromagnetic fields for staff that work in the scanner are unknown, and it is difficult to measure occupational exposure. However, it is thought that staff members are at risk of being exposed to higher than recommended levels of time-varying gradient fields. At present, there are moves to restrict occupational exposure.

There is a controlled safety area contained within the 5 Gauss line, over which unauthorized and unscreened personnel should not pass. There is a major and serious risk associated with ferromagnetic objects or equipment and their projectile capabilities. This is significant at the 50 Gauss line. The risk is minimized by strict management of the MR unit and thorough screening of equipment, staff and patients.

Noise

The noise emitted from an MRI scanner may average 95dB and is produced by the vibration of the wire loops that produce the gradient current. This is an issue for both the clinical staff and the patient and so auditory protection should be given to all patients, and staff within the scan room.

Quenching malfunction

Should there be a system fault or the staff are required to shut down the magnetic field, then the cryogenic gases that are used to cool the superconductor are rapidly expelled, in a process known as quenching. The venting normally occurs to the outside but should this fail then there is a potentially lethal hazard as the atmosphere will be deficient of oxygen. This places anyone including the staff and patient at risk of severe hypoxia and so emergency procedures must be in place to move to a place of safety should this occur.

Equipment safety considerations

Previously, equipment has been regarded as MR compatible or not. However, these terms have now been updated by the MHRA to MR *conditional*, MR *safe*, and MR *unsafe*. It is imperative to ensure that all equipment that is used is MR safe or conditional. This includes all monitoring equipment and ancillary equipment such as trolleys,

Monitors and anaesthetic machines that are MR safe are available commercially such that patients can be managed to the same level of safety as in the operating theatre. Safe vaporizers and gas cylinders can be placed within the scanner room. However, it is still recommended that monitoring equipment should be placed in the control room. This means that all cables need to pass through waveguide ports that are built into the Faraday cage, a radiofrequency shield that is built in to the fabric of the MR room.

Considerations for monitoring

Current burns

The radiofrequency currents that are used can induce currents and heating in monitor leads. There have been reports of burns when arms or legs are positioned in a way that creates a conductive loop pathway. MR safe systems use fibreoptic or carbon-fibre cabling to avoid this or foam pads can be used to insulate the cables.

Power supply

Mains power supply carries interference through the Faraday cage and so equipment should either be battery-powered or have a filtered and isolated power source. However, care must be taken as batteries are strongly ferro-magnetic and so equipment must be firmly secured.

Alarms

Since patients are inaccessible and usually in a different room to the anaesthetist, all alarms must be visual.

Pulse oximetry

Fibreoptic cable pulse oximetry is incorporated into MR-safe monitors to prevent the problem of current induction.

Blood pressure monitoring

Non-invasive monitors must have non-ferrous connectors. The oscillometric method is preferred. Invasive pressure monitoring is possible although the length of the pressure lines required increases the likelihood of damping.

ECG

MR-safe systems are appropriate to monitor rate and rhythm but not for ischaemia. This is due to Faraday's law of induction, which describes how a voltage can be induced by a conducting fluid passing through a magnetic field. When applied to blood flowing through the aorta, this concept can lead to ECG changes that mimic ischaemia. Also, the ECG is prone to interference; this can be reduced by using short leads, MRI-safe electrodes, and a narrow configuration.

Capnography

Side-stream capnography is possible; however, due to the long sampling time, there may be a delay of up to 20sec in obtaining the signal.

Temperature monitoring

Proprietary temperature monitoring using a fibreoptic surface sensor is possible.

Table 17.1 Implants and conditions of use for MRI	
Device	Conditions of use
Pacemakers & implantable defibrillators	See text
Neurostimulators	Most have batteries and implanted electrodes. MR is usually contraindicated
Implanted drug infusion pumps	Often contain ferromagnetic components and switches. MR is usually contraindicated
Programmable hydrocephalus shunts	Pressure seeing may be changed by the magnetic field. Programmer should be available to re-program the device following the MR scan
Cochlear implants	Usually ferromagnetic so usually contraindicated. MR can be performed under special conditions
Joint replacements	Large metallic implants may generate heat and degrade image quality. Must be carefully monitored
Heart valves	Have been safely scanned as low risk of displacement
Clips and staples	Nature of the clip/staple should be known and care taken
Aneurysm clips	Scanning must not proceed unless there is positive documented evidence that aneurysm clip is non-ferromagnetic
Intravascular devices	Non-ferromagnetic safe. Magnetic devices safe 6–8 weeks post-op as usually securely attached to vessel wall
Occular implants	High risk of movement of dislodgement. Refer to manufacturer's advice
Penile implants	Risk of dislodgement so MR not usually recommended
Tissue expanders and implants	Caution should be taken. Injection ports often metallic. Refer to manufacturer's advice
Intrauterine devices	Usually safe as contain plastic and copper

Patient safety considerations

The risks to the patient are related to effect of the magnetic field on metallic objects that are attached to or implanted in to the patient. All patients that are to undergo an MR scan should be thoroughly screened to determine the safety risks. All foreign objects including transdermal patches should be removed and the patient should be dressed in a gown.

Implanted devices

These fall in to two categories:

* *Active* which include pacemakers, defibrillators, neurostimulators, cochlear implants, and drug delivery devices whose operation depends on a power source.
* *Inactive* which includes joint replacements, heart valves, intracranial aneurysm clips, breast implants, and coronary stents.

Many medical devices contain ferrous metallic components which may cause artefact in the image, and may become dislodged, such as aneurysm clips. The manufacturer should provide patients and clinicians with accurate information; there are a large number of modern devices that are MR safe and MR conditional.

In most cases the manufacturer can be contacted for advice on MR safety. If this is not possible, then the device should be assumed to be MR-unsafe. However, in all cases the risk-benefit ratio of the MR scan should be assessed. See Table 17.1.

Pacemakers

Safety guidance specifies that anyone with a pacemaker or implanted defibrillator should not have an MR scan or enter within the 5 Gauss line. This is due to concerns that the magnetic fields could cause severe, and possibly life-threatening, disruption of the pacemaker's function.

However, pacemaker and MR technology is constantly evolving and MR-conditional pacemakers are now available.

Anaesthetic management

Preparation

Anaesthesia should be induced in a dedicated room outside the 5 Gauss line, where standard equipment can be used. This room should be close to the scanner so that the patient can be moved back there should an emergency arise. The patient is then moved in to the magnet area on a non-ferrous trolley and the anaesthetist ideally moves to the control room for the duration of the scan. There, they should have a clear view of the remote monitor, with visual alarms as necessary, the anaesthetic machine, and the patient. Care must be taken not to take any non MRI-safe equipment in to the inner MR controlled area.

Airway

In most cases, the airway is inaccessible once the patient is in the scanner. This mandates that the chosen airway device should be reliable, with all-plastic connections. An MRI-specific LMA is available, and is widely used. The use of the laryngoscope is not possible in the scanning room.

Maintenance

In the case of TIVA, most infusion pumps are strongly ferromagnetic and so often the pump is placed in the control room, with long infusion lines passing to the patient through the waveguide in the Faraday cage. MRI-compatible anaesthetic machines, vaporizers and ventilators are available, which limits the length of the breathing system. A co-axial Mapleson D circuit is usually used.

Future developments

The demand for MRI scans will increase as new techniques are developed. This is particularly true for intraoperative MR scanning which offers the advantage of real-time imaging guidance during surgery, especially neurosurgical procedures. The concerns are the same as those of a conventional MRI environment, with the additional focus on the neuroanaesthetic management of the patient.

Further reading

Reddy U, White MJ, & Wilson SR (2012). Anaesthesia for magnetic resonance imaging. *BJA CEPD Rev*, 12(3):140–4. doi:10.1093/bjaceaccp/mks002

17.3 Anaesthesia for electroconvulsive therapy

The use of electroconvulsive therapy (ECT) was first described in 1938, and was initially performed without anaesthesia. Although its exact mechanism of action is still unknown, it provides an important treatment modality for severe and medication resistant depression, mania, and schizophrenia.

It is commonly performed in remote locations and the conduct of anaesthesia can influence the efficacy of the treatment. Therefore, anaesthetists must have a good knowledge of the physiology of ECT, the effect of concurrent medications, and the effect of anaesthetic agents on the efficacy of ECT.

Administration of ECT

Generally, the acute phase of ECT is performed three times a week for up to 12 treatments. Maintenance therapy is performed from weekly to monthly to prevent relapses. During ECT, an electrical current is applied transcutaneously to the brain via two electrodes in order to provoke a generalized epileptic seizure. Although the optimal seizure length is not known, a well-modified seizure will manifest as minor tonic, followed by clonic activity of skeletal muscle lasting 10–120sec. This should be accompanied by characteristic EEG seizure activity, lasting from 25–50sec. Inadequate efficacy of ECT may result from missed or prolonged seizures.

Missed seizures

As many as 22% of ECT treatments result in either no seizure, or in one lasting 15sec or less. These may be due to insufficient stimulus, premature stimulus termination, hypercarbia, dehydration, or from the effects of current medication or excess anaesthetic agent. The patient may develop a marked bradycardia.

Prolonged or tardive seizures

A seizure lasting more than 2min or the late return of seizures even leading to status epilepticus, often in recovery, is the other main complication. Should this occur, the management is supportive along with the administration of agents to terminate the seizure.

Physiological responses to ECT

Central nervous system response

The generalized seizure results in a marked, but transient, increase in cerebral blood flow, intracranial pressure, and cerebral oxygen consumption. This can result in dizziness, confusion, agitation, and headaches. Also common is short-term memory loss lasting up to 6 months and cognitive dysfunction which may manifest as disorientation and attention deficits. Non-memory cognitive functions are unaffected. It is thought that unilateral ECT, performed on the non-dominant hemisphere, may limit these adverse effects.

More serious complications include transient ischaemic deficits, intracerebral haemorrhage, and cortical blindness.

Cardiovascular system response

This is twofold, and results from generalized autonomic nervous system activation. Initially, the parasympathetic response predominates resulting in bradycardia, and even asystole, lasting 10–15sec. This is immediately followed by the more prominent sympathetic response that results in tachycardia and hypertension lasting 5min or longer. During this time, cardiac arrhythmias may be seen.

Systolic blood pressure is typically raised by 30–40% and heart rate is increased by 20% or more thereby increasing the myocardial oxygen consumption. This is further compounded by hyperventilation-induced hypocapnia. Concurrently, seizure activity increases tissue oxygen consumption, potentially further reducing myocardial oxygen supply. Therefore, in elderly patients or in those with pre-existing disease, myocardial ischaemia and infarction can occur. Left ventricular dysfunction can persist for up to 6h post ECT, even in patients without cardiac disease.

Other responses

Previously, the generalized convulsion resulted in a high incidence of fracture-dislocations. However, these are now rare due to the modification of the fit with muscle relaxants. Side effects include headaches, myalgia, drowsiness, weakness, nausea, emergence agitation, and anorexia.

Intraocular and intragastric pressure increases, but this is transient and not usually clinically significant.

The mortality rate is comparable with minor surgical procedures at 1 per 10 000 patients. The most common causes of death are cardiovascular, pulmonary aspiration, and severe laryngospasm.

Preoperative assessment

In addition to a routine pre-assessment, medical history and examination any concurrent psychiatric medication should be noted. The anaesthetist should be particular aware of those drugs that have specific side effects, and the potential to interact with anaesthetic agents. These are shown in Table 17.2.

Investigations should be performed as clinically indicated. There are relatively few contraindications to ECT and none is absolute (see Box 17.2).

Table 17.2 Adverse effects of psychotropic drugs	
Drug	Side effect or interaction
Benzodiazepines	Anticonvulsant—avoid if possible
Tricyclic antidepressants	Proconvulsant Hypertensive crisis with indirect sympathomimetics
SSRIs	Reduce seizure threshold, can be associated with prolonged seizures Associated with SIADH Serotonin syndrome if given with tramadol or meperidine
Monoamine oxidase inhibitors	Increase seizure threshold Hypertensive crisis with indirect sympathomimetics
Lithium	Reduce seizure threshold. Levels should be 0.4–1mmol/L Associated with nephrogenic diabetes insipidus
SNRIs	Reduce seizure threshold Cause hypertension
Neuroleptics	Proconvulsant at low dosage Increase seizure threshold at high dosage

---

Box 17.2 Relative contraindications to ECT

- Uncontrolled cardiac failure
- Deep venous thrombosis until anticoagulated
- Acute respiratory infection
- Myocardial infarction in the last 3 months
- Stroke in the last month
- Raised intracranial pressure or unprotected cerebral aneurysm
- Unstable major fracture
- Untreated phaeochromocytoma
- Retinal detachment
- Cochlear implant.

In all cases, a balance must be struck between the risks of anaesthesia and ECT and the fact that ECT can be life-saving in some severe depressive states.

Special patient populations

Patients with pacemakers and implantable defibrillators
Patients with pacemakers can safely receive ECT. Skeletal muscle potentials may trigger pacemaker activity and so the pacemaker should be converted temporarily to fixed rate pacing before ECT. ICDs should have the defibrillator and antitachycardia functions deactivated prior to ECT.

Patients with cerebral aneurysms
ECT causes abrupt changes in systemic and cerebral haemodynamics which will increase the aneurysm wall stress. This can potentially lead to enlargement or rupture. If a patient needs ECT, then these changes should be attenuated by the use of nitroprusside and β-blockers prior to the procedure.

Conduct of anaesthesia

Anaesthesia should be administered by an experienced practioner who has a specialized knowledge of the issues affecting the administration of ECT, usually in a remote location.

The objective of anaesthesia is to provide rapid loss of consciousness and muscle relaxation, attenuation of the hyper-dynamic responses outlined, minimal interference with the seizure activity, followed by prompt recovery to full consciousness. This influences the choice of agents used and a balance should be struck between providing adequate anaesthesia without affecting the efficacy of the treatment.

Patients should be consented and fasted. Sedative pre-medications should be avoided. Patients should be given the opportunity to pass urine as incontinence is common.

Minimum monitoring should be as per AAGBI guidelines. Whilst an anaesthetic machine may not be required, there must be a flow-controlled oxygen supply, equipment for airway management including difficult airways, and emergency and resuscitation drugs and equipment.

The patient should be pre-oxygenated and generally intubation of the trachea is not necessary unless there are specific risk factors for aspiration of gastric contents. Following induction, ventilation can be performed using a face mask and a bite block should be inserted in order to protect the patient's teeth, lips, and tongue during the seizure. Hyperventilation lowers the seizure threshold and can cause tardive seizures. During the seizure, and subsequently, the patient can be gently ventilated until spontaneous ventilation resumes.

Induction agents
The dose of induction agent is initially calculated by the patient's weight but subsequently modified depending on the previous response to ECT and any changing seizure threshold. There are issues related to the use of all the induction agents. These are shown in Table 17.3. Since the demise of methohexital, propofol is the most commonly used agent, although there is no evidence that any of the agents have significant advantages over any other. Whichever one is chosen, it is unwise to alter that choice for the duration of treatment to avoid interfering with the seizure threshold.

By adding opioids, the dose of the induction agent can be reduced thereby potentially improving the quality of the seizure. Commonly, remifentanil (1mcg/kg) or alfentanil 10–25mcg/kg) are used due to their short-acting effects.

Table 17.3 Anaesthetic induction agents in ECT

Agent	Seizure	Advantages	Disadvantages
Propofol	Reduces seizure duration but usually acceptable	Reduced PONV, reduced haemodynamic response to ECT, good emergence profile	Pain on injection (ameliorated by adding lidocaine)
Etomidate	Longest seizure duration	Resistant seizures	Accentuated haemodynamic response, increased PONV, delayed recovery
Thiopental	Reduced duration; better than propofol	None over other agents	Haemodynamic response less well attenuated, post-op arrhythmias
Ketamine	Reduced seizure duration	Resistant seizures	Increased haemodynamic instability, increase ICP, emergence phenomena
Sevoflurane	Comparable with thiopental	Tocolytic, gas induction	Need appropriate equipment

Muscle relaxants
These agents are used to prevent myalgias and reduce the risk of musculoskeletal injury as a result of the seizure activity. However, it is not desirable to completely ablate muscle activity and an appropriate dose of neuromuscular blocking agent should still produce a classic, bilateral convulsion.

The most commonly used agent is *suxamethonium* (0.5–1mg/kg). The electrical stimulus should be given once fasiculations have ceased. It should not be used in the presence of pseudocholinesterase deficiency, neuroleptic malignant syndrome, a history of susceptibility to malignant hyperpyrexia, catatonia, or major burns.

If suxamethonium is contraindicated, then a non-depolarizing agent should be used. *Mivacurium* (0.15–2mg/kg) is most commonly used although it can be associated with clinically significant histamine release.

Adjunctive agents

Several agents can be used in order to attenuate the acute cardiovascular responses described.

Anticholinergic agents
Atropine and glycopyrrolate have both been used to control the parasympathetic effects. Although atropine pre-medication decreases the frequency of bradycardia, its routine use is not recommended due to the effects on myocardial oxygen demand. Glycopyrrolate (0.1–0.3mg IV) has become the drug of choice due to its superior antisialagogue effects in the absence of adverse central nervous system effects.

β-blockers
The acute sympathetic response to ECT may be controlled by intraoperative esmolol or labetalol. However, there is some controversy as to whether these drugs reduce seizure duration. For this reason, they should probably be administered immediately before or after the stimulation is applied.

Calcium-channel blockers
Effective control of the sympathetic response can also be achieved with nifedipine (sublingual), nicardipine, and diltiazem. However, the use of diltiazem has been associated with shortened seizure duration.

Direct vasodilators
Glyceryl trinitrate (GTN) is effective if given shortly before the administration of ECT without affecting the duration of the

seizure. It should be considered in patients at high risk of myocardial ischaemia.

Postoperative care

Standard monitoring should be continued in recovery and oxygen supplemented until full consciousness has been attained and the patient can maintain adequate saturations whilst breathing room air. The recovery area should be staffed by trained recovery personnel. The majority of patients make an uncomplicated recovery and can be discharged quickly.

The most common complaints in recovery are confusion, agitation, amnesia, and headache. Nausea and vomiting is rare. Emergence phenomena can be dramatic and titrated doses of midazolam may be necessary. The presence of a trained escort with whom the patient is familiar can be very reassuring.

The doses of all anaesthetic agents should be recorded.

Further reading

Ding Z & White PF (2002). Anesthesia for electroconvulsive therapy. *Anesth Analg*, 94:1351–64.

Scott AIF (2005). *The ECT Handbook* (2nd edn). Glasgow: The Royal College of Psychiatrists.

cc,
Adult i
there may .
lie still. The prc.

17.4 Sedation techniques

What is sedation?

There are several definitions of sedation. One common definition describes sedation as 'the use of drug(s) to produce a state of depression of the central nervous system enabling treatment to be carried out, but during which verbal contact with the patient is maintained throughout the period of sedation'. This emphasizes the key difference between the sedated state and general anaesthesia: the ability to maintain verbal contact with the patient throughout.

Given the high variability between patients, there is no one standard technique for all and here we consider the reasons for sedation, preparation of a patient, several techniques in current practice, after-care, and the potential risks and hazards involved when a patient presents for sedation.

Levels of sedation

The American Society of Anesthesiologists (ASA) defines levels of sedation as minimal, moderate, conscious, and deep sedation. Sedation is a continuum that can easily result in unintended loss of consciousness with consequences for cardiorespiratory function.

Minimal sedation

A drug-induced state where patients are awake and calm, respond normally to verbal commands with no effect on cardiorespiratory systems.

Moderate sedation

Patients are sleepy but respond appropriately to light touch or verbal commands. Haemodynamic parameters are usually unaffected and spontaneous ventilation is maintained without the need for airway adjuncts.

Conscious sedation

Similar to moderate sedation but verbal contact is always maintained. This technique is commonly employed in dentistry.

Deep sedation

Drug-induced depression of consciousness during which patients are asleep, cannot be easily roused but respond to repeated or painful stimuli. Ventilation may be impaired and airway assistance may be necessary. Cardiovascular function is maintained.

Situations where sedation is required

Sedation can be an appropriate and cost-effective alternative to anaesthesia for many diagnostic and therapeutic procedures (see Box 17.3). The aims of sedation are to reduce fear and anxiety, minimize movement, and provide an adjunct to analgesia.

Sedation in the theatre environment

Sedation may be used as an adjunct to a regional anaesthetic, e.g. total knee or hip replacements using a combined spinal and epidural technique as the primary mode of anaesthesia.

Sedation in the non-theatre environment

There is an increasing trend to expedite the stay of patients undergoing relatively short procedures such as CT/MRI scanning, radiotherapy, angiography, and intrathecal chemotherapy particularly in the paediatric population. In addition, procedures such as endoscopy and bronchoscopy are sometimes performed under sedation. Patients requiring sedation for these can be challenging—those with learning difficulties, claustrophobia, or an inability to [cooperate]. Problems of sedating patients in remote environments

notwithstanding, sedation is not without risk. As such, anaesthetists are increasingly involved in its delivery. Sedation is carried out throughout the hospital in A&E, radiology, oncology, nephrology and endoscopy.

Box 17.3 Procedures typically performed under sedation

Painful procedures
- Embolization of organs and tumours—hepatobiliary and renal interventions in particular are more painful than vascular procedures
- Angiography—cardiac, cerebral
- Percutaneous biopsy
- Drainage of abscess
- Insertion gastrostomy and nephrostomy tubes
- Central venous catheterization
- Endoscopy—oesophagoscopy, colonoscopy
- Dental procedures
- Suturing
- Orthopaedic manipulation
- Wound care—dressing changes.

Non-painful procedures
- Scanning: CT/MRI
- TTE in paediatrics
- Radiotherapy
- EEG.

Patient selection and preparation

Pre-assessment of patients is vital to identify any contra-indications to sedation and identify any risk due to the presence of comorbidities. Pertinent enquiry should be made with respect to the ability to lie flat without dyspnoea, a history of sleep apnoea, and cardiovascular comorbidity. An airway assessment is also important to carry out.

Fasting requirements are the same as those required for general anaesthesia: 2h for clear fluid, 4h for breast milk, and 6h for solids.

Informed consent must be provided to the patient. This may be in the form of information leaflets and attendance at a pre-assessment clinic. It is important that the patient understands that they are not receiving a general anaesthetic and that they will be aware of what is happening and their surroundings, depending on the level of sedation. Preparation of the child to improve cooperation is vital when considering sedation. Play specialists and experienced nursing staff have a vital role in achieving cooperation from children.

Contraindications to sedation have been described by SIGN (Scottish Intercollegiate Guidelines Network) specifically for sedation in children (see Box 17.4) but equally are applicable to adults.

Box 17.4 Contraindications to sedation in children

- Abnormal airway
- Raised intracranial pressure
- Depressed conscious level
- Sleep apnoea
- Respiratory failure
- Cardiac failure
- Neuromuscular disease

- Bowel obstruction
- Active resp. tract infection
- Known allergy to sedative
- Distress despite preparation
- Parental refusal
- Behavioural problems.

Consideration of general anaesthesia

Patients with certain conditions (see Box 17.5) should be considered for sedation in the presence of anaesthetist or consideration of a general anaesthetic.

Box 17.5 Conditions requiring anaesthetist-delivered sedation or GA
• Neonates—particularly ex-premature
• Infants <1 year or children <5 years
• Cardiovascular instability
• Impaired cardiac function
• Renal impairment
• Hepatic impairment
• Severe respiratory disease
• Impaired bulbar reflexes
• Gastro-oesophageal reflux
• Concurrent medication that may potentiate the effect of sedative medications or on other opioids or sedatives
• Emergency cases.

Sedation techniques

Intravenous access should be established before sedation is commenced. This may involve the use of topical local anaesthetic creams for children to aid the process of cannulation.

Drugs

A wide variety of drugs are used but largely rely on propofol (managed by anaesthetists), midazolam often combined with the use of an opiate, commonly fentanyl, alfentanil, or remifentanil. These drugs have a wide margin of safety to avoid unintended loss of consciousness. However, as multiple agents are used, the margin of safety of these drugs is narrowed and the risk for anaesthesia to ensue increases. This is particularly true in the paediatric population. The RCOA and AAGBI recommend that in such cases an experienced consultant paediatric anaesthetist with a specialist interest in sedation should be involved.

The benefit of using multiple agents is that the synergy of several agents providing amnesia, analgesia, and sedation together produces a better quality of sedation to allow procedures to be performed.

In paediatrics, ketamine is also used as is chloral hydrate, which is administered orally. Inhaled agents include nitrous oxide in the form of Entonox and also sevoflurane.

There is an increasing move for propofol to be used by non-anaesthetic medical practitioners but only where it is used as a single agent. The British Society of Gastroenterologists have published a statement in conjunction with the RCoA which allows the use of propofol administration without an anaesthetic machine or operating department practitioner outside the theatre environment in the case of ERCPs.

Delivery

Bolus sedation is a popular method of delivery of anaesthetic agents. This allows incremental dosing and careful titration to response. The use of multiple agents usually involves an anaesthetist. An alternative method is the use of target controlled infusions (TCI). In the case of remifentanil and propofol, pharmacokinetic models exist based on weight, sex, or height of adults. This allows fine control of plasma concentration of the agents, thereby reducing the risk of sedation progressing to anaesthesia. In the case of the use of sevoflurane, an anaesthetic machine is obligatory, including scavenging.

Airway management

Patients are able to maintain their own airway, requiring merely supplemental oxygen. The use of capnography is mandatory where deep sedation is required, in order to alert the operator to any reduction in respiratory rate or impending airway obstruction.

Monitoring

See Box 17.6.

Box 17.6 Parameters to be monitored
• Heart rate, electrocardiography,* and BP every 5min*
• Respiratory rate and pattern
• Capnography*
• Oxygen saturation by pulse oximetry
• Sedation level
• Discomfort—pain control, tolerance
• Perfusion- skin colour, warmth
• Hydration—IV fluids infused
• Urine output where catheterized.
*Required for deep sedation.

Equipment, personnel, and facilities

- Piped oxygen + suction.
- Appropriate equipment for maintaining airway and respiration (including airway adjuncts, LMAs, intubating equipment).
- Tilting trolleys.
- Monitoring.
- Full resuscitation facilities and reversal agents.
- Warming devices should be available so as to avoid the risks of hypothermia in patients. This is especially important in the young and the elderly.
- Adequately staffed recovery unit on-site.
- ALS trained staff.

Recovery

Patients ideally should undergo a period of close observation as seen in recovery after general anaesthesia. Often remote units have an area where patients can be monitored until the effects of sedative agents have subsided. This may not necessarily involve specifically trained recovery nurses. It is ultimately the responsibility of the anaesthetist or doctor involved to ensure that patients are fully recovered before discharge. Discharge criteria dictate that the patient must be easily rousable, able to tolerate oral fluids unassisted, be pain free, and not suffering from nausea or vomiting. Relevant instructions should be given to the carer.

As these cases are often performed as day cases, a responsible adult should be available to collect the patient, transport them home and remain with them for 24h. As with day-case recommendations, access to a telephone is also required. Driving should not be attempted until up to 48h post-sedation.

Further reading

Scottish Intercollegiate Guidelines Network (2004). *Safe Sedation of Children Undergoing Diagnostic and Therapeutic Procedures.* Edinburgh: SIGN.

Sury M (2004). Paediatric sedation. *CEACCP*, 4(4):112–18.

Chapter 18

Anaesthesia for orthopaedic surgery

341

18.1 Anaesthesia for orthopaedic surgery

Orthopaedic surgery

The patient cohort presenting for orthopaedic surgery represent a number of challenges to the anaesthetist:

- Ageing population
- Significant comorbidity (CVS, RS, renal)
- Higher BMI
- Polypharmacy
- Reduced exercise tolerance making cardiorespiratory function assessment difficult.
- Other affects of degenerative disease e.g. neck movement, lumbar spine disease

Perioperative considerations

Perioperative course may be complicated by haemorrhage, bone cement implantation syndrome and use of tourniquets.

Perioperative blood loss should be recorded and point of care haemoglobin measurement performed. Optimization of preoperative haemoglobin should occur at preassessment to reduce transfusion requirements.

Bone cement implantation syndrome is characterized by hypoxia and hypotension which occurs at the time of pressurized cementation or prosthesis insertion. It is thought to be due to microemboli (cement monomer, fat, fibrin, or marrow) and release of vasoactive mediators which cause pulmonary shunt, pulmonary hypertension, vasodilatation, low cardiac output and dysrhythmia. Surgical technique can be modified to reduce the risk; good haemostasis prior to cement insertion, medullary washout, retrograde cement insertion via a cement gun and venting the femur. Avoiding hypovolaemia and raising oxygenation may reduce the physiological effects but management is supportive with increased oxygen therapy, fluid resuscitation and vasoactive support.

Tourniquet use is common in orthopaedic surgery to reduce blood loss. Tourniquets are associated with a gradual increase in arterial pressure, possibly related to tourniquet pain. The tourniquet duration should always be minimized but a healthy adult should tolerate 1.5–2h. On deflation, a reperfusion syndrome occurs as ischaemic metabolites are released from the limb. Vasodilatation, myocardial depression, raised $ETCO_2$, potassium levels, and lactate all occur.

Regional (RA) versus general anaesthesia (GA)

The optimum anaesthetic technique for orthopaedic surgery should provide high patient satisfaction, reduce perioperative risks, provide good analgesia with few side-effects, and allow early mobilization. For many years there has been ongoing controversy regarding the potential benefit of RA on perioperative outcomes. Results of large meta-analyses often conflict and results have been affected by other changes in perioperative care and improved surgical techniques. Whilst RA is associated with potential problems (see Box 18.1), some of the benefits of regional anaesthesia may include:

Reduced Mortality

The orthopaedic subgroup of a large meta-analysis to compare RA and GA in 2000 showed reduced short term mortality with an OR 0.7 (95%CI 0.54 – 0.9).

Studies of adjusted mortality post hip fracture surgery suggest a 29% decrease with RA. This may be influenced by patient compliance and suitability for RA with higher risk patients requiring GA.

A large study of 382,236 joint arthroplasty patients also demonstrated reduced 30d mortality (0.1% with RA vs. 0.18% with GA). Interestingly the mortality of combined neuraxial block and GA falls between these values suggesting a protective effect of the neuraxial block.

Reduced pulmonary complications

Pulmonary complications such as pneumonia and respiratory failure are reduced with RA. This has been shown post primary arthroplasty and hip fracture.

No difference is seen relating to cardiovascular outcomes such as perioperative MI or cardiac failure. Hypotension is more common with combined neuraxial block and GA.

Reduced perioperative blood loss and transfusion

RA has been associated with reduced blood loss, higher postoperative haemoglobin levels, and reduced transfusion requirements.

Reduced thromboembolic risk

This is a very prominent finding in older studies. RA enhances venous blood flow and attenuates the prothrombotic stress response which was highly beneficial prior to contemporary thromboprophylactic regimes. There still appears to be a modest benefit in recent studies.

Reduced postoperative pain

RA has been associated with reduced postoperative pain scores, reduced opiate usage, and reduced nausea and vomiting. Peripheral nerve blockade and central neuraxial blocks provide a short-lived improvement. This is optimized by catheter techniques.

Joint range of motion and rehabilitation is optimized by good analgesia which has little motor effect.

Ambulatory patients benefit from earlier discharge, reduced nausea, and better postoperative analgesia when peripheral nerve block has been used.

Reduced operating time and length of stay

A reduced operating time associated with RA has been reported in some studies, but not always reproduced. Although length of stay is possibly slightly lower with RA, it is the incidence of prolonged stay that is most reduced.

Other potential benefits

RA has been linked in some studies with improved cognitive function postoperatively. This effect is not sustained to longer term differences or incidence of delirium.

RA has been linked with reduced infection rates in a number of studies.

RA has been associated with lower incidence of acute kidney injury postoperatively.

Elective Orthopaedic Procedures

Total hip arthroplasty

- Techniques include:
- Central neuraxial block i.e. spinal, CSE, epidural
- Central neuraxial block combined with sedation/GA
- General anaesthesia with systemic opiate

> **Box 18.1 Problems with RA**
>
> - Requires patient cooperation and consent
> - Contraindications e.g. coagulopathy, antiplatelet agents
> - Failure
> - Delay
> - Finite length of anaesthesia
> - May require combined sedation
> - Training and equipment required
> - Urinary catheter
> - Rare neurological injury
> - Prolonged motor block and delayed mobilisation
> - Respiratory depression—neuraxial opiates
> - Poor analgesia when block recedes—combine with peripheral nerve block (PNB)

- General anaesthesia with PNB
  - Femoral nerve block
  - 3 in 1 block
  - Fascia iliaca block
  - Lumbar plexus block
  - Local infiltration

When considering regional techniques for hip arthroplasty, all are found to reduce postoperative pain, opiate use, nausea and vomiting. Single shot femoral nerve block alone is usually not sufficient although continuous catheter techniques have good effect. A 3 in 1 block does not reliably block the obturator or lateral cutaneous nerves. Lumbar plexus blocks are the most reliable technique for blocking all three nerves and have a good effect for 8 hours, or prolonged with continuous catheter techniques. This is, however, a block associated with some serious complications such as psoas abscess/haemorrhage and renal trauma. Accessing these lumbar plexus nerves via the anterior fascia iliaca approach may increase safety. Continuous catheter techniques may provide postoperative analgesia comparable to epidural.

Total knee replacement

- Techniques include:
- Central neuraxial block i.e. spinal, CSE, epidural
- Central neuraxial block combined with sedation/GA
- General anaesthesia with systemic opiate
- General anaesthesia with PNB
  - Femoral nerve block
  - Femoral and sciatic block
  - Local infiltration

Total knee arthroplasty is associated with more severe pain related to the extensive osteotomy and splitting of the quadriceps involved in the procedure. Postoperative opiate consumption is increased and central neuraxial opiate doses may be insufficient. All central and peripheral techniques have an impact on postoperative pain levels and reduce opiate-related side-effects. Femoral block, either alone or combined with sciatic nerve block can provide good analgesia in the first 12–24 hrs. Sciatic nerve block may be associated with greater motor block and delay mobilization. A combination of femoral block and local infiltration into the posterior capsule of the knee may be optimal.

RA may make less impact on perioperative blood loss during knee arthroplasty as tourniquet use is usual. The impact of improved analgesia on time to mobilization, length of stay and length of rehabilitation is positive.

Further reading

Macfarlane AJ, Prasad GA, Chan VW, Brull R. (2009) Does regional anaesthesia improve outcome after total hip arthroplasty? A systematic review. *Br J Anaesth*, 103 (3): 335–345.

Macfarlane AJ, Prasad GA, Chan VW, Brull R. (2009). Does regional anaesthesia improve outcome after total knee arthroplasty? *Clin Orthop Relat Res,* 467; 2379–2402.

Menmtsoudis SG, Sun X, Chiu YL, *et al.* (2013). Perioperative comparative effectiveness of anesthetic technique in orthopaedic patients. *Anesthesiol,* 118 (5) 1046–58.

Rodgers A, Walker N, Schug S, *et al.* (2000). Reduction of postoperative mortality and morbidity with epidural or spinal anaesthesia: results from overview of randomised trials. *BMJ*, 321(7275): 1493.

18.2 Primary versus secondary arthroplasty

Arthroplasty is a common operation. According to figures from the National Joint Registry online over 114 000 arthroplasties were performed in England and Wales in 2010 and this is increasing annually. Arthroplasty encompasses quite a large range of operations, for example, hip arthroplasty may be subdivided as follows:

- Total hip arthroplasty, where the articular surfaces of the hip and acetabulum are replaced. For the femoral component this can be replacement of the femoral head and neck (conventional) or replacement of the surface of the femoral head (resurfacing).
- Hemiarthroplasty, where the articular surface of the femoral head is replaced. For unipolar only the femoral head and neck is replaced; bipolar is as for unipolar but with an acetabular cup that is not attached to the pelvis, resurfacing hemiarthroplasty where the femoral head is resurfaced.

Regarding surgical technique the most common classification is according to whether the prosthesis is cemented, uncemented, or hybrid—a cemented stem and uncemented cup. The type of arthroplasty and type of implant will all have a bearing on the anaesthetic choices and the potential difficulties encountered.

Patient populations will differ between primary and secondary arthroplasty. Generally patients for secondary arthroplasty will be older with more comorbidities. Additionally the reason for arthroplasty will potentially be different. The most common indication for primary hip or knee replacement is almost always osteoarthritis. In secondary arthroplasty, it may be due to any number or reasons including prosthesis failure, fracture, recurrent dislocation, or infection.

The complexity of revision surgery varies considerably: the procedure may be staged (initial removal of cement) with a later return to implant the prosthesis. If joint infection is present it invariably increases blood loss. Does a single component need replacing or the entire prosthesis? Procedures may need bone grafting and consideration of where bone graft will be taken from.

Preoperative assessment

It may be difficult to assess fully the patient's cardio-respiratory reserve as the limitation may be pain rather than exercise tolerance. Information gained from routine preoperative investigations may be limited as these will often reflect the patient at rest.

In general, in considering techniques for secondary versus primary arthroplasty, the requirements of patients undergoing secondary procedures are likely to be greater:

- Patients will probably be older, with increased comorbidities.
- Revision surgery will take longer: will a regional anaesthetic technique provide a sufficient duration of action?
- Blood loss may be significant: cross-matching will be required, as opposed to group and save.

- Increased postoperative pain—how will this be controlled? Supplementary analgesia over and above a simple PCA is almost de rigueur, especially after total knee replacement. Surgical dissection is likely to be more extensive, leading to increased swelling of soft tissues, increased pain, and decreased mobility.

Perioperative management

The anaesthetic technique must, of course, be tailored to each patient. In lower limb surgery, however, reviews have failed to show any difference in *long-term* morbidity or mortality between regional anaesthesia or general anaesthesia.

Patients will need appropriate monitoring. For secondary arthroplasty this may include arterial and central venous lines, with multiple large bore IV access if bleeding is anticipated.

For primary surgery a spontaneously breathing, laryngeal mask, general anaesthetic is suitable for most patients undergoing knee or hip surgery.

- Many anaesthetists will use a flexible laryngeal mask technique for primary shoulder surgery but access is potentially very limited should there be any airway problems. The patient may be moved significantly by the surgeons during the operation.
- Patient positioning is often critical. Revision surgery may increase operative time significantly, necessitating meticulous pressure point care, protection of peripheral nerves, and other structures.
- Where bleeding is anticipated cell salvage (see section 16.7) may be a useful adjunct.
- In secondary arthroplasty, blood loss can be considerable. It is important but very often difficult to monitor intra-operative losses. Drapes may mask many litres of blood loss. Fluids used for lavage can complicate matters further, necessitating careful monitoring of amounts used. If cell salvage is being used it is also likely that conventional suction will be in use: these losses need to be accounted for. The re-infusion of cell-salvaged blood will contain heparin—the effects of this should be anticipated. Blood loss can be increased by certain disease states, e.g. Paget's.
- The antibiotic prophylaxis/regimen may need to be altered. The timing of antibiotic delivery can be difficult. Vancomycin, for example, needs to be administered over 1h, and should ideally be started on the ward preoperatively.

Postoperative care

HDU/ITU care may be indicated. Long operative times combined with blood loss and comorbidities may produce hypothermia, acidosis, and coagulopathy.

18.3 Anaesthesia for fractured neck of femur

Hip fracture is extremely common, and the incidence is rising amongst an ageing population. The great majority of cases occur in females with the mean age at presentation being 80 years. 30 day mortality is around 10%, with significant interhospital variability, and 1 year mortality is as high as 25–35%. This high mortality, which is greatly influenced by perioperative care, has made hip fracture a national improvement target. The Hip Fracture Perioperative Network has been instituted to improve evidence-based anaesthetic care. The National Hip Fracture Database, a collaboration between the British Orthopaedic Association and the British Geriatrics Society, has been commenced to benchmark care and drive improvements in the UK.

The majority of fractures are treated either with conservation of the femoral head, most often via open reduction and interval fixation with the use of a dynamic hip screw (extracapsular fractures), or by replacement of the femoral head via hemi arthroplasty (cemented or uncemented) if the fracture is intracapsular.

Length of procedure can vary from 30min to 2h with potentially large blood loss. Pain is variable but often fracture reduction itself provides analgesia. Patients will be positioned either supine on the hip table or lateral. Techniques vary considerably but in a recent postal survey Sandby-Thomas et al. (2008) found in 75.8% of cases a regional technique was used (of these 95.5% using a spinal technique), 14.4% used a combined regional and general technique, and 9.8% used general alone. Postoperative analgesia regimens utilized paracetamol (either IV or orally) and a form of opioid adjunct with NSAIDs being used less frequently.

Many patients presenting with fractured neck of femur have significant comorbidities and this influences conduct of anaesthesia. With increasing age there is not simply a linear decline in physiological reserve but also the addition of various chronic conditions affecting all of the body systems. Cardiovascular disease, respiratory disease, renal dysfunction, neurological decline, and metabolic derangement are more common in the elderly.

Pathophysiological changes in ageing

See Table 18.1.

Patient management

Preoperative aspects

- Multidisciplinary preoperative assessment should occur, including orthogeriatric involvement.
- Patients with high perioperative risk should be identified early so that appropriate investigation and optimization can occur. These patients need geriatrician-led care with good communication between teams. 70% of patients will be ASA 3 or 4.
- Preoperative investigations should aim to identify anaemia, infection, renal and electrolyte disturbance, and ECG abnormalities which may be optimized.

Preoperative optimization

Careful resuscitation should begin immediately. It is important to recognize that blood loss may be minimal in intracapsular fractures but potentially in excess of 1L in multicomminuted extracapsular fractures. A sensible analgesic regimen should be instituted. Care should be given to restoring fluid balance and minimizing preoperative fasting. Rate control of tachyarrythmia, respiratory optimization with antibiotics, oxygen and chest physio, or rapid investigation of suspected cardiac disease may be undertaken.

Delays to surgery

Delays should occur only if there is a realistic prospect of improving the patient's condition prior to surgery. Investigation of suspected valvular heart disease may not alter outcome if an anesthetic technique assumes severe disease. Outcome is improved if surgery is performed within 36h of admission whilst delays past 48h show increased morbidity and mortality, mainly from pneumonia, pressure sores, and thromboembolic complications. Although some delay to optimize patients unfit for surgery may be beneficial, delays for non-medical reasons worsen outcome. Patients with three or more comorbidities have increased mortality. Patients with respiratory disease and renal disease predispose them to the most common and serious postoperative complications and this group justifies specialist referral.

Perioperative care

The patient will either be positioned supine on a hip table or lateral or supine on a normal operating table. For the hip table the patient will be elevated to the surgeon's shoulder height—potentially making access almost impossible.

Blood loss is variable and much dependent on the skill and speed of the operator. Significant haemorrhage may occur and transfusion may be necessary.

Outcome data to strongly support one form of anaesthesia over another are mostly equivocal although some studies do

Table 18.1 Pathophysiological changes in the elderly patient		
System	Common disease/ changes	Effects
CVS	Hypertension, ischaemic heart disease, valve disease, heart failure. Generalized decrease in elasticity and increase in stiffness	↓ CO, SV, ventricular compliance. Conduction defects, reduced maximal heart rate. Attenuated baroreceptor responses ↑ SVR
RS	COPD	Reduced chest wall compliance, closing volume surpassing FRC, leading to V/Q mismatch. Blunted response to hypoxia & hypercarbia. Reduced VC, FVC, FEV$_1$, peak flow
CNS	Alzheimer's disease, dementia, autonomic neuropathy.	↓ cerebral blood flow, cerebral oxygen consumption. Reduced neurotransmitters & receptors
ANS	Autonomic neuropathy Syncope	↑ sympathetic nervous system activity ↓ parasympathetic system activity Attenuated baroreceptor reflexes
Renal	Dehydration Hyponatraemia/ kalaemia Potential for fluid overload.	Impaired clearance of drugs ↓ GFR ↓ ability to conserve sodium, concentrate urine
Metabolic	Diabetes Hypothyroidism	↓ basal metabolic rate ↓ response to hypothermia
Musculo-skeletal	Rheumatoid arthritis Osteoarthritis	Osteoporosis Poor dentition

Adapted from AK Jandziol and R Griffiths, 'The anaesthetic management of patients with hip fractures', *Continuing Education in Anaesthesia, Critical Care and Pain*, 2001, 1, 2, pp. 52–55, by permission of Oxford University Press, *British Journal of Anaesthesia*, and Royal College of Anaesthetists.

suggest lower adjusted mortality and lower incidence of respiratory morbidity following regional anaesthesia. (Table 18.2). General anaesthesia, regional anaesthesia, and most forms of nerve blockade have all been used. If GA is used it should be combined with PNB as poor analgesia in the immediate postoperative period increases morbidity.

Invasive monitoring should be used if cardiac morbidity mandates and goal-directed fluid therapy using cardiac output monitoring has been shown to reduce length of stay.

Particular care with maintenance of normothermia and point of care haemoglobin measurement should be taken. Careful positioning and pressure point care is mandatory, elderly patients are particularly prone to pressure damage. Haemodynamic instability during cementing should be anticipated and managed appropriately.

Postoperative considerations

The most common postoperative complications are chest infection and cardiac failure (see Box 18.2).

Table 18.2 General vs regional anaesthesia for fractured neck of femur	
General anaesthesia	**Local anaesthesia**
More predictable duration of anaesthesia	Simplicity (e.g. spinal)
Greater haemodynamic stability	Lower incidence of systemic complications
Airway control	Provides intra- and postoperative analgesia
Tendency towards ↑ blood loss, MI incidence, postoperative confusion	↓ PONV
	↓ incidence of DVT and PE

Patients should receive supplemental oxygen for 12h post surgery and the following 3 nights as a significant number of patients will be hypoxaemic, irrespective of anaesthetic technique.

Box 18.2 Risk factors for common postoperative complications after hip fracture surgery
Cardiac failure
• Age >90 years
• Male gender
• History of cardiovascular disease.
Chest infection
• Pre-existing respiratory disease
• Use of oral steroids
• Increasing age.
30-day mortality
• Male gender
• Respiratory disease
• Renal disease.

Pain is often limited to the incision: some patients will report little pain; others will have significant analgesic requirements. Paracetamol, NSAIDs, and opioids have roles to play but great care is needed in the use of NSAIDs in the elderly.

Early mobilization and dietary supplementation have both been shown to reduce length of hospital stay.

AAGBI Guidelines for management of proximal femoral fracture

These guidelines were developed to drive service improvements by applying the following principles to care:
1. Protocol driven, fast track admission
2. Multidisciplinary team led by orthogeriatricians
3. Surgery is the best analgesia
4. Surgical repair should occur within 48h of admission
5. Surgery and anaesthesia must be undertaken by appropriately experienced surgeons and anaesthetists
6. High quality team communication is required
7. Early mobilization is key to management
8. Preoperative management should consider discharge planning
9. Measures should be taken to prevent secondary falls
10. Continuous audit and research should inform and improve.

Further reading

Jandziol AK & Griffiths R (2001). The anaesthetic management of patients with hip fractures. *BJA CEPD Rev*, 1(2):52–5.

Roche JJW, Wenn RT, Sahota O, et al. (2005). Effect of comorbidities and postoperative complications on mortality after hip fracture in elderly people: prospective observational cohort study. *BMJ*, 331(7529):1374.

Sandby-Thomas M, Sullivan G, Hall J (2008). A national survey into the peri-operative anaesthetic management of patients presenting for surgical correction of a fractured neck of femur. *Anaesthesia*, 63:250–5.

18.4 Scoliosis surgery

Patients presenting for corrective spinal surgery form a challenging group, presenting over a spectrum of ages and with a range of comorbidities. Scoliosis is a lateral curvature and rotation of the thoracolumbar vertebrae, resulting in an associated rib deformity.

Aetiology

Scoliosis occurs in approximately 2.5% of most populations, with a female preponderance of 4:1. 70% of cases are termed idiopathic, as there is no identifiable cause, whilst the remainder may be due to congenital changes, secondary changes related to neuropathic or myopathic conditions, or occur later in life from degenerative spondylosis (see Box 18.3).

Box 18.3 Classification of scoliosis aetiology

- *Idiopathic:* infantile(onset <4 years), Juvenile(4–9 years), Adolescent(10 years+)
- *Congenital:* abnormal spinal cord/vertebral development
- *Neuromuscular:*
  - *Neuropathic:* cerebral palsy, syringomyelia, poliomyelitis
  - *Myopathic:* muscular dystrophies, neurofibromatosis, Friedreich's ataxia
- *Mesenchymal:* Marfan's, rheumatoid arthritis, osteogenesis imperfecta
- *Malignancy:* primary/secondary tumours
- *Trauma:* fracture/surgery/radiotherapy
- *Infection:* TB, osteomyelitis
- *Degenerative:* osteoarthritis.

Natural history

Smaller curves may not progress and may even resolve. Larger curves (>30%) are more likely to progress and may result in greater cosmetic deformity and back pain. More severe curves correlate with the presence of respiratory symptoms and a restrictive lung defect. If left untreated, respiratory failure, pulmonary hypertension, and right heart failure may develop.

Surgical procedure

Surgical intervention is indicated for a variety of reasons and is dependent on the predicted natural history of the deformity. Adult idiopathic curves tend to progress slowly and the main indication is often for cosmetic improvement.

In contrast, in juvenile or adolescent idiopathic patients, the aim is to halt progression and to at least partially correct the deformity, preventing further respiratory and cardiovascular deterioration. In neuropathic scoliosis secondary to cerebral palsy/spina bifida, curves may interfere with posture and sitting, therefore correction can facilitate general care.

Surgery tends to be considered when the Cobb angle exceeds 50% in thoracic and 40% in the lumbar regions.

Surgical correction involves mobilization of the spine, correction of the deformity and subsequent fusion to maintain correction and limit progression. The approach may be anterior, posterior or combined depending on the cause and the severity of the curvature.

An anterior approach involves a thoracotomy incision to allow access to the spine. Lumbar and thoracolumbar curves are often correctable via this approach. It may also be the first part of a staged correction of thoracic, stiff or multiple curves. In this instance the procedure is called an anterior release and allows mobilization of the vertebrae aiding subsequent correction via a posterior approach. One-lung ventilation is rarely necessary and a single-lumen endotracheal tube is appropriate. Surgical lung retraction may lead to intraoperative and postoperative pulmonary complications if prolonged.

In the more commonly used posterior approach, the spine is accessed via a single longitudinal incision in the prone patient. The paraspinal musculature is reflected, the facet joints excised, and vertebrae decorticated. Bone graft is packed over the decorticated surfaces and correction achieved using stainless steel rods, which provide stability for subsequent spinal fusion.

Posterior correction may be performed at the same operation or may be performed several days later. The decision to perform these stages as combined or separate operations obviously has many anaesthetic implications.

Anaesthetic considerations

Preoperative assessment

Consideration should be made to the aetiology, location, and degree of scoliosis. All patients require a full history, physical examination, and appropriate investigations focusing on the cardiorespiratory systems:

Respiratory system

History

- Frequent respiratory tract infections
- Poor cough + chronic aspiration
- OSA
- Inability to cooperate with physiotherapy.

Aetiology

Myopathic conditions have a greater degree of pulmonary dysfunction for equivalent angle curves.

Cerebral palsy: risk of aspiration and unlikely to cooperate with assessment and post op therapy.

Spirometry

Scoliosis causes a restrictive lung defect, with reduced vital capacity and reduced total lung capacity. Pulmonary dysfunction is related to the degree of scoliosis (especially if >100°), the number of vertebrae involved, a cephalad location of the curve, and a loss of normal thoracic kyphosis.

If preoperative FEV_1 or FVC values are less than 20–30% predicted, postoperative ventilation becomes more likely. An anterior approach should be avoided unless surgically mandatory.

Arterial blood gases

There is increased V/Q mismatching. Apical blood flow is relatively increased in both lungs and distribution of ventilation abnormal, particularly in the lung on the concave side of the curve.

Sleep studies

Particularly useful in patients with poor spirometry results and also in those unable to perform simple spirometry. Significant night time disordered breathing and dependence on nocturnal

CPAP also indicates reduced physiological reserve and plans should be instituted for postoperative support.

Minimum investigations should include a plain chest film and spirometry.

Cardiovascular system

Cardiac dysfunction may be secondary to scoliosis: cor pulmonale can occur secondary to chronic hypoxaemia and pulmonary hypertension.

Cardiac disease may also be related to the underlying pathology, e.g. in muscular dystrophies.

Minimum investigations include 12-lead ECG and echocardiography to assess left ventricular function and PA pressures.

NB: patients with marked respiratory dysfunction should have RV assessment.

Anaesthetic technique

The aim is for a stable anaesthetic to allow optimal surgical, physiological conditions and also to allow for neurophysiological monitoring.

Positioning

For an anterior approach, the patient will be in lateral position with the convex side uppermost.

A posterior approach will require the patient to be prone often for a prolonged period of time. Care should be taken to ensure free abdominal and chest movement to allow adequate ventilation and minimize venous congestion.

Care with peripheral pressure areas especially: eyes, chin, elbows, hands, knees, ankles, breasts, and genitalia.

Monitoring

Scoliosis surgery can be associated with significant blood loss, therefore in addition to standard monitoring the following are recommended:

- Invasive arterial blood pressure monitoring—mandatory
- Urinary catheter
- ×2 large-bore IV access
- CVP line—if significant comorbidity
- Temperature monitoring, use fluid warmers and warm air blankets.

Haemostasis

At least 2 units of blood should be cross-matched. A posterior approach is associated with significant blood loss, while blood loss maybe as little as 100mL with an anterior approach.

Principles of controlled hypotension, use of cell salvage, use of antifibrinolytics, point of care coagulation testing (e.g. TEG®), maintenance of normothermia should be considered and employed where appropriate.

Neurological monitoring

Intraoperative spinal cord monitoring allows continuous monitoring of spinal cord function, providing an early marker of any compromise which may occur through direct cord or nerve damage by instrumentation, distraction injury, or reduced spinal cord perfusion leading to ischaemia.

The nervous system is stimulated and the response detected distal to the area of cord at risk. This may be done using either somatosensory evoked potentials (SEPs) or motor evoked potentials (MEPs). In SEP monitoring stimulation is applied peripherally, often via the posterior tibial nerve and the response is then detected either via a scalp or epidural electrode. Nerve injury may be indicated by a decrease in amplitude or increased latency. In MEP, stimulation is applied via transcranial electrodes to the motor cortex and the response detected by epidural electrodes or from muscle as compound muscle action potentials (CMAPs).

Anaesthetic technique impacts upon spinal cord monitoring (see Table 18.3).

Table 18.3 Effects of anaesthetic drugs on evoked potentials		
Drugs	**SSEP**	**MEP**
Thiopentone, propofol, midazolam	Neutral	Suppression
Inhalational agents	Neutral	Suppression
Nitrous oxide	Neutral	Suppression
Opioids	Neutral	Neutral
Ketamine, etomidate	Enhancement	Enhancement
NMBAs	Neutral	(Neuromuscular blocking agents prevent CMAP recording, but not the transmission of MEP)

Wake up test

This is a clinical test to assess spinal cord function, in which the patient is briefly woken during surgery and asked to move their hands and feet. The patient can then be immediately re-anaesthetized. These tests have the advantage of requiring no specialist equipment or personnel for their application. They provide only a snapshot picture and demonstrate only motor function, thus a sensory deficit may be missed. They are not applicable to children or those with diminished mental capacity.

Analgesia

Good postoperative analgesia is essential to allow early mobilization and compliance with physiotherapy. A multimodal approach is best, combining simple analgesics, systemic opioids, and regional anaesthetic techniques. An epidural or paravertebral catheter can be placed intraoperatively after an anterior correction. After initial neurological assessment a loading dose can be given, followed by continuous infusion.

Postoperative care

Most patients are extubated immediately and monitored overnight in a high-dependency area to allow continuation of invasive monitoring and neurological assessment. Some patients may require a period of either invasive or non-invasive ventilation postoperatively.

Further reading

Cooper MA & Edge G (2001). Pre-operative assessment of patients for corrective spinal surgery. *Curr Anaesth Crit Care*, 12:130–8.

Entwistle MA & Patel D (2006). Scoliosis surgery in Children. *CEACCP*, 6(1):13–16.

Raw DA, Beattie JK, & Hunter JM (2003). Anaesthesia for spinal surgery in adults. *Br J Anaesth*, 91(6):886–904.

Chapter 19

Regional anaesthesia

351

19.1 Regional anaesthesia

Local anaesthetic pharmacology

Local anaesthetic (LA) reversibly inhibits neural transmission by crossing the phospholipid neuronal membrane and binding to intracellular fast sodium channels. Sodium entry during depolarization is prevented and the threshold potential is therefore not reached. This stops propagation of the action potential and transmission of the nerve impulse.

Only the unionized form of LA can cross the membrane and this proportion is dependent upon the extracellular pH and the drug's pK_a (Table 19.1). The pK_a equates to the pH at which 50% of the drug's molecules are unionized. LAs are weak bases, therefore the lower the pK_a the greater the proportion of the drug which exists unionized at physiological pH (7.4).

Table 19.1 Important LA pharmacodynamics

Pharmacodynamic	Property
Potency	Lipid solubility
Duration of action	Degree of protein binding Total dose injected Rate of removal from the site of action
Speed of onset	Amount of unionized free base at the site of action—itself dependent upon: • the drug's pKa • the pH of the tissue • concentration of the solution

Choice of local anaesthetics

LAs can be divided into esters (amethocaine, cocaine) and amides (lidocaine, bupivacaine, levobupivacaine, ropivacaine, prilocaine; see Table 19.2). Amide LAs are used for regional anaesthesia as they are more stable in solution and, unlike esters, are usually heat stable so can be sterilized.

The choice of LA is usually dependent upon the speed of onset and the duration of action required for the clinical situation. A mixture of two different LAs, however, may be injected to utilize each drugs properties, e.g. lidocaine and bupivacaine—the former for rapid onset, the latter for prolonged duration. Finally, the relative safety of each drug is also a consideration. Levobupivacaine is the safer, less toxic, pure S-enantiomer of bupivacaine (a racemic mixture of S- and R-enantiomers) but is otherwise clinically similar. Ropivacaine is also supplied as a pure S-enantiomer and has an even better toxicity profile than levobupivacaine.

Differential block occurs when a LA produces more selective blockade for sensory than motor fibres. For example, ropivacaine has lower lipid solubility but a similarly high pK_a to bupivacaine.

When used at a low concentration, it blocks small, sensory C fibres more avidly than larger, myelinated, motor A fibres.

Local anaesthetic additives and adjuvants

See Table 19.3.

Table 19.3 Role of additives and adjuvants

Adrenaline	Localized vasoconstriction decreases vascular absorption—reduces peak plasma levels and prolongs duration of action More effective if used with short-acting, lipophobic LA, e.g. lidocaine Marker of intravascular injection Concentrations >1:200,000 (5mcg/mL) may have hemodynamic side effects NB Max safe dose of adrenaline is 4mcg/kg
Bicarbonate	Raises the pH of a solution, increasing the unionized proportion, and speed of onset Can reduce pain on injection as LAs are stored as hydrochloric salts in an acidic solution to prolong shelf life Risk of precipitation Use 1mL of 8.4% sodium bicarbonate per 10mL LA
Clonidine	Prolongs duration of action Additional peripheral analgesic action due to release of encephalin-like compounds Systemic absorption may cause hypotension and sedation Doses up to 150mcg can be used peripherally without side effects
Dexamethasone	May increase duration of analgesia
Midazolam	Early evidence suggests it may prolong sensory block
Neostigmine	Little consistent evidence for its use in peripheral nerve blocks Numerous side effects, especially GI
Opioids	No current evidence for their use in peripheral nerve blocks over systemic administration

Nerve localization

Successful and safe regional anaesthesia depends on accurate localization of nerves and deposition of LA solution. Available techniques are:

Eliciting paraesthesia using surface anatomical landmarks only. This is painful, with an increased risk of nerve damage and no longer advocated as a safe technique.

Nerve stimulation using anatomical landmarks and eliciting either paraesthesia (sensory nerves) or muscle contraction (motor nerves).

Table 19.2 Properties of local anaesthetics

	pK_a	Onset	Lipid solubility (relative)	Potency (relative)	Protein binding %	Duration	Max. safe dose (with adrenaline) mg/kg
Prilocaine	7.9	Fast	50	2	55	Short	6.0 (9.0)
Lidocaine	7.9	Fast	150	2	70	Medium	3.0 (7.0)
Ropivacaine	8.1	Medium	300	6	94	Long	3.5 (3.5)
Bupivacaine	8.1	Medium	1000	8	95	Long	2.0 (2.5)
Levobupivacaine	8.1	Medium	1000	8	95	Long	2.5 (3.0)

Ultrasound-guided needle placement within appropriate anatomical landmark areas.

Peripheral nerve stimulation (PNS)

Peripheral nerve stimulators induce nerve membrane depolarization via electrical impulses and cause either muscle contraction or paraesthesia. The nearer a needle tip (cathode) is placed in proximity to a nerve, the stronger the response elicited (based on Coulomb's law).

Features of modern nerve stimulator features
- Constant current generator, irrespective of variable resistance of surrounding tissue.
- Linear current output range (0.01–0.5 mA).
- Digital display.
- Facility to vary pulse duration (0.05–1.0msec).
- Monophasic rectangular output (unidirectional).
- Stimulating frequency of 1Hz and 2Hz.
- Disconnect indicator.
- Colour coded leads. Cathode (black) only connectable to the needle, anode (red) attached to the patient.

Advantages of PNS
- Low-cost equipment requiring little training to use.
- Avoids use of larger, cumbersome equipment.

Disadvantages of PNS
- Indirect evidence of nerve localization.
- Only useful when a motor response can be elicited.
- Evidence of correct needle position (e.g. motor response) disappears immediately upon injection.
- Stimulation at <0.5mA does not guarantee correct needle position.

Ultrasound

Ultrasound-guided regional anaesthesia (USRA) is used either alone or in combination with a PNS. Common components and features are:
- Transmitter: generates pulsed US in brief bursts.
- Transducer: piezoelectric crystals convert electrical energy into acoustic pulses and vice versa.
- Receiver: detects, compresses, and amplifies signals returning to the transducer.
- Display: shows the signal in the brightness B-mode, the motion M-mode, and the amplitude A-mode.
- Colour flow Doppler: identifies directional flow in relation to the transducer.
- Contrast adjustment: controls gain of image.

Advantages of USRA
- Identifies nerves and their surrounding structures.
- Real-time visualization of needle allows accurate adjustments of needle direction and depth.
- Images LA spread during injection.
- Volume of LA required may be reduced.

Disadvantages of USRA
- Costly equipment requiring training to use.
- Direct visualization creates a false sense of security.
- Learning curve to develop hand–eye coordination.

Practical aspects of USRA

Ergonomics
Successful USRA requires careful positioning of the operator, patient, and screen to facilitate manipulation of the probe and needle. To improve control both hands and arms should be comfortable and supported. The probe should be held close to the transducer contact surface with the operating hand resting on the patient.

Probe selection
Most US machines deliver US at 3–12MHz depending upon the probe used. *Linear probes* generate a higher frequency with a rectangular field of view. *Curvilinear probes* generate a lower frequency and are linear in shape but produce a curved view. Higher frequencies provide greater resolution, however lower frequencies have better tissue penetration. High-frequency linear probes are therefore best used to image superficial structures, e.g. the brachial plexus, whereas low-frequency, curved probes are best used to image deep structures e.g. psoas major muscle.

Use of gel
Gel is required to prevent air existing between the probe and the patient to allow US transmission.

Normal sonoanatomy of individual nerves
High-frequency US allows the visualization of the epineurium, perineurium, and neurons. When imaged proximally (e.g. above the clavicle) nerves appear dark grey (hypoechoic) as there is a high proportion of neurons. More distally (e.g. below the clavicle), the proportion of connective tissue increases so nerves appear white (hyperechoic). In longitudinal section the internal echotexture consists of continuous hypoechoic longitudinal bands (neural fascicles) interspersed with hyperechoic perineural connective tissue. Fluid and air do not reflect US and appear black (anechoic). See Table 19.4.

Anisotropy refers to a change in echogenicity of tissues as a result of transducer angle. A hypoechoic structure can appear hyperechoic when the angle of insonation changes from 45 to 90°, e.g. the sciatic nerve.

Table 19.4 Ultrasound appearance of various tissues	
Tissue	**Ultrasound appearance**
LA	Anechoic (spread from needle can be seen)
Veins	Anechoic (compressible)
Arteries	Anechoic (pulsatile)
Fat	Hypoechoic with irregular hyperechoic lines
Muscles	Hyperechoic lines within hypoechoic tissue
Tendons	Predominantly hyperechoic
Bone	Very hyperechoic lines with hypoechoic shadow

Needling techniques

In-plane
The needle is placed in-line, and parallel to, the ultrasound beam from the transducer so that the full length of the shaft and tip of the needle are visualized. The position of the needle relative to the nerve and surrounding structures can be followed in real time.

Out-of-plane
The needle is inserted perpendicular to the ultrasound beam from the transducer. The needle shaft and tip are seen as a hyperechoic dot. An echogenic needle tip aids location.

Needle position relative to angle of insonation

The angle of the insonation is a major determinant of US reflection. An US wave hitting a smooth, mirror-like interface at a 90° angle is reflected back perpendicular to that interface. An incident US wave hitting the interface at <90° will be deflected from the interface at an angle equal to the angle of incidence but in the opposite direction (angle of reflection). This weakens the signal of the returning echo so the image is darker. This is why it is difficult to visualize a needle inserted at a steep angle (>45° to the skin surface). Imaging of the needle is best when the shaft of the needle is perpendicular to the US beam (parallel to the probe).

Hydrodissection

Injection of fluid (saline or dextrose) can be used to 'dissect' out the intermuscular or fascial plane in which a nerve lies to aid its visualization.

Local anaesthetic spread

Perineural injection

Perineural injection is seen as an expanding collection of hypoechoic fluid around the nerve. Circumferential spread is generally desired but is not essential.

Recognition of incorrect LA spread

Even as little as 1mL LA injected intraneurally can expand a nerve. Movement of the nerve towards the needle on withdrawal also suggests intraneural needle placement. Arteries and veins are seen as anechoic circular or tubular structures. Although colour Doppler can be used, these vessels can be distinguished by varying the contact pressure on the probe to collapse veins. Inadvertent venous puncture may go unrecognized if contact pressure is too high. Aspiration prior to injection of LA and visualization of its spread is important to prevent intravascular injection. Intravascular injection results in rapid clearance of LA from the site of administration.

Peripheral nerve catheter techniques

Catheters can extend anaesthesia and analgesia into the postoperative period (24–72h). However, catheter placement is more difficult than standard nerve blocks, requires larger needles and less familiar equipment. The failure rate is high (>25%). LA intermittent dosing or infusion pumps may be used but require specialized nurse intervention and monitoring to ensure safety. This may be expensive and labour intensive.

Like standard nerve blocks, peripheral nerve catheters may be positioned using US, nerve stimulation or both. The spread of LA can be assessed to determine the best position for the catheter. If appropriate dressings are used the spread of LA can be assessed daily with US.

The catheter should be positioned parallel to the nerve being blocked. The needle must be carefully positioned to facilitate this. Prior to passing the catheter, the space is distended with 10–20mL saline/LA. The catheter is threaded 3–5cm into the space. The catheter is flushed after insertion to avoid obstruction with clotted blood, and secured carefully away from the site of surgery. The most common cause of failure is displacement.

Interscalene, supraclavicular, infraclavicular, and axillary catheters can be used for the upper limb. Mid-thigh femoral and sciatic catheters can be performed for the lower limb.

Advantages and disadvantages

Major limb blocks can be used as a sole anaesthetic technique or be combined with general anaesthesia (GA). The choice depends on patient preference and expected duration of the surgical procedure. Unless a catheter is used, peripheral nerve blocks have a limited duration.

Advantages of major limb blocks

• Avoids GA
• Attenuates stress response to surgery
• Improves postoperative analgesia
• Reduces use of other analgesics (and side effects)
• Less immunosuppressive (vs GA and opiates).

Avoiding the adverse effects of GA, such as cardiovascular compromise, may be highly desirable in certain patients. Obtunding the stress response to surgery may improve glycaemic control in diabetics and avoid perioperative tachycardia in those with ischaemic heart disease.

Good quality analgesia for up to 24h can be provided by single-shot techniques. This can be extended to 2–3 days with catheter insertion. The benefits of non-opiate-based analgesia are numerous and include reduction in postoperative nausea, vomiting, and bowel dysfunction, and less confusion and sedation with earlier hospital discharge. Although there remains inconclusive evidence that neuraxial anaesthesia reduces postoperative cognitive dysfunction there may be a role for major limb blocks.

Disadvantages of major limb blocks

• Appropriate equipment required
• Specialist training
• Time required performing the block
• Patient discomfort when needling
• Finite duration of single-shot technique
• Prolonged motor block
• Potential block failure
• Recognized complications.

Contraindications and anticoagulation

Absolute contraindications

• Patient refusal
• Infection at site of injection
• Allergy to LA (rare).

Relative contraindications

• Bleeding disorders and anticoagulation
• Pre-existing peripheral neuropathies.

Few guidelines exist regarding major limb blocks and anticoagulation, however the ASRA (American Society of Regional Anesthetists) recommend that the same precautions for neuraxial regional anaesthesia should be used for deep plexus and peripheral limb blocks. Although major limb blocks don't pose the same risk as neuraxial blocks of bleeding into a confined, non-compressible space with resulting nerve injury, accidental or unrecognized vascular puncture can cause significant blood loss if patients are anticoagulated.

Complications and side effects

Complications can essentially be divided into either those due to the insertion of the needle (or catheter), or due to the injection of LA and adjuvants (Table 19.5).

Table 19.5 Generic complications of peripheral nerve blocks	
Due to needle insertion	Due to the injection
Immediate	
Neuronal trauma	LA toxicity ± intravascular injection
Vascular puncture	Anaphylaxis
Damage to surrounding tissues	Ischaemia (due to vasoconstrictors)
Pneumothorax	Central neuraxial spread
Delayed	
Infection	LA toxicity absorption from vascular site/overdose
Haematoma	Prolonged motor block

Depending on the individual peripheral nerve block there are also recognized side effects which are specific to the site of injection (see sections 19.3 and 19.4). Side effects are reversible, undesirable consequences of a block which usually subside as the LA wears off, e.g. Horner's syndrome and phrenic nerve paralysis following an interscalene block. However, the latter could be considered a complication if it resulted in respiratory compromise significant enough to require intervention such as intubation.

Peripheral nerve injury

Mild paraesthesia following peripheral nerve blocks occurs in up to 15% cases. However, over 95% are likely to resolve within 4–6 weeks and >99% will resolve within 1 year. Serious, permanent neurological injury occurs in 0.01-0.04% of cases.

The difficulty in estimating the exact incidence of Peripheral nerve injury (PNI) following nerve block is that patient and surgical factors also play a role in development. Patient risk factors contribute to the 'double-crush' phenomenon. This is where an already compromised axon is less able to tolerate an insult and is therefore more prone to developing a deficit. Surgical causes for PNI may be compounded by a prolonged or dense block.

Patient risk factors for perioperative PNI

• Pre-existing neurological disorder
• Extremes of body habitus or deformity
• Severe peripheral vascular disease
• Diabetes mellitus
• Advanced age
• Male gender.

Surgical risk factors

• Prolonged surgery
• Direct surgical trauma or stretch
• Compressive dressings or casts
• Use of tourniquets
• Haematoma or abscess formation

- Perioperative inflammation
- Improper patient positioning.

The pathophysiology of PNI can be divided into 5 causes
- *Trauma*—from needles, catheters, or surgical incision.
- *Ischaemia*—vascular injury, tourniquet, vasoconstrictors.
- *Drug toxicity*—LAs and adjuvants.
- *Compression*—haematoma, postoperative oedema.
- *Stretch*—prolonged traction, improper positioning.

Traumatic PNI requires the protective epineurium and perineurium to be breached leaving individual nerve fascicles transected or exposed and vulnerable. Even when nerves are impaled, the needle often only disrupts the connective tissue which constitutes up to 70% of a nerve's cross-sectional area. Only if the fascicles containing nerve fibres are penetrated may damage occur, either by transecting them or exposing the neurons to potentially neurotoxic LA. Damage associated with LA is dependent upon both the duration and concentration of LA the fascicle is exposed to.

Following a PNI, prognosis is dependent upon whether the axon is disrupted or, more favourably, only compromised. Neuropraxia, where the myelin sheath is damaged but the axon is preserved, is commonly due to compressive or stretch injuries and is likely to resolve more rapidly.

Infection

Strict asepsis is important whilst performing a peripheral nerve block. A single-shot block has less risk of introducing infection than the use of peripheral nerve catheters. These may become colonized and cause localized inflammation (0–13.7%), infection (0.3–2%), abscess formation (0–0.9%) and very rarely sepsis. The exact frequency of infectious complications is related to both the site of injection or catheter placement (femoral and axillary catheters having the highest incidence) and the presence of patient risk factors.

Patient risk factors for developing infection
- Significant trauma
- Diabetes mellitus
- IV drug use
- Malignancy
- Pregnancy
- Immunocompromised states.

Local anaesthetic toxicity

LA toxicity occurs when either the maximum recommended dose of LA is exceeded (insidious onset) or there is accidental intravascular injection (rapid onset). The most likely mechanism is non-neural sodium channel inhibition. Other mechanisms proposed include the antagonism of oxidative phosphorylation within cell mitochondria. This would explain why the organs most affected are those most dependent upon aerobic metabolism (heart and brain). With regard to cardiac sodium channel binding, bupivacaine binds more rapidly and is longer acting than lignocaine. 'R' isomers bind more avidly than 'S' isomers (levobupivacaine and ropivacaine).

Toxicity classically causes central nervous system, and then cardiac, excitement then depression. Those most at risk are at the extremes of age (<4 months, >70 years) and those with pre-existing cardiac (especially conduction defects and ischaemic heart disease), renal, or hepatic dysfunction.

Features of LA toxicity
- CNS excitement:
  - Agitation, auditory changes, metallic taste
  - Peri-oral tingling
  - Tonic–clonic seizures
- CNS depression: drowsiness, coma, respiratory arrest
- Cardiac toxicity: hypertension, tachycardia, ventricular arrhythmias
- Cardiac depression: bradycardia, conduction block, asystole, decreased contractility.

For management, see Box 19.1.

Box 19.1 Management of LA toxicity
- Stop injecting LA.
- Call for help.
- Maintain airway and ventilation, 100% oxygen.
- Benzodiazepines first-line for seizure management.
- Vigilance for evidence of cardiovascular compromise.

If cardiac arrest:
- Standard ALS protocols.
- Arrhythmias can be resistant to treatment.
- Use of lipid emulsion whilst continuing CPR.
- Prolonged CPR (>1h) is required if LA toxicity is suspected.
- Avoid vasopressin, calcium channel and β-blockers.
- Consider use of cardiopulmonary bypass.

Using 20% lipid emulsion (Intralipid®):
- Bolus 1.5mL/kg over 1min.
- Infuse at 0.25mL/kg/min.
- Repeat initial bolus twice, 5min apart if still low BP.
- If no improvement, increase infusion to 0.5mL/kg/min.
- Continue infusion for >10min once cardiovascularly stable.

Further reading

AAGBI. Guidelines: management of LA toxicity: <http://www.aagbi.org/publications/publications-guidelines/M/R>

Jeng CL, Torrillo TM, & Rosenblatt MA (2010). Complications of peripheral nerve blocks. *Br J Anaesth*, 105(S1):i97–i107.

Neal JM, Bernards CM, Hadzic A, et al. (2008). ASRA Practice Advisory on Neurologic Complications in Regional Anesthesia and Pain Medicine. *Reg Anesth Pain Med*, 33:404–15.

Neal JM, Weinberg GL, Bernards CM, et al. (2010). ASRA practice advisory on local anaesthetic systemic toxicity. *Reg Anesth Pain Med*, 35:152–61.

Wiles MD & Nathanson MH (2010). Local anaesthetics and adjuvants—future developments. *Anaesthesia*, 65(suppl. 1):22–37.

Upper limb

Motor and sensory nerve supply to the upper limb is via a single brachial plexus. It is superficial, originating from the anterior primary rami of C5 to T1 spinal nerves in the neck, and passes laterally and caudally over the 1st rib to enter the axilla. In its course from origin to target organs the brachial plexus is organized into roots, trunks, divisions, cords, and major nerves (Fig. 19.1).

Anaesthesia and analgesia of the upper limb can be provided by injecting LA solutions at different sites of the brachial plexus and/or peripheral nerves depending on the site of surgery. In clinical practice different approaches are used, each having its own indication and unique complications. It is important to consider infiltration to areas outside the region of the primary block, e.g. interscalene block is used for shoulder surgery but may need supplementary infiltration to C3–C4 and/or T1–T3 dermatomes.

Interscalene block (ISB)

Indications: shoulder and proximal humeral surgery.

Limitations: C8 and T1–T3 segments not blocked, requiring supplementary subcutaneous injection. C3–C4 segments spared if low volumes of injectate used.

Patient position: supine, head turned contralaterally, arm by side of the body.

Nerve stimulator technique (see Fig. 19.2)

Landmarks: interscalene groove at the posterior border of sternocleidomastoid muscle and level of the cricoid cartilage (C6).

Depth: 0.5–2.5cm (use 50mm insulated needle).

Needle direction: medial, dorsal, caudad (i.e. towards contralateral elbow).

Stimulation end-points: shoulder abduction or elbow flexion. Diaphragmatic stimulation (phrenic nerve) indicates the needle is too anterior. Retraction of the scapula (dorsal scapular nerve) indicates needle is too posterior.

LA volume: 20–30mL.

Ultrasound-guided technique (see Fig. 19.3)

Probe position: axial, oblique plane at the level of cricoid cartilage so as to obtain the best transverse view of the roots/trunks between the scalene muscles.

Needle direction: out-of-plane or in-plane.

LA volume: 20mL or less.

Block specific complications/side effects

- Phrenic nerve palsy
- Recurrent laryngeal nerve palsy
- Stellate ganglion block (Horner's syndrome)
- Extradural/intrathecal injection (loss of consciousness, severe hypotension)
- Intravascular injection (especially vertebral artery)
- Spinal cord injury.

Supraclavicular block

Indications: elbow, forearm and hand surgery. A single injection can provide rapid onset, dense anaesthesia of the entire limb.

Limitations: may spare C8–T1 segments (i.e. ulnar distribution) and T2.

Patient position: as for ISB. (A semilateral position can aid the in-plane insertion of the needle.)

Nerve stimulator technique

This technique is now rarely used because of an unacceptably high incidence of pneumothorax (up to 10%).

Ultrasound-guided technique (see Fig. 19.4)

Probe position: posterior and parallel to the clavicle in the supraclavicular fossa. The divisions/trunks are lateral and superior to the subclavian artery (SA). See Fig. 19.5.

Depth: <2.0cm from the skin surface.

Needle direction: commonly in-plane, aiming lateral to medial.

LA volume: 20–30mL.

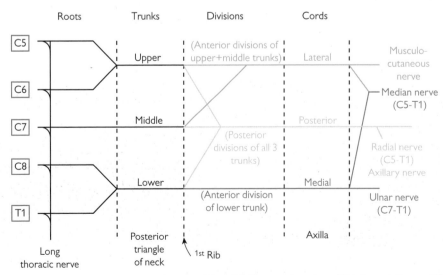

Fig. 19.1 The brachial plexus. Reproduced from Catherine Spoors and Kevin Kiff, *Training in Anaesthesia*, 2010, Figure 6.19, page 119, with permission from Oxford University Press.

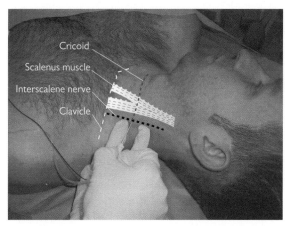

Fig. 19.2 Anatomical landmarks for ISB. Reproduced from Catherine Spoors and Kevin Kiff, *Training in Anaesthesia*, 2010, Figure 6.21, page 121, with permission from Oxford University Press.

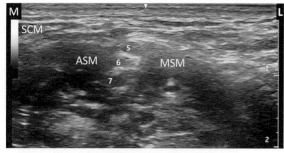

Fig. 19.3 Ultrasound view of interscalene block. SCM: sternocleidomastoid muscle. The C5 (5), C6 (6) and C7 (7) nerve roots run in the interscalene grove between the anterior (ASM) and middle scalene muscles (MSM).

Block specific complications/side effects
- Pneumothorax
- Intravascular injection (subclavian artery)
- Phrenic nerve palsy
- Recurrent laryngeal nerve palsy
- Stellate ganglion block (Horner's syndrome).

Axillary block

Indications: distal arm, forearm and hand surgery.

Limitations: musculocutaneous and intercostobrachial (T2 dermatome) nerves spared and require separate infiltration.

Patient position: arm abducted at 90° with elbow either straight or flexed.

Nerve stimulator technique
Landmarks: anterior to axillary artery at the level of pectoralis major muscle insertion (and posterior to the artery for the multi-injection technique).

Depth: 1.0–1.5 cm.

Needle direction: 30–45° aimed cranially and tangentially along the long axis of the artery.

Stimulation end-points: flexion of lateral digits (median nerve); flexion of 5th digit and adduction of the thumb (ulnar nerve); thumb abduction/extension of the wrist (radial nerve); elbow flexion (musculocutaneous nerve).

LA volume: 30–50mL.

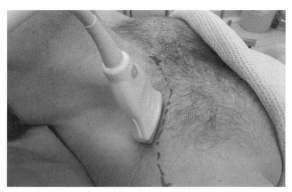

Fig. 19.4 Probe and needle position for in-plane US guided supraclavicular block. The patient is positioned supine or sat up at 30o. The probe is placed in the supraclavicular fossa; posterior & parallel to the clavicle (dashed line). The divisions/trunks of the brachial plexus are lateral and superior to the subclavian artery. The needle is inserted in the plane of the US aiming lateral to medial as shown. As the brachial plexus is usually within 2.0 cm of the skin surface a 50 mm needle is usually adequate. The 100 mm needle shown (for illustrative purposes) would be too long and flexible in practice.

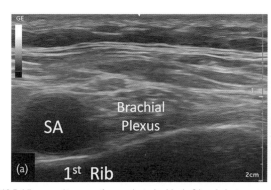

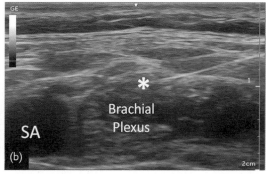

Fig. 19.5 Ultrasound images of supraclavicular block. SA: subclavian artery. (a) The brachial plexus. (b) The whole shaft of the needle is seen in-plane. The tip (*) is within the brachial plexus. Infiltrated LA can be seen around the plexus.

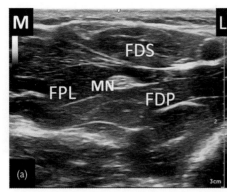
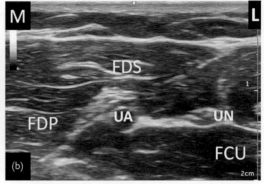

Fig. 19.6 (a) Median nerve in the forearm. The median Nerve (MN) is sandwiched between flexor digitorum superficialis (FDS) and flexor digitorum profundus (FDP) in the forearm. Proximal to the wrist it is more superficial and lies between FDS and Flexor carpi radialis (FCR). Flexor policis longus (FPL); Palmaris longus (PL). (b) Ulnar nerve in the forearm. Medial (M); Lateral (L). The ulnar nerve (UN) separates from the ulnar artery (UA) in the forearm. Flexor carpi ulnaris (FCU); flexor digitorum superficialis (FDS); flexor digitorum profundus (FDP).

Ultrasound-guided technique

Probe position: transverse plane as cranial in the axilla as possible to obtain the best cross-sectional view of the blood vessels and the four nerves.

Needle direction: in-plane (frequently practised) from the anterior to posterior part of the axilla, or out-of-plane (infrequently practised). The musculocutaneous nerve is usually located deeper, between the biceps and coracobrachialis muscle and is blocked separately.

LA volume: 15–25mL.

Block-specific complications

Intravascular injection.

Peripheral nerve blocks

Various nerves can be blocked at multiple sites distal to the axilla to provide either lone anaesthesia/analgesia or to augment and expedite brachial plexus blocks. The advent of ultrasound has further expanded the number of sites that nerves can be identified.

Radial nerve

The radial nerve can be identified with ultrasound above the elbow, lateral to the insertion of biceps tendon, as it passes posterior to the distal humerus.

Median nerve

The median nerve can be identified in the:

- Antecubital fossa, medial to the brachial artery.
- Middle of the forearm, where it lies between the muscles of flexor digitorum profundus, flexor digitorum superficialis, and flexor pollicis longus (Fig. 19.6a).
- At the wrist, between the tendons of flexor carpi radialis and palmaris longus.

Ulnar nerve

- Above the elbow, the ulnar nerve can be visualized proximal to the medial epicondyle before it descends into the ulna sulcus.
- In the distal to mid-forearm it runs along the medial border, medial to the ulnar artery (Fig. 19.6b).
- At the wrist it lies deep to flexor carpi ulnaris.

19.4 Lower limb blocks

Lower limb

The lower limb is innervated by both the lumbar and sacral plexi. Complete analgesia of the lower limb cannot be provided by a single nerve block. In clinical practice many approaches are used, each having its own indication and unique complications. The technique chosen must be appropriate for both the patient and surgical procedure. Supplementation may be required with infiltration to areas outside the region of the primary block, e.g. analgesia for total knee replacement may be provided using femoral nerve block and intraoperative LA infiltration of the posterior capsule of the knee by the surgeon.

The lumbar plexus

The lumbar plexus is formed by the anterior divisions of L1–L4 (Fig. 19.7). The L1 root often receives a branch from T12. After emerging from the intervertebral foramina the nerves lie within the psoas major muscle and its sheath, anterior to the transverse processes of the lumbar vertebrae.

The branches of the lumbar plexus are:

- Ilioinguinal (L1)
- Iliohypogastric (L1)
- Genitofemoral (L1–L2)
- Femoral (L2–L4)
- Lateral-cutaneous nerve of the thigh (L2–L4)
- Obturator nerve (L2–L4).

All except the obturator emerge laterally between the psoas and quadratus lumborum. The obturator passes medially before descending under the iliac vessels.

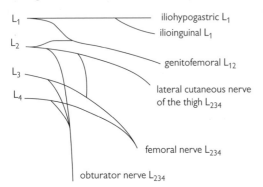

Fig. 19.7 The lumbar plexus. Reproduced from Catherine Spoors and Kevin Kiff, *Training in Anaesthesia*, 2010, Figure 6.45, page 135, with permission from Oxford University Press.

Lumbar plexus block

Indications: operations involving the groin, neck/shaft of the femur, anterior thigh and knee.

Limitations: systemic absorption of LA can occur from this highly vascular region. Minimize risk of LA toxicity with slow injection and frequent aspiration. Not generally used as a sole anaesthetic technique.

Patient position: lateral, side to be blocked uppermost with hip and knee flexed.

Table 19.6 Response to nerve stimulation for lower limb blocks		
Target	Required response	Muscle
Lumbar plexus & femoral nerve	Patella twitch (L3/4)	Quadriceps Femoris
Sciatic nerve:		
Tibial nerve	Plantarflexion	Gastrocnemius
Peroneal nerve	Dorsiflexion	Peroneal

Nerve stimulator technique

Landmarks: needle insertion is perpendicular to the skin of the back to locate the transverse process of L3. This is 3–4cm lateral to the lumbar spine. The needle is advanced angling cephalad over the transverse process to penetrate the fascia of quadratus lumborum and psoas sheath (<4cm beyond transverse process). Stimulation may not detect the plexus because the nerves are separated and embedded within the body of the muscle. A loss of resistance technique using a Tuohy needle can also be performed. A catheter may be inserted to provide continuous analgesia and radio-opaque contrast can confirm placement.

Depth: 8–12cm (use 100mm insulated needle).

Needle direction: perpendicular to the skin of the back.

Stimulation end-points: Patella twitch (see Table 19.6).

LA volume: 20–30mL

Ultrasound-guided technique

Probe position: paramedian on the back at the level of L3 transverse process to obtain transverse view of the psoas muscle.

Needle direction: out-of-plane or in-plane.

LA volume: 20–40mL.

Block-specific complications/side effects

- Intra/retroperitoneal bleeding and haematoma
- Epidural/intrathecal injection
- Trauma to intraperitoneal organs/blood vessels.

Femoral nerve block; 3-in-1 block

Indications: operations on shaft of the femur, anterior thigh, knee and medial side of the lower leg (saphenous nerve). The '3-in-1' block is a single injection, which aims to block the femoral, obturator, and lateral cutaneous nerves. Firm distal pressure is applied during injection of a large volume of LA. Although in theory this spreads the LA rostrally back to the psoas compartment to block all three nerves, this rarely occurs in practice.

Limitations: need for sciatic (popliteal nerve) and possibly obturator (medial thigh) to provide complete analgesia for the knee. Lateral cutaneous nerve of the thigh often requires supplementation.

Produces motor weakness of quadriceps limiting mobility.

Relatively contraindicated in ilioinguinal surgery and femoral vascular graft surgery.

Patient position: supine.

Nerve stimulator technique

Landmarks: 1cm lateral to femoral artery below inguinal ligament.

Depth: 2–4cm (use 50mm insulated needle).

Needle direction: 45° rostrally.

Stimulation end-points: patella twitch.

LA volume: 10–15mL femoral nerve, 30mL 3-in-1.

Ultrasound-guided technique (see Fig. 19.8)

Probe position: parallel to inguinal crease to obtain transverse view of femoral artery, femoral nerve, fascia lata, fascia iliaca, and iliacus muscle.

Needle direction: out-of-plane or in-plane.

LA volume: 10–20mL femoral nerve; 20–40mL 3-in-1.

Block-specific complications/side effects

Trauma to intraperitoneal organs and blood vessels.

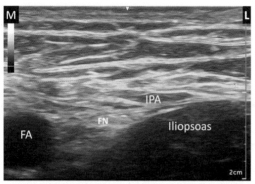

Fig. 19.8 Ultrasound appearance of the femoral nerve. Iliopectineal arch (IPA) The femoral nerve (FN) lies lateral to the femoral artery (FA). It is invested in the fascia iliacus above the iliopsoas muscle.

The sacral plexus

The sacral plexus is formed from the ventral rami of L4–5 (lumbosacral trunk) and S1–3 within the ventral surface of piriformis (Fig. 19.9). The most important branches for regional anaesthesia are the sciatic nerve and the posterior cutaneous nerve of the thigh.

The sciatic nerve is the largest in the body, and provides sensory and motor innervation to the lower limb. The sciatic nerve exits the pelvis via the greater sciatic foramen below the piriformis muscle. It descends into the thigh between the ischial tuberosity and greater trochanter. In the gluteal region, the sciatic nerve is deep (anterior) to the gluteus maximus muscle and is superficial (posterior) to the inner muscle layers (superior and inferior gemellus muscles, obturator internus muscle, quadratus femoris muscle).

The sciatic nerve continues down the midline of the posterior thigh behind the femur and branches into the tibial and common peroneal nerves at a variable location along its course in the thigh above the popliteal fossa.

Sciatic nerve block; posterior, anterior, and popliteal approaches

The sciatic nerve can be blocked proximally using an anterior or posterior approach or distally using a lateral approach.

Indications: operations on the knee and lower leg.

Limitations: femoral nerve block is also required to provide complete analgesia for the knee. Saphenous nerve block is also needed to provide complete analgesia for ankle and forefoot.

LA volume: 20mL.

Stimulation end-points: dorsi/plantar flexion and inversion/eversion of the foot.

Block-specific complications/side effects

Proximal approach will cover tourniquet pain but causes hamstring weakness and can block the parasympathetic nerves that control bladder emptying. Adrenaline should be avoided in LA.

Posterior sciatic nerve block (Raj)

Patient position: supine with leg flexed to 90° at hip and knee.

Nerve stimulator technique

Landmarks: mid-point of a line joining the greater trochanter to the ischial tuberosity. Usually the groove between hamstrings and adductors.

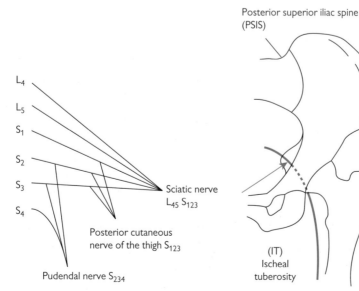

Fig. 19.9 The sacral plexus and the course of the sciatic nerve. Reproduced from Catherine Spoors and Kevin Kiff, *Training in Anaesthesia*, 2010, Figure 6.49, page 137, with permission from Oxford University Press.

Depth: 4–8cm.

Needle direction: perpendicular to the skin.

Posterior sciatic nerve block (Labat)

Patient position: lateral decubitus position with the leg to be blocked uppermost and flexed to 90° at hip and knee.

Nerve stimulator technique

Landmarks: mid-point of a line joining the greater trochanter to the sacral hiatus.

Depth: 5–10cm.

Needle direction: perpendicular to the skin.

Ultrasound-guided technique

Patient position: prone.

Probe position: parallel to subgluteal crease and inferior to ischial tuberosity to obtain transverse view of sciatic nerve lateral to biceps femoris and semitendinosus muscles.

Needle direction: in-plane or out-of-plane.

Anterior sciatic nerve block (Beck)

Limitations: in about 15% of patients the sciatic nerve lies immediately posterior to the femur and cannot be blocked using the anterior approach.

Patient position: supine.

Nerve stimulator technique

Landmarks: a line joining the anterior superior iliac spine to the pubic tubercle. A parallel line is drawn from the greater trochanter. The needle is inserted at the intersection of a perpendicular joining the junction of the medial third and lateral two-thirds of the upper line, to the lower line.

Depth: 2–3cm inferior to femur (8–10cm).

Needle direction: perpendicular to the skin to contact medial shaft of the femur, then redirected medially to advance beyond the femur.

Ultrasound-guided technique

Probe position: 8cm distal to inguinal crease to obtain transverse view of sciatic nerve medial to femur.

Needle direction: in-plane.

Popliteal sciatic nerve block

Patient position: prone, lateral decubitus position with the leg to be blocked uppermost or supine with the leg flexed to 90° at hip and knee.

Nerve stimulator technique

Landmarks: 1cm lateral to a point 7cm proximal to the mid-point of the skin crease of the popliteal fossa.

Depth: 3–8cm. Use100mm insulated needle.

Needle direction: perpendicular to the skin.

Stimulation end-points: plantar flexion or inversion of the foot indicates successful location of the posterior tibial nerve. Dorsiflexion may result from stimulation of the common peroneal nerve alone; the sciatic nerve may have already branched.

LA volume: 10–20mL.

Ultrasound-guided technique (see Fig. 19.10)

Probe position: parallel but proximal to skin crease of popliteal fossa proximal to division of sciatic nerve. The tibial nerve lies posterior and medial to popliteal artery.

Needle direction: in-plane or out of plane.

Ankle blocks (see Fig. 19.11)

Indications: operations on the forefoot.

Limitations: five nerves must be blocked to provide analgesia to the whole forefoot but this is rarely necessary. The saphenous nerve is a terminal branch of the femoral nerve. The other four are branches of the sciatic nerve. Generally not used as a sole anaesthetic technique.

Patient position: supine.

Saphenous nerve (supplies medial foot and ankle)

Landmarks: 1cm proximal and anterior to the medial malleolus close to the saphenous vein.

Volume: 2–3mL subcutaneous infiltration.

Ultrasound-guided technique

Probe position: medial aspect of lower leg below knee to seek nerve lateral to saphenous vein.

Needle direction: in-plane.

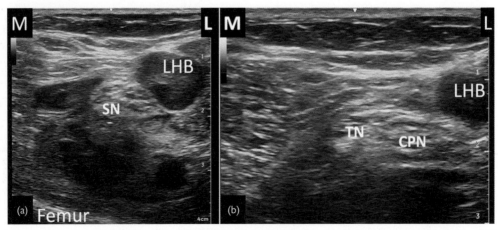

Fig. 19.10 Ultrasound appearance of the distal sciatic nerve. Medial (M); Lateral (L). (A) The sciatic nerve (SN) in the popliteal fossa. (B) Slightly more distally the SN begins to divide into the tibial nerve and the common peroneal nerve (CPN).

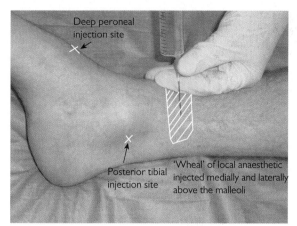

Fig. 19.11 Ankle block—anatomical landmarks. Reproduced from Catherine Spoors and Kevin Kiff, *Training in Anaesthesia*, 2010, Figure 6.53, page 137, with permission from Oxford University Press.

Posterior tibial nerve (supplies plantar surface)

Landmarks: medial malleolus either side of the posterior tibial artery.

Volume: 3–5mL.

Ultrasound-guided technique

Probe position: medial leg above the medial malleolus to seek nerve posterior to tibial artery.

Needle direction: in-plane.

Deep peroneal nerve (supplies dorsum of 1st webspace)

Landmarks: line joining malleoli, just medial to the dorsalis pedis artery.

LA volume: 3–5mL.

Ultrasound-guided technique

Probe position: anterior leg above the medial malleolus to seek nerve lateral to dorsalis pedis.

Needle direction: in-plane.

Superficial peroneal nerve (supplies dorsum of foot)

Blocked by lateral superficial infiltration along the line between the malleoli.

LA volume: 5mL.

Sural nerve (lateral border of foot)

Landmarks: between lateral malleolus and Achilles tendon.

LA volume: 3–5mL.

Chapter 20

Core topics in intensive care medicine

20.1 Recognition of critical illness

There have been many observational studies showing that a high proportion of patients suffering cardiac arrest have preceding warning signs in the form of physiological and biochemical instability, often up to 6–8h before the cardiac or respiratory arrest.

The poor identification, review, and treatment of deteriorating patients on the wards leads to poor outcomes in patients who sustain in-hospital cardiac arrests. This led to the concept of early warning scores (EWS) and rapid response teams (RRT).

Many of the 'care bundles' that are effective in critical care medicine rely on timely interventions, e.g. optimum fluid resuscitation, manipulation of oxygen delivery, and the administration of antibiotics, but this requires early recognition of illness. In this early phase of impending critical illness, many patients may be in the emergency department or on a hospital ward, rather than an ICU. It is here that organ failure begins to develop and patients admitted from a general ward have a considerably higher mortality rate than those from the emergency department or operating theatre. Thus the skills of the intensivist are required outside of the ICU: 'critical care without walls.' Table 20.1 shows early and late signs of a deteriorating patient.

Table 20.1 Early and late signs of acutely deteriorating health in hospital patients	
Early signs	Late signs
Partial airway obstruction	Complete airway obstruction
SpO$_2$ 90–95%	SpO$_2$ <90%
Respiratory rate 20–30 breaths/min	Respiratory rate >30 breaths/min
Mild hypotension (SBP >80mmHg)	Severe hypotension (SBP <80mmHg)
Urine output <0.5mL/kg/min	Anuric
Confusion/agitation	Unresponsive to voice/pain
Base deficit −5 to −8	Base deficit <−8
pH 7.2–7.3	pH <7.2
Lactate 0–4mmol/L	Lactate > 4mmol/L

Rapid response teams and outreach

Several names have been used to describe the teams that now actively seek patients with deteriorating conditions on general wards in order to intervene early: medical emergency teams (MET), RRTs, or critical care outreach (CCO). The structure of the team may vary but all focus on the early identification and treatment of acutely ill patients. The principle of the MET team is that they are called by ward staff once a patient's vital signs become abnormal. Small, single-centre studies consistently have shown that early detection and treatment of the critically ill patient improves patient outcome.

The decision as to when to call the MET has been simplified by the introduction of scoring systems that summate abnormal vital signs leading to a threshold value above which help is sought. Implementation of EWSs such as 'Track and Trigger' has been widespread across the UK. Interestingly, a prospective randomized controlled study (The MERIT study) showed no difference in mortality in RRT versus cardiac arrest teams. But this may be due to poor compliance with the criteria to call RRTs (a MET was only called to 30% of patients who fulfilled the criteria) and over-use of cardiac arrests teams (50% of calls were peri-arrest situations). Post hoc analysis of the MERIT data and subsequent smaller single-centre studies all reveal that the rate of peri-arrests increases as the rate of unexpected cardiac arrests and death decreases. Therefore the MET does have an impact on patient care and early recognition and treatment of the acutely ill patient remains important.

Clinical assessment of an acutely unwell patient

Clinical assessment of an acutely unwell patient is best done using the 'Airway Breathing Circulation' (ABC) approach used in the ALS or ATLS guidelines. Once the 'ABC' assessment is complete and the patient has been stabilized, a more thorough assessment should be undertaken to include a detailed history, review of observation, fluid and drug prescription charts as well as an secondary survey, i.e. a more extensive and detailed examination of each organ system.

A: Airway assessment

Ensure the patient does not have a compromised airway; signs include grunting, snoring, stridor, and wheeze. This could be due to several factors; obstruction could be due to the tongue obstructing the oropharynx secondary to trauma, anaphylaxis, or decreased GCS score. The airway may require clearing and an airway adjunct or definitive airway may be required.

B: Breathing assessment

Assessment of respiration may reveal the following concerning signs:

- Abnormal respiratory rate (<8 or >35 breaths/min)
- Low oxygen saturation (SaO$_2$ <85%)
- Use of accessory muscles of respiration
- Wheeze/dyspnoea
- Acute increase in supplemental oxygen requirement (>50% or non-rebreathing oxygen facemask).

Each EWS has different criteria set by local RRTs. A high respiratory rate >35 breaths/min is one of the most sensitive markers of acute illness and may be either due to hypoxia or metabolic acidosis as a result of poor tissue perfusion.

C: Circulation

Listed are some of the cardiovascular criteria used in EWS:

- Heart rate <40 or >140bpm
- SBP <90 or >200mmHg
- DBP <50 or >110mmHg
- Signs of tissue perfusion—CRT, peripheral skin temperature
- Oliguria and a decline in GCS score will occur as MAP falls precipitously.

When investigating the cause of shock, the following should be considered:

- Hypovolaemia (dehydration and haemorrhage)
- Sepsis (leading to distributive shock and vascular endothelial leakage)
- Cardiac failure
- Neurogenic shock (neurological and spinal injury)
- Outflow obstruction (tension pneumothorax, cardiac tamponade)
- Anaphylaxis.

The Surviving Sepsis Campaign and early goal-directed therapy (EGDT) studies state that for improved patient outcome fluid resuscitation should be commenced within 6h of the onset of the symptoms of shock.

It should be remembered that oliguria (urine output <0.5mL/kg/h) may be as a result of hypovolaemia, hypotension, or direct renal injury (endotoxins, drugs) leading to renal failure.

D: Disability

A patient's conscious level can be assessed using the GCS or AVPU scoring system (**A**lert, responds to **V**oice, responds to **P**ain, **U**nresponsive). Conscious level may vary from mild confusion and agitation to unresponsive requiring airway protection. The cause of neurological dysfunction in an acutely unwell patient may be due to several factors including hypotension, hypoxaemia, metabolic acidosis, acute liver failure, acute kidney injury, and severe sepsis or localized infection (meningitis). Hypoglycaemia is frequently forgotten as a cause of reduced conscious level; it should be treated promptly with IV dextrose.

E: Environment

After initial resuscitation and stabilization, further information regarding the patient should be gathered and appropriate tests ordered. Arterial blood gases will show information regarding ventilation ($PaCO_2$), oxygenation (PaO_2) and tissue perfusion (lactate concentration). Additional information should include the A–a gradient, base deficit, bicarbonate, sodium, potassium, and glucose levels. Lactate has shown to be an excellent prognostic marker in poor outcomes in severe sepsis. The Surviving Sepsis campaign uses a lactate >4mmol/L as part of its bundle to commence prompt EDGT. A complete top-to-toe examination should be conducted to look for any factors that could contribute to a patient's acute deterioration, e.g. bleeding, bruising, infection, and inflammation. Further investigations should be based upon these findings.

Predictors and scoring systems for the acutely unwell patient

EWSs were developed to help to identify patients that are at risk of deterioration at an early stage and who may benefit from critical care. Morgan et al. developed an EWS in 1997 to be used at the bedside that was based on the evaluation of five physiological parameters: SBP, pulse rate, respiratory rate, temperature, and AVPU score. Subbe et al. in 2001 validated a modified early warning system (MEWS) that showed this was a simple tool that could be used by nurses at the bedside. Most hospitals now use a MEWS to trigger the RRT. The use of a MEWS has been shown to improve the documentation of vital signs on the bedside chart.

The SOCCER trial attempted to identify early and late predictors of adverse outcomes and stated the failure of studies such as MERIT to demonstrate efficacy of MET may be due to these teams using late signs of deterioration rather than early signs.

National guidelines

An acutely deteriorating patient on the ward represents one of the sickest patients in the hospital. They require prompt management by senior and experienced staff if morbidity and mortality are to be reduced in this vulnerable patient cohort. Communication is the key to effectively managing these patients, particularly 'out of hours' and a recent NICE guideline highlighted this along with the need for:
- Physiological observations recorded at the time of the admission.
- Clearly documented monitoring plans.
- Physiological track and trigger systems should be used.
- Appropriate staff competencies/education/training.
- A graded response strategy for patients identified as being at risk of clinical deterioration.
- Consultant involvement for critical care admissions.

Further reading

Dellinger RP, Levy MM, Carlet JM, *et al*. (2008). Surviving Sepsis Campaign: international guidelines for the management of severe sepsis and septic shock 2008. *Crit Care Med*, 36:296–27.

Hillman K (2002). Critical care without walls. *Curr Opin Crit Care*, 8(6):594–9.

Morgan RJM, Williams F, Wright MM (1997). An early warning scoring system for detecting developing critical illness. *Clin Intens Care*, 8:100.

NICE (2007). *Acutely Ill Patients in Hospital: Recognition of and Response to Acute Illness in Adults in Hospital*. London: NICE.

Subbe CP, Kruger M, Rutherford P, *et al*. (2001). Validation of a modified Early Warning Score in medical admissions. *QJM*, 94:521–6.

20.2 Pathophysiology of sepsis

Definition

Sepsis remains one of the leading causes for admission to ICU, as high as 25%, and despite recent advances in medical treatments it continues to have a high mortality (30–50%). Sepsis is a clinical syndrome that represents a systemic inflammatory response to an infection. In 1991 the American College of Chest Physicians/Society of Critical Care Medicine (ACCP/SCCM) consensus conference committee introduced the concept of systemic inflammatory response (SIRS) and the definition of sepsis. Table 20.2 outlines the definitions for SIRS and sepsis.

Table 20.2 Definitions related to sepsis
Infection
Inflammatory response to the presence of a microorganism
Bacteraemia
The presence of viable bacteria in the blood
Systemic inflammatory response syndrome (SIRS)
A non-specific clinical response including two or more of the following: • Temperature >38°C or <36°C • Heart rate >90 beats/min • Respiratory rate >20/min • White blood cell count >12 000/mm³ or <4000/mm³ or >10% immature neutrophils As well as infection, SIRS can also be caused by trauma, burns, pancreatitis, and other insults
Sepsis
SIRS with a presumed or confirmed infectious process
Severe sepsis
Sepsis with signs of at least one acute organ dysfunction: • Renal • Respiratory • Hepatic • Haematological • Central nervous system • Unexplained metabolic acidosis • Cardiovascular
Septic shock
Severe sepsis with hypotension refractory to adequate volume resuscitation
Hypotension
A SBP <90mmHg or a reduction of >40mmHg from the baseline in the absence of other causes for hypotension
Multiple organ dysfunction syndrome (MODS)
Presence of altered organ function in an acutely ill patient such that homeostasis cannot be maintained without intervention

Pathophysiology

Sepsis results in a complicated immunological, metabolic, and cardiovascular response. The host's response and premorbid state determines the severity of the infection rather than the infecting organism alone.

The innate immune system is initiated by the pattern recognition receptors (PRRs) in response to pathogens of which there are three main families:

• Toll-like receptors (TLRs)

• Nucleotide-oligomerization domain (NOD) leucine-rich repeat proteins

• Retinoic acid-inducible gene-I (RIG-I).

A major advancement in understanding the early events of sepsis has been the recognition of Toll-like receptors (TLRs). These have 13 distinct receptors capable of recognizing organisms from bacteria, fungi, and viruses.

In Gram-negative infections, lipopolysaccharides (LPS) from endotoxins binds to lipopolysaccharide binding protein (LBP) in plasma and this complex then binds to the CD14 receptor found on macrophages. This receptor in turn presents the LPS to a TLR-4 causing macrophage activation and subsequently the production and release of inflammatory cytokines such as, tumour necrosis factor (TNF), interleukin (IL)-1, IL-6, and IL-8. Other systems and pathways activated include arachidonic acid pathway (leukotrienes, thromboxane, and prostaglandins), coagulation, complement and kinin systems. The peptidoglycan protein of Gram-positive organisms binds to CD14 and TLR2 activating the pathway.

T-helper lymphocytes are also activated in sepsis and secrete either pro-inflammatory or anti-inflammatory cytokines. Type 1 T-helper cells respond to the initial injury by secreting pro-inflammatory cytokines (TNF, interferon, and IL-2). This initial response then evolves into an anti-inflammatory phase with type 2 T-helper cells secreting IL-4 and IL-10.

Genetic polymorphisms

Genetic factors are thought to play a large role in determining the outcome and mortality from sepsis more so than in any other common condition. Genetic variability within the population can lead to a wide range of responses to sepsis or injury, for example, individuals that are TNF-β_2 homozygotes have been shown to mount a more aggressive inflammatory response to an organism with higher circulating TNF levels but also have higher mortality compared to the heterozygous TNF-β_1/TNF-β_2 patients.

Coagulation

Sepsis causes the activation of the coagulation system. Disseminated intravascular coagulation (DIC) and thrombocytopenia has been shown to be an independent predictor of organ failure and mortality. In patients with sepsis and DIC the mortality rises to 43%, versus 27% in patients with sepsis and no DIC.

In acute inflammation, activation of the endothelium at the site of inflammation occurs, permitting the localization of cells of the innate immune system. This leads to the release of pro-inflammatory cytokines (IL-6, TNF, and IL-1) and to inflammation-induced activation of the coagulation system.

Tissue factor plays a major role in inflammation-induced coagulation. In sepsis, mononuclear cells will express tissue factor when exposed to pro-inflammatory cytokines activating the coagulation pathway.

Tissue factor leads to the formation of thrombin (factor IIa) via factor VIIa, and factor X. Thrombin converts fibrinogen to fibrin and also acts as a platelet activator. This leads to clot formation, which is further enhanced by the downregulation of the anticoagulant pathways. The three main pathways are:

• Antithrombin (AT)

• Protein C

• Tissue factor pathway inhibitor (TFPI).

All three possess anti-inflammatory properties independent of their anticoagulation activities.

AT is a serine protease inhibitor and it is the main inhibitor of thrombin and factor Xa. Heparin is known to interact with

AT resulting in a 1000-fold enhancement of its activity. During severe sepsis, AT levels are low due to marked impairment of synthesis. AT anti-inflammatory properties include inducing prostacyclin release from endothelium, which in turn inhibits platelet activation and aggregation. It also prevents leucocyte migration and adhesion to endothelial cells therefore limiting capillary leakage. *The use of heparin in DIC has not been shown to improve outcome and may have a detrimental effect on AT, protein C activation, and TFPI.*

There has been a great deal of literature regarding activated protein C (APC) and it is thought to play a central role in promotion of fibrinolysis and inhibition of thrombosis and therefore prevention of clot formation and multiorgan dysfunction. APC works with protein S to degrade factors Va and VIIIa therefore acting as an anticoagulant. Its anti-inflammatory properties include inhibition of leucocyte chemotaxis and adhesion of leucocytes to endothelium, inhibition of platelet-derived growth factor in the lung, preventing the disruption of the endothelial barrier, and finally the inhibition of endothelial cell apoptosis.

TFPI is the main inhibitor of tissue factor–factor VIIa complex thus preventing thrombin formation.

All three pathways are downregulated in severe sepsis and levels of AT and APC are reduced.

Fibrinolysis is activated in sepsis but fails to keep up with the increased thrombin activation and fibrin generation further contributing to microvascular thrombosis and organ dysfunction despite adequate oxygen delivery.

Organ dysfunction

Sepsis and SIRS can affect all organs as a result of direct or indirect injury. Direct injury is usually due to endotoxins or the organism involved in the infection. Indirect injury can be a consequence of hypovolaemia, haemodynamic instability, and the inflammatory response leading to hypoxia and low cardiac output as well as microthrombi causing organ dysfunction.

Cardiovascular

In sepsis, cardiovascular dysfunction results from:
• Myocardial dysfunction
• Increased capillary permeability leading to hypovolaemia
• Shunting and blood flow redistribution (distributive shock)
• Decreased systemic vascular resistance (SVR)
• Increased pulmonary vascular resistance (PVR)
• Increased venous capacitance
• Abnormal microcirculatory blood flow.

Hypovolaemia in sepsis may be relative or absolute due to poor oral intake, diarrhoea, increased insensible losses or decreased SVR, increased venous capacitance, and increased permeability of cell membranes. The reduction in SVR is primarily caused by vasodilatation secondary to increased nitric oxide production from the vascular endothelium via inducible nitric oxide synthase (iNOS).

Myocardial dysfunction is common in severe sepsis and is associated with an increased mortality. It is characterized by biventricular systolic and diastolic dysfunction with an increase in both end diastolic and systolic volumes. This results in a reduction in ejection fraction despite a rise in cardiac index.

Other physiological changes seen include vascular hyperreactivity to catecholamines, thought in part due to excess production of nitric oxide and also adrenoceptor desensitization and downregulation due to high levels of endogenous catecholamines.

Renal

Sepsis and septic shock account for 50% of acute kidney injury (AKI) episodes. Pre-renal and reversible causes of AKI in sepsis include: hypovolaemia due to vasodilatation, capillary leak, venous pooling, and insensible losses.

Normotensive ischaemic causes of AKI are thought to be due to diminished or impaired autoregulation of renal blood flow and is seen in patients with atherosclerosis, hypertension or taking ACEIs and NSAIDs.

Acute tubular necrosis (ATN) is the most frequent mechanism of AKI in ICU accounting for 75% of cases of AKI. ATN is seen in low-flow states such as cardiogenic or haemorrhagic shock. There is no evidence of ATN seen in septic shock patients with AKI.

There have been many hypotheses including abnormal efferent and afferent vasodilatation leading to reduced GFR, LPS, and TNF causing direct kidney injury and renal tubular cell apoptosis but the true cause of kidney injury in septic shock remains unclear and may be a combination of these.

Respiratory

The lung is often involved in sepsis as either the primary source of infection or as a consequence of severe sepsis presenting as acute lung injury (ALI). ALI presents as hypoxia and diffuse alveolar infiltrates due to the influx of neutrophils, causing inflammation and damage to the alveolar-capillary barrier and therefore interstitial oedema, loss of surfactant and alveolar damage. This can lead to decreased lung compliance and impairment of gas exchange.

Patients with shock present with global hypoperfusion and lactic acidosis, resulting in hyperventilation and therefore increased use of the respiratory muscles.

The respiratory muscles use up to 30% of oxygen in shock. Work of breathing is increased and leads to acute respiratory failure requiring intubation and ventilation early in septic shock patients.

Central nervous system

Sepsis-associated encephalopathy may be as a direct consequence of sepsis or secondary to sepsis-related liver or renal failure, acidosis, or hypoperfusion. The neuroendocrine and autonomic systems modulate the immune response. For example, stimulation of the vagus nerve decreases the release of cytokines from macrophages. And although the blood–brain barrier prevents the entry of circulating inflammatory mediators, systemic inflammation can still be detected via the vagus nerve.

Direct causes of sepsis-associated encephalopathy include cerebral endothelial cells being activated by LPS and pro-inflammatory cytokines. One of the consequences of endothelial activation is the breakdown of the blood–brain barrier allowing the passage of neurotoxic factors.

Further reading

Bone RC, Grodzin CJ, & Balk RA (1997). Sepsis: a new hypothesis for pathogenesis of the disease process. *Chest*, 112:235–43.

Balk RA (2000). Pathogenesis and management of multiple organ dysfunction or failure in severe sepsis and septic shock. *Crit Care Clin*, 16:337–52.

20.3 Management of sepsis

Sepsis is the innate host response to infection and its successful management is a universal challenge around the world. It should be remembered that it is a syndrome (i.e. a collection of recognizable signs) rather than a distinct disease and the underlying causes are highly variable. This is the likely reason that specific 'magic bullet' therapies have repeatedly failed and the major treatment advances have come about through guidelines that tackle treatment of the causative infection and management of haemodynamic and systemic oxygen delivery deficiencies.

The Surviving Sepsis Campaign

Septic shock has a high mortality. Early treatment and resuscitation is essential to prevent multiple organ failure. The 'Surviving Sepsis Campaign' was an international process of consultations aiming to standardize the care of septic patients. It uses a care bundle format and the evidence is graded using the GRADE system. The management is condensed into two bundles: an acute 'initial resuscitation' bundle to be completed in the first 6h followed by an ongoing 'haemodynamic support' bundle to be completed in the first 24h (Table 20.3). Some authors argue that there is a lack of evidence to support parts of the guideline and the same protocol is used for sepsis of differing origins.

Table 20.3 Recommendations of the Surviving Sepsis Campaign

Initial resuscitation and infection issues

- Early goal-directed resuscitation within 6h of recognition of sepsis
- Blood cultures before antibiotic therapy
- Imaging studies performed promptly to confirm source of infection
- Administration of broad-spectrum antibiotics within 1h of diagnosis of septic shock or sepsis
- Reassessment of antibiotic therapy with microbiology
- Source control, i.e. surgery when appropriate

Haemodynamic support and adjunctive therapy

- Fluid resuscitation with crystalloid or colloid
- Fluid challenge to restore mean circulating filling pressure and to reassess when no improvement in tissue perfusion
- Noradrenaline is the first choice vasopressor
- Maintain MAP ≥65mmHg
- Dobutamine for myocardial dysfunction
- Stress dose steroid therapy only in septic shock unresponsive to fluid and vasopressors.
- Maintain haemoglobin concentration 7–9g/dL
- Lung protective ventilation
- Conservative fluid strategy for patients with ALI/ARDS
- Glycaemic control
- Venous thromboembolism prophylaxis
- Stress ulcer prophylaxis

Antibiotics

The Surviving Sepsis Campaign guidelines recommend administration of IV antibiotics as early as possible, certainly within the first hour of diagnosis. Appropriate cultures (particularly blood) should be taken prior to antibiotics being given; however, this should not delay treatment. Delays in antibiotic therapy increase mortality. Initially, empirical treatment should be commenced and rationalized if and when positive cultures reveal the infective organism. The specific choice of antibiotic will depend upon the suspected source of infection and local patterns of infective organisms and antibiotic resistance. In some circumstances antifungal agents may also be required. Following this, source control is a vital component of effective sepsis management; eradication of the source by physical means (e.g. via surgery or percutaneous drainage) can be life-saving.

Early goal-directed therapy

Rivers et al.'s landmark study in 2001 showed EGDT in the first 6h of severe sepsis and septic shock resulted in a reduction in 28-day and 60-day mortality. The algorithm used the following targets:

- Central venous pressure: 8–12mmHg
- Mean arterial pressure: ≥65mmHg
- Urine output: ≥0.5mL/kg/min
- Central venous oxygen saturations: ≥70%
- SpO_2: ≥93%
- Haematocrit: ≥30%.

These were achieved by the administration of crystalloid, colloid, vasoactive agents, red blood cells, and inotropic agents according to an algorithm that has now been emulated in many ICUs. The administration of blood in critically ill patients remains controversial; the risk:benefit balance of immunological injury and infective potential versus improved systemic oxygen delivery must be weighed up. The optimum haemoglobin concentration in septic patients is unclear.

Studies using EGDT have shown a delayed need for vasopressors, no difference in overall fluid requirement at 72h, less end-organ dysfunction, and decreased mortality. EGDT is also thought to modulate pro- and anti-inflammatory pathways as well as apoptosis and coagulation.

Inotropic and vasoconstrictor support

Distinction must be made between agents that induce vasoconstriction to maintain blood pressure (α-adrenergic activity) and agents that are primarily inotropic (β-adrenergic activity) to augment cardiac output. There is little evidence that any one agent is superior to another and like much of medicine, it is the manner in which an agent is used rather than the agent itself that is paramount.

Renal replacement therapy

Renal failure is common in sepsis therefore renal replacement therapy (RRT) is frequently required. There is much literature surrounding the details of when to commence RRT and the 'dose' a patient should receive. RRT should be initiated according to standardly accepted criteria (Box 20.1).

Box 20.1 Criteria for commencing RRT

- Hyperkalaemia (K^+ >6.5mmol/L)
- Uraemia (>36mmol/L)
- Severe acidaemia (pH <7.1)
- Fluid overload
- Oligo-anuria.

The dose should not exceed 25mL/kg/h for renal failure as evidence suggests increasing the dose further is of no benefit. However, high-volume RRT (>45mL/kg/h) has been shown to improve outcome in septic patients due to the removal of pro-inflammatory cytokines and toxins.

Steroids

There has been much controversy regarding the use of corticosteroids in severe sepsis and septic shock. The initial study by

Annane et al. was a large multicentre RCT that demonstrated low-dose hydrocortisone (200mg/day) reversed shock faster and more often than the control group, the study also showed a survival benefit. The subsequent CORTICUS trial did not demonstrate improved survival after hydrocortisone therapy was used in patients with septic shock. Most physicians now only use corticosteroids using the recommendations set out the 2008 update of the Surviving Sepsis Campaign, i.e. steroids are administered in patients poorly responsive to fluid resuscitation and vasopressors therapy.

Recombinant human activated protein C

In 2001 the PROWESS study reported a significant benefit in mortality (24.7% vs 30.8%) in patients with severe sepsis treated with activated protein C. The proposed action and benefits of the drug was promotion of fibrinolysis and inhibition of thrombosis and therefore less end-organ dysfunction.

Subsequent trials have failed to reproduce a survival benefit and shown significant bleeding complications. In October 2011, Eli Lilly withdrew activated protein C from the market.

Vasopressin

Studies have shown some benefit with use of vasopressin in patients with refractory septic shock. However the VASST trial showed no difference in 28-day mortality when compared to noradrenaline. The role of vasopressin in patients with septic shock therefore remains unclear.

Other essential components of treatment

Like other conditions treated on the ICU, attention to detail has as much influence on outcome as the drugs that are investigated in major trials. Deep vein thrombosis prophylaxis, nutrition, and stress ulcer prophylaxis are vital in reducing morbidity and mortality in sepsis.

A note on lactate in sepsis

Hyperlactataemia remains an excellent indicator of poor prognosis in septic shock and is not only due to hypoperfusion. Accelerated aerobic glycolysis due to catecholamine release and the inflammatory process results in the increased production of pyruvate which exceeds the oxidative capacity of the mitochondria resulting in production of lactate.

The presence of a high lactate in a resuscitated septic patient should not be taken as proof of oxygen debt. But other causes should be considered including diminished hepatic clearance, increased production by the lung in ALI, and the use of lactate buffered solutions in RRT.

Hyperlactataemia is the commonest cause for metabolic disturbances and acidosis in a septic patient, but other causes include hepatic and renal dysfunction, bicarbonate losses from the intestine, iatrogenic hyperchloraemia, and drug toxicity. Therefore given the varied causes of a base deficit, it is not recommended as an end-point during resuscitation.

Further reading

Abraham E & Singer M (2007). Mechanisms of sepsis-induced organ dysfunction. *Crit Care Med*, 35:2408–16.

Bone RC, Balk RA, Cerra FB, *et al.* (1992). Definitions for sepsis and organ failure and guidelines for the use of innovative therapies in sepsis. The ACCP/SCCM Consensus Conference Committee. American College of Chest Physicians/Society of Critical Care Medicine. *Chest*, 101:1644–55.

Dellinger RP, Levy MM, Carlet JM, *et al.* (2008). Surviving Sepsis Campaign: international guidelines for the management of severe sepsis and septic shock 2008: *Crit Care Med*, 36:296–327.

Rivers E, Nguyen B, Havstad S, et al. (2001). Early goal-directed therapy in the treatment of severe sepsis and septic shock. *NEJM*, 345:1368–77.

20.4 Acute lung injury and acute respiratory distress syndrome

Definitions

Acute lung injury (ALI) and acute respiratory distress syndrome (ARDS) were formally defined in 1967 but had been described long before this, by names that referred to the injurious origin of the condition (e.g. shock lung). ALI and ARDS are characterized by acute onset (<7 days) of hypoxaemia in association with bilateral lung infiltrates on the CXR, but without left atrial hypertension (i.e. not due to hydrostatic/cardiogenic pulmonary oedema). There must also be an identifiable cause to the injury, which may be direct or indirect (Table 20.4). ARDS simply represents a more severe form of lung damage than ALI in terms of hypoxaemia (Box 20.2). It must be remembered, however, that ALI/ARDS is only a collective term for a highly heterogeneous group of critically ill patients rather than a distinct disease. The term ALI is often used to describe the entire spectrum of injury.

Table 20.4 Common direct and indirect causes of lung injury	
Direct	Indirect
Pneumonia	Sepsis
Gastric aspiration	Blood product transfusions
Near-drowning	Shock
Fat and amniotic-fluid embolism	Salicylate or narcotic overdose
Pulmonary contusion	Acute pancreatitis
Alveolar haemorrhage	Multiple trauma
Smoke and toxic gas inhalation	
Reperfusion (pleural effusion drainage, embolectomy)	

Box 20.2 ALI/ARDS definitions

- Acute onset (<7 days)
- Bilateral infiltrates on CXR
- Absence of LV dysfunction (PAOP <18mmHg)
- Oxygen gradient:
  - PaO_2/FiO_2 <40kPa for ALI
  - PaO_2/FiO_2 <26.7kPa for ARDS.

Incidence and outcome

The reported frequency of ALI depends upon definition and varies widely throughout the world, being higher in developed countries (1.5–75 cases per 100 000 population). Outcome following ALI is influenced by factors such as age, comorbidities, concomitant organ failure, and shock. Paradoxically, for a disease defined by hypoxaemia, the initial degree of gas-exchange impairment is a relatively poor predictor of outcome. The mortality for ALI has declined with time and now lies between 25% and 30% in most published trials. Lung function tends to return to normal 6–12 months after the acute illness in survivors.

In non-survivors the commonest causes of death are multiple organ failure, sepsis, and the underlying triggers for ALI rather than hypoxaemia per se.

Pathophysiology

Early in the course of the injury (the exudative phase) there is a diffuse neutrophilic alveolar infiltrate along with an accumulation of protein-rich pulmonary oedema and blood in the alveoli. An inflammatory response ensues and surfactant production is prevented. Damage occurs to the respiratory membrane and elastase release injures the lung parenchyma. There is also a shift towards a prothrombotic state, leading to the formation of microthrombi in the alveolar circulation. A fibro-proliferative phase follows the exudative phase in some patients, consisting of chronic inflammation, fibrosis, and neovascularization.

There is widespread V/Q mismatch due to pulmonary oedema, inflammation, haemorrhage, and atelectasis. The resulting hypoxaemia can induce hypoxic pulmonary vasoconstriction and raised pulmonary artery pressure. Thoracic compliance becomes reduced due to the presence of pulmonary oedema in collapsed alveoli.

Diagnosis

Patients invariably present with dyspnoea and will be hypoxaemic. CXR will assist with radiological diagnosis although determination of diagnostic signs can be subjective. A trigger cause must be sought and differential diagnoses, such as cardiogenic pulmonary oedema, acute interstitial pneumonia and lymphangitis carcinomatosis, must be excluded. A CT scan usually demonstrates heterogeneous parenchymal involvement and dense opacification of dependent areas.

Treatment

Like many situations in critical care medicine, the mainstay of treatment for ALI is supportive, whilst ensuring no additional damage is caused to the lungs and other organs. Volutrauma and cyclical opening–closing of damaged lung units (atelectatrauma) can exacerbate the inflammatory damage of ALI whilst barotrauma (excessive pressure) risks physical damage to the airways including pneumothorax. High concentrations of oxygen are also highly toxic to lung tissue through the release of intracellular reactive oxygen species. Treatment of the underlying cause of ALI is imperative; although once the lung injury is initiated it may persist long after the original trigger has abated.

Respiratory

The provision of supplemental oxygen to restore normoxaemia is common, although lower levels of arterial oxygenation that may be tolerated to avoid the detrimental consequences of aggressive ventilatory strategies. Hypoxaemia in ALI rarely responds to supplemental oxygen alone and other measures are usually required to support ventilation. Some patients may tolerate non-invasive ventilation (via a tight-fitting mask); however, the majority eventually require intubation and mechanical ventilation.

Ventilator settings

No one mode or pattern of ventilation appears beneficial over another. It is common practice to use pressure (rather than volume) generated inspiration and a tidal volume of 5–7mL/kg ideal body weight, to reduce volutrauma. PEEP is usually applied, using increasing levels as hypoxaemia worsens (commonly 5–15cmH$_2$O. A pressure–volume curve can be used to identify the optimum PEEP required, by identifying the lower inflection point of the curve. The purpose of PEEP is to prevent collapse of alveoli during expiration, thus maintaining a better gas exchange area and reducing atelectatrauma. Maintaining an inspiratory plateau pressure of <30cmH$_2$O will help to reduce barotrauma. The inspiratory:expiratory ratio can also be adjusted to increase the length of inspiration in cases of refractory hypoxaemia. Such a ventilation strategy may result in raised PaCO$_2$, but this has not been shown to lead to any untoward outcomes so is tolerated as long as pH remains above 7.2 (permissive hypercapnia). Neuromuscular blocking agents have been shown to improve outcome if used early in ARDS despite their possible association with critical illness polyneuropathy and myopathy.

Alternative respiratory approaches

Recruitment manoeuvres and nursing patients in a prone position have been advocated to improve gas exchange but their overall effectiveness is debatable. Likewise, some centres titrate nitric oxide into the inspired limb of the ventilator circuit; whilst this improves oxygenation, no clear mortality benefit exists. High-frequency oscillatory ventilation and extracorporeal membrane oxygenation (ECMO) have gained recent favour, particularly during the influenza H1N1 pandemics. Whilst there have been some encouraging results, large-scale multicentre trials are awaited to fully evaluate these treatments.

Steroids

Early use of high-dose systemic glucocorticoids does not appear to modify the outcome of ALI although their administration later in the course of the illness may be of benefit (although conflicting evidence exists).

Fluid management

Damaged lungs tend to accumulate water more readily than in health. Whilst adequate intravascular volume is necessary to prevent organ hypoperfusion, excessive administration of IV fluids may be harmful. A more conservative approach in patients with ALI is advised.

ICU 'housekeeping'

Other general good practice measures all contribute to better outcomes

- Nursing in the 30° head-up position
- Appropriate nutrition (preferably enteral)
- Deep vein thrombosis prophylaxis
- Oral hygiene
- Sterile insertion technique for indwelling catheters
- Goal-directed sedation
- Careful blood glucose control.

Further reading

Bernard GR, Artigas A, Brigham KL, et al. (1994). The American European consensus conference on ARDS: definitions mechanisms, relevant outcomes and clinical trial coordination. *Am J Respir Crit Care Med*, 149:818–24.

Wheeler AP & Bernard GR (2007). Acute lung injury and the acute respiratory distress syndrome: a clinical review. *Lancet*, 369:1553–64.

20.5 Management of sedation in critical care

Sedative and analgesic drugs are used widely in intensive care to enable patient comfort, alleviate anxiety, facilitate nursing care, and enhance tolerance of supportive procedures, e.g. mechanical ventilation, suctioning, and mobilization. Communication should be retained with the patient if possible. The critical care environment itself can be frightening and is a potent source of patient stress. Stress can be physical or psychological and factors involved include pain, discomfort, inability to communicate, anxiety, disturbed sleep/wake cycles, depression, and an increased basal metabolic rate.

A range of drugs is utilized incorporating analgesics, anxiolytics, anaesthetics, antipsychotics, and amnesics. Multiple agents in varying combinations may be required and the appropriate depth of sedation varies during the course of any patient's illness from admission to recovery. Patients whose only problem is weaning via a tracheostomy can usually be managed with either intermittent oral sedation or no sedation at all. Providing appropriate sedation has assumed greater visibility and importance in the management of critically ill patients (see Box 20.3).

The recommended method to initiate sedation is to administer a loading dose, which is titrated to effect, and then to start an infusion. Increases in infusion rate should follow the same principle, i.e. a bolus, titrated to effect should be administered and the infusion rate increased by a small amount.

With modern ventilators, synchronization problems are relatively uncommon. Paralysis is occasionally needed, however, particularly in those with severe gas exchange problems because it is impossible to stop inter-breathing with sedatives alone without exposing the patient to serious overdosage. During these situations neuromuscular blockade should be monitored with a nerve stimulator. Patients must not be paralysed and awake.

Analgesia

All patients must be comfortable and pain free. Analgesia is thus the primary aim and opiates such as fentanyl are still first line in this approach. High doses of opioids can be sedating in their own right and the philosophy behind their use should be 'comfort without coma'. Some patients can be managed with intermittent analgesia alone. The theoretical advantage of a solely analgesia-based sedation scheme is to have more patients awake and cooperative with neurological assessment and rehabilitation therapy. Early rehabilitation after admission is an independent primary goal and is linked with improved outcomes including survival. Patients who retain some factual memory for ITU will experience a reduced incidence of post-traumatic stress disorder after discharge—being more awake should enhance factual memories. Such approaches contrast with historical regimens where the majority of practitioners preferred patients to be sedated deeply and unaware of their surroundings. Excess sedation is in most cases unacceptable.

Ideally an objective evaluation of pain should be undertaken in patient context. This is difficult as most critical care patients are unable to self-report. Physiological variables such as heart rate, blood pressure, respiratory rate, and pupil size in response to painful stimuli are non-specific within intensive care and may be affected by medication. A behavioural pain scale based on facial expression, upper limb posture, and compliance with ventilation has been demonstrated as able to differentiate between nociceptive and non-nociceptive procedures in contrast to a standard sedation scale.

Assessment of sedation

It is mandatory to accurately and continuously assess patients' sedation needs by utilizing a sedation scale to ensure optimal benefit of the drugs used. An example is the Richmond Agitation–Sedation Scale (RASS), which has been validated for its ability to detect changes in sedation status against constructs of level of consciousness and delirium. It is a 10-point scale that can be rated briefly using three defined steps and has discrete criteria for levels of sedation and agitation (Box 20.4). A unique feature is that it uses the duration of eye contact following verbal stimulation as the principal means of titrating sedation. The majority of ventilated patients require light to moderate sedation and RASS offers multiple levels (0 to −3) within this range. RASS embraces the principles of an ideal sedation scoring system in that it is accurate, reproducible, minimally invasive, relevant to the individual, and not time consuming to perform. By targeting a RASS score in patient context, individualized goal-directed sedation therapy is possible.

Box 20.3 Consequences of poor sedation

Under-sedation
- Agitation
- Hyperventilation
- Pain
- Hypertension
- Catheter displacement
- Tachycardia

Over-sedation
- More ventilator days and longer overall ITU stay
- More frequent periods of hypotension ± bradycardia
- Greater immobility (predisposing to DVT and critical illness polyneuropathy)
- Higher incidence of paralytic ileus and nosocomial infection
- More drug side-effects (including problems of withdrawal and tolerance)
- Increased costs and poor use of resources

Box 20.4 Procedure for RASS assessment

Step 1: observe the patient:
- Alert/restless/agitated (score 0 to +4).

Step 2: if not alert, address by name and ask to open eyes and look at speaker:
- Patient wakes with sustained eye-opening and eye contact (score −1).
- Patient wakes with eye opening and eye contact but not sustained (score −2).
- Patient makes any movement in response to voice but not eye contact (score −3).

Step 3: if no response to verbal stimulation, physically stimulate patient by shaking shoulder and/or rubbing sternum:
- Patient makes any movement (score −4).
- Patient makes no movement (score −5).

Interest in more objective tools of assessment when deep sedation and paralysis are required has focused on the EEG and Bispectral Index (BIS).

Sedation holidays

This concept involves stopping the sedative infusions on a daily basis and allowing the patient to wake. The infusions should be restarted at a reduced level once the patient is deemed uncomfortable or agitated. This strategy has been shown in some studies to decrease the duration of mechanical ventilation and length of stay on the ICU with no increase in adverse events. Daily interruption of sedation (DIS) may not be effective in all patient populations however, for example, those with a history of alcohol and drug abuse prior to admission to intensive care. Such initiatives are an attempt to counter the problems of continuous infusion of sedatives resulting in drug accumulation delaying weaning.

Tolerance and withdrawal

Tolerance exists when decreased pharmacological effects are seen with repeated administration of a drug. Dependence is an obsessive craving for a drug after taking it repeatedly and can be classified as either physical or psychological. In physical dependence distinct symptoms manifest after the drug is stopped, termed a withdrawal syndrome. Tolerance, physical dependence, and withdrawal are all biological phenomena that are readily apparent in the context of administration of sedative infusions in ITU. Various classes of drugs are associated with specific withdrawal symptoms and these can be severe, for example, rebound insomnia, depression, acute anxiety state, frank psychosis, and even haemodynamic instability. Managed and systematic withdrawal of sedatives within ITU may take weeks and must be complemented by careful and regular monitoring of abstinence symptoms and emergence phenomena.

Delirium

This is defined as a disturbance of consciousness associated with new-onset changes in cognition. It has a fluctuating course and is characterized by inattention and disorganized thinking. It is common in intensive care patients and often goes unrecognized. Delirium is important in that it is an independent predictor of mortality, ITU length of stay, and cognitive impairment at hospital discharge. Benzodiazepines are particularly implicated, providing another reason to limiting their use where possible. Delirium screening should take place and a valid and reliable tool, CAM-ICU (Confusion Assessment Method for the Intensive Care Unit), has been developed which all members of the multidisciplinary team can use.

Delirium can be either agitated in nature, or of the hypoactive variety (the latter often misdiagnosed as depression). Once identified, it should be treated and a variety of agents have been used in such cases including haloperidol, olanzapine, and quetiapine. When haloperidol (usually first line) is prescribed, the QT interval should be monitored regularly and if prolonged should prompt cessation of the drug as torsade de pointes may be induced.

Non-drug measures

These include provision of quality care and compassion for all patients (see Box 20.5).

> **Box 20.5 Non-drug approaches to improve well-being**
>
> - Ensure that thirst is alleviated.
> - Provide greater access to friends and relatives.
> - Provide aids to communication.
> - Aim to preserve the normal sleep–wake cycle:
>   - A clock should be visible if patient is awake.
>   - Manipulation of lighting.
>   - Clustering of activities/routine interventions to allow adequate rest periods.
> - Complementary therapies, e.g. massage.
> - Limit the use of physical restraints wherever possible.
> - Early tracheostomy formation: allows liberation from sedation and increases patient autonomy.

Sedative drugs

The ideal sedative drug (see Box 20.6) does not exist.

> **Box 20.6 Properties of the ideal sedative drug**
>
> - Cheap.
> - Stable in solution.
> - Short acting and non-cumulative.
> - Fast offset time—independent of renal or hepatic metabolism.
> - No active metabolites.
> - No adverse physiological side effects (e.g. hypotension).
> - Simple to administer.
> - No interactions with other medication.

Examples of specific problems include the following:

- **Etomidate infusions** have been implicated in increased mortality, possibly through adrenal suppression and an increased propensity to infection.
- **Propofol infusion syndrome (PRIS)** is a rare, but often lethal complication. See section 7.1.
- **Thiopentone infusions** are required occasionally for therapeutic coma in head injured patients or in those with refractory status epilepticus. This may cause hypokalaemia and when thiopentone is ceased abruptly, rebound hyperkalaemia may occur which can be fatal. The mechanism is unclear.
- **Morphine** metabolites include morphine-6-glucuronide. This is metabolically active, renally excreted, and considerably more potent than morphine itself. Morphine infusions should be avoided in patients with renal impairment and pronounced respiratory depression has been reported in such patients.

Pharmacokinetic changes in critical illness should influence sedative choice and dosage, for example, altered drug clearance, reduced serum proteins affecting drug binding and varying volumes of drug distribution.

The future

α-2 agonists such as clonidine and the more selective dex-medetomidine are being used increasingly for sedation in ITU, particularly when conventional sedatives are being withdrawn. Sedation is combined with arousability and the incidence of delirium is reduced. They are not suitable, however, in situations of cardiovascular instability and bradycardia.

Remifentanil has also shown initial promise, sometimes as sole agent.

Further reading

Fraser GL & Riker RR (2007). Comfort without coma: Changing sedation practices. *Crit Care Med*, 35:635–7.Intensive Care Society 2007. *Sedation guidelines.* <http://www.ics.ac.uk/>

Medical ethics may be defined as a system of moral principles that applies values and judgement to the practice of medicine. Nowhere more than in the critical care setting do clinicians apply ethical principles to everyday decision-making.

Guiding principles of medical ethics

The 'Four Principles'
One of the most widely used frameworks is that of Beauchamp and Childress. Their 'Four Principles' are general guides that allow room for judgement in specific cases:

Autonomy: respects the decision-making ability of patients, acknowledging the right of an individual to have control over his/her life. Patients should be enabled to make reasoned informed choices, and have the right to refuse or accept treatment. This principle can be difficult in the critical care setting as many patients lack the capacity to be involved in decision-making.

Beneficence: clinicians should act to serve the best interests of the patient; treatments should only be given if they are likely to benefit the patient. Often, it is not possible to foresee whether there will be a benefit from initiating treatment. Problems may arise in critical care when aggressive treatment is commenced but later deemed 'futile' and the question of withdrawal of treatment arises.

Non-maleficence: avoiding the causation of harm to the patient ('primum non nocere'). All treatments involve some harm, even if minimal or a by-product of eventual healing. Harm should not be disproportionate to benefits.

Justice: fair distribution of benefits, risks and costs—patients in similar positions should be treated in a similar manner; treatment should not be given if it deprives others of a greater benefit. This is an extremely difficult and uncertain area of medicine and the law.

The doctrine of double effect
This argues that a moral distinction exists between acting with the *intention* to bring about a patient's death, compared to performing an act intended to provide *benefit* (e.g. using opioids to provide relief from pain) but which has foreseeable adverse effects (e.g. respiratory depression and death).

The sanctity of life
Established principles, both ethical *and* legal, require that decisions concerning potentially life-prolonging treatment must start from a presumption in favour of prolonging life, and must not be motivated by a desire to bring about a patient's death. It is crucially important to engage the expertise of fellow clinicians when making decisions aimed at being in the patient's best interests. A responsible body of clinicians will need to concur that continuation of therapy is futile, irresponsible or unnecessarily burdensome.

Acts and omissions
The 'acts and omissions' distinction argues that there is a difference between actively ending someone's life as opposed to refraining from an action that may preserve life. A moral difference is proposed, for example, between administering a lethal dose of morphine and signing a 'do not resuscitate' order.

UK law has sought to clarify the situation, but in many religions, withdrawal of treatment is seen as a positive act to bring about death, which would be unlawful. Such issues commonly arise in ITU, when decisions are taken to extubate a patient or withdraw haemofiltration.

Whilst religious law is not recognized in UK courts, it must arguably be considered as part of an attempt to explore the patient's wishes and beliefs under the Mental Capacity Act. The danger for clinicians is that negotiations with relatives and friends may unintentionally lead to discrimination—for example, the family which quietly accepts a decision to withdraw treatment versus the family which objects: leading to another 48h of active treatment before attempting the discussion again. These scenarios contradict the principles of beneficence and justice.

The legal position

Despite the frequent moral dilemmas encountered in the critical care setting, the following principles are set down in *law*:

1. An act by which the doctor's primary intention is to bring about a patient's death would be unlawful.
2. Life-prolonging treatment can be lawfully withheld or withdrawn from a patient who lacks capacity, when starting or continuing treatment is not in the patient's best interests
3. There is no obligation to give treatment that is futile or burdensome
4. When the court is asked to reach a view about withholding or withdrawing treatment, it will have regard to whether what is proposed is in accordance with a responsible body of medical opinion. The court will, however, determine for itself whether treatment or non-treatment is in the patient's best interests.

The Mental Capacity Act (MCA)
The Mental Capacity Act (England and Wales, 2005) provides a statutory framework for people who lack the capacity to make decisions for themselves, or who have capacity but wish to make provisions for a time when they may lack capacity in the future.

It incorporates five key statutory principles that *must* be considered when working with or providing care or treatment for those who lack capacity:

1. A person must be assumed to have capacity unless it is established that they lack capacity.
2. A person is not to be treated as unable to make a decision unless all practicable steps to help him do so have been taken without success.
3. A person is not to be treated as unable to make a decision merely because he makes an unwise decision.
4. An act done, or decision made, under the Act for or on behalf of a patient who lacks capacity must be done, or made, in his or her best interests.
5. Before the act is done, or the decision made, regard must be had as to whether the purpose for which it is needed can be effectively achieved in a way that is less restrictive of the person's rights and freedom of action.

In respect of an incapacitated patient, most day-to-day decisions are taken by the clinical team in his or her best interests. Inserting arterial or central lines, performing CT/MRI scans, and administering medications are but a few. Difficulties arise when 'serious' treatment decisions need to be taken, such as performing major surgery or withdrawing treatment.

In cases of an immediately life-threatening emergency, clinicians may proceed to treat patients under the common law doctrine of necessity or under Section 5 of the MCA.

Where time permits, however, the Act requires the decision-maker to consult other people close to the person. These may include carers, close relatives and friends. Has the patient signed a Living Will or Advance Directive? If so, this is binding. The views of those close to the person are important factors to be taken into consideration and clinicians should explore the past wishes, beliefs, views and values of the incapacitated person. Where there is no one to consult, an Independent Mental Capacity Advocate (IMCA) must be instructed.

Ultimate legal responsibility for making a best interest decision for a patient who lacks capacity lies with the individual who carries out the intervention. Where there a dispute between the decision maker and the next friend or relative, legal advice should be sought and the matter may need to go before the Court of Protection for a ruling.

Perhaps the most challenging scenario in the critical care setting is where the patient has fluctuating capacity. It may be that the patient can consent to a tracheostomy being suctioned but perhaps would not be able to understand and weigh up the risks versus benefits of surgery or chemotherapy. The clinical team may consider using professionals with specialist skills in verbal and non-verbal communication, and also perhaps adjusting sedative medication to assist the patient to arrive at a decision.

It is important to thoroughly document the capacity assessment, discussions with friends or relatives, risks versus benefits assessment, and the best interests decision in the patient's notes. A Consent Form IV must be completed prior to invasive procedures or treatment and theatre.

General Medical Council guidance

The General Medical Council (GMC) has produced detailed guidance that should be adhered to by all clinicians:

Doctors have an ethical and legal duty to take all *reasonable* steps to prolong life. Where escalation is deemed futile, patients approaching the end of their life must receive the same quality of care as all other patients. End-of-life decision-making is the most ethically demanding area of medical practice and often subject to legal challenge.

A practical framework for end-of-life decisions

The guidance is clearly set out. The following practicalities may be useful:

- Make an overall assessment of the patient's condition. It is *essential* to consult peers when taking the decision to withhold or withdraw treatment.

- Document all conversations *and* ensure that peers document their views.

- Establish capacity (as set out earlier).

- Where the patient has capacity, take time to discuss the decision with them, ask for their views, what support can be offered and ensure there is time for the patient to absorb the information and ask questions.

- Where the patient lacks capacity, the next friend or relative must be consulted or an IMCA instructed.

- Where there is a dispute, legal advice should be sought. It may be appropriate to approach the Court of Protection but this must always be a last resort. Consider an external opinion or mediation in the first instance.

Careful and detailed documentation is *essential*, and makes any future challenges easier to respond to.

Consent

Case law surrounding consent is voluminous, but the fundamental principles are thus:

1. If a patient asks for treatment that a clinician has not offered, and the clinician concludes that treatment to be inappropriate, the clinician is not obliged to provide it, but should offer to arrange for a second opinion.

2. An adult patient who has capacity may decide to refuse treatment, even if refusal may result in harm or death.

3. If an adult patient has lost capacity, a refusal of treatment made when he or she had capacity (e.g. a Living Will or

Advance Directive) must be respected, provided it is clearly applicable to the present circumstance and there is no reason to suspect the patient has changed his or her mind.

4. In the case of a child, if clinicians and the child's family are in fundamental disagreement over treatment, then the views of the Court should be sought.

In conclusion

The requirement to weigh up apparently contradictory ethical principles amidst a complex legal framework is an exceptionally challenging aspect of critical care medicine, and assisting patients and their loved ones requires skill, patience, and experience. Effective communication is essential, together with a readiness to ask for help. The decision-making process should be clearly documented, and second opinions sought if needed. See Box 20.7 for a case study.

Box 20.7 Case study

Patient A, a 47-year-old male, presented via A&E with an acute subdural haematoma following a high-speed motor vehicle accident. Despite an emergency craniotomy, his ICP and inotrope requirements continue to rise. The neurosurgical team advise that they cannot offer any further intervention, supporting the view that further treatment is futile.

The police advise you that they can't trace any relatives. Can you proceed to withdraw treatment?

No. When a patient lacks capacity, and there is no next friend or relative to consult, yet serious treatment decisions must be made, an IMCA must be instructed. You can, however, complete a DNAR order, and there is no obligation to resuscitate the patient whilst awaiting the IMCA review.

Whilst you are documenting your decision, the police present to the unit with A's wife and two teenage children. A's wife is adamant that A would not want to 'give up', and she refuses to allow you to withdraw treatment. What do you do?

If after careful and sensitive discussion A's wife does not accept your decision nor your senior colleague's input, then an independent second opinion should be offered and documented. If she is not in agreement, you must offer her an opportunity to seek independent legal advice. If she does not engage in the opportunity to challenge your decision then you can proceed in the patient's best interests.

Whilst you are discussing the decision with your colleague, A's solicitor faxes an Advance Directive signed by A 6 months ago. In it he states that he does not wish to be kept alive if he has limited brain function or his condition is burdensome. The Trust's solicitor confirms it is valid and applicable. A's wife still refuses to accept your decision to withdraw treatment. Can you proceed to withdraw treatment?

Yes. Under the MCA, a valid Living Will or Advance Directive is legally binding.

Further reading

General Medical Council (2010). *Treatment and care towards the end of life: good practice in decision making.* http://www.gmc-uk.org/End_of_life.pdf_32486688.pdf.

General Medical Council (2008). *Consent: patients and doctors making decisions together.* <http://www.gmc-uk.org/guidance/ethical_guidance/consent_guidance_index.asp>.

http://www.ics.ac.uk/intensive_care_professional/standards_and_guidelines/mental_capacity_act>.

Kinsella J & Booth MG (2007). Ethical framework for end of life decisions in intensive care in the UK. *J Natl Inst Public Health*, 56:387–92.

Chapter 21

Trauma and stabilization

383

21.1 Pathophysiological changes in trauma

The pathophysiology of trauma, and particularly polytrauma, is a complex phenomenon that may disturb organ homeostasis and threaten life in a variety of ways (Fig. 21.1). There is currently no internationally accepted definition of the term polytrauma, although it may be thought of as severe injury in at least two body regions associated with the development of a systemic inflammatory response syndrome (SIRS). The degree of organ dysfunction is largely determined by the injury load. The most reliable indicator of this remains the injury severity score (ISS), with an ISS of 15 or greater indicating major or severe traumatic injury.

There is a clear biphasic pattern of death following major trauma: early deaths tend to occur within the first 24h following the primary injury. This is usually due to severe primary traumatic brain injury, or less commonly due to uncontrolled blood loss following either blunt or penetrating injury. There has been a reduction in death due to haemorrhage in the last decade. Late mortality is due to secondary brain injury and host defence disorder and failure, evidenced by a SIRS response, sepsis, and multiple organ failure (MOF), and usually occurs after 3–7 days.

Traumatic injury should therefore be viewed as an initial primary injury, which triggers the release of inflammatory mediators and effector cells resulting in a subsequent secondary injury. The SIRS response, along with tissue and endothelial damage, as well as microcirculatory dysfunction and coagulopathy perpetuate a hyper-immune response. Treatment (e.g. surgery) and complications of treatment may contribute to this second 'hit'. This may in turn be followed by a hypo-immune phase, the compensatory anti-inflammatory response syndrome (CARS). Imbalance between pro- and anti-inflammatory factors may result in apoptosis, organ dysfunction, MOF, or death.

Primary injury (first hit)

The degree of primary injury is related to the mechanical or thermal force applied to the body, the amount of organ, tissue, and bony disruption caused, as well as the distribution of the injuries. The higher the injury load, the greater the likelihood of early death or subsequent organ dysfunction.

Brain injury
Brain injury is present in 60% of cases of multiple injury with an ISS >15, and is a major contributor to mortality and morbidity. Significant primary brain injury may result in acute bleeding, either extradural, subdural, subarachnoid, or intraparenchymal, as well as acute cerebral oedema. Rising intracranial pressure causes a reduction in cerebral perfusion pressure (CPP). The Munro–Kelly hypothesis means that this can rapidly result in a lethal compartment syndrome. The rapid rise in intracranial pressure may also result in brain herniation and early death. Airway compromise following brain injury, if not adequately managed, can cause death or exacerbate secondary brain injury.

Haemorrhage
Haemorrhage accounts for a high percentage of deaths in the first 24h of trauma care. This is due to large vessel disruption, either from penetrating or blunt injury. In the UK pelvic and visceral bleeding following blunt trauma is the most common site of haemorrhage. Haemorrhagic shock also has a significant contribution on brain injury mortality, as an untreated fall in mean arterial pressure reduces CPP.

Shock is defined as a state of end-organ or tissue hypoperfusion, with an imbalance between oxygen supply and demand. Shock may be covert and compensated following blood loss of up to 15%, with activation of the sympathetic nervous system defending against the fall in intravascular volume, and causing only a slight tachycardia (see section 1.14). As the percentage of intravascular depletion increases to 30%, clinical features of shock become overt, with tachycardia and pallor. It is only with ongoing losses >30–40% that overt, decompensated shock occurs, as evidenced by a reduction in pulse volume, tachycardia, a fall in mean arterial pressure, and signs and symptoms of tissue and organ hypoperfusion (Table 21.1).

Table 21.1 Categorization of shock			
	Covert compensated hypovolaemia: 0–20% blood loss	Overt compensated: 20-30% blood loss	Decompensated (shock): >30% blood loss
Pulse	Slight tachycardia	Tachycardia	Tachycardia, eventual terminal bradycardia
BP	Normal	Normal	Low
End-organ perfusion	Normal	Reduced	Critically reduced

The imbalance between oxygen delivery and oxygen consumption that occurs during shock results in anaerobic tissue metabolism, and the subsequent development of acidaemia associated with hyperlactataemia. A lactate level of >2.5mmol/L is suggestive of hypoperfusion, though caution should be exercised in interpretation, as intoxication or fitting can also cause an elevated lactate. Of greater importance is the rate of lactate clearance, which is predictive of outcome, with persistent elevation associated with increased mortality. It is less clear whether this can be used to guide therapy. Tissue perfusion is further compromised by microvascular flow abnormalities that occur early following severe trauma.

Severe injury also results in the development of a primary coagulopathy, the acute coagulopathy of trauma shock (ACoTS). It used to be believed that the coagulopathy seen after major trauma was dilutional, but evidence suggests that initial coagulopathy is related to the traumatic insult, and patients present to hospital with abnormal coagulation parameters. Prolongation of the prothrombin time (PT) is most commonly seen, and these patients are more likely to require massive transfusion and to die.

Secondary injury (second hit)

Following injury or trauma the biological response is that of a host-immune response. It is now possible to characterize this response, and to quantify both the molecular mediators and effectors involved in this dynamic process. These inflammatory mediators are initially released locally at the site of the primary injury. Their subsequent systemic amplification, and the balance between pro- and anti-inflammatory mediators results in the development of the SIRS response.

Mediators
Cytokines are pleiotropic molecules that can act in an autocrine or paracrine fashion. There are hyperacute inflammatory cytokines such as tumour necrosis factor alpha (TNF-α) and interleukin 1β (IL-1β) that act immediately following injury, and subacute cytokines, the most important of which is interleukin

6 (IL-6). IL-6 levels have been shown to correlate with the ISS, as well as the degree of organ failure, ARDS, and death. Interleukin 8 (IL-8), a chemokine, has also been shown to be elevated in trauma, and to relate to outcome. Following injury, anti-inflammatory cytokines such as interleukin 10 (IL-10) are synthesized by lymphocytes and monocytes, and acts to modulate the production of TNF-α, IL-6, and IL-8.

The complement system is also activated following trauma, resulting in the release of biologically active peptides. It can be activated via either the classical, alternative, or lectin pathway, and the active peptides alter levels of pro-inflammatory peptides such as C3a, C3b, C4b, and C5b-9 according to the severity of the insult. C3a, C4a, and C5a are anaphylotoxins, and help to promote a pro-inflammatory microenvironment through causing chemotaxis of leukocytes and degranulation of phagocytic cells. They also cause increased vascular permeability and smooth muscle contraction, contributing to reductions in microvascular perfusion. C5b-9 (the membrane attack complex) causes disruption of cellular membranes and lysis of target cells. Complement activation also results in the production of oxygen free radicals.

Damage-associated molecular patterns (DAMPs) are a general term used to describe the interaction of endogenous danger signals on antigen-presenting cells such as T cells, including CD4+ and CD8+ cells, neutrophils, monocytes and macrophages, natural killer cells, and dendritic cells. These represent the effector limb of the inflammatory process. DAMPs include high mobility box group 1 (HMBG-1) proteins released from necrotic cells and activated effector cells, which causes epithelial and gut dysfunction, and has been implicated as a key mediator in haemorrhagic shock and ischaemia-reperfusion. The inflammatory action of HMBG-1 occurs through the interaction with Toll-like receptors (TLR), particularly TLR-4.

Effectors

Polymorphonuclear neutrophils (PMNs) are important effectors following trauma. They are primed by the pro-inflammatory mediators and attracted to the site of injury by chemokines such as IL-8. The PMNs adhere to damaged endothelium via adhesion molecules like L-selectin, and then transmigrate into tissue, where they degranulate, releasing toxic enzymes. These proteases and reactive oxygen species (ROS) produced during the respiratory burst including myeloperoxidase and nitric oxide (NO) result in remote tissue injury. Second hit priming of leukocytes results in increased and persisting levels of IL-6, with associated MODS.

Ischaemia/reperfusion can cause damage on both a systemic and local tissue level, depending on the extent of injury. Ischaemia results in an influx of sodium into cells depleted of ATP, causing cellular swelling and damage. Following reperfusion, the reaction of oxygen with hypoxanthine results in the production of ROS and NO, causing cellular apoptosis and tissue necrosis.

Depending on the severity of injury and subsequent interventions, a state of relative immune suppression can supervene, CARS. IL-10 is involved in suppressing the action of transcription factors such as NFκB (nuclear factor kappa-light-chain-enhancer of activated B cells), which is essential for the production of inflammatory cytokines. It may represent a homeostatic mechanism to reduce organ damage, while still enabling repair and prevention of the action of micro-organisms. The balance between pro- and anti-inflammatory reactions is influenced by interventions including either definitive or damage control surgery, blood transfusion, and the potential for infection of intravascular catheters. The incidence of post-traumatic hyperinflammation appears to be falling, which may reflect improvements in trauma care.

The complex interactions of the multiple pathophysiological processes at work following major injury, and the potential for secondary injury and death, are influenced by our decisions during anaesthesia and intensive care, and an understanding of these processes may help to improve outcome.

Further reading

Dewar D, Moore FA, Moore E, *et al* (2009). Postinjury multiple organ failure. *Injury*, 40:912–18.

Keel M & Trenz O (2005). Pathophysiology of polytrauma. *Injury*, 36:691–709.

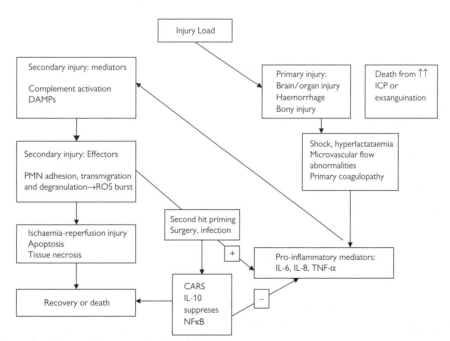

Fig. 21.1 Pathophysiology of trauma.

Triage is a concept that involves the prompt assessment of a patient's clinical condition in order to prioritize treatment requirements.

Single patient triage

When only one patient is involved, the purpose of triage is to ensure that life-saving treatments are initiated immediately and that the patient is taken to the most appropriate hospital, with activation of a trauma team (Fig. 21.2).

The advanced Adult Trauma Life Support (ATLS) system is commonly used around the world to harmonize a team approach to rapidly and effectively assessing and simultaneously treating trauma patients. This is often initiated at the scene of the trauma and the process repeated, or continued, on arrival to hospital; conducted by a dedicated team of specialists.

ATLS follows a pattern of primary, then secondary surveys which are repeated if the patient deteriorates or fails to respond to treatment.

Primary survey

Aims to identify and immediately treat life-threatening injuries according to the 'ABCDE' approach to resuscitation:

- Airway (with cervical spine stabilization)
- Breathing
- Circulation (including the control of haemorrhage)
- Disability or neurological status
- Exposure or undressing of the patient while also protecting the patient from hypothermia.

Secondary survey

If stabilization of the patient has been successful, a thorough medical history is obtained from the patient or witnesses and a 'head to toe' examination performed to document all associated injuries.

Multiple patient triage

Triage may also be used in the context of a major incident when multiple patients require rapid assessment to focus resources on those in whom intervention is most likely to result in a favourable outcome. A number of formalized systems are in existence for the triage of mass casualties and most have their origins from a military setting. In this setting, patients are classified based upon the priority with which they require treatment:

- P1 = immediate
- P2 = delayed
- P3 = minor

Initial triage is performed using the 'triage sieve' (Fig. 21.3). Triage status must be reviewed at intervals (for example on arrival at hospital) and the 'triage sort' tool, which is a version of the Trauma Score (see 'Trauma scoring'), may be used to refine triage. Discussion of major incident management is outside the scope of this text.

One might reasonably ask why triage is necessary at a major incident. Clearly one objective is to ensure the right patient reaches the right care at the right time. However, simply taking all injured patients to a major trauma centre will result in significant numbers of patients arriving with only minor injuries; this is referred to as over triage and is not benign especially during major incidents.

Trauma scoring

It is important to have an understanding of trauma scoring systems as they underpin a number of key definitions in injury care and research. Scoring allows comparison of outcome between different institutions along with the appropriate allocation of resources. A number of scoring systems exist, each with inherent limitations.

Abbreviated injury scale (AIS)

The AIS grades injuries anatomically, according to a detailed schema, from 1–6 with 1 being minor, 5 being critical and 6 being unsurvivable; six body areas are scored.

Injury Severity Score (ISS)

The ISS is made up of the highest three body area AIS scores squared and thus ranges from 0–75. Major trauma is defined as an ISS >15. A worked example of AIS and ISS calculation is shown in Table 21.2.

Revised Trauma Score (RTS)

The RTS is a physiological score based on the GCS, systolic blood pressure, and respiratory rate and is commonly used in the pre-hospital setting.

In the UK, the Trauma Audit and Research Network (UK TARN) calculates probability of survival using ISS, RTS and age, weighted to improve accuracy.

Table 21.2 Example of ISS calculation			
Region	Injury description	AIS	Square top three
Head & neck	Cerebral contusion	3	9
Face	No injury	0	
Chest	Flail chest	4	16
Abdomen	Minor contusion liver.Complex laceration spleen	5	25
Extremity	Fractured femur	3	
External	No injury	0	
	Injury Severity Score		50

Initial perioperative management

The perioperative management of the major trauma patient requires a dynamic assessment of the injuries present and the proposed procedures as well as the patient's physiological status and response to resuscitation and surgery. Most patients will benefit from an approach that provides definitive management for all injuries at one sitting—early total care. A smaller group will require a 'damage control' approach as described next.

Preoperative

It is essential to fully understand the proposed surgical procedures and their sequence, as well as alternative options should the patient's condition change. A comprehensive pre-operative assessment is essential and, in addition to the standard anaesthetic assessment, should address the following trauma-specific issues:

Airway and cervical spine

- Has the cervical spine been cleared?
- Are there potential airway problems related to direct trauma, spinal injury, or immobilization?

London Major Trauma Decision Tool (children under 12)

Children's Vital Signs

Respiratory rate

Age	Breaths/min
<1 year	30–40
1–2 years	25–30
2–5 years	25–30
5–11 years	20–25

Pulse rate

Age	Beats/min
<1 year	110–160
1–2 years	100–150
2–5 years	95–140
5–11 years	80–120

Glasgow Coma Score

Eye opening	
Spontaneous	4
To speech	3
To pain	2
None	1

Verbal response	
Orientated	5
Confused	4
Inappropriate words	3
Incomprehensible sounds	2
No verbal response	1

Motor response	
Obeys commands	6
Localised pain	5
Withdraws pain	4
Abnormal flexion	3
Extensor response	2
No response	1

Modified verbal response >4 years old	
Appropriate words, social smiles, fixes and follows objects	5
Cries but is consolable	4
Persistent irritable	3
Restless, agitated	2
Silent	1

Step 1

Assess vital signs and level of consciousness

- **6A** Glasgow coma score less than 14
- **6B** Inappropriate behaviour post injury (too quiet or inconsolable)
- **6C** Abnormal vital signs not explained by other cause for example crying, pain responses

Yes to any one → Convey to nearest **Major** Trauma Centre. Ensure pre alert call is passed on PD09.

Step 2

Assess anatomy of injury

- **7A** Significant bruising to chest or abdomen
- **7B** Traumatic amputation/mangled extremity proximal to wrist/ankle
- **7C** Penetrating trauma below the head above the knees (not arms)
- **7D** Suspected open and/or depressed skull fracture
- **7E** Suspected pelvic fracture
- **7F** Significant degloving (soft tissue) injury
- **7G** Spinal trauma suggested by abnormal neurology
- **7H** Open long bone fracture (with significant soft tissue injury)
- **7I** Multiple fractures (long bone)
- **7J** Burns/scald greater than 20 percent
- **7K** Facial burns with complete skin loss to lower half of face
- **7L** Circumferential burns from a flame injury

Yes to any one → Convey to nearest **Major** Trauma Centre. Ensure pre alert call is passed on PD09.

Step 3

Assess mechanism of injury

- **8A** Traumatic death in same passenger compartment
- **8B** Uninterrupted fall over twice the patient's height (not bouncing down stairs)
- **8C** Person trapped under vehicle or large object (including 'one unders') crying, pain responses
- **8D** Bullseye to the windscreen and/or damage to the 'A' post of the vehicle by impact of individual outside of the vehicle
- **8E** Bicycle injury resulting in abdominal and / or groin pain (thrown from or impacted on handle bars)
- **8F** Ejection from inside car, van or lorry
- **8G** Fall from or trampled by large animal

Yes to any one → Convey to nearest **Major** Trauma Centre. Ensure pre alert call is passed on PD09.

Step 4

Assess special patient consideration. Patients who have sustained trauma but do not fit any of the above criteria but do not fit any of the above criteria but are:

- **9A** Known to have bleeding disorder or receiving current anticoagulation therapy e.g. warfarin or novel oral anticoagulant agent

Yes to any one → Patient **may** benefit from going to a **Major** Trauma Centre. Contact The Clinical Hub on PD09.

Step 5

Assess system consideration. Patients who have sustained trauma but do not fit any of the above criteria but there is:

- **0A** Significant crew concern only when discussed with a Trauma Paramedic within EOC

Yes to any one → Patient **may** benefit from going to a **Major** Trauma Centre. Contact The Clinical Hub on PD09.

CHAPTER 21 **Trauma and stabilization**

Fig. 21.2 LTO trauma tree. Reproduced with permission from: Faulkner M, Parr T, Moore F P et al. (2013) *London Major Trauma Triage Decision Tool* 2nd Ed. London Trauma Office and London Ambulance Service.

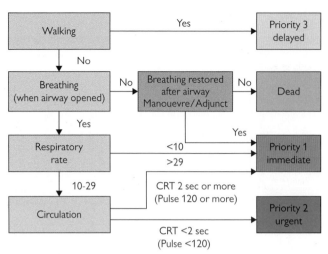

Fig. 21.3 Triage sieve. Reproduced from Advanced Life Support Group, *Major Incident Medical Management and Support: The Practical Approach*, BMJ Publishing Group, p. 121–122, copyright 2001, with permission from Wiley.

Breathing

- Has pneumothorax been excluded or drained? It is reasonable to consider not draining a small apical pneumothorax visible only on CT, especially if the patient was ventilated at the time of the CT.
- Is there evidence of pulmonary contusion or aspiration? Will postoperative ventilation be required?

Circulation

- Is the patient bleeding? At what phase of diagnosis and resuscitation is the patient?
- Is the patient euvolaemic? Is damage control resuscitation being employed? Should it be instigated or discontinued?
- Is there adequate IV access and availability of blood and blood products?

Disability

- Is there a head injury? Or has head injury been excluded by CT scanning?
- Has the thoraco-lumbar spine been cleared?
- What analgesia has the patient received so far and is it effective?

Exposure

Has normothermia been achieved?

Perioperative

Induction of anaesthesia

Due to aspiration risk, endotracheal intubation is required in all seriously injured patients and should usually be undertaken by either rapid sequence induction (RSI) or awake fibre optic approaches. RSI may require considerable modification in the trauma patient due to the competing problems of hypovolaemia and potentially raised ICP.

Maintenance of anaesthesia

A balanced anaesthetic technique should be used; no one technique has superiority over another. The principle objective during this phase is to continue resuscitation while deepening anaesthesia as tolerated. Early institution of cardiac output monitoring should be strongly considered especially in unstable/damage control patients or those with comorbidities.

Emergence from anaesthesia

A careful decision must be made regarding the appropriateness of extubation at the end of surgery, considering the patient's physiological state, intended analgesia, and the need for further imaging or intervention. Where extubation is deemed appropriate this should be with the patient fully awake.

The chronological age of a patient accounts for only a small increase in overall perioperative risk; therefore, in isolation age is a poor predictor of complications. However, increasing age is associated with accumulating comorbidities, each of which requires careful consideration preoperatively and may contribute to increased risk. The prevalence of cardiovascular disease increases with age along with a decline in respiratory and renal function.

Strategies to reduce secondary brain injury

Primary brain injury is common in trauma patients and discussed in detail in section 22.11. Prevention of secondary brain injury during the perioperative period is crucial. The clearest link between secondary brain injury and outcome exists for hypoxia and hypotension, with the latter being responsible for a 150% increase in mortality. The following are also at least *correlated* with worse neurological outcome or with neuronal damage or ischaemia in animal or radiological studies and should be avoided:

- Hypoglycaemia
- Hyperglycaemia
- Pyrexia
- Untreated seizures
- Raised ICP
- Hypocarbia.

Severe burns

Burns are a common form of trauma, with 0.5% of the population of the UK suffering from one each year (250 000 burns). Of these, 10% will require hospitalization, and of those hospitalized 10% will have severe, life-threatening burns. Burns may be classed as severe either if they involve a large surface area, or include airway burns or significant smoke inhalation. Most UK burns centres are currently not co-located with major trauma centres to which severely injured patients will be taken for initial treatment, so a thorough knowledge of burns management is essential even for those working outside burns centres.

Anaesthetists are intrinsically involved in the assessment and resuscitation of severely burned patients, as well as providing anaesthesia, sedation, analgesia, and critical care. They are also responsible for the transfer of severely burned patients to specialist centres for definitive care. It is important to be alert to the possibility of coexisting injuries, and to adopt a methodical approach to management. The principles of primary and secondary survey and simultaneous resuscitation should be followed. Burns centres commonly distribute pro-formas locally, which aid effective discussion, documentation, and initial management of patients.

Primary survey of the burns patient
This should consist of rapid identification and management of life-threatening conditions.

Airway maintenance with C-spine control
- It is important to be alert to the possibility that either thermal or chemical injury as a result of the burn can result in airway oedema. An altered voice, brassy cough, or stridor should prompt early consideration of intubation. If you think about it, do it!
- Be aware of possible C-spine injury following a fall to escape fires.

Breathing and ventilation
- Always give supplemental oxygen.
- Perform a blood gas and beware of carbon monoxide (CO) poisoning—HbCO >16% is enough to cause symptoms.
- Circumferential burns to the chest will require escharotomy to aid ventilation.
- Burned nostril hairs and soot in the hypopharynx should warn of the possibility of an inhalational injury. Mechanical ventilation may be necessary, and is likely to be complicated by reduced pulmonary compliance.

Circulation with haemorrhage control
- There is loss of fluid into both the burned and unburned areas, and inflammatory activation results in the development of capillary leak and interstitial oedema. Estimation of the area of burned skin helps to guide resuscitation strategy.
- Early shock is should be considered as due to a missed injury (e.g. pelvic) until proved otherwise.

Disability—neurological status
- Use the Awake Vocal Pain Unresponsive (AVPU) scale, or GCS to assess conscious level. Beware of hypoxaemia, CO poisoning, and cyanide poisoning causing confusion or decreased level of consciousness.

- Analgesia titrated to effect using incremental boluses of morphine or ketamine, but only *after* assessment of consciousness.

Exposure with environmental control
- Remove all clothing and jewellery, and wrap in clingfilm.
- Keep patient warm! Hypothermia is common in severe burns, and may exacerbate coagulopathy.
- Estimate burned area using rule of 9's (see Fig. 28.4 in Chapter 28). Differentiate between full-thickness and partial thickness burns, and take particular note of circumferential burns.
- Of note, a burn is a dynamic tissue process, and will continue evolving over the hours following the initial injury, commonly leading to under-estimation of the burn area.

Fluid resuscitation proportional to burn size
- Two large-bore venous cannulae, preferably through unburned skin.
- Take blood for FBC and clotting, U&E (including CK if electrical injury), amylase, and carboxyhaemoglobin.
- Fluid resuscitation using warmed fluids:
  - There is no evidence to support colloid use over balanced crystalloid use.
  - Parkland formula provides a useful *estimation* of the volume required—if in doubt, flow monitoring may be useful.
  - 3–4mL/kg/% burned, + maintenance for children. Half of the calculated fluid is given in the first 8h, and the rest over the following 16h.
  - The time of injury marks the start of fluid resuscitation.
- Insert a nasogastric tube, as gastroparesis is common following severe burns

Following initial resuscitation, a detailed secondary survey should be performed.

Definitive anaesthetic care
The issues involved in initial resuscitation also pertain to subsequent surgical procedures. It is essential to closely liaise with the surgeon to ascertain the extent of likely procedure, and the potential for blood loss and subsequent coagulopathy. Be aware of the possible need for repositioning the patient during surgery to access multiple surgical sites, and position and secure cannulae and monitoring equipment accordingly. The environmental temperature should be increased, to avoid hypothermia.

There is no induction agent of proven superiority for burns anaesthesia. Of importance is the avoidance of suxamethonium, as skeletal muscle depolarization can cause life-threatening hyperkalaemia. The increased number of acetylcholine receptors on skeletal muscle also results in resistance to the effects of non-depolarizing muscle relaxants.

Significant pain should always be anticipated, and pre-emptive, multimodal analgesia should be employed. Thought should be given prior to the use of NSAIDs, as though while very useful they have the potential to cause renal injury and gastric erosions. Also use NSAIDs with caution in elderly or hypovolaemic patients. Ketamine, often co-administered with benzodiazepines or opioids, is widely used in burns care.

Ongoing care on critical care and during transfer should conform to standards of practice, with particular attention to the increased risks of infection and hypothermia.

Electrical injuries

Electrical burns and injuries account for 3–4% of admissions to burns units, and occur most commonly in young males. These are typically occupation-related, though 20% occur in children, usually involving wall sockets or cable extensions. The mechanism of injury can be due to thermal burns, muscle contraction and subsequent trauma, and cardiac arrhythmia. The extent of the injury will depend on the current, the voltage (type and magnitude), the resistance to travel and the contact duration.

Low voltage (<1000 volts)

The typical domestic voltage used in the UK is 240 volts alternating current (AC) at 50 cycles per second (50Hz). This can result in tetanic contraction, making letting go of items difficult, and can cause small, deep entrance and exit wounds. The amount of current and the current path will determine the extent of the injury, potentially resulting in respiratory difficulties and cardiac dysrhythmias. Skin offers reasonable impedance to flow in low voltage shocks that is lost at higher voltages. Wet skin reduces the body's impedance and aids current flow.

High voltage (>1000 volts)

Typically 11 000–33 000 volts is encountered in high-tension transmission cables, and commonly causes extensive tissue damage and limb loss. Most shocks above 11 000 volts are in fact fatal.

Voltage type

Alternating and direct current (DC) shocks result in different responses. High-voltage DC tends to cause a single large skeletal muscle contraction that throws the victim away from the electrical source. A similar AC voltage results in muscle tetany and in the hand this tends to prolong grip on an electrical source and exacerbate injuries.

Thermal tissue damage

This is a function of the resistance of the tissue, the duration of the contact and the square of the current. It more closely resembles a crush injury at cellular level, and rhabdomyolysis is common. The generation of heat is a function of tissue resistance—the greater the resistance, the greater the thermal injury. In order of decreasing resistance, tissue may be listed as: bone, skin, fat, nerve, muscle, blood, and body fluids. Current will always pass along the path of least resistance, causing necrosis within tissues and organs between the entry and exit surface wounds. These wounds may be complicated by flame burns from clothing. As electrical current can pass so easily throughout the body, it must be remembered that even if a surface electrical burn appears superficial, there may be extensive underlying tissue damage. Surface burns may also be found at the point of electrical grounding (earth point) on the body.

Cardiac arrhythmias

The risk of dysrhythmia depend on the type and magnitude of current; 60mA of 50Hz AC or 300–500mA of DC can lead to significant ventricular fibrillation. This makes domestic electrical supplies particularly dangerous. Application of the current directly to the chest increases this likelihood, as does the presence of an assisted pathway to the heart such as a central IV catheter or pacemaker wire. Microshock can occur when a very small current passes directly to the heart via such a false pathway.

The possible arrhythmias following electrical injury include ventricular fibrillation (VF), right bundle branch block (RBBB), and non-specific ST and T wave abnormalities. Acute MI has been reported therefore cardiac monitoring should be instituted, as delayed arrhythmias may occur.

Alterations in resting membrane potential can also result in respiratory arrest and altered mentation. Spinal cord injury and complex regional pain syndrome have been reported. Renal injury is common, both as a result of haemochromogenuria and the development of compartment syndrome. Adequate fluid resuscitation and early fasciotomy may be required.

Conducted electrical weapons

Tasers are an electrical weapon designed to stun victims, and have been used by the police. They emit a series of low-amplitude DC shocks at approximately 50 000 volts and 2mA for approximately 5sec. They are thought to be safe in healthy volunteers but deaths have occurred around the time of their use.

Management of electrical injury

In the immediate management of an electrical injury it is imperative that the electrical current is switched off prior to approaching the patient. Assessment and resuscitation should then proceed in the 'ABCDE' manner described earlier for trauma triage. Serial creatinine kinase and troponin measurement may assist in the detection of rhabdomyolosis and cardiac damage respectively. According to the British Burns Association Criteria, all electrical burns should be admitted to a burns centre for definitive management.

Further reading

Brusselaers N, Monstrey S, Vogelaers D, et al. (2010). Severe burn injury in Europe: a systematic review of the incidence, aetiology, morbidity and mortality. *Crit Care*, 14:R188.

Gueugniaud P-Y, Carsin H, Bertin-Maghit M, et al. (2000). Current advances in the initial management of major thermal burns. *Intens Care Med*, 26:848–56.

Monafo WW (1996). Initial management of burns. *NEJM*, 335:1581–6.Papini R. (2004). ABC of burns: Initial management of burn injuries of various depths. *BMJ*, 324:158–60.

21.4 Drowning and hypothermia

Drowning

Current WHO terminology defines drowning as 'the process of experiencing respiratory impairment from submersion/immersion in liquid'. The majority of drowning accidents occur in fresh water (e.g. swimming pools, lakes, and rivers), usually within only a few metres of safety and in the company of other people.

Young males are the commonest presenting demographic group but children also form a significant proportion. Alcohol is the single most common factor in drowning accidents and its consumption is noted in approximately 75% of adult cases.

Patients may present with a spectrum of severity from asymptomatic (after rescue) to death; the principal problems are respiratory failure, hypoxic brain injury, and cardiovascular compromise. Multiorgan failure may supervene. Respiratory failure is due to surfactant depletion and dysfunction, aspiration of particulate matter such as sand, and later pneumonia and ARDS. Differing electrolyte problems are not found in drowning in salt versus fresh water.

Physiology of drowning

When immersed in water, subjects tend to go through a series of stages:

1. *Panic*: victim struggles to keep their head above the water; heart and respiratory rate rise markedly.
2. *Breath holding*: victim tires and can no longer remain above the water and frequent submersion occurs.
3. *Terminal gasp*: usually results in pulmonary aspiration or laryngospasm may occur resulting in hypoxaemia.
4. *Unresponsiveness:* may occur within a minute of the previous stage, due to cerebral hypoxia.

If water has caused laryngospasm at an early stage, therefore reducing the water load in the lungs, outcome may be favourable if there has been no cerebral damage.

Immersion into water <21°C initiates the diving reflex in most mammals, resulting in bradycardia and vasoconstriction. The reflex is more pronounced in younger individuals and may contribute to better outcomes via a process of reduced oxygen consumption.

Otherwise, for those victims who are immersed in cold water, a response called cold water shock occurs that leads to a gasp reflex, hyperventilation, and tachycardia. Gasping and hyperventilation in this scenario can significantly increase the risk of pulmonary aspiration.

Management of drowning

History from pre-hospital care personnel is essential and should address immersion time if known, duration of CPR and potential for other injuries for example, due to jumping or diving into shallow water.

Patients who are unconscious, agitated, or hypoxaemic require intubation and ventilation, though in cases of borderline respiratory failure continuous positive airway pressure (CPAP) ventilation may be considered. Volume expansion is often required to achieve haemodynamic stability but caution should be taken in the presence of lung injury. Hypothermia often coexists and may be neuroprotective. Where cerebral hypoxic injury is likely, strong consideration should be given to either therapeutic hypothermia or not rewarming above 34°C.

Hypothermia

Hypothermia is defined as a core temperature <35°C and may be classified as:

- Mild: 32–35°C
- Moderate: 28–32°C
- Severe: <28°C.

Primary hypothermia is due to exposure to a cold environment, as is commonly seen intraoperatively and in trauma patients. Secondary hypothermia results from an underlying illness such as hypothyroidism. Therapeutic (iatrogenic) hypothermia is used post-cardiac arrest and in the management of intractable raised intracranial pressure.

Symptoms will depend upon the temperature on presentation and duration of hypothermia. Mild hypothermia results in shivering, dysarthria, tachycardia, tachypnoea, and cold diuresis. Moderate hypothermia leads to a reduction in conscious level heart rate, cardiac output, and oxygen consumption. Severe hypothermia induces profound acid–base disturbance, profound bradycardia and hypotension, loss of consciousness and reflexes.

Management of hypothermia

Axilla and tympanic temperature measurement can be inaccurate in hypothermia and insertion of an oesophageal or rectal thermometer will give more accurate readings. Electrolytes, blood gases, and coagulation must be regularly monitored during treatment as all may deteriorate rapidly.

The ECG may show prolongation of the PR and QT intervals and QRS complex, which can lead to ventricular arrhythmias. Characteristic J-waves (Osborn waves) may be seen after the QRS complex. As hypothermia becomes more severe, ventricular fibrillation (33–28°C) or asystole (<25°C) may occur. Cardiac output also declines with increasing hypothermia. Careful observation of blood glucose concentration will be required and insulin may be required to control hyperglycaemia.

Priorities in the hypothermic patient should be:

1. Maintenance of tissue oxygenation:
   - Adequate circulation
   - Adequate ventilation
   - Identification of primary versus secondary hypothermia.
2. Thermal stabilization:
   - Conduction
   - Convection
   - Radiation
   - Evaporation.
3. Rewarming.

Current consensus in the management of hypothermia favours active warming to maintain normothermia, particularly in trauma patients, except in haemodynamically stable patients with an isolated head injury, where early rewarming above 34°C is relatively contraindicated. Rewarming should usually proceed at a rate similar to the suspected rate of cooling (0.5°C/h is a common target). During active rewarming, close monitoring is mandatory in order to avoid complications associated with arrhythmia and hypotension.

The method of rewarming will depend upon the severity of hypothermia and availability of local resources:

1. Passive rewarming with blankets in a warm environment is adequate for mild hypothermia when patients are conscious and without serious complications.

2. Active rewarming is required for moderate and severe hypothermia, and mild hypothermia with complications:
   - External—radiant heat, warm air blowers.
   - Minimally invasive—warmed, IV and nasogastric fluids, bladder irrigation.
   - Invasive—warmed peritoneal or pleural lavage, intravascular catheters.
   - Extracorporeal
     - Cardiopulmonary bypass
     - CVVH
     - Extra-corporeal membrane oxygenation (ECMO).

Fluid resuscitation will be required due to cold induced diuresis and reversal of vasconstriction. 'Rewarming collapse' describes the fall in blood pressure that accompanies vasodilatation as temperature rises. 'Core afterdrop' refers to a further fall in core temperature sometimes occurs during warming; it is thought to occur when the temperature gradient from core to periphery is reversed during warming. It tends to occur during rapid rewarming from severe hypothermia.

Prognostication after drowning or hypothermia

While the adage that a patient is 'not dead until they are warm and dead' is widely promulgated it must be remembered that many patients are 'cold because they are dead'. Where the history clearly implies death *before* hypothermia has occurred and initial attempts at resuscitation are unsuccessful serious consideration should be given to stopping resuscitation. Adult patients who drown in UK waters do not become hypothermic rapidly enough to achieve neuroprotection. Case reports of neurologically intact survivors relate principally to infants who have succumbed to primary hypothermia in conditions much colder than those commonly found in the UK.

Prolonged immersion time, prolonged time without CPR, asystole, prolonged resuscitation, and profound hyperkalaemia are all markers of very poor survival and outcome, although exact time limits are difficult to establish from the literature. The lowest recorded temperature a human has survived accidental hypothermia is 13.7°C in a Swedish skier who was trapped in water under an ice sheet for 80min, the latter 40min of which she had no cardiac output. Cardiopulmonary bypass and then ECMO was used in her resuscitation; she made a full recovery to normal function.

Further reading

Danzl D, Pozos RS, & Hamlet MP (1995). Accidental hypothermia. In PS Auerbach (ed), *Wilderness Medicine: Management of Wilderness and Environmental Emergencies*, 3rd edn, p. 70. St Louis, MO: Mosby–Year Book, Inc.

Gilert M, Busund R, Skagseth A, *et al.* (2000). Resuscitation from accidental hypothermia of 13.7°C with circulatory arrest. *Lancet*, 355:375–6.

21.5 Management of blood loss, coagulopathy, hypothermia, and acidosis

Major changes in resuscitation after injury have occurred in recent years with increasing emphasis placed on control of haemorrhage rather than fluid administration. Damage control surgery (DCS) has become a widely accepted concept and subsequent work has developed the concepts of damage control resuscitation and anaesthesia.

Following recognition of significant blood loss, urgent attempts should be made to identify and control the source and to establish vascular access. Wide-bore peripheral access is most desirable; alternatives include central venous access with an introducer sheath or via the intraosseous route (even in adults).

Prior to expedited control of haemorrhage, a low volume resuscitation strategy should be employed. In patients without a head injury permissive hypotension can be used, accepting SBPs of around 80mmHg. In the presence of a significant head injury a SBP of 100mmHg should be targeted but this should be achieved using 250mL fluid challenges. Animal work suggests this approach is safe for around 1h.

In patients with polytrauma, major torso trauma or who are transient or non-responders to fluid, an early switch to blood and blood products should be made as outlined in the following sections. A hospital policy that allows for urgent release of uncrossmatched blood products is needed.

Major objectives of damage control surgery

- Control of bleeding.
- Prevention of contamination
- Planned re-operation for definitive treatment.

There are three distinct phases to the damage control approach to care of trauma patients: initial abbreviated surgery or interventional radiology, postoperative resuscitation on the ICU, and subsequent definitive surgery.

For DCS to be effective, the anaesthetist must understand the lethal triad of events that accompany massive haemorrhage: coagulopathy, hypothermia, and metabolic acidosis. If performed effectively, DCS will prevent or mitigate this vicious triad.

Hypothermia

Hypothermia in massive blood loss will exacerbate coagulopathy, acidosis, and organ failure. It also results in a left shift of the oxygen–haemoglobin dissociation curve, reducing tissue oxygen release. Hypothermia is therefore associated with worse outcome in trauma and must be avoided.

Coagulopathy

It is now recognized that coagulopathy during trauma may occur via two distinct mechanisms:

Acute coagulopathy of trauma shock

Acute coagulopathy associated with trauma, present on admission, is seen in approximately one in four trauma patients and is associated with a fourfold increase in mortality. Active treatment of this coagulopathy results in improved outcomes. This coagulopathy is identified prior to any fluid administration (so is not the result of haemodilution) or the development of hypothermia.

This is thought to be driven by endothelial exposure and activation of the protein C pathway.

Haemodilution

The second mechanism is due to a combination of haemodilution following IV fluid administration, which is compounded by hypothermia. Dilution of clotting factors plays a major role in trauma coagulopathy; some colloids also have a direct negative impact on clot formation. Packed red blood cell (PRBC) transfusions also dilute clotting factors, hence the necessity to administer plasma (FFP) concomitantly.

It must also be remembered that standard laboratory tests that are calibrated to 37°C may overestimate true *in vivo* coagulation.

Retrospective data from recent military conflicts appears to demonstrate an improved mortality with the use of PRBCs and FFP in ratios of 1:1 or 1:2 from the outset, in the most seriously injured. The exact ratio of PRBC:FFP and indications for this approach in civilian practice remain to be fully elucidated. High ratio platelet transfusion (1:1:1) from the outset may also be of benefit, though the evidence base is less established. Cryoprecipitate transfusion should ideally be guided by near patients testing, or to maintain a normal fibrinogen level.

Adjuncts to haemostasis

The CRASH 2 trial demonstrated that tranexamic acid administration in shocked trauma patients was associated with a reduction in the risk of death (relative risk 0.91). A dose of 1g initially followed by 1g every 8h is recommended.

Recombinant factor VIIa (rfVIIa—Novoseven®) has been used on a rescue basis for trauma patients with refractory bleeding and coagulopathy. In an RCT it has been shown to be associated with reduced blood transfusion but not reduced mortality. It should be understood that rfVIIa use in trauma is at supra-physiological concentrations with the intention of producing a thrombin burst at the site of injury. This is only likely to be effective if adequate substrate has been administered in the form of platelets and FFP, and if the patient is not profoundly acidotic or hypothermic.

A growing range of novel haemostatic agents e.g. Celox™ and Quickclot® is available for both local wound application as well as surgical use. Limb tourniquets are now accepted for severe haemorrhage if direct pressure is ineffective. None of these replaces good quality direct pressure to bleeding points, splintage of injured limbs, and minimal patient handling.

Near patient testing

Near patient testing is essential for the management of massive transfusion in the major trauma patient. Blood gases should be monitored and in addition to standard parameters must include lactate, potassium, calcium, and haematocrit or haemoglobin concentration. Coagulation should be monitored using thromboelasotography (TEG) or rotational thromboelastometry (ROTEM®). Near patient monitoring of whole blood coagulation using one of these viscoelastic methods allows faster and more targeted product replacement resulting in more rapid correction of coagulopathy, reduced morbidity and potentially less blood and product use overall. Prolongation of the time taken to initiate clot formation should prompt the administration of FFP. Reduction in clot strength indicates the need for platelets with or without cryoprecipitate. Both platforms have reagents available that allow the relative contribution of fibrinogen and platelets to clot strength to be elucidated, and hence guide therapy. In the absence of this fibrinogen should be maintained above 1.5g/L.

Metabolic acidosis

Hypoperfusion and hypoxaemia can result in anaerobic metabolism of tissues and subsequent development of metabolic acidosis. The clearance of lactate from the circulation is a good indicator of tissue perfusion and is closely related to patient outcome. Metabolic acidosis should therefore be treated by restoration of hypovolaemia.

Damage control resuscitation

Immediate management of hypovolaemia, hypothermia, and coagulopathy along with judicious permissive hypotension, minimal patient handling, and rapid senior decision-making to expedite control of haemorrhage may be considered as damage control resuscitation.

The anaesthetist has a crucial role in the damage control resuscitation team, and with modern trauma care concepts may be required to manage ongoing resuscitation not just in theatre but in the angiography suite, CT scanner, ICU and during both intra- and inter-hospital transfer. Effective communication with the operating surgeon throughout this process is imperative for patient survival. A list of important considerations for the anaesthetist is shown in Box 21.1.

Following the initial surgical control of bleeding, aggressive resuscitation with blood and blood products should occur; these will need to be warmed with a device capable of doing so effectively at high flow rates. At the conclusion of surgery the patient should remain sedated, intubated, and ventilated to assist normalization of physiology, and assessment of any ongoing bleeding. If the patient's physiology is borderline for definitive surgery a brief halt to operating should be called, the abdomen temporarily packed and covered, and resuscitation continued. If the response is good further surgical intervention can continue—otherwise the patient should be transferred to the ICU.

Trauma patients are at high risk of acute lung injury (ALI) and ventilation should be modified to minimize further lung damage (tidal volume of 6–8mL/kg, adequate PEEP, maximum plateau pressure of $30cmH_2O$). Use of cardiac output monitoring will greatly aid fluid resuscitation in this cohort of patients.

If at any point during resuscitation the patient begins to deteriorate haemodynamically, one should reassess systematically using the ABCDE approach to resuscitation and consider the factors outlined in Box 21.2.

Box 21.1 Objectives of damage control anaesthesia

- Safe rapid establishment of a definitive airway.
- Controlled ventilation: early use of lung protection.
- Low volume resuscitation prior to control of bleeding.
- Early use of blood and blood products.
- Management of electrolytes: Ca^{2+} >1.2 and K^+ <6.
- Rapid shock reversal after control of bleeding.
- Adequate analgesia and sedation.
- Progression to deep anaesthesia as soon as possible.
- Avoidance of hypothermia/rewarming: core temp >35°C.
- Safe transfer for further imaging and critical care.
- Neuroprotection if indicated.

Box 21.2 Failure to respond to resuscitation: reassess ABCDE

- Missed injury:
  - Tension pneumothorax
  - Tamponade
  - Pelvic or retroperitoneal bleeding
- Myocardial contusion
- Myocardial infarction
- Addisonian or myxoedema crisis
- Septic shock
- Profound electrolyte disturbance
- Co-ingestion of drugs or exposure to toxins.

Further reading

CRASH-2 trial collaborators (2010). Effects of tranexamic acid on death, vascular occlusive events, and blood transfusion in trauma patients with significant haemorrhage (CRASH-2): a randomised, placebo-controlled trial. *Lancet*, 376(9734):23–32.

Rossaint R, Bouillon B, Cerny V, et al. (2010). Management of bleeding following major trauma: an updated European guideline. *Crit Care*, 14:R52.

Sagraves SG, Toschlog EA, & Rotondo MF (2006). Damage control surgery--the intensivist's role. *J Intens Care Med*, 21(1):5–16.

21.6 Management of children with multiple injuries

Trauma is the leading cause of death in children over the age of 1 year old. Children are at particular risk of trauma due to their lack of experience, lack of awareness of danger, and ignorance of threats posed to them. Most of the injuries are due to blunt trauma. One must also consider the risk of trauma due to non-accidental injury in children.

Major paediatric trauma is not a common presentation to most hospitals and, as a result, there will be relative inexperience in dealing with seriously injured children. The injured child presents difficulties to the trauma team because he or she may be:

- Unable to describe pain
- Unable to cooperate
- Frightened.

However, although these factors might cause problems for the team, a structured approach to the injured child remains critical and ATLS principles should be followed and treatment priorities remain the same. A Broselow tape can be a useful tool to estimate the child's weight and to provide a reminder of paediatric drug doses.

Changes in a child's vital signs can be subtle. The increased physiological reserve of a child allows maintenance of most vital signs in the normal range, even in the presence of shock (Table 21.3).

Table 21.3 Normal vital signs in children			
	Pulse (beats/min)	SBP (mm Hg)	Respiration (breaths/min)
Newborn	95–145	60–90	30–60
Infant	125–170	75–100	30–60
Toddler	100–160	80–110	24–40
Preschool	70–110	80–110	22–34
School age	70–110	85–120	18–30
Adolescent	55–100	95–120	12–16

Airway and cervical spine control

Airway management should follow the standard ATLS sequence. There might be an early requirement for intubation to allow safe assessment and management of the multiply injured child if the child is particularly distressed and unable to cooperate.

If a child is uncooperative or combative, the C-spine should have only a hard collar applied rather than full immobilization, so thrashing around does not cause leverage on the neck.

Spinal cord injury without bony injury is more likely in children than in adults due to the increased flexibility of the cervical spine and a more tenuous bloody supply to the cord. It is more common in children under the age of 8 years. This is known as SCIWORA (spinal cord injury without radiological abnormality). It is reported in 10–20% of children with spinal cord injury.

Breathing

Infants and small children are primarily diaphragmatic breathers; their ribs lack the rigidity and configuration present in adults. As a result, any compromise of diaphragmatic excursion significantly limits the child's ability to ventilate.

A child might have significant pulmonary injury without bony injury due to the softer, thinner chest wall. Pulmonary contusion and pneumothorax are frequently present without rib fractures.

The heart and great vessels are more mobile than in adults, so chest injuries are more poorly tolerated, particularly a tension pneumothorax.

Circulation

Early intraosseous access should be established if it is not possible to site an IV cannula.

A child with hypotension represents decompensation and indicates severe blood loss.

The abdominal wall is thinner and the liver and spleen are lower-riding resulting in greater incidence of injury.

Fluid and blood administration guidelines are under frequent review and consensus is elusive. Current recommendations are for a fluid bolus of 20mL/kg according to ATLS guidelines and 10mL/kg under APLS guidelines. If 40mL/kg of fluid has been administered to a child who remains unstable, blood should be used for further fluid replacement.

Disability

Children have a greater susceptibility to parenchymal structural damage and secondary brain injury due to hypovolaemia, as well as having a greater susceptibility to the effects of raised intracranial pressure. The AVPU score or GCS should be used. The GCS is modified for infants (see Table 21.4).

Table 21.4 Paediatric Glasgow Coma Scale	
Score	Eyes
4	Opens eyes spontaneously
3	Opens eyes to speech
2	Opens eyes to pain
1	Does not open eyes
	Voice
5	Interacts appropriately, smiles, fixes and follows, orientates to sounds
4	Inappropriate interactions, cries but is consolable
3	Moaning, inconsistently inconsolable
2	Inconsolable, agitated
1	No verbal response
	Motor
6	Moves spontaneously or purposefully
5	Withdraws from touch
4	Withdraws from pain
3	Abnormal flexion
2	Abnormal extension
1	No motor response

Data from Jennett & Teasdale, *Lancet* 1977;i:878–881, James & Trauner, *Brain insults in infants and children*, Orlando: Grune & Stratton, 1985:179–182; Sharples et al., *Journal of Neurology, Neurosurgery and Psychiatry*, 1995;2:145-152; and Tatman, Warren, Williams, Powell, Whitehouse, *Archives of Disease in Childhood*, 1997;77:519–521.

Exposure

Children become cold very quickly due to the high ratio of body surface area to body mass. Preventing hypothermia is critical.

Multiply injured children requiring surgery should be managed by a surgical team familiar with dealing with the paediatric patient and may require input from several different specialties. Seriously injured children are more likely to require secondary transfer from the receiving hospital than adults. Some areas of the country have dedicated paediatric retrieval teams who will carry out transfer to a specialist unit.

A child with life-threatening problems who presents to a unit without paediatric surgeons and anaesthetists must have those problems dealt with before transfer.

Further reading

Schmitz B & Albrecht S (2002). Pediatric trauma anesthesia. *Curr Opin Anaesthesiol*, 15(2):187–91.

21.7 Use of regional anaesthesia in patients with multiple injuries

Neuraxial, plexus, and nerve blocks can play an important part in the anaesthetic management and the control of peri-operative pain in the multiply injured patient. Regional anaesthesia can be used at any stage after evaluation in the Emergency Department to provide analgesia or as an adjunct to general anaesthesia.

The use of regional anaesthesia in trauma patients is considered to be contentious by some colleagues who believe the techniques used may mask the development of compartment syndrome, or due to concerns over the safety of blocks performed on an anaesthetized or sedated patient and concerns about the risk of haematoma formation in patients with trauma coagulopathy.

Compartment syndrome

Compartment syndrome occurs when increased pressure within a closed compartment compromises the circulation and function of the tissues within that space. Most commonly, it occurs in an osteofascial compartment of the leg or forearm, but it may occur in the upper arm, thigh, foot, buttock, hand, and abdomen. The commonest cause of compartment syndrome is trauma and, most usually, after a fracture, but it can follow reperfusion of an ischaemic limb. It requires prompt diagnosis and treatment with fasciotomy to avoid the potentially disastrous sequelae of neurological deficit, muscle necrosis, amputation, and death.

The clinical signs and symptoms of compartment syndrome are unreliable (Box 21.3). Pain is subjective and variable; pulselessness is uncommon and implies a late stage. Compartment pressure monitoring is recommended as an adjunct to clinical examination in high-risk patients and a high index of suspicion should be maintained.

> **Box 21.3 Symptoms and signs of compartment syndrome**
> - Pain out of proportion to injury
> - Paraesthesia
> - Pallor
> - Pulseless
> - Paralysis.

Mar et al.'s systematic review (2009) revealed no evidence that postoperative regional anaesthesia resulted in a delayed diagnosis of acute compartment syndrome, and in fact may help facilitate the diagnosis when the patient experiences breakthrough ischaemic pain.

Regional blocks under anaesthesia

Many anaesthetists perform major regional blocks on anaesthetized patients as a matter of routine despite the views of some medical experts who strongly advise against the practice. Anaesthetists increasingly recognize the benefits of regional anaesthesia in the perioperative period and may justify performing the block on anaesthetized patients for several reasons: greater patient acceptance (especially children), less impact on the throughput of the operating list, easier positioning of the patient, easier performance of the block, and better conditions for teaching and supervising trainees. Others argue that by removing verbal contact with the patient the most useful warning of impending nerve contact is lost and that no potential benefit to the patient is worth the risk of serious nerve damage. However, there is insufficient published data to lend support to the views of either side.

There are no prospective randomized controlled studies which compare the relative risks of regional anaesthesia performed on anaesthetized or conscious patients. The existing data comes from retrospective qualitative studies (critical incident reporting, closed claim analysis, and case reports), where there has been a negative outcome. This has inherent weaknesses with reporting bias, incomplete voluntary reporting, and the increase of medicolegal litigation.

The increased use of ultrasound for guiding the placement of the needle for regional blocks has meant many colleagues feel more able to place blocks on an anaesthetized or sedated patient. The exception to this is the interscalene block where many anaesthetists feel this block should only be performed on an awake patient because there have been a number of case reports detailing permanent neurological damage and total spinal anaesthesia due to the complications of the block. The most useful regional blocks are:

Lower limb
- Femoral nerve block
- Lateral popliteal approach for sciatic nerve block.

Both of these blocks can be done with minimal repositioning of the patient.

Upper limb
- Supraclavicular brachial plexus block.
  This block is known as the 'spinal of the arm'.

Torso blocks
- Transversus abdominis plane (TAP) block.

Useful for providing analgesia for a midline laparotomy incision when the patient is unsuitable for an epidural.

Neuraxial blocks
- Thoracic epidural, e.g. to provide analgesia for a damage control laparotomy.
- Lumbar epidural, e.g. to provide analgesia for pelvic fracture reconstruction.

Regional anaesthesia and coagulopathy

Trauma patients may be coagulopathic for a variety of reasons:
- Acute coagulopathy of trauma shock
- Anticoagulant medications
- Massive transfusion
- Pre-existing clotting disorder.

Any of these can make the patient more likely to develop a haematoma following regional block.

The most worrying and most damaging to the patient complication would be the development of a vertebral canal haematoma. When this occurs, it is more likely to occur in the epidural space. The incidence is small with the incidence of permanent harm being 1 in 20 000 with perioperative epidural. The classic finding of intense back pain is less common than neurological deficit of the legs, so to aid early diagnosis of this potentially catastrophic complication epidural infusions should minimize the degree of lower limb block.

The use of near patient testing, such as TEG® or ROTEM®, is exceptionally helpful in addition to normal laboratory tests of clotting to aid anaesthetists with the decision on when and whether to use regional anaesthetic techniques in the trauma patient. For example, a patient who has had a trauma laparotomy may not be suitable for an epidural before leaving the operating theatre, but it might be possible to perform the epidural before the patient is woken up on the ICU.

Further reading

Mar GJ, Barrington MJ, & McGuirk BR (2009). Acute compartment syndrome of the lower limb and the effect of postoperative analgesia on diagnosis. *Br J Anaesth*, 102:3–11.

Royal College of Anaesthetists (2009). *National Audit Project: National Audit of Major Complications of Central Neuraxial Block in the United Kingdom*. London: Royal College of Anaesthetists.

Ulmer T (2002). The clinical diagnosis of compartment syndrome of the lower leg: Are the clinical findings predictive of the disorder? *J Orthop Trauma*, 16:572–7.

Chapter 22

Neuroanaesthesia and neurocritical care

The control of intracranial pressure (ICP) is described in section 6.4. Raised ICP may lead to brain injury and death through two distinct mechanisms: (1) global hypoxic-ischaemic injury secondary to reduced cerebral perfusion pressures (CPPs), and (2) mechanical compression and herniation of brain tissue secondary to mass effect. Successful management techniques for ICP are thus essential, and involve not only the immediate treatment of raised ICP, but also equally importantly, circumvention of precipitating and provoking factors (see Table 22.1). General, medical, and surgical measures should be considered.

Table 22.1 Causes of raised ICP

Intracranial (primary)	Extracranial (secondary)
Tumour	Hypoxia
Haemorrhage	Hypercarbia
Infarct	Hypertension
Hydrocephalus	Posture
Benign ICP	Seizures

Treatment of raised ICP

An ABC approach may be adopted to remember the methods used to prevent and reduce raised ICP. For anaesthetists, the commonest reason for needing to treat raised ICP is following severe traumatic brain injury (TBI). ICP should generally be maintained below 20mmHg in this cohort of patients.

Airway

Intubation may be necessary, and tubes should be taped or tied loosely to minimize disruption in venous drainage. C-spine immobilization may be necessary depending on the nature of the pathology.

Breathing

Intubation and ventilating a patient allows precise titration of their gaseous parameters. Hypoxia and hypercapnia both dramatically increase ICP secondary to cerebral vasodilatation and subsequently increased cerebral blood flow.

Current guidelines suggest that a normal $PaCO_2$ (4.5–5.0kPa) should be maintained following TBI, however, hyperventilation to achieve a $PaCO_2$ 4.0–4.5kPa may be necessary to reduce cerebral blood flow and ICP in some cases. PaO_2 should be >12kPa and SpO_2 >96%. The usefulness of hyperventilation to create a respiratory alkalosis is time limited (10–20h), for as the CSF pH equilibrates to the achieved $PaCO_2$ level, cerebral arterioles dilate resulting in hyperaemia and subsequent increased ICP. Mechanical ventilation per se may also have adverse effects as can PEEP: increasing ICP through impeding venous return, increased cerebral venous pressure, and decreased systemic blood pressure.

Circulation

Given that hypotension is a leading cause of secondary brain injury in trauma, maintenance of an adequate blood pressure is essential. A MAP high enough to ensure a CPP >60mmHg should be the target (CPP = MAP – ICP). In the absence of a measurable ICP in an acutely brain injured unconscious patient, use IV fluid boluses and vasopressors (if necessary) to maintain MAP >90mmHg.

In the presence of severe systemic hypertension, antihypertensive agents should be considered with caution; α-blockers (clonidine) or β-blockers (esmolol, labetalol) are preferred as they have minimal effect on ICP whilst achieving the desired fall in systemic blood pressure. Calcium channel blockers, and nitrates dilate intracerebral vessels and will further increase ICP.

Pharmacological interventions

A variety of pharmacological agents may be used to minimize raised ICP.

Sedatives and analgesics

Both agitation and pain are liable to raise ICP if not treated appropriately; however, the drug of choice remains a debate. The effect on ICP, CPP, and cerebral metabolic rate of oxygen consumption ($CMRO_2$) must all be considered, and also the need for sedation breaks to assess neurological status. Commonly an opiate and a benzodiazepine are used. Seizures, seen in 20% of patients with TBI, must be immediately treated (section 6.3), and a role for seizure prophylaxis (with phenytoin) for patients with severe brain injury has been proposed for the immediate 7 days post insult. The requirement for barbiturate sedation presently tends to be reserved only for cases of refractory raised ICP, for whilst it decreases CBF, ICP, and $CMRO_2$, adverse effects include hypotension, hypokalaemia, hepatic and renal dysfunction, and neurological examination is impossible for a number of days.

Muscle relaxants

Muscle paralysis is not routinely indicated and does not reduce ICP per se. However, in the event that the patient is coughing or straining against mechanical ventilation, muscle relaxation should be considered.

Hypertonic solutions

Mannitol 20% 0.25–1.0g/kg and hypertonic saline (NaCl 3–23.4%) 1–2mL/kg are used as hyperosmolar therapies. Mannitol lowers ICP within 5–20min, with a peak effect 20–60min later, and duration of action of up to 6h. Its effects are biphasic. Initially the osmotic effect, through increased tonicity, creates an osmotic gradient and draws water from the brain parenchyma into the intravascular compartment, thus lowering ICP. Its secondary diuretic effect leads to excessive free water clearance. This may occur to such an extent that it may necessitate fluid replacement to maintain intravascular volume and is relatively contraindicated in hypotensive patients.

Adverse effects include, hyperosmolarity (keep <320mOsm/L), congestive cardiac failure, electrolyte disturbances, acute tubular necrosis, and rebound raised ICP with vasogenic oedema. Hypertonic saline, potentially equally or more effective than mannitol in reducing ICP, demonstrates advantages in that it treats hypovolaemia and raises blood pressure. It is also not without risks and creates electrolyte abnormalities (hyperchloraemic acidosis) and may affect coagulation.

Steroids

Steroids (particularly dexamethasone) are used to decrease vasogenic cerebral oedema associated with intracerebral tumours or abscesses. An improvement in neurology may be seen within hours and ICP decreases over 2–5 days. They provide no benefit in TBI or haemorrhage.

Exposure and positioning

To minimize venous outflow resistance and aid CSF drainage from the intracranial cavity, as long as the patient is not profoundly hypotensive, the head should be elevated at 30° in the neutral position. Care must be taken to place pressure monitoring devices (MAP and ICP), at the same level (usually taken at the level of the foramen of Monro) to adequately assess CPP. Head elevation >45° should be avoided as paradoxical increases in ICP may occur in response to sudden excessive CPP reduction.

Normothermia to mild hypothermia should be maintained, pyrexia, a potent vasodilator, will increases $CMRO_2$ and systemic metabolism by 10% per degree rise, and should be treated aggressively with paracetamol and active cooling. Moderate systemic hypothermia (approximately 34–35°C) has been used to treat intractable raised ICP and can be achieved through the infusion of cold IV fluids and cold air or fluid blankets.

Appropriate antibiotic cover should be instigated if SIRS/sepsis is present.

Fluids, glucose and haematology

IV fluids should be commenced in patients, and the traditional practice of 'dehydration therapy' avoided. This habit of restricting total fluid intake with the aim of reducing extracellular fluid volume has proven to be of no benefit. Isotonic fluids such as 0.9% saline should be used in preference to hypotonic solutions (e.g. Hartmann's solution or 5% glucose) as the lower tonicity of these fluids may worsen cerebral oedema and subsequently increase ICP.

Insertion of a urinary catheter and will aid fluid balance assessment, as will central line placement. Normoglycaemia should be maintained, as both hypo- and hyperglycaemia are associated with adverse effects. To ensure adequate oxygen delivery, anaemia should be avoided (Hb >10g/dL).

Surgical intervention

The requirement for surgical interventions should be continuously evaluated, and in the case of intracranial masses, acute haematomas, pneumocephalus, and brain abscesses may reduce the mass effect on ICP. In the event of a sudden rise in ICP, or pressure that is refractory to medical management stratagems, surgery should be the initial consideration. In the latter, a decompressive craniectomy, through the creation of a window in the cranial vault, effectively reduces ICP in most patients (85%), and furthermore cerebral tissue oxygenation and CBF are improved. Complications include infection, hydrocephalus, haemorrhage, and subdural hygroma. CSF drainage may also be used to lower ICP, however in a severely swollen cerebrum, the ventricles may be effaced and thus limit drainage of CSF.

Further reading

Gupta A & Gelb A (2008). *Essentials of Neuroanaesthesia and Neurointensive Care*. Philadelphia, PA: Saunders Elsevier.

22.2 Positioning for neurosurgery

General considerations for positioning

Neurosurgical procedures require patients to be positioned to allow surgical access. Other than supine, positions commonly used are prone, lateral, park bench, and sitting position. Procedures may be lengthy and patients are at risk of nerve, joint and skin injury. Minimizing the risk of injury requires knowledge of the particular pressure areas and complications associated with each position.

Prone position

In the classic prone position, the patient rests face down on the ventral aspect of the torso. A log roll technique is used to turn the patient. The legs are extended and the arms can either be raised beside the head on padded arm boards or ideally retained at the sides of the body. Placing the arms above the patient's head can cause a stretch injury to the lower trunks of the brachial plexus. Great care must be taken when the arms are raised to rotate the shoulder and not to force the joint. In some individuals it will not be possible to rotate the shoulder and raise the arms. In this situation the arm may be placed on an arm board, abducted to <90° with the elbows flexed and the palms facing downwards. The forearms should be lower than the torso to avoid stretching the brachial plexus and its related vascular structures. The face can be supported in a neutral position with a contoured face pad or turned gently and minimally to one side on a suitable support. Alternatively the head can be secured with pins attached to a frame (Mayfield). Females with large breasts should have them displaced laterally and in males the genitalia should hang freely with no compression or torsion.

The head-elevated prone position is used frequently for neurosurgical operations. The head is held in pins and elevated above the heart to improve venous drainage of the head and neck. This requires strapping across/under the buttocks to support the trunk and prevent sliding down the table. This could cause pressure on the chin from the mattress or excessive traction on the cervical vertebrae. Additional support is provided by flexing the knees with a wedge and/or pillow beneath the lower legs.

Considerations for prone position

The major pressure points in a prone patient are the ears, eyes, cheeks, acromial processes, breasts, iliac crests, male genitalia, patellae, and toes.

- Ensure that the Montréal mattress does not press in to the axilla and cause damage to the neurovascular bundle in the patient whose arms are raised.
- Avoid pressure directly on the ulnar nerve at the elbow as the raised arm is placed on the arm rest.
- Reduce tension in the leg extensor muscles and sciatic nerve by bending the legs and raising the feet to give minimal flexion at the hips and knee.
- Special consideration should be given to eye protection. The relative positions of the eyes and the head ring should always be checked before, during and after the procedure. Head movement may result in direct pressure on the eye.

The frequency of eye injury during anaesthesia and surgery is very low (<0.1%), but the spectrum of injury ranges from mild discomfort to permanent loss of vision. Corneal abrasions are most common and generally are avoidable with appropriate eye protection. In the prone position, direct pressure on the eye is more likely. If the weight of the head and the pressure within the globe exceeds arterial pressure then arterial inflow may be reduced, resulting in potentially devastating retinal ischaemia. Perioperative ischaemic optic neuropathy may relate to compromised blood flow to the optic nerve. In nearly all reported cases, affected patients have experienced intraoperative or postoperative anaemia, hypotension, prone or lateral position, lengthy procedure times, and significant intraoperative hydration.

Lateral position

By convention a patient in the left lateral decubitus position is positioned with the left side down.

Most often the patient is turned such that a 90° angle is established between the patient's back and the table surface. The head is supported so that the cervical spine is in neutral alignment. The lower leg is flexed to stabilize the torso against tilt, while the upper leg is extended and a pillow is placed between the legs. The patient is secured to the table and a suitable padded mattress is used to relieve pressure over bony prominences and around supports.

A pad or roll may be placed just below the axilla, supporting the area of the upper rib cage to reduce the pressure on the down-side shoulder. Following placement of the axillary pad/roll the radial pulse on the dependent arm must be checked.

Considerations for the lateral position

Pressure points in the lateral position include the dependent ear, shoulder, the acromial process, olecranon, ribs, iliac crest, greater trochanter, medial and lateral condyles and medial and lateral malleoli.

- The common peroneal nerve should be protected with padding. It is often compressed against the head of the fibula as the fibula is pressed against the operating table.
- Compression of the brachial plexus can occur between the thorax and the humeral head.
- Stretch on the brachial plexus is reduced by supporting the head to keep the cervical and thoracic spine horizontal along the long axis of the spine.
- The arm should not be abducted beyond 90° as the radial nerve may be compressed between the edge of the operating table and the humerus.

Park bench position

The park bench position is used most frequently in neurosurgery and has superseded the sitting position as a safer position with less risk of air entrainment. It is used most often for posterior fossa surgery and is so called because it resembles the posture adopted by an individual sleeping on a park bench after a 'late night' (Fig. 22.1).

The patient is log rolled in to the lateral position. The head is held in pins attached to a Mayfield frame. The basic position is similar to the lateral position, but in order to access the base of skull/posterior fossa, the head is tilted towards the lower shoulder. The cervical spine is, therefore, curved down from the shoulders. The upper arm is pulled towards the feet and secured. A chest pad or axillary roll is placed under the chest wall below the axilla. The patient is secured in this position with padded supports, strapping and/or a 'beanbag' mattress. The pressure and skin contact area are all generously padded as procedures may be long.

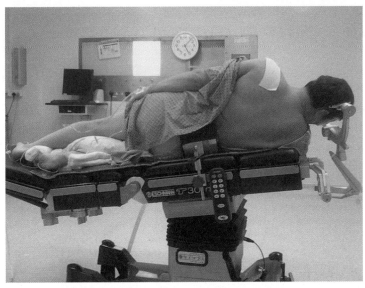

Fig. 22.1 Picture of park bench position.

Considerations for park bench position

The main pressure areas are the shoulder, chest wall, iliac crest/pelvis, and dependent lower limb. Most of the weight is transferred through these areas and they must be protected with a combination of pressure relieving/absorbing padding, e.g. gel-filled pads and Gamgee.

- Care must be taken not to 'open up' the gap between the skull base and the shoulder to the point that excessive tension is placed on the skin and the brachial plexus. As well as brachial plexus injuries, nerve pressure palsies, stretch injuries, and thoracic outlet obstruction of the subclavian artery are all potential risks during park bench positioning.
- The eyes need to be protected; eyelids taped closed, yellow soft paraffin applied, and a gauze pad held in place with a clear plastic adhesive dressing. Rigid eye shields may cause damage to the supra-orbital branch of the trigeminal nerve.
- A degree of facial and corneal oedema develops in some patients.
- Antisialagogue drugs or effective skin covering may be used to prevent saliva from the mouth damaging surrounding skin.

Sitting position

The possibility of air embolism in this position has discouraged its use when suitable alternative positions are acceptable. Adequate surveillance for venous air embolism is crucial as early detection and treatment have significantly reduced its associated morbidity and mortality (see section 22.9).

The sitting position is used almost exclusively by neurosurgeons for posterior fossa craniectomies, foramen magnum decompression, and, rarely, cervical spine operations. The legs are gently flexed at the thighs and the feet are supported at right angles so that they are approximately at the level of the heart. Subgluteal padding must be used to protect the sciatic nerve. The frame of the head rest holder is fixed to the side rails of the table. The head is flexed and secured to the head rest. In the event of an air embolism, the patient's head can be lowered simply and rapidly by lowering the back section of the table while reverse Trendelenburg will encourage good venous return and raise the venous pressure. The arms are placed in a neutral position in front of the body.

Pressure on the common peroneal nerve is a particular concern in the sitting position.

Further reading

Contractor S & Hardman JG (2006). Injury during anaesthesia. *CEACCP*, 6(2):67–70.

Knight DJW & Mahajan RP (2004). Patient positioning in anaesthesia. *CEACCP*, 4 (5):160–3.

22.3 General aspects of neuroanaesthesia

Preoperative considerations

As in all cases, a systematic approach is required, covering the patient's acute physiology, general medical history, regular medications, and allergies whilst establishing a rapport with the patient. Explanation of the sequence of events that the patient will experience in the anaesthetic room or X-ray suite is especially important if the procedure requires patient cooperation, for example, awake fibreoptic intubation.

Airway and respiratory considerations

In anaesthesia for neurosurgery particular attention should be paid to assessing cervical spine range of movement and vertebral column stability. Relevant radiology may need to be reviewed.

Neuropathology may affect the integrity of the cough and gag reflexes, which should be specifically assessed in patients at risk of bulbar weakness.

Respiratory muscle function can usually be adequately assessed at the bedside by asking the patient to demonstrate a forced vital capacity. If in doubt formal lung function tests may be indicated.

Prolonged immobility, depressed conscious level or obtunded protective reflexes predispose patients to pulmonary atelectasis/aspiration/infection. Perioperative physiotherapy may be indicated.

Cardiovascular system

Baseline blood pressure should be noted and the specific neuropathology considered regarding the integrity of the blood–brain barrier, cerebrovascular autoregulation, or the possibility of cerebral vasospasm. ICP and the CPP should be discussed with the neurosurgeon in order to establish the optimal target range for blood pressure throughout the procedure.

ECG changes may occur secondary to intracranial events. Coronary spasm with cerebral ischaemia should be suspected in all patients with acute intracerebral events.

Renal/endocrine function

Considerations pertinent to neurosurgery and neuroradiology are:

- Planned use of osmotherapy: ensure renal function intact prior to use.
- Disturbance of the hypothalamic–pituitary axis: diabetes insipidus, syndrome of inappropriate anti-diuretic hormone (SIADH), cerebral salt wasting.
- Hyponatraemia and hypoglycaemia: increase the risk of seizures.
- Hyperglycaemia: increases cerebral susceptibility to damage in hypoperfusion states. May be caused by steroid treatment.

Neurological assessment

The GCS score and specific neurological deficits must be documented in detail prior to the procedure. The size, site, and nature of the neuropathology determine many aspects of the patient's care including:

- Airway control and intubation technique.
- Need for intra-arterial blood pressure monitoring and its timing either pre or post induction.
- Positioning on the operating table.
- Safe limits for blood pressure during the procedure.
- Risk of intraoperative haemorrhage and cardiovascular instability.

- Risk of postoperative seizures, cerebral oedema, or haemorrhage.
- The need for planned admission to ITU or HDU postoperatively.

It is of paramount importance that these issues are discussed with the surgeon before the procedure.

Haematology

It is prudent to check the full blood count and clotting screen for defects in the coagulation pathway prior to any neurosurgical procedure. The possible need for blood transfusion should also be considered and planned for appropriately.

Medications

Steroids should be continued perioperatively and cover for suppression of adrenal function should be prescribed. Anticonvulsant medications may induce liver enzymes, shortening the action of many hepatically metabolized drugs such as steroidal muscle relaxants. Drugs which interfere with coagulation (aspirin, clopidogrel, NSAIDs, anticoagulants) should be stopped preoperatively and coagulation and platelet function checked.

Sedative premedications are generally discouraged.

DVT prophylaxis

Prolonged immobility or lower limb weakness predisposes patients to DVT, however neurosurgical patients cannot be safely anticoagulated as part of their DVT prophylaxis. It is therefore especially important to examine for lower limb oedema, warmth, and calf tenderness and ensure that patients wear graduated compression stockings, maintain mobility perioperatively if possible, and wear pneumatic compression boots throughout their procedure.

Infection risk

Antibiotic prophylaxis is routine in most centres.

Preoperative pyrexia may result from intracranial non-infective pathology. A raised white cell count may result from treatment with steroids. These two factors complicate the process of excluding or confirming infective aetiology.

Intraoperative management

Most intracranial surgery is performed under general anaesthesia, but for minor procedures, such as burr hole evacuation of a chronic subdural haemorrhage, infiltration of the scalp with local anaesthetic can provide adequate analgesia in a cooperative patient. Specialist techniques such as awake interval anaesthesia, awake fibreoptic intubation, and specialized patient positioning may be required, and must be planned for carefully when appropriate.

The main objective of a neurosurgical anaesthetic is to maintain stable cardiovascular status within well-defined limits throughout the procedure. Whilst desirable in most specialities this is essential in neuroanaesthesia as even short-lived compromise of cerebral or spinal perfusion can have a significant impact on operating conditions and patient outcome.

Monitoring, vascular access, and set-up

In addition to routine monitoring it is worth emphasizing the importance of a few specific aspects of care:

- *Reinforced endotracheal tube*: exact positioning in order to avoid endobronchial migration when the head is optimally positioned for surgery. Fastidious attention must be paid to securing the tube as there is no opportunity to adjust it during the surgery.

- *End-tidal CO_2 monitoring*: to ensure normocapnia, and assist in detection of air embolism.
- *Large-bore IV access*: always prudent.
- *Intra-arterial blood pressure monitoring*: to detect and manage abrupt changes secondary to surgical stimulation; also to assist in detection and management of air embolism/acute haemorrhage.
- *Central venous cannulation*: is not usually required unless indicated by pre-existing comorbidities. Although a carefully placed internal jugular cannula will not raise the ICP, many anaesthetists prefer subclavian or femoral approaches to the central circulation.
- *Urinary catheter*: mandatory in prolonged surgery or if osmotherapy is planned.
- *Peripheral nerve stimulator*: should always be used at induction to ensure complete paralysis prior to intubation. Intracranial surgery requires relatively light anaesthesia, therefore maintaining profound neuromuscular blockade is advisable to ensure that there is no coughing or straining.
- *Temperature probe*: normothermia should be maintained.
- Consideration should be given to siting a *nasogastric tube* after induction if the bulbar reflexes are impaired.

Induction

A smooth induction without any coughing, straining, or major fluctuations in the blood pressure is required for all intracerebral procedures. Methods used to obtund the pressor response to laryngoscopy include:

- 2–3mcg/kg of fentanyl
- TCI remifentanil
- β-blockers
- IV lidocaine.

Propofol is the most commonly used induction agent although thiopentone is a suitable alternative as both agents reduce the $CMRO_2$, CBF, and ICP. Induction agents must be given carefully to prevent a fall in blood pressure and hence CPP. It is often prudent to insert the arterial line under local anaesthesia prior to induction.

A non-depolarizing muscle relaxant is used to facilitate intubation. Suxamethonium is relatively contraindicated as it causes a small rise in ICP. Management of the unstable cervical spine is discussed in section 22.8.

The eyes must be carefully protected, particularly if the patient is to be placed in a prone position. Surgical cleaning solution must not soak into the eye protection when the surgical area is prepped.

Particular issues related to positioning of the neurosurgical patient are covered in section 22.2.

Maintenance of anaesthesia

There is no clear benefit of any specific modern anaesthetic agent or TIVA technique. Remifentanil has an ideal pharmacological profile for neuroanaesthesia as it allows rapid titration during stimulating periods and still ensures a rapid wake up. All volatile anaesthetic agents uncouple cerebral blood flow and $CMRO_2$: reducing $CMRO_2$ but causing a rise in cerebral blood flow secondary to their capacity to dilate the cerebral circulation and obtund autoregulation. This effect is dose dependent; isoflurane and sevoflurane have minimal cerebrovascular effects

<1MAC. Nitrous oxide should be used cautiously as it is a potent cerebral vasodilator and can also expand air filled spaces creating a pneumoencephalocele postoperatively.

If a Mayfield clamp is to be used, adequate depth of anaesthesia should be ensured and an additional bolus of analgesia may be required, as pinning is particularly stimulating.

Ensuring a motionless surgical field is critical during any neurosurgical procedure and this can be achieved with a remifentanil infusion, small boluses of non-depolarizing muscle relaxant guided by a peripheral nerve stimulator, or an infusion of muscle relaxant.

Intermittent positive pressure ventilation should be used intra-operatively in order to ensure control of the partial pressure of CO_2. A $PaCO_2$ of 4.5–5kPa is ideal for routine neurosurgery or 4–4.5kPa for cases of traumatic brain injury. PEEP should generally be avoided.

In general the blood pressure should be maintained, with vasoconstrictors if necessary, to ensure a CPP of at least 60mmHg. However, specific neuropathology may require a higher CPP and this should be discussed with the surgical team preoperatively. Occasionally a lower mean arterial pressure will be requested in order to achieve a less haemorrhagic surgical field. This can be achieved either by increasing the depth of anaesthesia or analgesia or with small boluses of an antihypertensive agent such as labetalol.

Dextrose solutions should not be used as the free water will worsen any cerebral oedema and hyperglycaemia exacerbates brain injury in hypoperfusion states.

Appropriate warming devices should be used for all but the shortest of procedures. Although hypothermia can reduce ICP it does not improve outcome in TBI.

In terms of analgesia, although stimulating intraoperatively, many neurosurgical procedures are not particularly painful postoperatively. Local anaesthetic infiltration by the surgeon into the skin and subcutaneous tissues can be very helpful.

Extubation

Prior to awakening all patients should be monitored for any residual neuromuscular blockade and reversed. The use of sugammadex may be particularly helpful in neuroanaesthesia.
Ideally all patients should be woken and extubated at the end of a procedure to enable neurological assessment. If the patient is to remain sedated ICP monitoring should be considered. There is little consensus as to whether extubating deep or awake is the safer option.

Postoperative care

Postoperative intensive care admission should be organized for all cases where cerebral oedema is expected, the procedure is prolonged, or massive haemorrhage is experienced. For other patients a high dependency area is required, where they can be monitored for a drop in GCS score, respiratory insufficiency, or the development of any neurological deficits. In all cases careful handover of care should occur and all pre-existing neurological deficits should be meticulously documented.

Further reading

Dinsmore J (2007). Anaesthesia for elective neurosurgery *Br J Anaesth*, 99(1):68–74.

22.4 Anaesthesia for specific neurosurgical procedures

Shunt surgery

Shunt surgery is used to treat hydrocephalus. The most common procedure performed is the ventriculoperitoneal (VP) shunt, which is used to drain CSF from the lateral ventricle to the peritoneal cavity. Other types of shunt include ventriculopleural, ventriculoatrial, and lumbar-peritoneal. This is usually a relatively elective procedure without the concerns of an acutely raised ICP. A high proportion of cases may be paediatric patients. Considerations include:

- The position of the patient will depend on the procedure, usually prone or lateral.
- The ICP may be normal or raised.
- Invasive monitoring is not usually required.
- The tunnelling process is very stimulating, but significant postoperative pain is unusual.
- Intracranial haemorrhage is possible if there is a rapid CSF shift.

Evacuation of intracranial haematoma

Intracranial haematomas may be extradural, subdural, or intracerebral (Box 22.1). Depending on the rate of haematoma development, a rapid increase in ICP may result. The limited compliance of the dura/skull is unable to compensate for rapid increase in intracranial contents. This is consequently detrimental to perfusion and may lead to coning (the Munro Kellie doctrine).

The overriding priority in intracranial haematoma management is the maintenance of cerebral perfusion. This requires prevention of significant changes in both arterial and intracranial pressure. Further considerations include:

- Invasive monitoring is essential, with the transducer at head level.
- Adequate venous access and blood products.
- Ensure smooth induction and normotension throughout.
- If ICP is not being measured, assume it is 20mmHg and maintain an adequate MAP.

Box 22.1 The intracranial haematomas

Extradural haematoma
- Between periosteum and dura.
- Usually due to tear in middle meningeal artery or dural sinuses.
- Usually associated with fracture and has a Lentiform appearance on CT scan.
- After loss of consciousness there is a lucid period prior to further deterioration.

Subdural haematoma
- Between pia and arachnoid mater due to tearing of bridging vessels at subdural space.
- Acute SDH requires early evacuation.
- Chronic SDH often occurs in the elderly even after trivial injury.
- Crescent-shaped appearance on CT scan.

Intracerebral haematoma
- Most commonly due to trauma or haemorrhagic stroke.
- May be a complication of anticoagulation therapy.

- Ventilate to achieve a PaCO$_2$ of 4.0–4.5kPa.
- Mannitol (0.5–1g/kg), furosemide (0.25–1mg/kg), and hypertonic saline may be used to lower ICP temporarily.
- Postoperative ventilation is usually required for patients with high ICP or those obtunded preoperatively.

Supratentorial surgery

Elective craniotomies are commonly performed for excision or debulking of tumours, for drainage of an abscess, or treatment of a vascular lesion. Patient position is either supine or lateral depending on the surgical approach.

- Invasive monitoring is usually indicated, with the transducer at head level.
- Neck flexion or rotation is minimized to preserve venous drainage.
- Surgical pins for skull positioning are very stimulating and require adequate depth of anaesthesia.
- Site of the pathological lesion will determine duration of surgery and blood loss.
- Adequate venous access and blood products are required.
- Neuromuscular blockade is maintained.
- Stimulation is often reduced once craniotomy is performed and the dura is open. MAP is maintained with vasopressors.

Vascular lesions are usually aneurysms or arteriovenous malformations (AVMs), the site of which will determine the surgical difficulty (Box 22.2). Cerebral protection with barbiturates or hypothermia may be indicated if a vessel needs prolonged clamping to allow surgical control. Profound neuromuscular blockade is prudent during clipping of the aneurysm. Tight BP control is essential to prevent aneurysm rupture (with high BP) or vasospasm (low BP). Intraoperative rupture requires immediate BP suppression and cerebral protection (e.g. propofol or thiopentone bolus) to aid surgical control, but mortality is high. Any increases in BP on emergence or in recovery are treated effectively with labetalol boluses (10mg).

Box 22.2 Intracerebral vascular lesions

- Berry, saccular, and congenital aneurysms occur in the anterior circulation. Arteriosclerotic and fusiform aneurysms occur in the vertebrobasilar circulation.
- Most common sites include internal carotid, anterior/posterior communicating and middle cerebral arteries.
- AVMs are dilated arteries and veins without an interconnecting capillary network. High-flow AVMs may cause surrounding cerebral ischaemia and high-output cardiac failure.
- The majority of vascular lesions are now treated by interventional radiology.

Posterior fossa surgery

Pathology within the brainstem or cerebellum tends to have a profound physiological impact due to the concentration of ascending/descending pathways, cranial nerves, CSF outflow, and cardiovascular and respiratory control centres.

Surgery to this area is hazardous intra- and postoperatively, with anaesthetic challenges throughout.

- Preoperative assessment is vital with regard to conscious level, airway reflexes (and potential chronic respiratory changes), ICP, fluid and electrolyte status.
- Meticulous patient positioning is necessary; sitting position has a number of potential consequences (see section 22.3). Prone and lateral positions are becoming more commonly used.
- Many pathological conditions occur predominantly in paediatric patients (Arnold–Chiari malformation and medulloblastoma).
- Electrophysiological monitoring may be employed to detect nerve track damage.
- Lumbar CSF drainage may be required to improve surgical conditions.
- Rapid cardiovascular changes may occur with surgical traction, including arrhythmias.
- Initiation of suction on surgical drain postoperatively may also cause significant cardiovascular changes such as bradycardia.
- Respiratory drive may be impaired as a consequence of medullary surgery; postoperative ventilation may be required.

Emergency surgery for traumatic brain injury

The priority in TBI management is to prevent secondary brain injury. Damage to the *penumbra* (the area around the primary brain injury) is potentially reversible and all efforts must be made to optimize conditions for recovery. This can be summarized by maintaining the five 'Ns':

1. Normotension: a single pre-hospital episode of SBP <90mmHg has been shown to increase mortality significantly.
2. Normoxia: any hypoxic periods (SaO_2 <90%) will worsen outcome.
3. Normocapnia: hyperventilation may rescue high ICP in the acute setting, but causes regional ischaemia.
4. Normothermia: CBF changes 5–7% per °C. Avoid hyperthermia. Temperature <35°C also shown to be detrimental.
5. Normoglycaemia: the brain is an obligate glucose user. High glucose increases $CMRO_2$ and has osmotic consequences.

The severity of injury is most commonly assessed using the GCS, with the motor component giving the greatest predictive power of outcome. A head injury may result in cerebral contusions, diffuse axonal injury, and/or subarachnoid, subdural, or extradural bleeding. Regardless of the injury pattern, maintaining perfusion and appropriate physiological parameters is essential.

- Assessment and documentation of extracranial injuries must not be overlooked.

- Airway management must take into account potential spinal injury.
- Seizures need aggressive and immediate treatment; most cases will require loading with phenytoin, regardless of a history of seizure.
- Once intubated, adequate sedation is required to minimize $CMRO_2$.
- Vasopressors are invariably necessary to maintain a CPP >60–70mmHg.
- Transfer to a neurosurgical centre should not occur until life-threatening extracranial injuries have been stabilized.
- Mannitol is often used to treat intracranial hypertension with pupillary signs. Preserving optimal volume status may be complicated thereafter, especially with any ongoing blood loss.
- In a polytrauma case there will inevitably be conflict between maintaining an adequate CPP and controlling BP to prevent massive intra-abdominal/thoracic haemorrhage. This needs full consideration by all teams involved.

Spinal column surgery

There are essentially four indications for spinal surgery: decompression of cord or nerve roots, correction of spinal deformity, excision of tumour, and stabilization following trauma.

Spinal surgery can involve any site from the atlanto-occipital joint to the coccyx. A posterior surgical approach is most common and requires prone position. Anterior approaches may be used at cervical and thoracic levels. Combined approaches are infrequently used. Important considerations for spinal surgery include:

- Careful documentation of preoperative neurological deficit.
- Pathology at the cervical level will require careful airway management, and potentially fibreoptic intubation.
- Antisialagogue administration may prevent excessive drooling which can compromise ETT security when prone.
- One-lung ventilation via a double-lumen tube is required if an anterior thoracic approach is employed.
- Spinal cord monitoring may be required by the surgeon. Interpretation by the neurophysiologist requires a constant depth of anaesthesia and potential avoidance of neuromuscular blockade.
- Spinal cord damage has been reported due to surgery, poor positioning and inadequate spinal cord perfusion pressure (SCPP = MAP − CSFP).
- Blood loss can be excessive in multilevel fusion, tumour excision and deformity correction.

22.5 Anaesthesia for interventional neuroradiology

The practice of interventional neuroradiology encompasses a range of invasive endovascular procedures used predominantly to treat vascular disorders of the central nervous system. In particular, endovascular treatment of intracranial aneurysms is now a well-established therapy, offering proven advantages over surgical clipping in the majority of cases.

Certain important anaesthetic considerations apply to all procedures (see Box 22.3).

> **Box 22.3** Important anaesthetic concerns for all interventional neuroradiology procedures
>
> - Maintaining complete immobility during the procedure.
> - Ensuring rapid emergence from anaesthesia to permit assessment of neurological function.
> - Managing anticoagulation therapy.
> - Responding to sudden procedure-related complications, e.g. vascular occlusion or haemorrhage.
> - General concerns related to:
>   - Remote site anaesthesia (section 17.1)
>   - Transfer of critically ill patients (section 23.2)
>   - Radiation safety (section 10.3).

Preoperative considerations

It is especially important to establish the patient's baseline blood pressure and cardiovascular reserve.

After acute intracranial catastrophes, cerebral autoregulation is impaired (Fig. 22.2), and perfusion of the ischaemic penumbra becomes directly pressure-dependent. Defective autoregulation may persist for days or weeks.

Below the lower limit of autoregulation, vessels passively collapse, and ischaemia results. Above the upper limit or 'breakthrough zone', increased intravascular volume and pressure results in vasogenic oedema and further ischaemia.

In patients with acute brain injury, therefore, cerebral blood flow becomes pressure passive in ischaemic areas.

Preoperative calcium channel blockade with nimodipine is often employed in an attempt to reduce vasospasm and prevent cerebral ischaemia, but may itself affect haemodynamic management during the interventional procedure.

Invasive beat-to-beat monitoring of arterial pressure is desirable. This can be achieved via a dedicated peripheral arterial line or, more commonly, via a side port of the femoral arterial introducer sheath.

Other aspects of preoperative evaluation are intuitive: a careful airway assessment is mandatory, to predict the ease of laryngoscopy, both planned but also emergent if the procedure is to be undertaken under sedation (noting the potential limitations of airway access, table, room, etc.).

Secure IV access is essential, with an adequate length of extension tubing to allow administration of drugs and fluids at a safe distance from the image intensifier during fluoroscopy.

A thorough appreciation of radiation safety (see section 10.3) is crucial. Digital subtraction angiography (DSA) is commonly used during interventional procedures, and delivers more radiation than conventional fluoroscopy. Vascular anatomy is visualized by contrast injection into the circulation to obtain a 'road map' of the vasculature. By superimposing the road-mapped image onto real time fluoroscopy, the radiologist is enabled to follow the progress of the catheter tip. All staff members should take maximal precautions by increasing their distance from the X-ray source and/or moving behind a glass shield. Recent data highlight the particular importance of adequate *eye protection* amongst anaesthesia and other personnel working in the interventional neuroradiology suite.

Anaesthetic technique

Most centres use *general anaesthesia* for complex interventional procedures. The primary reason is to eliminate movement (which degrades image quality and is potentially hazardous

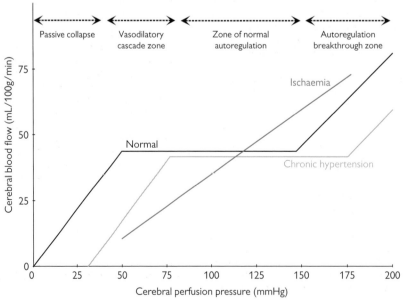

Fig. 22.2 Changes in cerebral autoregulation in disease.

during intravascular manipulations). IPPV to maintain relative normocapnia should be maintained unless intracranial pressure is a concern, when mild hypocapnia may be indicated.

It is fundamentally important to avoid wide swings in blood pressure both during induction and subsequently. Propofol is usually used in conjunction with an opioid (fentanyl, alfentanil, or remifentanil) to induce anaesthesia. It is important to confirm full neuromuscular blockade before laryngoscopy (electrode position should ideally be verified after induction but before administration of muscle relaxant). Some authorities recommend further pressor response obtundation with IV lidocaine or esmolol.

The general considerations for maintenance of neuroanaesthsia apply to these interventional cases (see section 22.3).

The major benefit of *IV sedation* is that it allows continuous monitoring of neurological function during the procedure. The technique must achieve the important goals of alleviating anxiety, pain, and discomfort, whilst promoting immobility and rapid recovery. Contrast injection may cause a burning sedation, whilst vascular distension and traction causes headache. The requirement for prolonged immobility may cause significant discomfort. A variety of sedation techniques may be used. In all cases, there is an obvious need to avoid airway obstruction. α_2 agonists have been used on account of their analgesic, sedative, and anxiolytic properties (with a relative lack of respiratory depression), but they may have adverse effects on cerebral perfusion.

Anticoagulation

Careful anticoagulation is required to prevent thromboembolic complications during the procedure. It is usual to obtain a baseline activated clotting time (ACT), then to administer IV heparin (approximately 70 units/kg), aiming for an ACT of 2–3 times baseline. Heparin is then given by intermittent top-up boluses, with frequent monitoring of the ACT. At the end of the procedure, or if a haemorrhagic complication occurs, heparin may be reversed with protamine.

Blood pressure management

The importance of careful blood pressure monitoring in respect of maintaining cerebral perfusion has already been alluded to. Occasionally, it may be necessary to manipulate the blood pressure during an interventional procedure, either raising it to improve collateral vertebral blood flow, or lowering it to test cerebrovascular reserve, or to slow cerebral flow prior to glue injection.

During acute arterial occlusion or vasospasm, increasing systemic blood pressure may improve collateral cerebral blood flow to otherwise ischaemic areas, via the circle of Willis and other collateral pathways (e.g. the leptomeningeal pathways). IV phenylephrine is typically used, to increase BP by perhaps 30% above baseline. The risks of causing haemorrhage must always be balanced against the benefits of improving perfusion, but in acute ischaemic states, raising the blood pressure is usually advantageous.

The primary indication for induced hypotension is to slow flow in the feeding artery to an AVM prior to glue injection. It may sometimes be used in an awake patient to test cerebrovascular reserve before carotid artery occlusion, or in the presence of an unsecured or incompletely treated aneurysm. A variety of agents has been used: labetalol is commonly employed by intermittent bolus or infusion. IV adenosine has been used to achieve a transient cardiac pause and flow arrest.

Management of intraoperative catastrophes

The anaesthetist must be alert to the constant possibility of a sudden crisis during the procedure, usually either haemorrhage or vascular occlusion.

It is obvious that the primary goals are to maintain oxygenation and ventilation, and to maintain effective communication with the interventionist in respect of the likely underlying problem and the appropriate action.

In an awake or sedated patient, haemorrhage will usually produce headache, nausea, vomiting, seizures, or, in some cases, sudden loss of consciousness. In the anaesthetized patient, a Cushing's response may ensue (bradycardia and hypertension), but often the only clue to developing haemorrhage will be contrast extravasation.

The usual response will be to reverse heparin therapy with protamine (1mg for each 100 units of the initial heparin dose that produced therapeutic anticoagulation). Blood pressure should be lowered to pre-bleed values. An attempt will usually be made to seal the rupture site endovascularly. The patient will require an urgent CT scan, and will sometimes proceed to external ventricular drain (EVD) insertion or craniotomy.

In cases of vascular occlusion, the aim is to increase cerebral perfusion by blood pressure augmentation. Thrombolytic therapy may be administered locally via the endovascular catheter.

Specific neuroradiology procedures

Cerebral aneurysms

These are present in 1.5–8% of the population, and are multiple in 20% of cases. Those with a neck diameter <4mm are suitable for endovascular occlusion, but improvements in stent technology now allow for more complex lesions to be considered. Data from the International Subarachnoid Aneurysm Trial (ISAT) report a better outcome in patients undergoing coiling compared to surgical clipping.

Arteriovenous malformations

These are complex lesions with abnormal feeding and draining vessels, and patients may present with subarachnoid haemorrhage (SAH), seizures, or focal neurological deficits. During embolization, BP should be lowered to reduce flow and allow time for the embolic material to set.

Carotid artery stenting

The SAPPHIRE (Stenting and angioplasty with protection in patients at high risk for endarterectomy) trial compared carotid artery stenting with surgical endarterectomy. Stenting is of comparable efficacy, and although performed under LA, experienced anaesthetic input is required to deal with potential problems such as bradycardia during stent manipulation. Postoperatively, restoration of blood flow to a chronically ischaemic vascular bed may overwhelm normal autoregulatory capacity (entering the 'breakthrough zone,' see Fig. 22.2), resulting in oedema or even haemorrhage. Tight control of blood pressure is essential, with continued high-dependency care for patients judged to be at risk.

Post-procedure management

The patient must be monitored in an appropriate setting during the immediate postoperative period to observe for signs of haemodynamic instability or neurological deterioration.

Further reading

Dorairaj IL & Hancock SM (2008). Anaesthesia for interventional neuroradiology. *CEACCP*, 8(3):86–9.

Lee CZ & Young WL (2012). Anesthesia for endovascular neurosurgery and interventional neuroradiology. *Anesthesiol Clin*, 30:127–47.

Schulenburg E & Matta B (2011). Anaesthesia for interventional neuroradiology. *Curr Opin Anesthesiol*, 24:426–32.

Varma MK, Price K, Jayakrishnan, V, *et al*. (2007). Anaesthetic considerations for interventional neuroradiology. *Br J Anaesth*, 99(1):75–85.

22.6 Anaesthetic implications of pituitary disease

Considerations pertinent to the perioperative care of patients undergoing pituitary surgery should include factors related to the anatomical site and size of the lesion, and its endocrine function.

Anatomy

The pituitary gland lies within the pituitary fossa, (the 'sella turcica') a depression in the skull base lined with dura mater. At its lateral margins lie the cavernous sinuses containing the carotid arteries and cranial nerves III, IV, and VI. The pituitary stalk enters the roof of the pituitary fossa (Fig. 22.3) transmitting hypothalamic control of the anterior pituitary endocrine function, and posterior pituitary hormones formed in the hypothalamus and stored in the posterior pituitary. The sphenoid air sinus forms the floor of the fossa through which the surgeon can gain access to the pituitary.

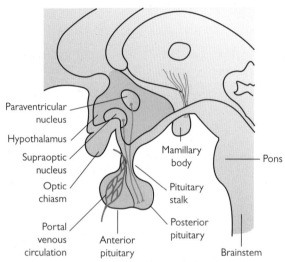

Fig. 22.3 Anatomical relations of the pituitary gland. Reproduced from Catherine Spoors and Kevin Kiff, *Training in Anaesthesia*, 2010, Figure 18.3, Page 445, with permission from Oxford University Press.

The anterior pituitary is composed of specialist secretory cells secreting growth hormone, prolactin, adrenocorticotrophic hormone (ACTH), thyrotropin (TSH), and the gonadotrophs, together with functionally inert cells. See section 5.3.

The posterior pituitary stores and releases oxytocin and vasopressin.

Pathology

Most pituitary tumours arise from the anterior pituitary, and are usually benign, accounting for 10–15% of intracranial neoplasms. The majority are asymptomatic (and can be found in 10–27% of postmortem studies or in about 10% of patients undergoing coincidental cranial imaging). About 75% of symptomatic pituitary tumours are secretory, presenting with hypersecretion of prolactin, growth hormone, or ACTH. TSH secreting tumours are extremely rare, and gonadotroph tumours usually present as inactive adenomas.

25% of pituitary tumours are non-functioning, and present with visual disturbance secondary to pressure on the optic chiasma,

headache secondary to increased ICP, secondary amenorrhoea, or are discovered fortuitously.

Macro-adenomas (functioning or non-functioning) may cause failure of anterior and/or posterior pituitary function due to direct pressure, or pressure on the pituitary stalk.

Secretory tumours: anaesthetic implications

Prolactin-secreting tumours account for more than half of functioning pituitary tumours. Prolactin hypersecretion has no specific anaesthetic implications, but first-line treatment may include a dopamine antagonist (e.g. bromocriptine).

Excess growth hormone produces acromegaly in adults, usually with insidious onset and characterized by increased soft tissue growth. Acromegaly is associated with difficult intubation secondary to enlargement of the tongue and jaw. The pharyngeal and laryngeal tissues, vocal cords and peri-epiglottic folds may be thickened and enlarged, and there may be a reduction in the size of the laryngeal aperture. Sleep apnoea may result from these changes.

Despite these upper airway effects, bag–valve–mask ventilation is usually straightforward although a large oropharyngeal airway may be required. Tracheal intubation can usually be accomplished with a long-bladed laryngoscope and a gum-elastic bougie, but difficult intubation equipment should be available to hand. Fibreoptic intubation is rarely necessary.

Cardiovascular effects of acromegaly may include hypertension, cardiomegaly, and impaired left ventricular function. A careful history and examination of the electrocardiograph are mandatory.

Impaired glucose tolerance or overt diabetes may result from the excess circulating growth hormone. Plasma glucose should be checked regularly in the perioperative period.

ACTH-secreting tumours account for only 4% of functioning pituitary adenomas, mostly in women, mostly micro-adenomas. High circulating levels of cortisol from a pituitary adenoma cause Cushing's disease characterized by the effects listed in Box 22.4.

Box 22.4 Typical features of Cushing's disease

- Centripetal redistribution of body fat
- Proximal myopathy
- Osteoporosis which may lead to vertebral collapse
- Easy bruising, fragile skin, purple striae
- Impaired glucose tolerance/diabetes
- Hypertension, left-ventricular hypertrophy
- Hypernatraemia/hypokalaemia/alkalosis
- GI reflux
- Renal calculi
- Sleep apnoea.

Non-secretory tumours

Hormone replacement therapy should be continued into the operative period.

General perioperative considerations in pituitary surgery

In addition to considerations pertinent to the endocrine function the anaesthetist should establish preoperatively the size and extension of the tumour, and the surgical approach which is planned.

The trans-sphenoidal route is preferred for all but the largest of tumours. Supra-sellar extension may require insertion of a lumbar drain, through which 10mL aliquots of normal saline can be administered in order to produce prolapse of the supra-sellar component of the tumour into the surgical field.

Tumours may erode in to the cavernous sinus to surround the carotid arteries. On those rare occasions where carotid puncture occurs during the surgery, haemorrhage may be brisk, but is usually controllable by packing and controlled hypotension.

Mass effects are more commonly caused by non-functioning macro-adenomas (>1cm diameter). Compression of the optic chiasm characteristically results in a bitemporal hemianopia. Large tumours may also impede the circulation of cerebrospinal fluid with hydrocephalus and raised intracranial pressure, and cause endocrine failure of the adjacent gland.

Induction and set-up

Trans-sphenoidal surgery is carried out with the patient in the supine position, with slight head-up tilt. The head may be turned slightly towards the surgeon. For the anaesthetist access to the patient during surgery is very limited.

Airway management should include the insertion of a reinforced endotracheal tube and a throat pack, secured carefully but allowing unimpeded surgical access to the nose (for the endonasal approach) or upper lip (for the sublabial approach).

Preparation of the nasal mucosa with a vasoconstricting agent is essential. Mixtures of cocaine and adrenaline (e.g. Moffett's solution) are effective, but carry a risk of tachyarrhythmias and myocardial infarction, so should be used with caution especially in the presence of ischaemic heart disease. It is vital to avoid cardiac irritant anaesthetic agents, hypercapnia, or endogenous surges of catecholamines if such solutions are used.

Neuromuscular blockade should be confirmed with a nerve stimulator, and controlled ventilation to normocapnia should be established.

Insertion of an arterial cannula for intra-arterial pressure monitoring is routine, and large-bore peripheral venous cannulation is prudent.

Short-acting agents are preferred. There are periods of intense surgical stimulation during the trans-sphenoidal access to the pituitary fossa. Short-acting opioids such as remifentanil or alfentanil allow maintenance of stable conditions throughout surgery and rapid emergence at the end.

Prophylactic antibiotics are advisable because it is almost impossible to achieve a sterile field in the endonasal route.

Careful protection of the eyes is necessary to ensure that cleaning solution does not run up the nasolabial fold in to the eye, and to limit the risk of inadvertent pressure upon the eye by surgical assistants.

Monitoring

Routine monitoring should include intra-arterial blood pressure monitoring. Manipulation around the optic nerves may provoke intense bradycardia, the risk of puncture of the carotid arteries is always present, and in steep head-up position the potential for air embolism should be considered.

Emergence

Spontaneous respiration must be established prior to extubation because bag–valve–mask ventilation cannot be safely applied in the presence of a transnasal route to the pituitary fossa and the potential for pneumocephalus, or the possible presence of blood and mucus in the oropharynx/nasal passages. Postoperative CPAP is contraindicated for the same reason, increasing the challenge posed by sleep apnoea.

It is essential to carefully remove the throat pack and apply gentle pharyngeal suction under direct vision prior to extubation, to avoid the risk of aspiration of blood, mucus, or debris which may have fallen into the nasopharynx during surgery.

A smooth and rapid emergence is preferable, with early return of laryngeal and pharyngeal reflexes. Short-acting agents are therefore optimal, but pre-emptive analgesia should be administered to ensure that cardiovascular stability is maintained in to the recovery room.

Laryngeal and pharyngeal reflexes should be established before the patient is returned to the recovery room, where slight head-up posture and careful analgesia may help to reduce the risk of postoperative haemorrhage or CSF leak.

Patients often find the presence of nasal packs distressing, and may need to be encouraged to breathe through the mouth.

Postoperative care

Careful attention should be paid to fluid and hormone replacement, glucose homeostasis, analgesia, and monitoring for complications. It is safest to assume that all patients require cortisol replacement in the short term pending a thorough endocrine review.

Diabetes insipidus should be suspected if the patient is passing >250mL of dilute urine per hour for 4 consecutive hours associated with hypernatraemia.

Inappropriate antidiuretic hormone secretion (SIADH) and cerebral salt wasting are rarely the result of pituitary surgery. More commonly hyponatraemia is secondary to injudicious fluid management or over-enthusiastic administration of desmopressin (DDAVP) in suspected diabetes insipidus.

Further reading

Benjamin E, Wong DKK, & Choa D (2004). Moffett's solution: a review of the evidence and scientific basis for the topical preparation of the nose. *Clin Otolaryngol*, 29:582–7.

Menon R, Murphy PG, & Lindley AM (2011). Anaesthesia and pituitary disease. *CEACCP*, 11(4):133–7.

Moffett AJ (1941). Postural instillation: a method of inducing local anaesthesia in the nose. *J Laryngol Otol*, 56:429–36.

Smith M & Hirsch NP (2000). Pituitary disease and anaesthesia. *Br J Anaesth*, 85(1):3–14.

22.7 Anaesthesia for trigeminal neuralgia

Trigeminal neuralgia is characterized by paroxysms of severe facial pain within the area of the sensory distribution of the trigeminal nerve. The annual incidence is 5–10 per 100 000, and it is slightly more common in females. The condition becomes more frequent after middle age.

Clinical presentation

The diagnosis remains very much a clinical one, based on a history of sudden shooting episodes of unilateral facial pain, typically lancinating or electric in quality. These are separated by pain-free intervals, although some patients report a more sustained aching or burning sensation in addition to the acute attacks.

Daily activities such as talking, eating, or shaving may produce unbearable pain, and attacks are often provoked by a cold wind.

The maxillary (V_2) and mandibular (V_3) divisions are affected with equal frequency: symptoms isolated to the ophthalmic division (V_1) are rare, accounting for only 4% of total cases.

Summary of trigeminal nerve anatomy

Amongst cranial nerves, the anatomy of the trigeminal nerve is complex (Fig. 22.4). It has a large sensory and small motor root, and three divisions. It provides sensation to most of the face and scalp in addition to the oral mucosa and anterior two thirds of the tongue. Its motor component serves the muscles of mastication.

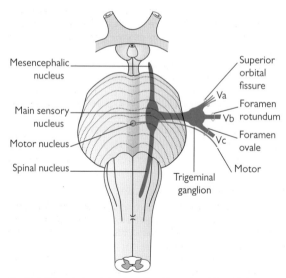

Fig. 22.4 Trigeminal nuclei and ganglion. Reproduced from Catherine Spoors and Kevin Kiff, *Training in Anaesthesia*, 2010, Figure 7.7, page 145, with permission from Oxford University Press.

The *motor nucleus* is situated in the upper pons, beneath the floor of the 4th ventricle.

The *sensory nucleus* is in three parts:

- *Mesencephalic nucleus*: resides in the central grey matter of the midbrain and is concerned with proprioception.
- *Superior (or principal) sensory nucleus*: lateral to the motor nucleus: mediates touch.
- *Nucleus of the spinal tract*: runs caudally from the principal sensory nucleus and transmits pain and temperature.

Central fibres relaying from each sensory nucleus decussate, then ascend in the trigeminal leminiscus to the lateral thalamus, thence to the sensory cortex.

The two *roots* of the trigeminal nerve emerge from the ventro-lateral aspect of the upper pons:

- The larger *lateral root* is sensory.
- The smaller *medial root* is motor.

After a course of about 1cm, the sensory root swells into the trigeminal (or Gasserian) ganglion, which is equivalent to the dorsal root ganglion of a spinal nerve. It lies within a pocket of dura in a hollow near the apex of the petrous temporal bone.

The three divisions of the trigeminal nerve, ophthalmic (V_1), maxillary (V_2), and mandibular (V_3) pass from the ganglion to exit the skull respectively through the superior orbital fissure, foramen rotundum and foramen ovale. The first two divisions are purely sensory; the mandibular division has both motor and sensory components. The divisions are illustrated in Fig. 22.5.

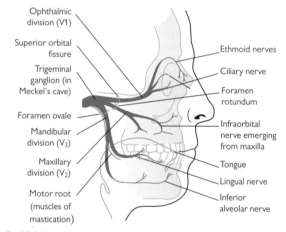

Fig. 22.5 Divisions of the trigeminal nerve. Reproduced from Catherine Spoors and Kevin Kiff, *Training in Anaesthesia*, 2010, Figure 7.8, page 145, with permission from Oxford University Press.

Aetiology and pathogenesis of trigeminal neuralgia

The evidence suggests that a major causative factor in many cases of trigeminal neuralgia is *nerve root compression* by a blood vessel at or near the dorsal root entry zone in the pons. Several observations are taken to support this:

- Observations from both MRI and surgery consistently show an aberrant blood vessel loop (usually an artery, less commonly a vein) in contact with the nerve root (80–90% of cases).
- Intraoperative recordings show immediate improvements in nerve conduction following decompression, and most patients wake up pain free.
- Most patients gain long-term relief when the compression is eliminated.

As a consequence of ageing, intracranial vessels become elongated, forming redundant loops that lead to increased neurovascular contact within the compactness of the posterior fossa. Pulsatile vascular indentation of the trigeminal root leads to focal demyelination. The demyelinated nerve fibres may then generate ectopic impulses, either spontaneously, or in response to normally innocuous afferent impulses.

In respect of other aetiologies, there is a well-established association between trigeminal neuralgia and multiple sclerosis (MS). Up to 5% of patients with MS develop trigeminal neuralgia, and a similar proportion of patients with trigeminal neuralgia may be diagnosed with MS. Occasionally, trigeminal neuralgia may be the first manifestation of MS. Such patients are typically younger than most trigeminal neuralgia patients, and the symptoms are more frequently bilateral.

Posterior fossa tumours are found in 2% of patients who present with typical symptoms of trigeminal neuralgia.

Investigations and differential diagnosis

Trigeminal neuralgia is essentially a *clinical* diagnosis. Investigations serve two purposes:
- To clarify the differential diagnosis.
- To exclude identifiable causes (e.g. tumours or AVMs).

Other causes of facial pain are more common than trigeminal neuralgia. Many of these can be distinguished by a careful history and physical examination (see Box 22.5).

Box 22.5 Common differential diagnoses of trigeminal neuralgia symptoms
• Dental infection • Temporomandibular joint pain • Persistent idiopathic ('atypical') facial pain • Migraine • Temporal arteritis.

In 5–10% of cases of trigeminal neuralgia, an identifiable cause is present, such as a tumour, skull base abnormality, MS or AVM, and the threshold for MRI should be relatively low (Box 22.6).

Box 22.6 Indications for MRI in trigeminal neuralgia
• Younger age at presentation. • Atypical clinical features (sensory loss or persistent dull ache between paroxysms). • Patients who respond poorly to initial medical therapy.

Approaches to treatment

Little is known of the natural history of the condition without treatment, since the severity of symptoms is usually sufficient to warrant intervention.

Interventions may be medical or surgical (see Box 22.7).

Box 22.7 Treatment options in trigeminal neuralgia

• Medical therapies:
  • Carbamazepine
  • Other drugs: gabapentin, lamotrigine, baclofen
• Surgical interventions:
  • Ablative procedures
  • Microvascular decompression.

Medical therapies in trigeminal neuralgia

Drug treatments remain the approach of first choice, despite only a small body of evidence from randomized trials.

Carbamazepine remains the drug of first choice, and has a good initial effect in approximately 70–80% of cases, reducing to 50% over the longer term. A range of important side effects may require dose limitation or even cessation of therapy.

Common, and often self-limiting, side effects include drowsiness, nausea, dizziness, ataxia and diplopia. Less common, but potentially more serious reactions include rashes, bone marrow suppression (including aplastic anaemia), hepatotoxicity and the Stevens–Johnson syndrome.

Oxcarbazepine is an analogue of carbamazepine without the potential for bone marrow or hepatic toxicity. Other side effects are similar to those of carbamazepine.

Gabapentin has emerged as a useful alternative to carbamazepine, even as first-line therapy. Although less efficacious, it has the considerable advantage over carbamazepine of a relative lack of significant side effects. It may, therefore, be particularly advantageous in an elderly patient with multiple comorbidities.

Baclofen may be introduced alone or in combination with carbamazepine or gabapentin for recurrent or persistent cases. Common side effects include dizziness, drowsiness, weakness and gastrointestinal discomfort.

Lamotrigine may be tried in patients not responding to other drugs. Side effects again include diplopia, ataxia and dizziness, and, rarely, Stevens–Johnson syndrome.

Surgical interventions

These are usually reserved for patients with debilitating symptoms that have not been controlled with medical therapy.

Ablative procedures

One of the commonest interventions is **percutaneous radiofrequency ablation** (RFA) of the trigeminal (Gasserian) ganglion. Initial pain relief occurs in over 90% of cases, with recurrence rates of 10–25%.

Glycerol injection into the ganglion is slightly less efficacious, and with higher rates of recurrence.

Both procedures carry a small risk of *anaesthesia dolorosa* (persistent facial pain and numbness) for which there is no effective treatment.

Peripheral nerve ablation procedures (e.g. alcohol injection) are reserved for patients whose comorbidities render them unsuitable for other interventions, and are associated with high recurrence rates.

Microvascular decompression (MVD)

MVD of the trigeminal nerve root through a posterior fossa craniotomy carries the highest success rates in respect of both initial response and long-term efficacy. A good outcome is more likely in cases with typical symptoms.

MVD was previously reserved for younger patients, but more recent reports of risks and benefits suggest that carefully selected older patients may also be suitable.

Further reading

Bennetto L, Patel NK, & Fuller G (2007). Trigeminal neuralgia and its management. *BMJ*, 334:201–5.

Cheshire WP (2005). Trigeminal neuralgia: diagnosis and treatment. *Curr Neurol Neurosci Rep*, 5(2):79–85.

Nurmikko TJ & Eldridge PR (2001). Trigeminal neuralgia – pathophysiology, diagnosis and current treatment. *Br J Anaesth*, 87:117–32.

22.8 Recognition and management of the unstable cervical spine

Unstable cervical spine (C-spine) injuries represent a significant diagnostic challenge for all clinicians that if missed or inappropriately managed may result in significant morbidity and mortality. Pertinent issues for any anaesthetist involved in the care of patients with unstable C-spine injuries include recognition, immobilization, potentially difficult airways, pathophysiological consequences of spinal cord injuries, and any associated injuries.

Aetiology

Although the majority of C-spine injuries will be traumatic in origin (Box 22.8), there are a number of potential non-traumatic causes including Down's syndrome, neoplasia, degenerative disease, rheumatoid arthritis, ankylosing spondylitis, infectious processes, and post-laminectomy kyphosis.

C-spine injuries occur in 1.5–3% of all major polytrauma (0.5% in paediatric group) and at least 50% of these injuries are potentially unstable. The age frequency peaks are 15–35 years and >65 years of age and are seen more commonly in males (7:3).

Typical mechanisms of injury include road traffic collision (50–70%), falls (6%-10%), blunt head and neck assault, penetrating neck injuries, and contact sports injuries.

> **Box 22.8** High-risk parameters for C-spine injury: the presence of any one parameter places a patient at >5% risk of a C-spine fracture
>
> - High velocity road traffic collision >35mph
> - Death at scene (road traffic collision)
> - Fall >10ft
> - Cervical spine pain, spasm, deformity, or neurology
> - Significant closed head injury
> - Pelvic or multiple extremity fractures.

Initial assessment and management

The initial management of any patient who has sustained multi-system trauma follows the universal structure set out in the Advanced Trauma Life Support (ATLS) course. The *primary survey* seeks to rapidly identify any life-threatening injuries and aggressively treat in a structured manner. At this stage, a C-spine injury is assumed to be present and the aim is simply to stabilize the C-spine to limit the risk of a secondary spinal cord injury (SCI). The *secondary survey* is made up of a focused SAMPLE (Signs & symptoms, Allergies, Medications, Pertinent past medical history, Last oral intake, Events leading to the illness or injury) history and detailed examination and appropriate radiological investigations (see Chapter 21).

Airway with C-spine immobilization

Airway interventions may be required as an emergency during the primary survey (for threatened/actual airway obstruction, inadequate oxygenation/ventilation, or as part of the management of a traumatic brain injury) or later during induction of anaesthesia for surgical management of other injuries. Until the C-spine has been 'cleared' and a spinal injury has been excluded, the C-spine must be immobilized at all times, especially during airway manoeuvres. A C-spine is considered to be protected when continuous immobilization of the patient occurs with either the combination of a semi-rigid cervical collar, head blocks and tape/straps or manual in-line stabilization (MILS). Although there will inevitably be some movement of the C-spine during airway manoeuvres and direct laryngoscopy, MILS is now established as the superior and safest technique. MILS and direct laryngoscopy may be electively combined with a gum elastic bougie, which allows inferior laryngoscopic views to be accepted thereby limiting the forces transmitted to the C-spine.

The aim of cervical immobilization is to prevent secondary damage to the spinal cord in unstable injuries. This is vital because a reported 6% of inpatients experience deterioration in neurological symptoms following a C-spine injury. However, a delay in C-spine clearance is not without risk and can contribute to increased patient morbidity due to prolonged immobilization (Box 22.9).

> **Box 22.9** Potential complications of C-spine immobilization
>
> - Difficult laryngoscopy
> - Exacerbation cervical spinal injuries
> - Airway obstruction
> - Increased ICP as well as obstructed access to the neck for central venous access
> - Aspiration risk
> - Risk of deep vein thrombosis
> - May cause significant skin breakdown and decubitus ulcers.

Breathing

The main muscles of inspiration are the diaphragm (C3–C5), the external intercostal muscles (T1–T11), and the accessory muscles. Although expiration is predominantly a passive process, the abdominal muscles (T6–T12) play a vital role for forced expiration and coughing.

Respiratory complications are the most common cause of morbidity and mortality with SCI. The risk of respiratory failure is associated with the level and completeness of the SCI. In a 5-year prospective analysis of 261 SCIs Jackson et al. found that respiratory failure occurred in 40% of individuals with C1–C4 injuries, 23% in C5–C8 injuries, and 9.9% in thoracic-level SCI.

There are few absolute indications for intubation in patients with a SCI (such as apnoea) and the decision to intubate will be based on a number of factors (see Box 22.10). When the clinical status of the patient allows, aggressive physiotherapy and non-invasive ventilation should be utilized prior to a decision to intubate, thus hopefully avoiding unnecessary invasive ventilation.

> **Box 22.10** Indications for intubation in SCIs
>
> - Complete C-spine injuries, especially C5 and above, at the first sign of respiratory distress.
> - Rising $PaCO_2$ and falling PaO_2.
> - Forced vital capacities <15mL/kg ideal body weight.
> - Increasing oxygen requirements and increasing respiratory rate with low tidal volumes.
> - Signs of atelectasis.
> - Failure to clear secretions.
> - Presence of other injuries, e.g. head and chest injuries.

Circulation

The immediate cardiovascular response to a SCI is that of massive sympathetic stimulation and reflex parasympathetic activity that usually lasts for 3–4min. After this period, the loss of descending sympathetic outflow below the cord transection level results in loss of vasomotor tone, vasodilatation, and severe hypotension, which may last up to 8 weeks. This so-called 'neurogenic shock' may be associated with a bradycardia if the injury level falls above T1–T4. The explanation for this bradycardia is an interruption of the cardioacceleratory fibres and hence sympathetic afference coupled with unopposed vagal activity. Neurogenic shock is a diagnosis of exclusion and all other causes for hypotension (particularly bleeding and hypovolaemia) should be sought first. Initial management should be targeted at fluid resuscitation until pre-load/stroke volume responsiveness is lost. Refractory hypotension and bradycardia may necessitate inotropic and chronotropic support. The end point for resuscitation in SCIs remains controversial, but there is some evidence that ongoing ischaemia and secondary SCI is successfully treated by maintaining a MAP >90mmHg for up to 7 days.

Autonomic dysreflexia is a late manifestation which occurs weeks to months after a SCI usually above T10, which is characterized by the occurrence of paroxysmal hypertension and bradycardia in response to a stimulus occurring below the level of the spinal cord injury.

Disability
10% of patients with C-spine injuries will have a second, non-contiguous vertebral column fracture. So in any trauma patient with a high-risk mechanism of injury, if a C-spine injury is found it is imperative to actively search for and delineate any associated injuries.

Search for a therapeutic intervention in SCI patients has been an area of much interest and controversy: however, thus far results have been disappointing. The use of methylprednisolone in the treatment of acute SCI is not proven as a standard of care. In the over 60s, it is associated with increased morbidity as a result of pneumonia and sepsis. Targeted temperature management (therapeutic hypothermia) is gaining some popularity but as yet there are no randomized control trials to suggest any benefit.

Exposure
Other considerations will be the maintenance of an adequate haemoglobin and glycaemic control. Unfortunately the absolute level and range for these are not well defined and will be governed frequently by local policy.

Secondary survey

SAMPLE history and examination
A full history and documentation of the main presenting neurological symptoms and deficits should be undertaken. Any signs or symptoms must be assumed to indicate a potentially unstable injury and further examination should be avoided until imaging is complete.

Clearance and radiological investigation of C-spine injuries
Timely yet complete examination of the cervical spine is a key component of the secondary survey. Rigid C-spine collars and immobilization should be removed as soon as feasibly possible. The mechanism of injury is vital in assessing the likelihood of a C-spine injury. In penetrating trauma to the neck and head, C-spine immobilization is not necessary unless a direct C-spine injury is suggested by the trajectory.

The Eastern Association of the Surgery for Trauma (EAST) 2009 guidelines suggest that clinical assessment can safely exclude spinal injury. If all criteria are fulfilled and there is no bruising, deformity, midline tenderness, and a pain-free range of movement the C-spine can be cleared clinically (Box 22.11). Those patients that do not fit the criteria should be imaged.

Box 22.11 Criteria to be fulfilled for imaging not to be performed

- Fully alert with no neurological deficit
- No drugs or alcohol
- No neck pain/mid-line tenderness
- No abnormal neurology
- No significant distracting injury.

The use of whole-body CT in early trauma care has significantly increased the probability of survival in patients with polytrauma. Current evidence suggests the principal imaging modality to evaluate the presence of a C-spine injury should be an axial CT from C0 to T1, with sagittal and coronal reconstructions. Plain radiography has a low sensitivity for identifying injuries and should not be used to clear the C-spine.

Clearance of the C-spine in the unconscious trauma patients has been a contentious issue for many years and the relative paucity of good evidence has resulted in uncertain guidance. However, the increasing availability of multi detector CT and MRI has helped move trauma care forward. In patients who are unconscious, have a high-risk mechanism/injury, or in those who are undergoing CT to evaluate other injuries, a CT of the C-spine should be performed. A normal CT in an unconscious trauma patient has a negative predictive value approaching 100%.

Patients with focal neurological signs, equivocal CT, evidence of cord or disc injury, and patients whose surgery requires preoperative cord assessment should be imaged with MRI. The use of MRI in unstable polytrauma may be limited because of the difficulties in monitoring patients, the remote site and the prolonged scan/transfer times.

Ongoing management and anaesthesia

Neuromuscular blockade
Suxamethonium is safe to use in the first 3 days and after 9 months following a SCI. During the intervening period the risk of hyperkalaemia due to denervation and up-regulation of nicotinic acetylcholine receptors precludes its use.

Airway management options
Despite the increased incidence of difficult intubation and risk of C-spine movement with cricoid pressure, if deemed necessary and the assistant is appropriately trained, bimanual cricoid pressure can be applied safely.

Thromboembolic complications
Patients with a SCI are high risk for developing thromboembolic complications; the incidence in untreated patients could be >40%. Prophylaxis should be reviewed regularly and all the means of prevention should be considered.

Others
Other issues include stress ulceration, upper gastrointestinal bleeding, ileus, and occult peritonitis. Such sequelae should be anticipated and appropriate management instigated.

Further reading
Como JJ, Diaz JJ, Dunham CM, *et al.* (2009). Practice management guidelines for identification of cervical spine injuries following trauma: update from the eastern association for the surgery of trauma practice management guidelines committee. *J Trauma*, 67(3):651–9.

22.9 Recognition and management of air embolism

Vascular gas embolism is uncommon but is a mainly iatrogenic and potentially life-threatening event. It is defined as the entrainment of air (or gas) into the vasculature producing systemic effects. The majority are venous air emboli although arterial and paradoxical emboli can also occur. The gas in question may be air, carbon dioxide, or nitrous oxide. The morbidity and mortality can be substantial and is related to the amount and rate of air entrainment. A fatal dose can easily be administered through a 14G cannula (300–500mL) and 43% of survivors have neurological sequelae at time of ICU discharge.

Pathophysiology

Any air entering the venous system is carried to the right atrium and subsequently the right ventricle.

Air lock
This is seen with a large bolus of air (5mL/kg). Air, unlike blood, is compressible and so causes obstruction to right ventricular ejection resulting in rapid cardiovascular collapse.

Arteriolar obstruction
Slower infusions of air get trapped at the level of the pulmonary arterioles directly impeding flow. This results in pulmonary hypertension and right heart failure.

Microemboli
Very slow infusions of air allow microbubbles to enter the pulmonary circulation. In addition to obstructing flow, they cause an inflammatory response in the vessel wall. The resultant structural damage to the vessel leads to pulmonary oedema, bronchoconstriction, and V/Q mismatching.

Transpulmonary shunting
This is seen when sufficient pressure builds up on the right side of the heart to push the gas through the pulmonary circulation to the left atrium. A paradoxical air embolism results, without a patent foramen ovale (PFO).

Arterial and paradoxical air emboli cause end-organ damage in the cerebral and cardiac circulations.

Aetiology

For a venous air embolism to occur, there are generally three common factors:

1. Source of gas.
2. Connection of gas to the venous system.
3. Pressure gradient causing ingress of gas into the venous system.

However, gas may also enter via the epidural space and tissue planes.

At-risk surgical procedures
The highest risk procedures (see Box 22.12) involve:
- Elevated position of the head relative to the heart.
- Numerous large, non-compressed, venous channels in the surgical field.

Box 22.12 At-risk procedures for air embolism

- Neurosurgical (incidence 10–80%):
  - Posterior fossa surgery
  - Sitting position craniotomies
  - Cervical laminectomy
- Head and neck:
  - Radical neck dissection
  - Thyroidectomy
- Cardiovascular:
  - Cardiac surgery
  - Cardiopulmonary bypass
  - Angiography
  - Carotid endarterectomy
- Orthopaedics:
  - Arthroscopy (esp. shoulder)
  - Total hip arthroplasty
- Obstetrics:
  - Caesarean section
  - Termination of pregnancy
  - Removal of placenta
- General/urology:
  - Laparoscopic procedures
  - Prostatectomy
  - Endoscopy
- Non-surgical:
  - Central venous catheterization
  - Positive pressure ventilation
  - Hydrogen peroxide
  - Thoracocentesis
  - Intra-aortic balloon rupture
  - Rapid infusor systems.

Presentation

A large air embolus will present with cardiovascular collapse, smaller emboli can present with a number of symptoms and signs (see Box 22.13).

Box 22.13 Signs of air embolism

Cardiovascular
- Chest pain
- Tachyarrhythmias
- ECG changes:
  - Right heart strain
  - ST-T changes
  - Myocardial ischaemia
- Decreased blood pressure
- Decreased cardiac output
- Increased pulmonary artery pressure
- Increased central venous pressure
- 'Mill-wheel' murmur.

(Continued)

Box 22.13 (Continued)

Pulmonary
- Acute dyspnoea and tachypnoea
- Coughing
- Wheeze
- Decreased ETCO$_2$
- Decreased PaO$_2$ and SaO$_2$
- Increased PaCO$_2$
- Increased PAP.

CNS
- Sense of impending doom
- Altered mental state
- Coma.

Detection

Mainly a clinical diagnosis and should be considered in the following circumstances:
- Any unexplained hypotension or decrease in ETCO$_2$ intraoperatively in the presence of surgical risk factors.
- Patients who complain of shortness of breath during or slightly after central venous catheter insertion.
- Patients undergoing LSCS with hypotension and hypoxia not explained by hypovolaemia alone.

Other methods of detection

Transoesophageal echocardiography

The most sensitive monitoring device and can detect as little as 0.02mL/kg of air. It can also show evidence of right heart failure. It is, however, invasive and requires expertise to interpret, which limit its use.

Precordial Doppler ultrasound

The most sensitive non-invasive monitor and can detect 0.05mL/kg of air. The probe is placed along the right heart border and air is picked up as a change in sound. Limitations of this modality include sound artefacts, problems in obesity, and position other than supine.

End-tidal carbon dioxide

The increase in physiological dead space and worsening of V/Q matching causes a fall in end-tidal CO$_2$. This is, however, non-specific, with similar findings in PE, cardiac arrest, and massive blood loss. It is the most practical monitor in most situations, being readily available.

Electrocardiography

The ECG typically shows a sinus tachycardia, right heart strain with peaked P waves, ST and T wave changes, or acute myocardial infarction.

Radiological investigations

CXR will usually be normal. CT may detect large air emboli in the central venous system, right ventricle, or pulmonary artery. Asymptomatic emboli can be found in 10–25% of CT scans if carefully sought.

Pulmonary angiography may also be normal since the air may be reabsorbed. Positive scans may reveal corkscrewing, tapering and delayed vessel emptying in the affected lung.

End-tidal nitrogen

End-tidal nitrogen (ETN$_2$) is the most sensitive gas detection method for air emboli. Changes occur 30–90sec earlier than changes in CO$_2$. Increased ETN$_2$ is due to an increase in physiological dead space. However, this is not routinely available and cannot be used in the presence of N$_2$O.

The best routine monitor remains a high index of suspicion and vigilance in at-risk situations.

Prevention

Preoperative

Identification of preoperative risks is important to allow appropriate preventative measures and monitoring to be instituted. Ideally, patients known to have a patent foramen ovale (PFO) should not undergo high-risk procedures.

Intraoperative

Reducing the height between the operative site and the right atrium will reduce the pressure gradient between the two. Increasing right atrial and central venous pressures (patient comorbidities permitting) will again reduce the pressure gradient. This can be achieved by IV fluid loading, PEEP, or jugular venous compression. Devices such as G suits or antishock trousers to elevate the venous pressure can also be used.

When inserting central venous catheters, a position should be used that keeps the right atrium above the level of the insertion site (e.g. Trendelenburg for internal jugular catheterization). Hypovolaemia can increase the risk of air embolism further and should be treated prior to catheter placement.

Ensure that all fluid giving sets (including pressure transducers) are free from air bubbles.

Avoidance of nitrous oxide will prevent an air bubble from increasing in size if a gas embolism does occur.

Surgical factors

The venous system should be left open to atmospheric pressure for the shortest time possible and meticulous haemostasis should be ensured to limit the amount of air–vascular interfaces.

Confirmation of correct positioning of needle prior to gas insufflations in laparoscopic surgery, with aspiration of the needle, will avoid intravascular gas insufflation.

Management

The aims are resuscitation of the patient, prevention of further air entry, reduction of the size of the embolism, and to overcome the mechanical obstruction.
- ABC approach and call for help.
- Secure the airway and administer 100% FiO$_2$, commence CPR if indicated. Chest compressions may help to force air out of the pulmonary outflow tract and high FiO$_2$ increases the rate of air reabsorption.
- Flood the operative site with saline and compress the wound edges.
- Eliminate the source of gas if possible (e.g. in laparoscopic surgery).
- Discontinue N$_2$O if using.
- If a central line is in place, it may be possible to aspirate air from the right atrium. Resuscitation should not be delayed to place a central venous catheter if not *in situ*.
- Left lateral decubitus (Durant's manoeuvre) or Trendelenburg positioning to move the air into a position within the right ventricle where it is least likely to obstruct the RV outflow.
- Consider inotropes, cardiopulmonary bypass, or thoracotomy if required/feasible.
- Consider hyperbaric oxygen therapy if stable for transfer.

Further reading

Muth C (2000). Gas embolism. *NEJM*, 342:476–82.

22.10 Principles of anaesthesia for patients with neuromuscular disease

Guillain–Barré syndrome

Guillain-Barré syndrome is an immune-mediated acute demyelinating polyneuropathy that often follows a viral or bacterial illness. Typically, there is an ascending symmetrical weakness from the legs and this may lead to respiratory compromise requiring intubation and ventilation in 15–20% of patients.

Anaesthetic technique

Autonomic instability may be profound; tracheal suctioning may provoke asystole, so invasive monitoring is beneficial.

Depolarizing neuromuscular blockers should be avoided after the first week of illness due to the development of extra-junctional acetylcholine receptors and the risk of severe hyperkalaemia and subsequent cardiac arrest.

There may be increased sensitivity to non-depolarizing neuromuscular blockers, avoid if possible.

Myasthenia gravis

Myasthenia gravis is an autoimmune disease, resulting from the production of IgG antibodies against the post-junctional acetylcholine receptors. These antibodies can be detected in 85–90% of patients.

It may be associated with other autoimmune disorders e.g., thyroid dysfunction and rheumatoid arthritis.

Preoperative

Careful history with evaluation of duration of disease, severity, and extent of bulbar and respiratory muscle involvement is important.

Preoperative lung function tests may be indicated to assess the extent of respiratory involvement and the need for postoperative ventilation.

Optimization with steroids, immunosuppressants, plasma exchange, or IV immunoglobulin may improve the medical status of the myasthenic patient and improve outcome.

Anticholinesterases should be withheld on the morning of surgery. They potentiate vagal responses and may predispose to bradycardias. They also inhibit plasma cholinesterase activity, altering the metabolism of other drugs such as local anaesthetics.

Premedication with sedatives is not recommended due to the risk of severe respiratory depression. Atropine can be given to avoid the risk of vagal potentiation.

Anaesthetic technique

Where possible, regional techniques avoid the majority of problems encountered during general anaesthesia in these patients.

Myasthenic patients have a variable response to muscle relaxants with resistance to depolarizng and sensitivity to non-depolarizing drugs (see section 6.7). If general anaesthesia is required, there are a number of techniques that can be used to avoid neuromuscular blockade.

Deep inhalational anaesthesia usually provides good intubating conditions, as myasthenic patients have a more pronounced response to the muscle relaxant properties of inhalational anaesthetic agents. However, adverse cardiovascular and respiratory side effects can be encountered using this technique.

The use of remifentanil can avoid the need for muscle relaxants to maintain anaesthesia; however, where neuromuscular blockers are required (e.g. for surgical reasons), smaller doses and constant neuromuscular monitoring should be used. Reversal of any neuromuscular block should be avoided due to the risk of potentiating a cholinergic crisis.

Postoperative

Monitor ventilatory function carefully, and sustained respiratory muscle strength should be confirmed prior to extubation. Criteria which may predict the need for postoperative ventilation include:

- Duration of myasthenia gravis for >6 years.
- A history of chronic respiratory disease.
- A dose of pyridostigmine >750mg/day.
- Pre-operative vital capacity of <2.9L.

Pyridostigmine should be restarted, initially at a reduced dose and building up as required with increasing mobilization.

Post thymectomy it is important to look for surgical complications such as pneumothorax and haemothorax, which may also cause postoperative respiratory failure.

Myasthenic syndromes

Eaton–Lambert syndrome

In contrast to myasthenia gravis, this is an acquired disorder of the motor nerve terminal in which quantal release of acetylcholine is reduced. Dysautonomia can also occur due to reduced ACh release at cholinergic sites leading to dry mouth, double vision, constipation, and urinary hesitancy.

There is an improvement in muscle strength with exercise, which is not readily reversed with acetylcholinesterase.

Anaesthetic technique

Patients are sensitive to both depolarizing and non-depolarizing neuromuscular blockers, but anticholinesterases can be safely given for reversal of blockade. Due to the generalized lack of acetylcholine, consider invasive monitoring in case of autonomic instability.

Congenital myasthenic syndromes

These are due to genetic defects within the neuromuscular junction itself and cause problems with acetylcholine formation, release or binding to the receptor. The anaesthetic management is as for myasthenia gravis.

Dystrophia myotonica

The most common of the myotonic syndromes with a prevalence of 2–5 in 100 000. It is inherited in an autosomal dominant manner with the responsible gene on the long arm of chromosome 19.

The main features of this multisystem disorder are myotonia (persistent muscle contraction after muscle stimulation), cataracts, distal muscle weakness, frontal baldness, cardiac conduction abnormalities, cardiomyopathy, central obstructive sleep apnoea, and respiratory muscle weakness.

A malignant hyperthermia-type syndrome does not occur in dystrophia myotonica, but is seen in myotonia congenita. Rhabdomyolysis, however, can occur with sustained myotonia and should be actively looked for.

Preoperative

Management and optimization of extramuscular manifestations of dystrophia myotonica are important. Cardiology input with consideration of pacing and optimization of cardiac medications may be considered.

A preoperative ECG should be performed.

Anaesthetic technique

It is important to avoid myotonia during anaesthesia, excessive muscle contraction can cause rhabdomyolysis and its associated complications. General principles are avoidance of drugs and factors which precipitate myotonia. This means maintenance of normothermia to avoid shivering, and avoidance of anticholinesterases, opioids, potassium, and propranolol.

There is a greatly increased risk of aspiration, premedication with prokinetic and antacid and a modified rapid sequence induction may be required. Non-depolarizing neuromuscular blocking agents are generally safe but suxamethonium should be avoided. Propofol has been implicated in causing myotonia, but is generally used safely. Consider the use of rocuronium to allow for the use of sugammadex for reversal, which has been described in case reports.

Myotonic contraction secondary to stimulation during surgical manipulation or diathermy use can be difficult to control. If initial attempts to minimize this with neuromuscular block, peripheral nerve blockade, or regional blockade do not work, phenytoin or procainamide can be considered in order to stabilize muscle membranes.

Postoperative

Maintain normothermia and avoid postoperative shivering.

Muscular dystrophy

Duchenne muscular dystrophy (DMD)

DMD is the commonest childhood muscular dystrophy with an incidence of 1 in 3500. It is an X-linked recessive disorder causing a lack of dystrophin. It presents in childhood with wasting and weakness of the proximal muscles. Affected males are often wheelchair bound with contractures, scoliosis with restrictive lung function deficits, and cardiomyopathy.

Becker's muscular dystrophy

In this form of muscular dystrophy, the dystrophin gene is only partially absent and so symptoms are milder than in DMD. It often presents in the teenage years and has a much more protracted course than DMD. Like DMD, patients suffer with restrictive lung deficits and cardiomyopathy.

Anaesthetic technique

There are serious risks of perioperative respiratory insufficiency and cardiac dysfunction. Preoperative assessment with ECG, ECHO, and lung function tests will help to guide optimization and the need for postoperative respiratory support.

Due to smooth muscle and platelet dysfunction, blood loss may be increased; consider methods such as hypotensive anaesthesia or cell salvage in order to minimize this loss. Hypovolaemia should be avoided due to a fixed cardiac output state due to non-compliant ventricles. Consider invasive monitoring.

Depolarizing neuromuscular blockers should be avoided due to development of extra-junctional receptors and the associated risk of hyperkalaemia. Rhabdomyolysis can also occur.

Non-depolarizing neuromuscular blocker use should be kept to a minimum: there is a delay in onset and offset which can lead to a prolonged block. Avoid where possible by using remifentanil if GA is required or regional techniques. Central neuraxial blockade may be technically difficult and should be used with extreme caution due to a fixed cardiac output state.

Inhalational anaesthetics have been implicated in causing rhabdomyolysis due to their effects on calcium. It may not be a true malignant hyperthermia but inhalational anaesthetics should be used with extreme caution. Consider TIVA as an alternative.

Paraplegia/chronic spinal cord damage

May be caused by trauma, vascular insult or compressive lesions. The extent of respiratory involvement depends on the level of the lesion:

- T1–T7 causes partial intercostal nerve paralysis, resulting in a poor cough and impaired chest movement.
- C5–C8 causes complete intercostal nerve paralysis but preserves diaphragm function, resulting in an ineffective cough, use of accessory muscles and a paradoxical respiratory pattern.
- C3–C5 causes partial paralysis of the diaphragm resulting in the same respiratory issues as in a C5–C8 lesion but usually requiring assisted ventilation.
- C3 or above causes denervation of the diaphragm and respiratory failure requiring full ventilation.

Anaesthetic technique

Patients may be at greater risk of aspiration and require appropriate premedication.

Postoperatively, increased respiratory support will often be necessary. Poor cough causes sputum retention and an increased risk of respiratory failure.

Previous spinal fixations may cause airway difficulties: careful airway assessment and planning with consideration of the need for awake fibreoptic intubation is needed.

Suxamethonium is contraindicated beyond the first few weeks of injury due to the development of extra-junctional acetylcholine receptors and the risk of causing hyperkalaemic cardiac arrest.

Autonomic disturbance may persist, causing hypotension and bradycardia and so consider invasive monitoring.

Patients may have associated problems with poor nutritional status and fluid balance, pressure ulcers may be present and if not, regular turning and meticulous care with pressure areas will prevent them forming.

22.11 Neurocritical care of traumatic brain injury

Traumatic brain injury (TBI) is responsible for 1% of all adult deaths in the UK. It is also a huge socioeconomic problem as it affects mainly adults in their most productive years and significantly contributes to the prevalence of long-term disability. Approximately 3500 patients per annum are admitted to a critical care unit following a head injury.

Brain injury

Severe TBI is defined as a post-resuscitation GCS score of ≤8. Primary brain injury is the direct result of mechanical trauma applied at the moment of impact and causes irreversible cell damage from physical disruption of neurons and axons. Primary brain injury includes pathologies such as extradural haematoma, subdural haematoma, traumatic subarachnoid haemorrhage, diffuse axonal injury, and haemorrhagic contusions and lacerations. These cannot be treated by medical intervention, but early surgical evacuation of expanding intracranial mass lesions reduces morbidity and mortality.

Secondary brain injury begins from the moment of primary traumatic injury and develops during the subsequent minutes, hours, and days, causing further neuronal damage and worsening of the ultimate neurological deficit. It represents additional insults to the neuronal tissue and is essentially ischaemic in nature. Secondary brain injury occurs as a result of a variety of intracranial and extracranial causes that can be influenced by clinicians throughout its course, particularly poor perfusion and tissue hypoxia.

Cerebral ischaemia is the dominant factor determining neurological outcome after severe TBI. It occurs when blood flow falls below a critical level, causing the delivery of oxygen and essential substrates to be insufficient for the brain's metabolic needs. Profound changes in cerebral blood flow (CBF) occur after TBI, and up to one-third of patients sustain significant cerebral hypoperfusion in the first few hours after injury.

Immediate resuscitation

Resuscitation according to the mantra of airway (with C-spine stabilization), breathing, and circulation followed by definitive surgical intervention of the primary brain injury within 4h of insult will usually be followed by a period in a critical care unit. Definitive diagnosis and resuscitation must occur simultaneously in order to avoid delay. Avoiding hypotension and hypoxaemia during resuscitation is crucial to a favourable outcome.

Ongoing critical care management

The essence of critical care management is the ongoing maintenance of adequate brain perfusion and avoidance of secondary brain injury. Specialist neurocritical care with ICP and CPP-guided therapy should be available for all patients with severe TBI and is likely to improve outcome.

Consensus guidelines for all stages of the management of patients after severe TBI have been published and those relevant to the critically ill patient are summarized as follows:

Sedation and analgesia
Sedation is an essential part of the management of severe TBI. Barbiturates were previously the mainstay of treatment; however, propofol is now the drug of choice because its favourable pharmacological profile allows easy titration of sedation levels and rapid wake-up. Propofol causes a dose-dependent reduction in cerebral metabolism, CBF, and ICP while maintaining pressure autoregulation and CO_2 reactivity. Barbiturates still have a place in selected patients for the management of refractory intracranial hypertension. Neuromuscular-blocking drugs have no direct effect on ICP but may prevent rises caused by coughing or straining on an endotracheal tube. Their routine use should be discouraged in favour of appropriate sedation with propofol, benzodiazepines (usually midazolam), and analgesia with opioids (such as fentanyl or morphine).

Ventilation
Controlled ventilation combined with adequate sedation is mandatory to maintain arterial blood gas targets. High inspired oxygen concentration and the use of PEEP may be necessary to maintain adequate arterial oxygenation (PaO_2 ≥13.0kPa); however, PEEP >10cmH$_2$O may impair venous drainage and lead to a secondary increase in ICP. Consensus guidelines recommend that $PaCO_2$ should be maintained between 4.5kPa and 5.0kPa to maintain normal CBF.

Hyperventilation was once the cornerstone of ICP control after TBI. A reduction in $PaCO_2$ causes cerebral vasoconstriction and a fall in CBF, cerebral blood volume, and ICP. However, hyperventilation only has short-lived effects on ICP, and empirical and excessive hyperventilation is associated with adverse neurological outcome. Hyperventilation to a $PaCO_2$ below 4.5kPa may be required to control severe intractable intracranial hypertension in patients in whom CO_2 reactivity is maintained; however, this should only be undertaken in conjunction with jugular venous oxygen saturation monitoring to ensure that hyperventilation itself does not precipitate cerebral ischaemia.

Cardiovascular support
Hypotension, MAP <90mmHg, is associated with an adverse neurological outcome and should be avoided. A higher MAP may be necessary to maintain an adequate CPP in the presence of raised ICP. This should be achieved by fluid resuscitation to normovolaemia and administration of a vasopressor as necessary thereafter. There is probably no 'best' fluid for patients with severe TBI although crystalloid and colloid are suitable. Isotonic crystalloids are widely used and 0.9% saline is a scientifically justified choice. Glucose-containing solutions should be avoided because the free water liberated following the metabolism of glucose can worsen cerebral oedema. Hyperglycaemia is associated with poor outcome following severe TBI and blood sugar should be maintained within the normal range.

ICP and CPP control
Conventional approaches to the management of severe TBI have focused on the reduction of ICP in order to prevent secondary brain injury. Although it has not been demonstrated in randomized controlled studies that lowering ICP improves outcome, an ICP >20mmHg is a powerful predictor of poor outcome after TBI and treatment should be initiated if ICP rises to >20mmHg. Over the last decade there has been a shift of emphasis from primary control of ICP to a multifaceted approach of maintenance of CPP, and the importance of maintaining cerebral perfusion and oxygenation throughout the entire management period is now accepted.

$$CPP = MAP - ICP$$

There is general agreement that CPP should be maintained between 50mmHg and 70mmHg by control of MAP and the treatment of intracranial hypertension. The risk:benefit ratio of ICP or CPP directed strategies should be assessed by appropriate monitoring techniques and therapy tailored to each patient individually.

CPP can often be improved by proper positioning of the patients that includes a neutral head position and 30° head-up tilt.

Monitoring of ICP can be via an intracranial catheter or if it has been necessary to insert one, extraventricular drain.

Osmotic therapy

Mannitol, an osmotic diuretic that causes a reduction in intracranial volume, may be used to lower ICP after TBI. A Cochrane review has concluded that 'high-dose' mannitol may be beneficial in the preoperative management of patients with acute intracranial haematomas; however, there is little evidence to justify its empirical and regular use in patients suffering raised ICP as a result of diffuse brain swelling. Under certain circumstances mannitol can cross the blood–brain barrier and cause a reverse osmotic shift, leading to a rise in ICP. Hypertonic saline solutions also have a place in osmotherapy after TBI.

Therapeutic hypothermia

Modest reductions in brain temperature reduce the release of excitatory amino acids, and moderate hypothermia (32–34°C) has been shown to ameliorate axonal damage in animal models. However, a prospective, randomized study of moderate hypothermia in TBI was terminated early because of increased morbidity in patients >45 years of age treated with hypothermia. Notwithstanding, moderate hypothermia remains a treatment option in many neurocritical care units because it is an effective means of reducing ICP. Pyrexia should certainly be avoided at all stages of management because elevations in temperature worsen outcome after TBI.

Surgical intervention

Timely removal of a space-occupying haematoma can be the most effective way to improve CPP and overall outcome in many instances. Sudden changes in neurological state or a rise in ICP may indicate on going intracranial haemorrhage and the need for further surgery should be considered throughout the course of recovery. Imaging is usually necessary to confirm this prior to the decision to proceed to surgery. Decompressive craniectomy involves the removal of a flap of bone to allow the brain to expand and reduce ICP. The long-term benefit of this procedure, however, has not been proven.

Other important management factors

A number of other key factors in the management of severe TBI include appropriate nutrition, maintenance of normal electrolyte values, prophylaxis for DVT (either pharmacological or mechanical), and prevention of systemic infection. Abnormalities of serum sodium may be particularly challenging and must be managed carefully to avoid further harm. Hypernatraemia may be due to diabetes insipidus or dehydration whilst hyponatraemia may be due to SIADH or cerebral salt wasting.

Agitation is common following reduction of sedation and this needs to be dealt with effectively to avoid harm to patients. Some patients may also experience sympathetic storming during the recovery phase and this can be treated with β-blockers or clonidine.

Further reading

Protheroe RT & Gwinnutt CL (2011). Early hospital care of severe traumatic brain injury. *Anaesthesia*, 66(11):1035–47. doi:10.1111/j.1365-2044.2011.06874.x.

Transfer medicine

427

Primary, secondary, and tertiary transfer

Anaesthetists frequently supervise the movement of patients within hospitals (e.g. from the anaesthetic room into the operating theatre or from the emergency department to the radiology suite) or between hospitals (e.g. for specialist treatment). Although the transfer of any patient even over small distances can cause significant complications, these risks and the significance of the potential complications are magnified in critically ill patients.

Transport of patients outside of the hospital environment can be considered to be:

- *Primary:* transfer of the patient from the scene of injury or onset of illness to an initial receiving medical facility, e.g. field hospital or first aid station.
- *Secondary:* transfer of the patient from an initial receiving medical facility to a hospital where higher level care can be provided.
- *Tertiary:* transfer of the patient from one hospital to another for the provision of specialist care unavailable in the referring hospital.

Primary transfer

In the UK transfer from the site of injury or illness to hospital is usually performed by trained paramedics using land ambulances. In some circumstances support may be provided to the ambulance crew by local medical teams from a nearby hospital or general practice. In remote locations, or when timely transportation cannot be achieved by land ambulance (e.g. inner city and rural areas) primary transfer may be undertaken by helicopter. In the UK, the primary receiving medical facility is often a hospital with the resources to provide the patient with all necessary on going care. In these circumstances no further transfer will be required.

Secondary and tertiary transfer

After resuscitation and stabilization in an initial receiving facility patients may require secondary or tertiary transfer. Indications for transfers to a tertiary centre or another secondary centre are:

Clinical

- Specialist intervention not available
- Specialist investigation not available
- Lack of staffed ICU bed
- Ongoing support not available.

Non-clinical

- Repatriation
- To create capacity for another admission
- Patient choice
- Between NHS and private hospitals.

Risk:benefit analysis

If a hospital lacks the resources to manage a patient that patient must be transferred to an appropriate centre.

The main risk to the patient is deterioration of their medical condition in an environment lacking the full resources of the referring unit. Deterioration may occur as a direct consequence of the underlying illness, but may also be precipitated by transfer. This may be induced by the physiological effects of movement (tipping, vibration, acceleration and deceleration forces) or changes in barometric pressure and temperature associated with air transport. These risks are increased in critically ill patients, who, even if 'stable', have limited physiological reserve. There are also risks to the patient and staff from accidents associated with any mode of transport.

It should not be forgotten that the transfer of critically ill patients in the UK often requires the participation of an anaesthetist from the referring hospital. For the duration of the transfer and return journey therefore, the referring hospital will be deprived of the services of the transferring anaesthetist.

Benefit to the patient is obvious if life-saving intervention is required, but is less clear if the patient is medically 'stable' and the primary indication is lack of resources (i.e. no staffed critical care bed) at the referring hospital.

Even minor complications in transit may be life threatening. Therefore whilst primary transfers are almost by definition in the patient's best interests, secondary transfers should only occur after a careful assessment of the risks and benefits.

Investigations should only be performed if the results will change management. If the performance of a particular investigation requires a patient to be transferred, its necessity must be confidently assured by a senior clinician. Interhospital transfers to create bed capacity should only be considered as a last resort. 'The most stable patient in the unit' certainly does not benefit and may even be harmed by being transferred to create space for a new admission. Careful clinical and ethical assessment of the situation and discussion with the affected patients and their families are required.

Transfer decisions

Transfer decisions involve many complex issues. Guidelines are available on the timing of transfer for some groups of patients (e.g. those with head injury). However in most cases the risk:benefit ratio and timing of transfer require discussion between senior staff. The decisions should therefore be made by consultants at the referring and receiving hospitals after full assessment and discussion. Decisions on how to send/retrieve a patient depend on urgency, available equipment, and the skill mix of available staff. Local policies should cover a broad spectrum of clinical scenarios, referral patterns, and available expertise.

Prevention of complications

The risks to patients and transport staff are reduced by careful planning, use of trained staff, appropriate equipment, and meticulous assessment and stabilization of patients prior to transfer. Everyone involved in the treatment of critically ill patients must understand the transport environment, staff, equipment, vehicles, and risks.

Although it is almost possible to reproduce the ICU environment during transport; monitoring is difficult and the ability to manage complications is limited. Ongoing treatment may be interrupted and the patient may be affected.

While there are distinct differences between interhospital and intrahospital transport, there are many common factors to consider. Reduce transport-related risks by only transferring patients when absolutely necessary. Ensure appropriate monitoring and clinical support before leaving. Patients often have several lines, drains, tubes, and mechanical support devices that must be managed before transfer. Any risk of cardiopulmonary instability is increased by movement. To ensure safe transport inadvertent interruption of monitoring or organ support must be avoided.

Any therapies to support the airway, breathing, and circulation in place prior to transport must be continued.

Airway

Securing and maintaining a patent airway during the transfer is the highest priority. Plans for airway management must be made before departure. In the absence of a definitive airway, consider securing the airway prior to transfer. Patients with a potentially unstable airway should be accompanied by a team with the skills and equipment required to intubate.

Intubated patients are at risk of accidental extubation, particularly during transfers between beds, trolleys, and vehicles. The endotracheal tube (ETT) or tracheostomy tube (TT) must be secured before transfer. Specific fixation devices are available. However, tapes or ties are usually sufficient. Physical restraint, sedation and paralysis with muscle relaxants further reduce the risk of accidental extubation.

Correct placement of the ETT or TT must be confirmed and documented before leaving and reassessed after each transfer (i.e. from bed to trolley, trolley to table, vehicle to vehicle, etc.). The airway and any equipment required to manage the airway must be easily accessible at all times.

Breathing

Adequate oxygenation and ventilation must be maintained in transit. Inappropriate ventilation strategies (over or under) may cause hypoxemia, hypocarbia, hypercarbia, and disturb acid–base balance.

Some routinely use a portable transport ventilator, while others perform manual ventilation with a bag-valve-mask (BVM). Manual ventilation is only safe if the pretransport FiO_2, PEEP, and minute ventilation can be provided by the person using the BVM. However, for long transfers, manual ventilation is not practical and portable mechanical ventilators are more consistent. Mechanical ventilation reduces the incidence of acid-base disturbance, cardiac arrhythmias, and hypotension. Although a BVM must be easily accessible during interhospital transfer, manual ventilation is not appropriate unless mechanical ventilation fails in transit.

Regardless of the ventilation strategy, establish the FiO_2, minute ventilation (i.e. tidal volume and respiratory rate), and PEEP required. Many (but not all) transport ventilators function almost as well as traditional ICU ventilators. Pressure limits prevent some transport ventilators from delivering high minute ventilation, airway pressures, or PEEP.

Although chest wall movement (rate, depth, and symmetry) should be assessed continuously, portable devices for monitoring oxygenation and ventilation are available. These include spirometry, end-tidal CO_2, transcutaneous PO_2, and pulse oximetry.

Several advanced therapeutic options are available to treat severe respiratory failure. These include inhaled nitric oxide (NO), high-frequency oscillation, and extracorporeal membrane oxygenation. Without portable systems to continue these treatments, patients may be severely compromised in transit and in some cases the risk of transfer would outweigh any potential benefit. For example, stopping NO therapy for acute hypoxemic respiratory failure may result in rebound worsening of gas exchange and cardiovascular instability.

Circulation

Patient transport may cause haemodynamic instability. The risk and severity of these changes during transport generally correlate with patient status prior to transfer.

Common complications include hypotension, hypertension, and arrhythmias. These are preventable. To reduce these risks correct electrolyte abnormalities prior to transfer and continue any vasoactive agents during the transfer.

When patients are moved, intravascular lines may dislodge or disconnect from drug infusions pumps. Battery-powered pumps can also fail. Most vasoactive drugs have short half-lives and so rapid decompensation occurs if these infusions stop. Careful preparation (e.g. spare batteries), attention, and supervision are required to prevent these problems.

Disability

The nervous system may be directly impaired if the airway, breathing or circulation are compromised. Cerebral ischaemia and secondary brain injury significantly increase mortality but may be preventable.

The most common complications during transfers which cause secondary brain injury include:

- Hypoxaemia
- Hypotension
- Reduced cerebral perfusion pressure (CPP).
- Raised intracranial pressure (ICP)
- Hypertension.

Appropriate pre-transfer ventilation, sedation, and analgesia may prevent increases in ICP whilst in transit. If possible, patients with increased ICP should be transported with the head elevated. Keep the heights of any transducers or ventricular drains at pre-transfer levels to prevent inaccurate readings or major cerebrospinal fluid shifts.

Training, evaluation, and coordination

Several specialist societies have developed guidelines on the transfer of critically ill patients. In the UK guidelines have been developed by the Royal College of Anaesthetists, the Association of Anaesthetists of Great Britain and Ireland, and the Intensive Care Society. These guidelines include recommendations on the minimum requirements for personnel, equipment, and medication for the transportation of critically ill patients. Specialist training in transfer medicine is provided at a national level by the Advanced Life Support group through regular courses, and locally for staff by expert teams such as London's Helicopter Emergency Medical Service (HEMS). Local and national incident reporting systems, together with formal audit processes exist to help maintain and improve standards of care. There are certain considerations that are specific to interhospital transport (e.g. vehicle selection and lack of immediate support), however the preparation and planning steps are broadly similar to those for intrahospital transport. (Box 23.1). Formal hospital and network policies aim to improve consistency and reduce errors.

Box 23.1 Example process for safe patient transport

- Plan for patient transfer and transport.
- Reduce delay by detailed coordination and communication.
- Appropriately select and use available resources (staff, vehicles, and equipment).
- Stabilize patient before transfer.
- Verify all tubes and lines are functional and well secured.
- Provide safe transport environment for patient and staff.
- Continuously monitor for changes in patient condition.
- Treat any changes in status.
- Safely transfer patient to receiving facility for further management.

Further reading

Advanced Life Support Group (2006). *Safe Transfer & Retrieval of Patients (sTaR): The Practical Approach* (2nd edn). London: Wiley.

23.2 Transfer of multiple trauma and neurosurgical patients

Multiple trauma patients

Whilst increasing numbers of multiply injured patients are now taken directly to regional trauma centres, the remainder may still present to the nearest district general hospital lacking specialist surgical services such as neurosurgery and cardiothoracic surgery. This arrangement commonly necessitates subsequent transfer to a larger tertiary facility. Early definitive surgery will often be required in order for optimal outcomes to be achieved, and transfers in these circumstances may be particularly urgent. It is important that essential transfer is not delayed by carrying out non-urgent investigations.

A logical and stepwise approach (ATLS protocol) facilitating thorough assessment and adequate resuscitation assists clinicians in determining the necessity, and degree of urgency of, secondary transfer in the multiply injured patient. Performance of a primary survey and initial resuscitation must occur before transfer, although occasionally it may become clear that this phase cannot itself be completed without transfer, e.g. uncontrollable bleeding requiring surgical intervention not available in that hospital. Multiple trauma has the potential to cause *massive blood loss* and subsequent cardiovascular instability. Targeted resuscitation with intravascular volume expansion and blood products should occur prior to transfer.

Indications for transfer for specialist services include:

- Neuroscience
- Mediastinal injury
- Spinal injury
- Pelvic injury
- Burns
- Paediatrics
- Liver injury
- Severe facial injury
- Polytrauma.

In the event that a secondary transfer is deemed necessary, the patient should be assessed with an ABC-type checklist. Any potential problems in transit must be identified and appropriate precautions taken prior to departure, e.g. insertion of intercostal catheters for decompression of pneumothoraces. Clear direct communication between referring and accepting clinicians must occur and the substance of this must be documented in the patient's notes.

Airway

A patent airway, not at risk of deterioration, is mandatory prior to transfer. If there is any doubt as to the security of the airway, the trachea should be should be intubated with a cuffed ETT. In multiply injured patients general anaesthesia and tracheal intubation facilitates immobilization and safe analgesia (requirements for which are likely to be high), and the majority of this group will require management in this manner. Unless contraindicated an oral or nasal gastric tube should be inserted to permit drainage of stomach contents. Immobilization of the cervical spine is indicated in these patients.

Breathing

All multiply injured patients should be breathing an appropriately oxygen-enriched gas mixture to maintain a suitable arterial oxygenation. Prior to transfer it must be confidently ensured that the patient's breathing is stable and that no possibility of deterioration in transit exists. Again, in the presence of any doubt the patient should be electively intubated and ventilated before departure. Pneumothoraces of any size should be drained prior to departure as these have the potential to worsen in transit, particularly if air transportation is to be used. A chest radiograph should be performed before departure to confirm positioning of the tracheal tube and assess the extent of chest injury. Arterial blood gas analysis should be performed in all ventilated patients and those with impaired breathing.

Circulation

Adequate IV access must be obtained; at a minimum this would consist of two large-bore peripheral cannulae. Central venous access will be an advantage in many patients, and will be essential if inotropic drugs need to be administered. Arterial access is also desirable to facilitate monitoring and control of blood pressure (e.g. in patients with traumatic brain injury) and should be sought in all ventilated patients. Hypovolaemic shock is very common in multiply injured patients and should be treated with IV fluids and blood products. External haemorrhage should be controlled wherever possible and fractures splinted to reduce the potential for further blood loss. Unless precluded by local trauma urinary catheterization should be performed to enable urine output to be assessed.

Deficits

Appropriate analgesia and antiemesis should be provided before transfer. Consideration should be given to the potential for motion sickness in awake patients. Measures should be taken to prevent heat loss and active warming should be provided where traumatic brain injury is not suspected. Blood tests including full blood count, urea and electrolytes, and blood glucose should be checked before transfer. In many cases important investigations will have been carried out at the referring hospital and it is crucial that the results of these be communicated to the accepting team as well as documented in the notes. Copies of any imaging performed must accompany the patient to the accepting hospital.

A final check of the patient, their documentation and investigation results, and transfer equipment should occur immediately before departure. Clinical responsibility remains with the referring hospital until the patient is physically taken over by the accepting facility.

Neurosurgical patients

It is well recognized that patients with severe neurosurgical injury have better outcomes, regardless of the need for operative intervention, when managed in neuroscience centres with the requisite expertise in caring for them. Because of the specialist nature of these services, and the relatively small number of patients who require admission to a neuroscience centre, they are organized on a regional basis. As a result it is often necessary to transfer brain-injured patients from a presenting facility to another hospital for definitive care. Patients presenting with isolated traumatic brain injury, polytrauma, or non-traumatic intracranial haematomata may fall into this group.

The essential goals of the medical team at the transferring facility are to resuscitate the patient before departure, and expedite transfer for definitive care while minimizing the risks of secondary brain injury. It is crucial for the outcome of these patients that hypoxia and hypotension be avoided, and that the balance between cerebral oxygen supply and demand be optimized. In order to properly manage patients with brain injury the caring personnel must have a thorough working knowledge of the cerebral circulation and the factors which determine cerebral blood flow (CBF). Careful attention to resuscitation, stabilization, and maintaining cerebral oxygenation are the keys to success:

- The decision to transfer a patient for specialist care at a neuroscience centre should be taken at consultant level after comprehensive communication between referring and accepting teams.
- All patients with serious brain injury should be anaesthetized, intubated, and ventilated prior to transfer. This will ensure control of the airway and optimization of gas exchange in transit, as well as reducing the cerebral metabolic rate for oxygen. Exceptions to this will necessarily be rare and the responsibility of senior clinicians at transferring and receiving facilities.
- The principles of ABCDE resuscitation protocols should be followed. No brain-injured patient should be transferred before they have been resuscitated and stabilized at the referring facility. To do so would be to invite potentially devastating secondary injury.
- To optimize cerebral perfusion and oxygenation, and intracranial volume, certain physiological parameters should be targeted and additional factors considered:

- Maintain PaO_2 >13kPa.
- Maintain $PaCO_2$ 4.5–5kPa.
- Maintain mean arterial pressure >80mmHg (volume loading and vasopressors).
- Frequent monitoring of pupillary size and reaction.
- Treat and prevent seizures and hyperthermia.
- Position patient >20° head-up.
- Maintain normoglycaemia.
- Avoid hypotonic IV fluids.
- Consider osmotic agents if evidence of severe intracranial hypertension.

It should be noted that it is not possible to adequately manage this group of patients without access to the full range of modern ITU monitoring equipment including $ETCO_2$ and invasive blood pressure measurement. In some circumstances the patient may have an ICP monitor inserted before transfer. This greatly facilitates optimization of the CPP.

Further reading

Association of Anaesthetists of Great Britain and Ireland (2009). *Recommendations for the Safe Transfer of Patients with Brain Injury.* London: AAGBI.

23.3 Transfer of spinal injury and pregnant patients

Spinal injury patients

Patients with known or suspected spinal injury all require spinal immobilization during transfer. Methods for achieving this range from a spinal board with cervical collar and blocks to sophisticated mechanical frame devices designed for aeromedical transport over long distances. The complications of immobilization include patient discomfort, venous thromboembolism, decubitus ulceration and pressure necrosis, diaphragmatic splinting, and respiratory embarrassment. All these problems become more severe with increasing duration of immobilization, and are lessened with the application of devices with softer yielding surfaces to be in contact with the skin. For all but the briefest transfers alternatives to a spinal board should be considered—well-padded scoops, semi-rigid mattresses, and vacuum mattresses are some of the options available. As soon as is practically possible after arrival the patient should be moved to a bed or trolley with a firm but cushioned surface.

The physiological effects of spinal cord injury depend on the severity and level of the trauma. Loss of muscular innervation and subsequent paralysis is highly relevant to the transferring team when it affects the muscles of respiration. Supplementary oxygen should be provided for all patients, and elective intubation carried out before transfer where there is clear respiratory insufficiency. During the initial stages of cord damage, as cord oedema spreads from the level of injury, the effective motor level may rise. If there is any doubt over the patient's ability to breathe adequately without assistance intubation and mechanical ventilation should be instituted prior to departure. Patients with concomitant chest trauma are especially at risk of decompensation. Any attempts at direct laryngoscopy should be performed with manual in-line stabilization of the cervical spine after temporary removal of the blocks and cervical collar. Given the suboptimal positioning of the patient's head and neck it is recommended to prepare for a difficult intubation at the first attempt.

After an initial outpouring of catecholamines, a period of vasodilatory shock may follow severe injury to the high thoracic or spinal cord due to the interruption of sympathetic outflow. Unopposed activity of the vagus may exacerbate this situation by causing bradycardia. Hypotension must be vigorously corrected to maximize perfusion of the injured cord. The potential for severe bradycardia or even asystole precipitated by vagally stimulating manoeuvres (e.g. instrumentation of the pharynx) must be considered and premedication with vagolytics used where appropriate.

In the case of conscious patients with spinal injury it must be borne in mind that pain, paralysis, numbness, and fear constitute a potentially devastating combination. Psychological support for these patients, combined with symptomatic relief, represents a particular challenge.

Pregnant patients

In principle the transfer of a pregnant woman entails the transfer of two patients. Transfer may be indicated by the need for specialist medical care of the mother, the baby, or both. Careful attention to optimization of maternal physiology is usually the most effective way to provide safe intrauterine conditions for the pre-term fetus. When considering how best to optimize the patients it should be borne in mind that the life of the mother takes precedence over that of the fetus. Sometimes it may be safer to deliver the baby prior to transfer, a decision that will require careful consideration by senior clinicians and the mother. The decision to transfer a pregnant patient involves a complex risk:benefit analysis and must be made at consultant level. Before transfer effective communication between teams at referring and accepting hospitals must occur. Obstetric, midwifery, paediatric, nursing, anaesthetic, and ITU teams are likely to be involved and communication must take place between all of them.

The important changes in maternal anatomy and physiology that occur during pregnancy must be appreciated to enable safe care by the transferring physician (see section 24.1):

- Aortocaval compression—relieve with wedge
- Aspiration risk
- Difficult airway risk

The pregnant patient should be accompanied during transfer by personnel with knowledge and experience of obstetric emergencies, in life-threatening cases this is likely to require an obstetrician rather than a midwife, and a doctor skilled in resuscitation and critical care (usually an anaesthetist). If there is a risk of delivery of a baby in need of special resuscitation (e.g. early pre-term fetus) a paediatrician should also be present.

In addition to the usual routine monitoring equipment required for the mother, some means of monitoring the fetal well-being is required. At the simplest level this may be a Pinnard stethoscope, though more commonly a handheld Doppler device is employed.

Further reading

Martin T (2001). *Handbook of Patient Transportation*. London: Greenwich Medical Media.

23.4 Equipment for transfer

General considerations

Medical equipment used during patient transfer includes that required for the monitoring of vital signs, devices for provision of treatment and life support (ventilators, infusion pumps etc.), and resuscitation equipment. Equipment used for patient transportation should be dedicated to this purpose, not used in any other situation. It should be stored in the minimum number of clearly identified locations and be readily available at short notice. Electrical equipment with battery power should be maintained in a fully charged state.

All medical electrical equipment must adhere to strict standards of safety and reliability. Electrical equipment used for patient transportation must satisfy additional criteria. Such equipment should be:

- Rugged and hardwearing.
- Able to withstand a drop from standing height without loss of functionality.
- Resistant to the ingress of water, dust, sand, and salt spray.
- Failsafe.
- As lightweight as possible.
- Able to operate effectively with low power consumption and for prolonged periods.

The range of equipment required to safely manage the transportation of the vast majority of patients is predictable. Checklists should be used to ensure that all equipment is available, fully charged and within its 'use by date'. In most institutions dedicated transport bags (rucksacks, 'grab bags' etc.) are employed to facilitate storage, carriage, and rapid access to the required equipment. Frequent and regular checking of all equipment should be undertaken by a designated individual.

Minimum equipment

Patients who are critically ill, or have the potential to become so during transfer, require a range of monitoring and therapeutic equipment to be immediately available during transportation. A suggested minimum complement is as follows:

- Three-lead continuous ECG
- Non-invasive BP measurement
- Pulse oximetry
- Stethoscope
- Self-inflating bag with valve and face mask
- Transport ventilator
- Capnography
- Portable suction
- Pressurized oxygen
- Advanced airway equipment
- Defibrillator
- Venous access equipment
- Resuscitation drugs
- Equipment for invasive BP monitoring
- Infusion devices for IV medications.

Specific equipment considerations

Electrocardiography

ECG monitoring provides real-time data about the patient's heart rate and rhythm as well as alerting transferring personnel to possible myocardial ischaemia. Standard lead positions may be employed, as may a 'CM5' position to increase the sensitivity to ischaemia of the left ventricle.

Electrical interference and motion artefacts are often troublesome during transfer. Techniques to minimize these problems include:

- The use of modern, heavily shielded monitors.
- Gentle abrasion of the skin prior to electrode application.
- Electrode placement over bony prominences when possible.
- Fixation of electrode leads to prevent movement.
- Placement of the monitor as far away from other electrical devices as possible.

Non-invasive blood pressure measurement (NIBP)

Modern automated BP measurement devices are reliable, accurate and easy to use with simple training. Manual sphygmomanometry using auscultation is often rendered impossible by extraneous noise. The convenience of NIBP devices is, however, offset by problems commonly encountered during transfer:

- The mechanical work inherent in the technique consumes large amounts of electrical power, usually considerably more than any other single monitor.
- Movement artefact is a major limitation.

For these reasons the use of NIBP during transport can only be recommended for intrahospital episodes, relatively well patients, and the very briefest of inter-hospital transfers. For all other scenarios invasive BP monitoring should be preferred.

Pulse oximetry (SpO$_2$)

Pulse oximetry is a simple, convenient method for estimating oxyhaemoglobin saturation and should be regarded as an essential monitor. Nonetheless its utility during transfer, as during stationary use in hospital is subject to certain limitations:

- Movement artefact degrades the quality of the measurement.
- Probe displacement may be difficult to rectify if access to the patient is limited.
- In patients with poor peripheral perfusion or cardiac dysrhythmia it may be difficult or impossible to obtain a measurement.
- Nail varnish can produce spurious readings.
- High concentrations of carboxyhaemoglobin cause overestimation of SpO$_2$.
- The accuracy of the measurement falls off below an SpO$_2$ of approximately 80%.
- Due to the shape of the oxyhaemoglobin dissociation curve, a marked reduction in PaO$_2$ may occur before a significant fall in SpO$_2$.
- SpO$_2$ provides no information about ventilatory adequacy.

Stethoscope

This most basic piece of monitoring equipment forms an essential part of any transfer kit. Even with the availability of modern, sophisticated electrical monitors, there is no substitute for listening to the patient's chest oneself. It is, however, undeniable that the stethoscope is rendered effectively useless in noisy environments. As a result the stethoscope has little effective role in aircraft, and even in land ambulances unless stationary with the engine off.

Oxygen

Oxygen is vital during transport both for providing an enriched atmosphere for the patient to breathe and also as a driving gas for certain types of transport ventilator. Oxygen supplies for use in transfer are nearly always provided in the form of cylinders of pressurized gas. Occasionally liquid oxygen cylinders may be encountered in situations where very large quantities are required, e.g. international repatriation. In principle oxygen concentrators could be used for transport purposes, but in practice the relatively low concentrations of oxygen they produce make them an unattractive alternative to pressurized gas.

Oxygen is stored in cylinders made from a variety of materials including robust, lightweight synthetic carbon fibre compounds (e.g. 'Kevlar'), which can be filled to very high pressures. In the NHS, however, by far the most commonly encountered material is molybdenum steel alloy. These cylinders are filled with gaseous oxygen such that the internal pressure is 137 bar at 15°C. The cylinder sizes typically used during transport are sizes D (340L when full), and E (680L when full). Because the oxygen is stored as a gas its contents are subject to Boyle's law, and therefore the amount of oxygen contained within is proportional to the internal pressure. The reading on an attached pressure gauge will reflect the amount of oxygen remaining in the cylinder.

By considering the expected duration of transfer, the properties of the oxygen delivery system used, the likely minute volume of the patient and their inspired oxygen concentration it is possible to estimate the total oxygen required for a given transfer episode. Many transport ventilators need a supply of pressurized oxygen to act as a driving gas (e.g. Oxylog ventilators) and this requirement typically uses an extra 1L/min of oxygen. A knowledge of the volume of oxygen contained within full cylinders of given sizes then allows the transferring personnel to calculate how many cylinders of particular sizes they should carry. It is considered standard safe practice to take approximately twice the amount of oxygen thought likely to be used during the transfer. This confers a wide margin of safety in case unexpected delays or patient deterioration should be encountered.

Electrical power supplies

All electrically powered devices designed for use in patient transportation have the facility to function on battery power, almost always via rechargeable batteries. The most commonly encountered type of rechargeable battery in medical transfer devices is the nickel-cadmium (Ni-Cd) battery. Ni-Cd batteries have the advantages of being affordable and able to be charged up relatively rapidly. The main problem with Ni-Cd batteries is their tendency to discharge very rapidly to zero voltage when out of condition through age and poor maintenance. This can lead to a situation where the battery may appear to hold 50% charge, and then be exhausted a few minutes later. Regular full discharge and recharge cycling, in line with the manufacturers recommendations, can reduce the severity of this problem.

Failure of battery power is probably the single most common cause of equipment problems during patient transfer. The spectre of power failure can be avoided by following a few simple guidelines. All personnel should be aware of the manufacturer's stated battery life for electrical equipment, and also know that this is likely to be, for practical purposes, an overestimate. Spare batteries are, therefore, absolutely essential for all but the briefest of transfers. All equipment should be kept fully charged when not in use, and the manufacturer's recommendations on charge and discharge cycling should be followed. Whenever the opportunity presents itself for connection to external or mains power this should be taken advantage of to maximize the duration of battery power. All transfers should be undertaken with sufficient battery power to supply all necessary devices for considerably longer than the expected duration of the journey. Aspects of equipment use that consume the most power (e.g. NIBP, monitor backlights) should be factored in to estimates of battery life.

The availability of electric power from an ambulance should not be relied upon except in long journeys under exceptional circumstances, e.g. international repatriation or military operations where prior familiarity with the vehicle is guaranteed. Although many modern ambulances do have the facility to supply some external power, it is common for incompatibilities to arise between this electrical supply (if any) and the needs of transfer equipment used by another team.

Further reading

Association of Anaesthetists of Great Britain and Ireland (2009). *Safety Guideline – Interhospital Transfer*. London: AAGBI.

Intensive Care Society (2011). *Guidelines for the transport of the critically ill patient* (3rd edn). London: WB Saunders.

23.5 Ventilation during transfer

Principles of ventilation during transfer

Traditionally ventilators used for transport purposes have been simple robust devices employing fluid logic circuits, often totally without the need for electric power. While there are some obvious advantages to these sorts of devices they are limited in their ability to deliver modern modes of ventilation such as pressure controlled and pressure support ventilation. Modern transport ventilators have become increasingly sophisticated in recent years with advances in microprocessor technology. Devices are now available which are capable of providing a wide range of ventilatory modalities catering to the individual needs of all but the most challenging of patients.

Even the simplest of transport ventilators should incorporate alarm mechanisms to alert personnel to high circuit pressure and disconnection from the pressurized gas supply, and these should be both audible and visual. Airway manometry should be regarded as essential. In terms of pure functionality, minimum requirements should be the ability to deliver PEEP, control the inspired oxygen concentration, the tidal volume, respiratory rate and inspiratory:expiratory ratio. The facility to provide pressure controlled ventilation greatly improves the management of patients with poorly compliant lungs, mitigating the potential harm inherent in separating them from the ITU ventilator for a prolonged period. For spontaneously breathing patients the possibility of providing synchronized intermittent mandatory ventilation, or pressure-supported breaths, dramatically improves the comfort and efficacy of ventilation, reducing the need for sedative and paralysing agents.

The latest transport ventilators are, in terms of functionality, nearly equivalent to a standard ITU ventilator. Comprehensive training before use is mandatory. Such training will necessitate familiarity with a broad range of ventilatory modes, an understanding of the lung pathology involved in many conditions, and experience with related techniques such as safe and effective sedation.

As with any environment in which general anaesthesia is provided, a means of manually inflating the patient's lungs in the absence of pressurized medical gas must be available. Self-inflating resuscitation bags with unidirectional valves are an essential item for any transfer.

Modes of ventilation during transfer

Modern transport ventilators have become increasingly sophisticated in recent years. It is now possible, even in transit, to provide patients with an advanced level of ventilatory support nearly equivalent to that provided by the ITU ventilator. Knowledge of a range of ventilatory techniques for managing commonly encountered respiratory pathology is essential if gas exchange is to be optimized and complications of ventilation minimized (e.g. ventilator-induced lung injury, cardiovascular compromise).

Asthma

- Characterized by high airways resistance: types 1 and 2 respiratory failure are common.
- Use pressure-controlled ventilation (PCV) or related modes (e.g. BiLevel, PRVC).
- Relatively high inspiratory pressure may initially need to be applied at the inspiratory limb to achieve adequate tidal volumes, but due to high airway resistance the true transalveolar pressure should be lower than this. Beware increasing plateau pressures over time, and aim to limit plateau pressure to ≤30cmH$_2$O.
- Severe limitation of airflow leads to dynamic hyperinflation, or 'breath stacking'. Intrinsic PEEP should be suspected where expiration is not completed before a subsequent inspiration; it can be estimated by an end-expiratory hold manoeuvre.
- Gas trapping worsens compliance and increases the risk of pneumothorax.
- Limit tidal volumes to 6–8mL/kg of ideal body weight and set long expiratory times. Use spirometry to check for emptying of the lungs in expiration.
- Set initial PEEP low, 0–5cmH$_2$O.
- Permit hypercarbia providing pH ≥7.20.
- Maximize bronchodilatory therapy.
- Assess for possible pneumothorax frequently, and always before transfer.

COPD

- Principles of ventilation in exacerbations of COPD are broadly similar to those in acute asthma.
- The presence of bullae in emphysematous patients places them at increased risk of developing pneumothoraces.
- Abnormal lung architecture makes the presence of occult intrinsic PEEP (difficult to detect with spirometry/manometry) more likely, and a high degree of clinical suspicion is recommended.

ARDS

- Characterized by poor pulmonary compliance and hypoxaemia.
- Evidence for improved outcome with adherence to ARDS ventilatory criteria.
- Use PCV.
- Limit peak airway pressure to 30cmH$_2$O or below.
- Limit tidal volume to 6mL/kg of ideal body weight.
- Use high levels of PEEP to maintain lung recruitment and oxygenation.
- Consider inverse ratio ventilation and recruitment manoeuvres.
- Permit hypercarbia providing pH ≥7.20.

Capnography

Capnography should be available in all areas where general anaesthesia is provided. Its use in ICUs for continuous monitoring of intubated patients is now also commonplace. As a component of transport monitoring it confers very significant advantages for safety as well as providing the usual diagnostic information. As well as confirming initial correct placement of the endotracheal tube should intubation become necessary in transit, capnography also provides a rapid indication in the event of circuit disconnection. Failure to ventilate for any other reason, such as displacement of the tube or obstruction of the circuit (e.g. kinking), will also be immediately apparent through changes in the capnograph. The relatively hostile environments encountered in transport situations make such complications more likely to occur and their rapid detection is greatly facilitated by vigilant attention to the capnograph.

Capnographs are available as side-stream and main-stream types. Mainstream sampling devices require the CO_2 sensor to be at the patient end of the breathing circuit, with electrical cables attached to it. This arrangement tends to be more cumbersome and can cause drag on the breathing circuit. It is becoming less common in modern practice and side-stream sampling capnographs are generally preferred for transport purposes.

A full discussion of the utility of capnography is beyond the scope of this chapter, however certain facets are particularly advantageous in the context of transfer and worthy of mention. It is unusual for arterial blood gas (ABG) analysis to be available in transit. Correlation of a measured ABG prior to departure with the contemporaneous capnometry will permit estimation of the patient's $PaCO_2$ during the transfer. A reduction in end-tidal CO_2 noticed en route can provide a useful clue to a fall in cardiac output that might otherwise be difficult to detect in the back of an ambulance. Changes to the capnography waveform plateau can suggest uneven ventilation or interbreathing, which can be similarly hard to spot initially without the aid of the capnograph. In patients with neurosurgical pathology, where intracranial hypertension is known or suspected, careful monitoring of the capnograph permits ventilatory adjustments to be made in transit.

Modern capnometers and capnography display units are relatively robust devices suffering less from vibration and movement artefact than other monitors. The processes of set-up and use are essentially the same as in the operating theatre environment.

Further reading

Martin T (2001). *Handbook of Patient Transportation*. London: Greenwich Medical Media.

Physiological effects of transport and noise

There is a range of adverse effects caused by the mechanical properties of various vehicles used to transport patients. Acceleration, deceleration, vibration, changes in ambient pressure, and time differences all contribute to physiological derangement in patients and staff.

Acceleration and deceleration

Humans have evolved to live in the earth's gravitational field with a constant accelerating force of 1G (approximately $9.8m/sec^2$) directed downwards toward the earth. Modern vehicles, particularly aircraft, are capable of producing accelerations many times this and, of course, these 'G-forces' are not something to which humans are adapted. All bodies possess inertia by virtue of their mass and will tend to resist a change in the state of their motion.

When subject to acceleration forces solid organs and fluids will tend to shift within the body in the direction opposite to the applied acceleration force. The degree to which this happens depends on the magnitude and direction of the accelerating force. For example, in an aeroplane during take-off considerable acceleration force is applied along the long axis of the vehicle (i.e. horizontally). For conscious individuals seated in the upright position this is experienced as being 'pushed back into the seat'. Internally solid organs move slightly towards the rear of the body cavity, dragging on their tissue attachments, intravascular fluid also tends to move in a similar fashion. However there should be no deleterious physiological effects of these movements. The same cannot be said of a patient lying horizontally on a transport stretcher. For the patient in this position significant fluid shifts result in changes to cardiac preload and afterload, with corresponding changes in cardiac output and activation of baroreceptor reflexes. The magnitude of these effects depends on the amount of force applied and the duration of application. Hypovolaemic, heavily sedated, and critically ill patients are less tolerant of acceleration than well patients. In practice sustained accelerating forces in transport aircraft are usually not of sufficient magnitude to cause any lasting harm to the patient but each case will need to be assessed on its own merits and appropriate limitations applied where necessary. Acceleration and deceleration, especially if repetitive, has the potential to cause motion sickness.

Rapid deceleration causes the opposite effects to those just described. In the most extreme case, that of a crash, brief but enormous forces can cause massive shear stress to internal organs leading to vascular disruption, perforation of organs, and serious injury or death.

The effects of acceleration and deceleration on equipment must always be borne in mind and care taken to ensure that all items are securely stowed in a position that minimizes risk to the patient and personnel should they move in transit.

Vibration

Vibration is an inescapable feature of travel in any vehicle whether a land ambulance or an aircraft. Land ambulances experience vibration through the interaction between the road surface and their shock absorber/suspension system. Aircraft experience vibration due to turbulence. Helicopter rotors produce considerable vibration. All vehicles experience vibration from their engines and gear boxes.

Vibration is uncomfortable for awake patients and staff and can be tiring over long periods as effort is required to maintain a stable position within the vehicle. Discomfort from vibration may increase sedation and analgesia requirements for some patients, particularly those with unfixed fractures. For patients and staff alike, vibration can lead to or worsen motion sickness. Major vibration may make interventions difficult or even impossible in transit, e.g. IV cannulation, and it is not always possible to stop the vehicle to facilitate these.

Monitoring equipment and infusion pumps can be adversely affected by vibration causing physical movement or electromagnetic interference. ECG and NIBP monitors are particularly likely to be hindered.

Ambient pressure

Changes in ambient pressure with ascent in aircraft have the potential to causes problems in two main ways.

Firstly the reduction in the partial pressure of oxygen in ambient air at altitude places patients and staff at risk of hypoxia. The cabins of most modern aircraft designed to operate at altitudes in excess of 10 000ft are pressurized. This pressurization mitigates against the hypoxic effects of ascent. The cabins of commercial aircraft are not pressurized to full atmospheric pressure at sea level however but only partially. The equivalent effective cabin pressures of these aircraft lie in the range of 4500–8000ft. At an altitude of 8000ft a healthy individual is likely to have an oxyhaemoglobin saturation of 92–95%. It can be seen rather easily, therefore, that an individual who is already hypoxic at sea level may become dangerously so at altitude even in the pressurized cabin of an aircraft. Any pathological process which impairs gas exchange or oxygen carrying capacity must be identified and treated prior to ascent, and a risk:benefit analysis made before air transfer. The availability of supplemental oxygen is essential for all patients.

The second way in which ascent to altitude can cause harm to patients during transfer, relates to the expansion and contraction of gas filled spaces. Boyle's law tells us that when temperature remains constant the volume of a fixed amount of gas is inversely proportional to the pressure. It follows therefore that any gas filled space will increase in volume with the drop in ambient pressure on ascent. Gas filled spaces within the body will expand with the potential to damage the patient:

- Gas in the sinuses within the skull and the middle ear will expand. Under normal circumstances gas will escape from these spaces via drainage tubes, the Eustachian tube in the case of the middle ear. Inflammation and oedema of these tubes may cause blockage and make it impossible to equalize the pressure in these spaces with ambient pressure. If this occurs, a sensation of pressure ('squeeze') results that can progress to severe pain and even perforation of the tympanum. In awake patients and staff holding the nose and blowing out (the Frenzel manoeuvre) may open the Eustachian tube and provide relief of ear pain (otic barotrauma), though it is not effective for sinus pain.

- Gas within the gastrointestinal tract may lead to nausea and discomfort on expansion. Diaphragmatic splinting may occur. A freely draining gastric tube will help to ameliorate this situation. Patients with pre-existing bowel obstruction may be at risk of perforation on ascent.

- Pneumothoraces that have been unidentified or inadequately treated before departure will expand at altitude, becoming pathologically more significant. It is essential to ensure that any pneumothorax has been fully drained prior to ascent. Mechanically ventilated patients should be observed closely and any suggestion of a developing pneumothorax should prompt swift intervention.

Noise

Noise is a problem in all vehicles to varying degrees. It has a nuisance value as well as more serious consequences for safety and health. Ambient noise is greater in aircraft than land ambulances and greatest of all in helicopters. Ear protection should be worn to protect patients and staff from hearing loss as well as temporary effects such as headache, nausea and fatigue. Ideally a headset should be employed to provide protection and a means of communication with other transfer staff, aircrew, and patient where appropriate. In a noisy environment audible alarms cannot be heard, nor can the tone of the pulse oximeter. Furthermore stethoscopes are nearly useless and alternative means of patient observation will be required.

Legal issues

Any doctor providing diagnostic or therapeutic services to a patient has entered into a contract with that patient and is legally obliged to provide care of a standard appropriate to the training and experience of the doctor. In the case of transfer medicine the transferring doctor has that responsibility. Commonly, however, the transferring doctor will be part of a team at the referring hospital, and under the indirect supervision of a senior colleague. In such cases, in addition to the aforementioned contract, overall clinical responsibility for the patient's care lies with the supervising doctor (often the consultant anaesthetist on call) at the referring facility until care is taken over by the receiving team. In the case of NHS organizations, ultimately the chief executive carries vicarious liability for the actions or inactions of all their staff when on duty. These distinctions are important because the exact timing of any act or omission that subsequently leads to legal action will determine which individuals and organizations are liable. Accurate, complete, attributable contemporaneous documentation is essential for successful legal defence.

Occasionally, despite the best efforts of the caring team, patients die during transfer. When this occurs on an international aeromedical transfer some difficult decisions have to be made. Death has legal implications, which often differ from country to country. The laws of the country in whose airspace the death occurs will apply. However when death occurs in international airspace the situation is less clear. Jurisdiction may fall to the country in which the airline or aircraft is registered, or where the aircraft most recently departed or overflew. When a death occurs the captain of the aircraft must be informed and a decision on how to proceed will be made based on the location of the aircraft at the time and the remaining flight plan. Options include returning to the originating airport, landing at a nearby airport, or continuing on to the destination. Any decision is likely to have significant practical implications for the deceased's family and a degree of discretion is usual.

All doctors undertaking transfer work should consider their need for personal indemnity and injury insurance. In the UK both the Association of Anaesthetists of Great Britain and Ireland, and the Intensive Care Society offer policies to members.

The national register of critical care beds

Before any patient transfer is planned and undertaken it is, of course, essential for there to be an identified bed available in the appropriate receiving facility. With the aim of facilitating the identification of suitable critical beds and reducing the time taken to complete the process of referral and acceptance, the National Intensive Care Bed Register is a vital resource. The register is updated several times per day and is maintained by London's Emergency Bed Service (EBS) in partnership with other agencies in the north of England. Contacting the local agency responsible for the register when a patient requiring transfer is identified has the potential to dramatically reduce time delays prior to departure.

Regional protocols, audit, and incident reporting

Currently in the UK individual trust ITUs are organized into regional cooperative groups known as critical care networks. These networks encourage standardization of care across regions and implementation of best practice. Issues that affect units across the region can be managed at a network level. The advantages for transfer medicine are that quality, documentation and equipment compatibility can be standardized across the network, improving care and helping to control some costs. Close cooperation with regard to bed capacity (always in short supply) enables transfer times and distances to be minimized with improved resource utilization and less inconvenience to patients and their families.

Audit of transfer practice is important to facilitate the maintenance of high standards and identify failings or areas in need of improvement. Local, regional, and national audit projects are now frequent and look certain to remain a vital part of the quality assurance process. Similarly the reporting of adverse incidents that occur during transfer is crucial to the development of transfer services. It is clear that patient transfer is a complex process with commensurate potential for mishap. Adverse events can and do happen relatively commonly in transit, but only by fostering a blame-free environment in which to report such incidents can their frequency and severity be properly identified. Where problems are found steps can then be taken to prevent recurrence. All staff involved in transfer should be aware of the local policies and mechanisms for reporting adverse incidents, and follow them when such incidents occur.

Further reading

Milligan JE, Jones CN, Helm DR, et al. (2011). The principles of aero-medical retrieval of the critically ill. *Trends Anaesth Crit Care*, 1:22–6.

Chapter 24

Obstetric anaesthesia

441

24.1 Physiological changes during pregnancy

Maternal physiology

Physiological changes during pregnancy support the developing fetus by optimizing uteroplacental circulation and maternofetal gas exchange in response to placental hormones. Many physiological changes occur as a protective measure for the mother to withstand delivery. A good understanding of these changes helps the anaesthetist to manage normal pregnancy and identify the abnormal.

Cardiovascular system

The maternal circulation is high flow, low resistance due to the endocrine stimuli (progesterone and oestrogen) and the low resistance of the uteroplacental circulation.

Increased blood volume

Blood volume increases are detectable very early in pregnancy with rapid expansion in the 2nd trimester reaching a plateau at about 35 weeks. Blood volume increases by 50%, representing an extra 2L volume. This is due to sodium and water conservation as a result of:

- Oestrogen activation of renin system
- Progesterone increasing aldosterone production
- Decreased MAP stimulating renin-angiotensin system.

Increased cardiac output

Cardiac output increases from 8 weeks reaching an extra 35% by the end of the 1st trimester and 50% by the end of the second trimester. It then remains stable until term.

This is a combined effect of:

- Increased heart rate—20% by end of the 1st trimester.
- Increased stroke volume—30% by end of 2nd trimester.

By term, the uterus receives 10% of the cardiac output with approximately 800mL/min blood flow.

Reduced systemic vascular resistance

Systemic vascular resistance (SVR) is reduced by 35% at 20 weeks but increases slightly to a final 20% reduction at term. Progesterone is responsible for vasodilatation, perhaps via modulation of prostaglandin-mediated vascular responsiveness. The low resistance uteroplacental circulation also reduces SVR.

Other changes

- Decreased blood pressure, SBP 5–10mmHg, DBP 10–15mmHg. Lowest in 2nd trimester, normalizes by term.
- Decreased pulmonary vascular resistance, therefore maintaining normal pulmonary occlusion pressure despite increased vascular volume.
- Increased left ventricular mass and ejection fraction.
- Increased oxygen consumption by 16%. Oxygen delivery is far in excess of consumption.
- Decreased colloid osmotic pressure to about 22mmHg (normal 26mmHg) due to reduced albumin. This increases the risk of pulmonary oedema.
- Aortocaval compression occurs (see Box 24.1).

Changes in labour

Rapid changes in cardiac output, preload and afterload occur in labour. During strong contractions placental autotransfusion increases maternal circulating volume by 300mL and cardiac output increases further by 30%. Epidural analgesia partly attenuates this increase by reducing the sympathetic response to pain. Following delivery, cardiac output remains elevated due to placental autotransfusion and mobilization of extracellular fluid. Within 2 weeks parameters have mostly returned to normal levels, although it may take 12 weeks for all changes to fully resolve.

Box 24.1 Aortocaval compression

- Obstruction of inferior vena caval flow sometimes with aortic compression, by the gravid uterus in the supine position. Venous return and cardiac output are reduced.
- Can occur from 16 weeks.
- Can occur semi recumbent and even standing.
- Exaggerated under anaesthesia as compensatory reflexes attenuated.
- Greater incidence with increased uterine size and obesity.
- 60% are asymptomatic due to collateral venous flow through paravertebral and azygous system.
- 10% result in supine hypotensive syndrome: hypotension, reduced uteroplacental flow and fetal distress.
- 15° left lateral tilt relieves compression.

Respiratory system

Mucosal oedema due to progesterone-mediated vasodilatation causes difficulty in nasal breathing and may lead to laryngeal oedema. As pregnancy progresses ventilation becomes predominantly diaphragmatic. The ribs splay and the diaphragm elevates.

Increased minute ventilation

Minute ventilation increases from early pregnancy to 40% at term. This is due to altered tidal volume (respiratory rate is largely unchanged). Progesterone lowers the respiratory centre threshold for response to CO_2 and may act as a direct respiratory stimulant. The hypoxic ventilatory response is also increased. High minute ventilation causes:

- Decreased $PaCO_2$ (3.6–4.3kPa) which facilitates excretion of fetal CO_2 across the placenta. There is metabolic compensation by renal excretion of bicarbonate.
- Slight increase in PaO_2.

Reduced functional residual capacity (FRC)

FRC reduces from the 2nd trimester, reaching 25% of pre-pregnancy values by term. This falls further when supine and as a result closing capacity is easily exceeded. The time to desaturation during apnoea is halved by the combination of reduced FRC and increased oxygen consumption. Preoxygenation is hence extremely important and should be performed with some head-up tilt.

Other changes

Total lung capacity and vital capacity remain normal—the increase in tidal volume is balanced by reduced FRC.

Airway resistance is unchanged (flow-volume loops normal).

The P50 of the oxyhaemoglobin dissociation curve increases, probably due to increased 2.3-DPG, facilitating oxygen delivery to fetal haemoglobin.

Changes in labour

Further increases in tidal volume and respiratory rate occur in labour, which correlate with pain levels. Marked hypocapnia can occur and cause hypoventilation and even apnoea between contractions, especially in the presence of parenteral opioids. The active second stage increases minute ventilation and oxygen consumption despite analgesia.

Renal system

Renal blood flow increases and glomerular filtration rate is raised by 50% in the 3rd trimester, reducing serum creatinine levels.

Excretion of bicarbonate is increased to compensate for respiratory alkalosis. A reduction in plasma bicarbonate means that metabolic acidosis may be poorly tolerated.

Urinary bacteraemia is more common and hypotonicity of the ureters causes dilatation and increased likelihood of reflux and ascending infection.

Gastrointestinal system

Gastric changes
Lower oesophageal sphincter pressure is reduced by the effect of progesterone on smooth muscle and a more horizontal gastric axis above the uterus. Combined with the increased intraabdominal pressure, this reduces barrier pressure and causes reflux. This resolves 24–48h post delivery.

Gastric emptying and gastric acidity is thought to be unchanged throughout pregnancy until active labour ensues.

Hepatic changes
Hepatic blood flow is unchanged but increased microsomal activity occurs raising liver enzyme measurements to the upper limits of normal. The elevated level of alkaline phosphatase is due to placental production. Gallstones are more common in pregnancy.

Pancreatic changes
Pancreatic beta cell insulin production is stimulated by oestrogen and in early pregnancy. This effect is then surpassed by the many 'anti-insulin' effects of cortisol, human placental lactogen, prolactin, progesterone, and oestrogen.

Haematological changes

Physiological anaemia of pregnancy
A mild relative anaemia is caused as the 50% increase in plasma volume outweighs the 25% in red cell mass. It is thought that the low haematocrit and viscosity confers protective effects for placental circulation. Other causes for anaemia should be investigated if haemoglobin levels are <11g/dL.

Hypercoagulable state
Fibrinogen levels double by term pregnancy despite evidence of increased fibrinolysis with elevated plasminogen and fibrin degradation products. Fibrinolysis may be balanced by plasminogen activation inhibitors produced by the placenta.

Most clotting factor levels rise (factors VII, VIII, IX, X, and XII) so there is a slight reduction in prothrombin time and partial thromboplastin time.

Although mild gestational thrombocytopaenia occurs in 8% of women at term, platelet activity and turnover is increased.

Other changes that have relevance to the conduct of anaesthesia are described in Boxes 24.2 and 24.3.

Box 24.2 Maternal changes of relevance to regional anaesthesia

- Increased lumbar lordosis
- Increased adipose tissue and oedema
- Difficulty flexing back
- Wider pelvis—in lateral position causes slight head-down position and increased height of block
- Softer ligaments—including ligamentum flavum
- Epidural venous engorgement:
  - Increased bloody tap
  - Increased spread of local anaesthetic
- Reduced dose requirement for block height by 25%:
  - Decreased CSF volume,
  - Increased cephalad spread,
  - Possible increased neural susceptibility.

Box 24.3 Maternal changes of relevance to GA

Intubation
- Reduced LOS barrier pressure
- Increased Mallampati class
- Upper airway oedema—smaller ETT
- Increased breast tissue
- Increased weight
- 10× failed intubation
- More rapid denitrogenation during preoxygenation (increased minute ventilation, decreased FRC)
- Rapid desaturation—decreased FRC and increased O_2 consumption.

Drugs
- Reduced MAC volatiles by 40%
- Reduced thiopentone dose by 35%
- Unchanged propofol dose
- Unchanged suxamethonium dose—reduced plasma cholinesterase but high volume distribution
- Increased sensitivity to aminosteroid muscle relaxants.

Further reading

Heidemann BH & McClure JH (2003). Changes in maternal physiology during pregnancy. *CEPD Review*, 3(3):65–8.

24.2 Labour analgesia and anaesthesia

Labour pain

In the first stage of labour, pain is due to muscle tension in the uterine body and fundus during contraction. Visceral afferent nerve fibres, which accompany the sympathetic nerves, transmit this painful stimulus to T10–L1 cord segments. The pain in the first stage of labour may respond to opiates.

In the late first and second stage of labour pain is transmitted via somatic nerve fibres from the cervix, vagina and perineum. These are carried via the pudendal nerve to S2–S4. Pain in the second stage of labour is opioid resistant.

Low-dose epidurals in labour

The use of low-dose or 'mobile' epidurals is now routine. Low-concentration, high-volume LA with addition of opiate is used, e.g. bupivacaine 0.1% + fentanyl 2mcg/mL. This provides good quality sensory block whilst reducing the LA dose and hence motor block. Evidence has shown that low-dose epidurals:

- Do not increase the risk of Caesarean section (CS).
- Do not increase the duration of first stage of labour (even if commenced early).
- May increase the rate of instrumental vaginal delivery (possible due to poor expulsive effort or less fetal rotation during descent).

Epidural analgesia delivery modes

The optimal method of delivery of labour epidural analgesia has been extensively investigated.

Continuous infusion of 'low dose mixture' (LDM) creates a stable analgesia level, may provide greater maternal cardiovascular stability, reduces staff workload, and reduces risk of toxicity provided the initial connection is correctly sited. It is associated with a greater total LA dose and hence increased motor block. This could be expected to increase rates of instrumental delivery.

Intermittent bolus of LDM is commonly used. This reduces the total LA dose but may result in regression of analgesia due to delays in drug administration and staff workload.

Patient-controlled epidural analgesia (PCEA) may offer the best combination. It is associated with reduced LA dose and low staff workload but allows good analgesia with the ability to escalate analgesia levels in the second stage of labour. Research into the optimal regimens suggests a background infusion in addition to bolus administration provides superior analgesia but rates >5ml/h result in greater motor block. A high volume, long lock-out bolus (such as 15mL, 30min) seems to provide better analgesia than low volume, high frequency bolus whilst reducing overall LA dose.

Combined spinal epidural for labour

CSE may be performed to provide labour analgesia using a low-dose intrathecal LA with or without opioid, followed by low-dose epidural. The optimal intrathecal dose is about 2–3mg bupivacaine. Advantages include:

- Faster onset
- High-quality analgesia
- Higher patient satisfaction in second stage of labour
- Reliable sacral block.

When compared to standard LDM epidural, CSE seems not to be associated with increased hypotension or significant motor block. A possible increase in fetal heart rate abnormalities may be attributable to intrathecal opiates.

Remifentanil PCA in labour

Remifentanil, a short acting μ-1 opioid receptor agonist, may have ideal characteristics to provide labour analgesia; onset within 30–60sec, peak effect in 2–3min and a short half-life. Remifentanil PCA may offer an alternative method of labour analgesia and may be especially useful in patients with absolute/relative contraindications to epidural analgesia.

When compared to other opiate regimens, remifentanil provides lower pain scores, lower conversion to epidural, and better neonatal APGAR scores. When compared to epidural analgesia, although pain scores are higher, patient satisfaction scores are similar.

Concerns over the safety of remifentanil PCA centre on the high frequency of maternal desaturation and the risk of apnoea. Monitoring requires:

- Continuous oximetry
- 1:1 nursing
- Availability of anaesthetic support.

Typical regimens are a bolus dose of 0.3–0.5mcg/kg with a lock-out of 2–3min. Analgesia is improved if a variable bolus can be used, with dose escalation as labour progresses.

Epidural top-up for emergency CS

A rapid onset epidural top-up for emergency CS may prevent GA and the associated airway morbidity/mortality. Lidocaine with adrenaline top-ups may be associated with faster onset when compared to bupivacaine/ropivacaine. Addition of opiate also increases the onset time.

Studies have also found that the addition of bicarbonate to a lidocaine/adrenaline mixture halved the onset time when compared to bupivacaine. Unfortunately, this drug mixture is not stable in solution for storage.

Although these top-up mixtures may allow the use of epidural extension to anaesthesia in Category 1 CS, this must be balanced with the time required for drug preparation and also the safety aspects of potential drug errors.

Rapid sequence spinal anaesthesia

In many emergency CSs, GA could be avoided by provision of rapid spinal anaesthesia. The patient is positioned laterally and can be preoxygenated concurrently. The original concept points for Category 1 delivery are:

- No touch
- No opioid
- Limited attempts
- Allow surgical start before full block
- Prepare for GA.

The preoxygenation time is used to site a spinal anaesthetic. It is important not to delay the start of surgery with multiple attempts and it can be useful to use the theatre timer. The block should be sufficient to allow the start of surgery and delivery. This technique may allow a surgical start within 6–8min.

The technique can be modified if time or staffing allows to include concurrent limited scrubbing and use of fentanyl.

Management of spinal-induced hypotension

Hypotension post-spinal anaesthesia, a reduction in maternal systolic blood pressure by 20–30%, occurs in about 60% of cases. Uteroplacental perfusion depends on maternal blood pressure and fetal distress can ensue. Maternal symptoms include presyncope, nausea and vomiting. Techniques to reduce hypotension include:

• Prevention of aortocaval compression
• Fluid preloading
• Fluid coloading
• Reduction in intrathecal dose
• Vasopressors—ephedrine, phenylephrine.

Phenylephrine has been found to correct spinal-induced hypotension equally to ephedrine and meta-analysis has shown that it is associated with higher umbilical artery pH in the neonate. This is in contrast to animal placental studies which showed that α-agonists cause increased resistance and decreased flow in the uterine and umbilical arteries. It is hypothesized that ephedrine may cross the placenta and increase fetal acidosis via sympathetic effects.

Phenylephrine is used optimally as a prophylactic infusion (starting at 50mcg/min) to achieve target maternal blood pressure of baseline values. It is fast becoming the vasopressor of choice in obstetric anaesthesia.

Difficult or failed intubation during GA

Failed intubation occurs in 1:300 obstetric cases yet there are no specific obstetric guidelines. Management should broadly follow the Difficult Airway Society guidelines.

Preoxygenation and positioning is especially important in the obstetric patient. A ramped position with 30° head-up improves preoxygenation and access to the airway. If intubation fails, optimization of the airway may require modification or reduction of the cricoid pressure. Videolaryngoscopes may be useful.

An emergency CS may proceed on facemask or LMA if necessary, preferably with cricoid pressure if it can be maintained. Each case requires assessment on an individual basis—see Fig. 24.1.

Further reading

Hillyard SG, Bate TE, Corcoran TB, *et al*. (2011). Extending epidural analgesia for emergency LSCS: a metaanalysis. *Br J Anaesth*, 107:668–78.

Loubert C, Hinova A, & Fernando R (2011). Update on neuraxial analgesia in labour. *Anaesthesia*, 66:191–212.

Rucklidge M & Hinton C (2012). Difficult and failed intubation in obstetrics. *CEACCP*, 2:86–91.

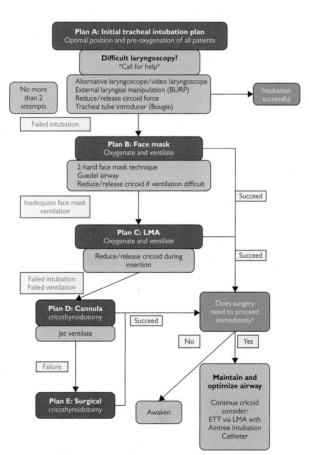

Fig. 24.1 Failed obstetric intubation drill. Reproduced from Rucklidge M and Hinton C, 'Difficult and failed intubation in obstetrics', *Continuing Education in Anaesthesia, Critical Care and Pain*, 2012, figure 2, 12, 2, p. 88, with permission from Matthew Rucklidge and Oxford University Press.

24.3 The parturient with medical disease

Cardiac disease

Indirect maternal death from cardiac disease during pregnancy is the leading cause of maternal mortality. The increased cardiac output during pregnancy and delivery, is tolerated poorly in some conditions.

Antenatal care

Early cardiology assessment and investigation, which may require invasive procedures, should be carried out. High-risk women (Box 24.4) may require referral to a tertiary unit. Frequent review is required to optimize maternal condition and monitor fetal growth.

Box 24.4 Low- and high-risk risk conditions

Low-risk condition
- NYHA class I or II—associated with <1% mortality
- No pulmonary hypertension
- Able to increase stroke volume
- Able to tolerate tachycardia.

High-risk condition
- NYHA class III or IV—associated with 30% mortality
- Left ventricular outflow obstruction or mitral stenosis
- Pulmonary hypertension
- Cardiomyopathy.

Delivery

Vaginal delivery is possible in most conditions and may be preferable to reduce blood loss, postdelivery pain, and immobility. Induction of labour uses drugs with many cardiovascular effects and should be avoided if possible. Labour and delivery are associated with profound haemodynamic changes and invasive monitoring may be required in addition to ECG and oximetry. Epidural analgesia attenuates the additional sympathetic increase in cardiac output, and low concentration epidural solutions are well tolerated. An assisted second stage of labour reduces further cardiac output rises.

Caesarean section may be required for maternal or fetal deterioration before term. Although this avoids the cardiovascular challenge of labour, Caesarean delivery also increases cardiac output and may result in greater blood loss. Regional techniques are now used in situations where GA was considered mandatory. Incremental epidural techniques or low-dose spinal anaesthesia with CSE have been used successfully in many cases. Single-shot spinal anaesthesia should be avoided. GA may require modified rapid sequence techniques using etomidate, remifentanil, and suxamethonium to enhance cardiovascular stability.

Oxytocin should be administered as an infusion rather than bolus to minimize the vasodilatation and hypotension caused. Both ergometrine and carboprost may precipitate pulmonary oedema in susceptible patients.

Postpartum

High-dependency obstetric care or intensive care should continue post delivery for at least 24–48h. Pulmonary oedema is more common in the postnatal period.

Ischaemic heart disease

IHD is an important cause of maternal mortality and must be considered in women with chest pain, especially in the presence of risk factors. The hypercoagulable state of pregnancy, increase in coronary artery spasm and dissection, combined with the high oxygen consumption cause susceptibility to ischaemia in the peripartum period. Management should be the same as a non-pregnant patient and angiographic coronary intervention may be performed. Thrombolysis carries greater risk. Where possible, delivery should be delayed for at least 2 weeks post infarction. Vaginal delivery with good epidural analgesia and an assisted second stage is the best way to reduce oxygen demand.

Congenital heart disease

Many patients have fully corrected congenital heart disease and have a normal cardiovascular response. Early assessment with echocardiography can confirm this. Patients with acyanotic congenital heart diseases, e.g. atrial or ventricular septal defects, generally tolerate pregnancy and delivery well. Regional analgesia/anaesthesia is suitable and helps to avoid high SVR which may increase left-to-right shunting. Patients with cyanotic congenital heart disease, e.g. Fallot's tetralogy, are high risk and should be referred to a tertiary unit. The low SVR associated with pregnancy worsens right-to-left shunting and cyanosis. Delivery is traditionally by Caesarean section under GA with full invasive monitoring, but regional anaesthesia may be used successfully.

Pulmonary hypertension

Where pulmonary hypertension is present, maternal mortality is high as the physiological changes of pregnancy are tolerated poorly in patients with a fixed right ventricular output. Termination of pregnancy should be considered. If pregnancy continues, tertiary referral is required.

Valvular disease

Mitral and aortic regurgitation are well tolerated in pregnancy. Patients with severe mitral or aortic stenosis, however, tolerate reduced SVR and high cardiac output poorly. Antenatal valvotomy may be considered. Good pain relief attenuates tachycardia. Stroke volume is fixed so sudden changes in preload or SVR should be avoided. Invasive monitoring should be used in severe disease, although vaginal delivery is possible with an assisted second stage. Post delivery, these patients are at high risk of developing pulmonary oedema due to placental autotransfusion and low colloid osmotic pressure.

Peripartum cardiomyopathy

Peripartum cardiomyopathy is the development of cardiac failure during the last month of pregnancy, or within 5 months of delivery, in the absence of precipitating causes or previous cardiac disease. It is associated with 50% mortality. A dilated cardiomyopathy causes fatigue, dyspnoea, tachycardia, and oedema. This is treated with diuretics, digoxin, and afterload reduction. Vaginal delivery with epidural analgesia is suggested.

The parturient with asthma

Asthma

Asthma occurs in about 1% of pregnancies and the clinical course is stable in half of the cases. 25% find their asthma improves and

25% show deterioration. It is often patients with more severe asthma, unfortunately, that worsen.

Factors that cause improvement of asthma:

- Progesterone-induced airway smooth muscle relaxation
- Increased levels of cortisol.

Factors that worsen asthma:

- Reduced sensitivity to β-agonists
- Increased bronchoconstricting prostaglandins
- Reduced sensitivity to cortisol (progesterone binds to receptors)
- Reluctance to take usual medication.

Women with asthma are more likely to have pregnancies complicated by preterm delivery, low birth weight, and pre-eclampsia.

Antenatal care

Women with severe asthma, or worsening symptoms should be seen urgently by a respiratory physician. All normal treatment should continue and there is no evidence of fetal harm from any asthma medication. Acute attacks may cause maternal hypoxia and hypocarbia which reduce fetal oxygen delivery (vasoconstriction of umbilical artery and left shift of oxyhaemoglobin dissociation curve). Regular home assessment of peak expiratory flow helps detect deteriorations early and women should have a plan for escalating treatment if necessary.

Acute attacks are managed in the same way as a non-pregnant patient. High intrathoracic pressure during an acute severe attack may reduce cardiac output and so relief of aortocaval compression and fetal monitoring is important.

Asthma may preclude the use of β-blockade for management of hypertensive disease. Patients on corticosteroids will need screening for gestational diabetes.

Delivery

Drugs used for induction of labour may precipitate asthma. All asthma medication should continue despite the possible uterine effects of β-agonists. Steroid cover may be required in patients on oral prednisolone or with recent steroid use. The high minute volume associated with pain in labour may precipitate an acute deterioration, and epidural analgesia is beneficial. Severe asthmatics should have oxygen therapy during labour.

If a Caesarean section is required, regional anaesthesia is preferable although a high motor block may reduce the ability to cough. GA may provoke bronchoconstriction. Severe asthmatics should be induced with propofol or ketamine. Non-steroidal analgesics may need to be avoided.

Oxytocin is the safest drug for management of the third stage, carboprost (PGF2α) causes bronchoconstriction as may misoprostol (PGE2).

The parturient with diabetes

Diabetes

Pre-existing diabetes complicates 0.3% of pregnancies and gestational diabetes (GDM) occurs in a further 2%. Pre-pregnancy optimization of diabetic control may reduce the incidence of fetal congenital anomalies. Good glycaemic control antenatally improves maternal and fetal outcomes.

Women with diabetes are more likely to develop pre-eclampsia and preterm labour. Perinatal mortality is five times higher and close fetal observation is required from 32 weeks of gestation. Congenital anomalies are more frequent, particularly cardiac and renal defects. Glucose crosses the placenta whereas maternal insulin does not. Fetal hyperglycaemia increases insulin production and the anabolic effects cause fetal macrosomia. This increases the frequency of difficult delivery, especially shoulder dystocia and the incidence of Caesarean section.

Antenatal care

Early multidisciplinary care is essential and insulin requirements change throughout pregnancy.

In the first 20 weeks:

- Oestrogen causes increased pancreatic secretion of insulin and increased peripheral utilization.
- Plasma glucose is lower.
- Insulin requirements are reduced.
- Increased risk of hypoglycaemia.

Between 20 weeks and term:

- Insulin resistance increases due to human placental lactogen, prolactin, cortisol, and progesterone.
- GDM develops if insulin secretion fails to increase and meet demands.
- Higher blood glucose levels.
- Increased insulin requirements (about 30%).
- Increased risk of hyperglycaemic episodes.
- Diabetic ketoacidosis may be precipitated by infection, steroids for fetal lung maturation.
- Near term, night time hypoglycaemia is common so evening insulin doses may need reducing.

GDM is more likely with older maternal age, obesity, family history of diabetes, previous GDM and glycosuria. High risk parturients should be screened with a glucose tolerance test. GDM can be managed with diet, metformin, or insulin.

Delivery

Insulin requirements reduce in the first stage of labour, then increase in the second stage. Sliding scale insulin infusion is required. There is little evidence that the sympathetic block from epidural analgesia changes glycaemic control. If elective Caesarean section is required, this should be performed first on the list after omitting morning insulin. GA risks are as per the non-pregnant diabetic population.

Following delivery, insulin requirements are hugely decreased for a few days. Neonatal hypoglycaemia may occur due to persistent elevation of insulin levels.

The obese parturient

Obesity in pregnancy

Obesity has been identified as a major risk factor for maternal morbidity and mortality. About 25% of UK pregnant women are obese.

Antenatal care

Women with a BMI >35 with medical comorbidity or a BMI >40 should be seen in the anaesthetic antenatal clinic. Physiological changes during pregnancy are compounded by obesity and cardiorespiratory complications are increased. Women should be encouraged to consider early epidural analgesia for labour but should be informed of the relative difficulties in performing regional techniques. Antenatally, obese women are at increased risk of GDM (10%), pre-eclampsia (20%), cardiomyopathy, thromboembolic disease, fetal macrosomia, fetal birth defects, and intrauterine death.

Delivery

Obese women are at increased risk of labour complications including failure to progress, malpresentations, shoulder dystocia, instrumental delivery, and Caesarean section. Emergency Caesarean section rate is 24–45%. For this reason, early labour epidural analgesia should be encouraged. This can then be extended to provide anaesthesia for an emergency situation. Epidural analgesia is more difficult and problems occur with identification of midline, level of insertion and catheter displacement. Failure rate may be as high as 40% and some morbidly obese women may require over three attempts to establish analgesia. There is an increased incidence of accidental dural puncture and neurological injury. The sitting position allows better identification of the midline and reduces depth to the epidural space when compared to the lateral position. Ultrasound and verbal direction may be required to identify the midline. Epidural depth is related to maternal weight rather than BMI. It is actually rare for the depth to exceed 8cm but long epidural needles should be available. The efficacy of analgesia should be frequently reviewed and the anaesthetist should ensure that they are informed early of any possibility of emergency delivery.

An elective Caesarean section should be performed under regional anaesthesia where possible as this reduces maternal morbidity and mortality. Experienced senior personnel should be involved. Spinal anaesthesia is more difficult to perform and high block is more common. This is perhaps as a result of reduced CSF volume from epidural venous engorgement, or relative head-down position from altered buttock to hip ratio. CSE techniques allow titration of block to avoid this problem as well as more gradual cardiorespiratory changes which are better tolerated. There is the added benefit of use for postoperative analgesia.

GA should be avoided where possible and an experienced anaesthetist must be involved. The risk of a difficult airway in the obese parturient is as high as 33%. Airway assessment is essential and awake fibreoptic intubation may be considered. A head-up ramped position will improve preoxygenation and successful airway management. A short-handled laryngoscope may be helpful and failed intubation pathways must be adhered to.

Perioperatively, cardiorespiratory compromise may occur due to increased aortocaval compression, and with retraction of the panniculus which may require vertical suspension. Maternal complication rate with Caesarean section is five times that of vaginal delivery. Anaesthetic and surgical complications, operative time, and blood loss are all increased.

Postpartum

Respiratory complications are common postoperatively with hypoxaemia due to atelectasis, pneumonia, obstructive sleep apnoea, and hypoventilation due to opioid analgesia. Ventricular dysfunction may present as pulmonary oedema. Thromboembolic risk is high and heparin doses should be adjusted for weight. Endometritis, wound infection, and dehiscence are more common.

The parturient with haematological disease

Thrombophilia

This includes the familial or acquired disorders of haemostasis such as antithrombin III deficiency, factor V Leiden mutation, protein C or S deficiency, and antiphospholipid syndrome. These conditions increase the risk of thromboembolism and cause antenatal complications due to placental thrombosis and insufficiency, e.g. pre-eclampsia, placental abruption, intrauterine growth retardation, and intrauterine death. Patients are managed with LMWH prophylaxis, sometimes in combination with aspirin. This must be stopped in labour or 12h before scheduled delivery to allow epidural analgesia (Box 24.5). Patients should receive thromboembolic stockings and pneumatic compression devices whilst immobile.

> **Box 24.5 Epidural procedure and LMWH**
> - For siting an epidural allow:
>   - 12h after prophylactic dose
>   - 24h after treatment dose
> - Prior to recommencing LMWH allow:
>   - 6–8h post surgery
>   - 4h post epidural catheter removal

Haemophilia

The most common disorder is von Willebrand's disease, occurring in 1% of the population. Von Willebrand factor forms a complex with factor 8 to mediate platelet adhesion. Reduced von Willebrand factor reduces both platelet and factor 8 function leading to prolonged bleeding time. Type 1 von Willebrand's is mild and more common. Due to a natural rise in factors during pregnancy, no treatment is usually required. Type 2 patients have more severe disease and bleeding tendency remains during pregnancy. Regular factor 8 levels are required during pregnancy. For labour, desmopressin (DDAVP 0.3mcg/kg every 12h) or factor 8/von-Willebrand concentrate is required if factor 8 levels are <50%. For Caesarean section levels must be >80%. A multidisciplinary team plan for delivery is essential and Haematology should advise if regional anaesthesia is contraindicated.

Immune thrombocytopaenia

Platelet counts may reduce further in pregnancy and should be closely monitored. High-dose steroids or immunoglobulin may be used. Regional anaesthesia is contraindicated if platelet count is <80 (if clotting normal). Caesarean section may require platelet transfusion.

Sickle cell disease

Sickling occurs with hypoxia, venous stasis, hypothermia, and acidosis. Antenatal exacerbations are common and maternal mortality is 1% due to sepsis (particularly renal tract infection) and thromboembolic disease. Pre-eclampsia, placental abruption, placenta praevia, intrauterine growth retardation, and preterm labour are all increased. Perinatal mortality is 20%. Patients must be kept warm, well-hydrated, oxygenated and appropriate analgesia used. It is important to relieve aortocaval compression to decrease venous stasis. Transfusion may be required for severe anaemia, hypoxia and surgery. The aim should be for Hb >8d/dL with >40% HbA.

The parturient with epilepsy

Epilepsy

Epilepsy complicates 0.5% pregnancies and 30% patients experience an increase in seizure frequency antenatally. This may be due to:
- Hormonal changes, hypocapnia, sodium, and water retention.
- Alteration in drug levels due to changes in volume of distribution and drug clearance.
- Poor compliance with medication.

Antenatal care

There is an increased incidence of congenital abnormalities and all anticonvulsants have been linked to teratogenic effects with associated facial, cardiac, neural tube, and limb defects. Maternal seizures are associated with maternal death, trauma, and fetal hypoxia. It is therefore best to continue anticonvulsant medication at the lowest dose of single agent which will adequately control seizures. Regular drug level monitoring and dose modification is necessary antenatally. Maternal seizures are treated with benzodiazepines or phenytoin. Fetal monitoring should be instituted. It is important to consider eclampsia.

Delivery

Pethidine has epileptogenic effects (mediated by its metabolite norpethidine) and should be avoided. There is no contraindication to epidural analgesia or regional techniques for operative delivery.

The parturient with back problems

Scoliosis and spinal surgery

Mild scoliosis is common and rarely leads to difficulty with epidural insertion. Severe scoliosis may require ultrasonography or even MRI to aid location of the epidural space. Patients may have had surgery for scoliosis or disc disease. Surgical details should be collated and the patient examined for scar position. Anatomy may be abnormal and the risks of difficult insertion, accidental dural puncture, abnormal spread of LA and failed analgesia are increased. Spinal anaesthesia may be more reliable than epidural. Where possible, the epidural should be performed away from the site of surgery.

Further reading

Burt CC & Durbridge J (2009). Management of cardiac disease in pregnancy. *CEACCP*, 9:44–7.

Gupta A & Faber P (2011). Obesity and pregnancy. *CEACCP*, 11(4):143–6.Saravanakumar K, Rao SG, & Cooper GM (2006). Obesity and obstetric anaesthesia. *Anaesthesia*, 61:36–48.

24.4 Management of premature delivery and fetal distress

Premature delivery

Premature delivery is defined as a delivery between 20 and 37 weeks' gestation. It is the most important single determinant of adverse neonatal outcome. Neonatal survival rate increases with gestational age and birth weight; it is almost 100% by 32 weeks' gestation.

Factors associated with premature delivery:
- Previous premature delivery
- Infection
- Cervical incompetence
- Obesity
- Pre-eclampsia
- Abnormal placentation
- Multiple gestation
- Polyhydramnios.

A fibronectin test may help predict premature delivery. Fetal fibronectin is not usually present in vaginal secretions until term but is present with imminent delivery. The test has a high negative exclusion rate.

The normal triggers for the onset of labour are not completely understood. Near term there is an increase in myometrial prostaglandin and oxytocin receptors and activation of ion channels. The fetal HPA axis appears to have a role in the final triggering of labour.

Tocolysis

Tocolytic therapy may be used to delay premature labour although no clear improvement in neonatal morbidity/mortality has been shown. Tocolysis may only create a 2–7 day delay, but this time allows maternal administration of corticosteroids to accelerate fetal lung maturity and improve outcome. It may also allow maternal transfer to deliver at a unit with appropriate neonatal facilities. Tocolysis is only used if infection and abruption are excluded and the cardiotocograph (CTG) is reassuring.

Tocolytic agents include:

Oxytocin receptor antagonists
Atosiban is a competitive inhibitor and does not alter the myometrial sensitivity to oxytocin following delivery which reduces uterine atony. A bolus dose is followed by an infusion. Nausea is the main side effect.

β-adrenergic receptor agonists
Ritodrine, terbutaline, and salbutamol may be used. β-2 receptor stimulation activates adenyl cyclase, increasing cyclic AMP and reducing intracellular calcium to relax smooth muscle. These agents are associated with significant maternal and fetal side effects. Maternal tachycardia and hypotension are common but cardiac arrhythmia; myocardial ischaemia, and pulmonary oedema have all been reported. Fetal tachycardia results and neonatal hypoglycaemia may be a concern.

Calcium channel antagonists
Nifedipine 20–30mg initially, followed by 10–20mg every 6h. Doses >60mg are associated with headache and hypotension. Comparative efficacy to atosiban and may be associated with the best neonatal outcome.

Glyceryl trinitrate (GTN)
GTN acts as a nitric oxide donor, activating cyclic GMP and reducing intracellular calcium to relax smooth muscle. It has the advantage of rapid onset and offset, reducing postpartum uterine atony, but may cause maternal hypotension.

Magnesium sulphate
Used in a similar regimen to pre-eclampsia protocol but is less effective in reducing premature birth. May reduce cerebral palsy rates.

Cyclooxygenase inhibitors
Indomethacin may be used to reduce prostaglandin E2 and F2α but may be associated with neonatal complications relating to premature ductus arteriosus closure and pulmonary hypertension.

Tocolytics should not be used in combination as the adverse effects increase. These drugs may also be used in other circumstances:
- External cephalic version
- Uterine hyperstimulation
- Delivery of second twin
- Intra-uterine resuscitation.

Anaesthesia for premature delivery

The premature fetus is more susceptible to acidosis and hypoxia during labour but Caesarean section does not improve overall survival. Labour epidural analgesia confers a number of benefits for obstetric management which may impact on perinatal mortality, as well as allowing conversion to provide anaesthesia for Caesarean section which is an increased risk. Benefits include:
- Reduction in maternal catecholamines
- Reducing early pushing and precipitous delivery
- Allowing controlled delivery of the head.

For Caesarean section, regional anaesthesia may be preferable for maternal reasons. In very premature infants mortality may be higher following spinal anaesthesia as compared to general and epidural anaesthesia.

General anaesthesia should be performed for the usual indications but the neonate may show increased depressant effect related to the immature blood–brain barrier and reduced metabolic function. The incidence of intubation and lower 5min Apgar score is increased.

If regional anaesthesia is used, an increased intrathecal dose may be required to provide adequate block. Maternal blood pressure should be maintained with fluid and phenylephrine infusion to optimize uteroplacental flow.

Fetal distress

Fetal distress is the result of inadequate oxygen delivery to the fetus. CTG abnormalities may suggest fetal distress:
- Abnormal baseline rate (normal 120–160bpm)
- Loss of variability (normal 10–15/min)
- Absence of accelerations
- Late decelerations (>20/min and occurring 10–30sec after a contraction).

Fetal scalp pH may be monitored if CTG is non-reassuring but there is no immediate indication for emergency Caesarean. A pH >7.25 is normal, <7.2 usually prompts delivery. Values between require repeat investigation.

Intra-uterine resuscitation aims to correct the causes of fetal distress and may be used concurrently to planning delivery. Resuscitation may create more time for anaesthesia provision. See Table 24.1.

Table 24.1 Cause and mechanism of reduced intra-uterine oxygen delivery	
Reduced arterial pressure:	Resuscitative measures:
Maternal hypotension	Relieve aortocaval compression IV fluids Vasopressors
Cord compression	Change maternal position Elevate fetal presenting part: Bladder dilation Amnio-infusion Manual (if cord prolapsed)
Cord vasospasm	Return prolapsed cord to vagina and keep warm
Increased uterine venous pressure:	
Aortocaval compression	Relieve aortocaval compression
Poor uterine relaxation	Stop oxytocin infusion
	Tocolysis: GTN IV 50–100mcg Salbutamol inhaler Salbutamol IV 25mcg
Increased uterine vascular resistance:	
Maternal catecholamines	Epidural analgesia
Pre-eclampsia	

Caesarean delivery for fetal distress

Good communication among the labour ward team is the key to managing an emergency delivery. It may be helpful for the obstetrician to convey a target delivery time as well as a category of Caesarean section. The anaesthetic options are determined by the time available and the presence of a functioning labour epidural. Intrauterine resuscitation and CTG monitoring should continue until the point of delivery.

Regional anaesthesia is associated with higher Apgar scores, earlier sustained respiratory function, reduced resuscitation requirement, and better neurobehavioural scores. Despite this a large meta-analysis demonstrates a significantly lower umbilical pH and higher base deficit with spinal anaesthesia as opposed to general anaesthesia.

Category 1 Caesarean—immediate delivery or within 30min

For example, cord prolapse, uterine rupture. This will usually necessitate a general anaesthetic. A 'rapid sequence spinal' anaesthetic may be attempted where the patient pre-oxygenates in a lateral position and the pre-oxygenation time is used to perform spinal anaesthesia.

Category 2 Caesarean—delivery within 30–60min

For example, serious CTG abnormality, fetal scalp pH <7.2, This situation will usually allow regional anaesthesia or extension of epidural analgesia with faster onset solutions:

• Lidocaine, adrenaline, bicarbonate

• Lidocaine, bupivacaine, adrenaline

• Lidocaine, bupivacaine.

Category 3 Caesarean—delivery within 2h

For example, failure to progress, pre-eclampsia. Regional anaesthesia may be instituted or labour analgesia extended to anaesthesia within this time frame.

Category 4 Caesarean—elective delivery

No restriction on mode of anaesthesia.

Further reading

Laudenbach V, Mercier FJ, Rozé JC, et al. (2009). Anaesthesia mode for caesarean section and mortality in very preterm infants. *IJOA*, 18:142–5.

Royal College of Obstetricians and Gynaecologists (2010). *Classification of urgency of caesarean section-a continuum of risk*. London: RCOG.

Royal College of Obstetricians and Gynaecologists (2011). *Tocolysis for women with preterm labour*. Greentop guideline. London: RCOG.

Reynolds F & Seed PT (2005). Anaesthesia for caesarean section and neonatal acid-base status: a meta-analysis. *Anaesthesia*, 60:636–53.

Multiple pregnancy

Monozygotic twins occur in 4/1000 maternities with dizygotic twins occurring in 3–14/1000, the incidence increasing with maternal age and parity. In the USA, 0.2% of births are now triplet or higher order pregnancies. This effect is due to the increase in assisted conception.

Multiple pregnancy causes increased maternal and fetal complications which may require anaesthetic management. The delivery of triplet or higher-order births is by Caesarean section but twin delivery may be performed vaginally which requires anaesthetic planning and supervision.

Maternal effects of multiple pregnancy

The physiological and anatomical changes associated with pregnancy are exaggerated further, largely as a direct effect of the greater uterine size.

CVS
- Blood volume is increased by an extra 500mL
- Relative anaemia is more common
- Greater effects of aortocaval compression.

RS
- FRC further reduced
- TLC further reduced
- Increased tendency to hypoxia
- Adequate preoxygenation is essential before GA.

GI
- Increased lower oesophageal sphincter incompetence
- Increased maternal weight (increased incidence of difficult intubation).

Maternal complications

The incidence of maternal complications increases with the number of fetuses carried.

Antenatal
- Pre-eclampsia
- Gestational diabetes
- Premature delivery
- Antepartum haemorrhage—placenta praevia and abruption.

Delivery
- Increased cord prolapse
- Increased operative delivery
- Increased uterine atony
- Increased obstetric trauma
- Increased postpartum haemorrhage—12%.

Fetal complications

Perinatal mortality is at least seven times that of a singleton pregnancy and increases with the number of fetuses present.

There is an increased risk of:
- Congenital anomalies.
- Intrauterine growth retardation—due to restriction by overall uterine size and other fetal sacs as well as vascular compromise.
- Twin–twin transfusion syndrome.
- Cord 'accidents'.
- Intrauterine death is increased.

Elective Caesarean delivery

In many cases, elective Caesarean delivery will be planned although the high rate of premature labour may necessitate more urgent delivery.

Regional anaesthesia
Regional anaesthesia is preferable and has been associated with improved outcome in the second twin. Patients may find upright positioning for an epidural difficult and it may cause aortocaval compression. The lateral position may be considered. Some studies have reported increased cephalad spread with standard spinal anaesthetic doses. Using a CSE technique may allow some reduction in intrathecal dose whilst ensuring adequate duration of block.

Special considerations
Large-bore IV access should be sited and, in view of the increased risk of postpartum haemorrhage, it may be appropriate to cross-match blood for patients with anaemia.

Patients with multiple gestation are very prone to hypotension relating to aortocaval compression following sympathetic block. Patients may require the full lateral position rather than tilt, as well as the standard techniques to prevent hypotension, e.g. fluid co-loading and vasopressor infusion.

Pulmonary oedema following delivery has been reported in many high-order multiple births. The increased volume of placental autotransfusion on delivery should be taken into account when administering intravenous fluids.

Uterotonic drugs are not given until all babies are delivered. Due to a high risk of atony, further uterotonic medications may be required.

Vaginal delivery of twins

If both twins are cephalic in presentation, vaginal delivery is possible. Unless the first twin is breech, no difference has been shown in morbidity or mortality for neonates or mother between vaginal delivery and Caesarean section. There is, however, an increased risk of instrumental delivery and emergency Caesarean section, particularly for the delivery of the second twin.

Labour epidural analgesia
Women having twin vaginal delivery should be counselled in the antenatal period as to the risks of delivery. Women should be encouraged to have epidural analgesia for labour, and the anaesthetist must ensure that this is working well. This allows extension to anaesthesia should an emergency situation arise.

Delivery
Many centres perform twin vaginal delivery in the operating theatre to allow rapid emergency delivery if fetal distress occurs. The

anaesthetist should ideally be present for the second stage of labour. A study has shown that 27% of patients require anaesthetic intervention and 6% require emergency Caesarean section for delivery of the second twin. Despite working epidurals, half of these cases required general anaesthesia for Caesarean due to profound fetal distress. Good communication between the multidisciplinary team is essential.

The epidural may be extended for Caesarean section at the time of delivery of the first twin. Between 15min and 30min are allowed before the second twin must be delivered and fetal heart monitoring is continued. If the second twin is breech, uterine relaxation may be required to facilitate internal cephalic version or delivery as breech. Sublingual or IV GTN 50mcg may be used and the procedure performed after 45sec. GTN is a short-acting tocolytic which avoids uterine atony following delivery.

Further reading

Carvalho B, Saxena A, Butwick A, *et al*. (2008). Vaginal twin delivery: a survey of location, anaesthesia and intervention. *IJOA*, 17:212–16.

Marino T, Goudas LC, Steinbok V, *et al*. (2001). Triplet Caesarean section. *Anesth Analg*, 93:991–5.

24.6 Pre-eclampsia

Pre-eclampsia

Pre-eclampsia (PET) is defined as the presence of:

1. Hypertension (two readings >90mmHg diastolic taken at least 4h apart or a single reading >110mmHg)
2. Proteinuria (>0.3g/L or two reagents strip tests 2+)
3. Hyperuricaemia
4. Oedema

after 20 weeks of gestation. Hypertension prior to 20 weeks is known as chronic hypertension. Isolated hypertension after 20 weeks is known as pregnancy-induced hypertension.

PET complicates about 3% of pregnancies and is associated with increased maternal and fetal morbidity and mortality. About 20% of cases present postpartum. See Box 24.6 for risk factors.

Severe PET is defined as the presence of one or more of the following features:

- SBP >160mmHg or DBP >110 mmHg
- Proteinurea >5g/24h or >3+
- Oliguria
- Cerebral problems—hyper-reflexia, visual disturbance
- Pulmonary oedema
- Hepatic dysfunction
- Thrombocytopaenia
- HELLP syndrome—Haemolysis, Elevated Liver enzymes and Low Platelets. Associated with rapid clinical deterioration, subcapsular haematomas of the liver which may rupture and high mortality. Hypertension may not be prominent.

Box 24.6 Risk factors for developing PET

- Maternal factors:
  - Primiparous
  - Extremes of maternal age
  - Previous PET
  - Family history of PET
  - Hypertension
  - Obesity
  - Diabetes
  - Renal disease
  - Thrombotic tendency
- Partner-related factors:
  - Short duration of sperm exposure
  - Father of a previous PET pregnancy
- Obstetric factors:
  - Multiple pregnancy
  - Molar pregnancy.

Pathophysiology of PET

Genetic or immune factors may be responsible for the development of PET. The first stage is of abnormal trophoblast invasion. The placenta remains shallow and does not penetrate into the myometrium. Myometrial segments of the spiral arteries remain relatively vasoconstricted and responsive to further vasoconstrictive stimuli. The high resistance reduces flow in the uteroplacental circulation. Arterial occlusion may occur by fibrin and platelets causing placental ischaemia. The second stage is that of widespread

maternal endothelial damage. Reduction in vasodilator substances leads to vasoconstriction and hypertension. Proteinuria develops due to increased glomerular permeability. Salt and water retention occurs due to reduced glomerular filtration rate. Coupled with the reduced colloid osmotic pressure, this causes oedema. Platelet aggregation reduces platelet number. See Box 24.7.

Box 24.7 Physiological effects of PET

- CVS:
  - Increased SVR
  - Reduced plasma volume
  - Increased LV work
  - Reduced cardiac output
- RS:
  - Pulmonary oedema
- Renal:
  - Reduced renal blood flow
  - Reduced glomerular filtration rate
  - Reduced urate clearance
  - Raised renin, angiotensin, and catecholamines
- CNS:
  - Loss of autoregulation of cerebral blood flow
  - Possible focal vasospasm
  - Cerebral oedema
- Hepatic:
  - Reduced hepatic blood flow
  - Raised transaminases
  - Periportal/focal necrosis
  - Subcapsular swelling and rupture
- Haematological:
  - Thrombocytopaenia
  - Coagulopathy
  - Haemolysis
- Fetal:
  - IUGR
  - Premature delivery
  - Placental abruption
  - Intrauterine death.

Management of PET (see Box 24.9)

Control of blood pressure

Control of hypertension reduces the risk of intracerebral haemorrhage, renal failure, and placental abruption. A blood pressure below 140/90 should be the target. Chronic management may be with oral methyldopa, labetalol, or nifedipine.

Acute blood pressure management in severe PET requires close monitoring and IV agents in accordance to local protocol. Labetalol and hydralazine are the commonly used agents. Hydralazine-induced vasodilatation may require concurrent fluid therapy to protect the uteroplacental flow. Labetalol has been shown to be as effective with fewer incidences of maternal side effects. The aim is to lower MAP by 15–25% but rapid changes may compromise uteroplacental blood flow.

Prevention of seizures

The Magpie Trial demonstrated that magnesium is of benefit for the prophylaxis of seizures in severe PET. It is not clear whether this effect is due to membrane stabilization or cerebral vasodilatation. Management with magnesium requires monitoring of tendon reflexes, respiratory rate, ECG, and oxygen saturations to detect signs of magnesium toxicity, especially in women with impaired renal function.

Magnesium has been shown to be more effective than diazepam or phenytoin in the treatment of eclamptic seizures. The Eclampsia Trial demonstrated good seizure control with less maternal need for ventilation and intensive care admission. Emergency management of eclampsia is described in Box 24.8.

> **Box 24.8 Management of eclampsia**
>
> - Maintain the airway.
> - Maintain oxygenation.
> - Avoid aortocaval compression.
> - Stop the seizure—magnesium 4g bolus over 10min.
> - Prevent subsequent seizures—magnesium infusion 1g/h.
> - Control hypertension.
> - Consider delivery when stable.
> - If seizures recur give a further 2g bolus of magnesium.
> - If prolonged seizure consider CT to exclude intracerebral haemorrhage.

Appropriate fluid management

Relative hypovolaemia and oliguria are common. Acute tubular necrosis associated with PET frequently recovers. Fluid resuscitation may precipitate pulmonary oedema (low colloid osmotic pressure, endothelial dysfunction and possible ventricular dysfunction all contribute) which carries a higher risk of maternal morbidity and mortality. Fluid intake should be restricted to 1mL/kg/h or about 85mL/h and fluid balance recorded. If 'fluid challenges' are considered this should be titrated against CVP or non-invasive cardiac output measurements. If pulmonary oedema occurs, frusemide should be given and respiratory dysfunction may require CPAP or ventilation to maintain oxygenation.

> **Box 24.9 Management of severe pre-eclampsia**
>
> - Management of severe hypertension:
>   - Labetalol 20mg IV, every 10min. Onset 5–10min. Max 220mg.
>   - Hydralazine 5mg IV, every 20min. Onset 10–20min. Max 20mg.
> - Prophylaxis of seizures:
>   - Magnesium sulphate. Bolus 4g over 10min. Infusion 1g/h.
> - Fluid management:
>   - 85mL/h (or 1mL/kg/h depending on local protocol).

Regional analgesia/anaesthesia in PET

Labour epidural analgesia is beneficial in PET. Further elevations in blood pressure due to the catecholamine response to pain are attenuated and there is a beneficial effect on placental blood flow. Labour epidurals can be extended to provide anaesthesia for Caesarean section if required, avoiding the concerns with general anaesthesia.

For Caesarean section, the concerns that spinal anaesthesia may cause cardiovascular instability have been disproved. Maternal blood pressure changes and maternofetal outcomes are similar using epidural and spinal anaesthesia. Maternal cardiac output is maintained following spinal despite a reduction in SVR. Pre-eclamptic women may actually have a reduced incidence of

spinal-induced hypotension and fewer requirements for vasopressor than controls.

Thrombocytopaenia and coagulopathy are a concern for regional procedures. Coagulopathy or a platelet count <50 preclude regional techniques. A platelet count >80 is generally considered acceptable but a recent result is required if the trend has been for a rapid drop in platelet number. Between 50 to 80, in the presence of normal PT and APTT, the risks and benefits of the individual patient must be assessed. TEG® may aid the decision by demonstrating overall clot formation.

General anaesthesia in PET

General anaesthesia may be necessary for emergency Caesarean section or if regional anaesthesia is precluded. There are three main concerns in performing general anaesthesia:

Difficult intubation

The incidence of difficult intubation is increased and careful airway examination is required. Airway oedema may occur which can increase traumatic bleeding during intubation and necessitate smaller diameter endotracheal tubes.

Hypertensive response to laryngoscopy

A further increase in blood pressure in response to laryngoscopy may cause intracerebral haemorrhage or pulmonary oedema. Blood pressure should be optimized prior to induction and invasive blood pressure monitoring should be considered. Remifentanil (1mcg/kg) is well suited to attenuating the response to laryngoscopy but labetalol, magnesium, alfentanil, and esmolol may all be used. Esmolol or labetalol are used to prevent hypertension during extubation where depression of airway reflexes must be avoided.

Effects of magnesium

Magnesium use interacts with neuromuscular junction transmission (Box 24.10). Non-depolarizing muscle relaxants are prolonged in action. The action of suxamethonium is unchanged but muscle fasciculation may be dampened.

Magnesium also causes reduction in uterine tone which is a risk for postpartum haemorrhage. Despite this, there is little evidence for increased blood loss at Caesarean in PET.

> **Box 24.10 Magnesium**
>
> *Effects*
> - Direct vasodilatation
> - Sympathetic block
> - Inhibition of catecholamine release
> - Bronchodilation
> - Cerebral vasodilatation
> - Sedation
> - Therapeutic level 4–8mmol/L.
>
> *Magnesium toxicity*
> - 6–10mmol/L—nausea, flushing, diplopia, slurred speech.
> - 10mmol/L—loss of patellar tendon reflexes, muscle weakness.
> - 15mmol/L—respiratory muscle paralysis, cardiac conduction defects.
> - 25mmol/L—cardiac arrest.
> - Treatment of toxicity is with calcium chloride 10mmol.

Further reading

Hart E & Coley S (2003). The diagnosis and management of pre-eclampsia. *CEACCP*, 3(2):38–42.

Polley L (2009). Hypertensive disorders. In D Chestnut (ed), *Chestnut's Obstetric Anesthesia Principles and Practice* (4th edn, pp. 975–1007). Philadelphia, PA: Mosby.

24.7 Major obstetric haemorrhage

Major obstetric haemorrhage

Major obstetric haemorrhage is an important cause of maternal morbidity. Mortality rates have decreased since CEMACH's emphasis on early senior input, good communication with specialists, management of clotting abnormality, and haemorrhage protocols and drills. Abnormal blood loss is considered to be >500mL following vaginal delivery and >1000mL following Caesarean section. Major obstetric haemorrhage is declared at >1500mL blood loss. There are many difficulties in assessing this in the obstetric setting.

Difficulties in blood loss assessment
- Underestimation of visible blood loss is common.
- Concealed blood loss—up to 1000mL in uterus.
- Amniotic fluid combined in volume.
- Young, fit women compensate well for hypovolaemia with late hypotension.
- Autotransfusion from placenta at delivery may mask early signs.

Causes of major haemorrhage

Antepartum haemorrhage (APH)
APH occurs in about 20% of pregnancies but only a fraction of these are life threatening. The greatest threat is to the fetus as uteroplacental flow has no autoregulation. The aim is to restore maternal blood volume and oxygen-carrying capacity, and to treat the underlying cause which usually requires immediate delivery of the fetus and placenta.

Causes of APH
- Placenta praevia—discussed in section 24.8.
- Placental abruption—complete/partial separation of the placenta causing maternal haemorrhage and fetal distress.
- Uterine rupture—rupture of previous uterine scar (usually due to trauma or inappropriate use of oxytocin) causing persistent pain, bleeding, and fetal compromise.

Postpartum haemorrhage
Postpartum haemorrhage occurs in 5% of pregnancies and is due to uterine atony in 80% of cases (see Box 24.11). Normally uterine contraction, stimulated by endogenous oxytocic agents and prostaglandins, compresses the vessels of the placental bed and uterine wall achieving haemostasis. This fails in an atonic uterus. Other causes include retained placental tissue, genital trauma, placenta accreta, and uterine inversion.

Management of major obstetric haemorrhage

Call for help
If major obstetric haemorrhage is confirmed, an immediate call for obstetric emergency team help is required. Many hospitals have an emergency bleep system to alert obstetricians, anaesthetists, neonatology, blood bank, and porters. Senior members of each team should be present.

Airway and breathing
- High flow oxygen via a non-rebreathing system.
- Ventilatory support may occasionally be required if maternal conscious level is reduced.

Circulation
If antepartum, left lateral tilt should be used to avoid aortocaval compression.

Two large-bore cannulae should be inserted and bloods taken for FBC, clotting, and cross-match of 8 units.

Fluid resuscitation should be commenced to restore circulating volume. Colloids may be used to replace estimated loss and provide a rapid, sustained increase in plasma volume, or crystalloids at about three times the volume of estimated loss. Blood transfusion should be commenced if blood loss is 2000mL and ongoing, or if anaemia is demonstrated by bedside haemoglobin measurement. Emergency group O negative blood may be used within the first 30min unless type-specific blood is available early. Vasopressors may be used to maintain blood pressure until intravascular volume is restored. Fluids and blood should be warmed.

Full monitoring should be instituted: ECG, NIBP, oximetry, and urine output. Invasive monitoring should be considered if there is a poor response to volume resuscitation or massive ongoing blood loss. Fetal monitoring is required if antepartum.

Treatment of underlying cause
A rapid assessment of the estimated blood loss (see Table 24.2) and likely aetiology will aid resuscitation and the management plan.

APH will often necessitate emergency delivery which will usually require general anaesthesia. Uterine atony is treated with oxytocin infusion and bimanual compression which is successful in most patients. Aggressive use of other uterotonic agents (ergometrine, carboprost and misoprostol) is associated with lower risk of hysterectomy (see Table 24.3).

Other invasive treatment options include:
- Uterine compression sutures, e.g. B-Lynch
- Intrauterine balloon tamponade
- Arterial embolization or ligation
- Emergency peripartum hysterectomy.

Box 24.11 Causes of uterine atony

Uterine overdistension
- Multiple gestation
- Macrosomia
- Polyhydramnios.

Poor contraction
- High parity
- Prolonged labour
- Augmented labour
- Use of tocolytics
- Chorioamnitis.

Table 24.2 Clinical signs in obstetric haemorrhage

% Blood loss	15–20%	20–25%	25–30%	>35%
Volume	1L	1–1.5L	1.5–2L	>2L
Signs	None	Anxious	Restless	Drowsy
RR	<16	16–20	20–30	>35
HR	<100	100	100–120	>120
BP	Normal	Raised diastolic	Reduced systolic	Systolic <60mmHg
Urine output	Normal	Normal	Oliguria	Anuria

Table 24.3 Uterotonic drugs

Dose	Action/use	Effects	
Oxytocin	Bolus 5U IV	Acts on oxytocin receptors	↓SVR, ↑HR
	Infusion 10U/h		↓MAP, ↑PAP
			Less in infusion
Ergometrine	250–500mcg	Acts on α adrenergic	↑↑SVR, ↑BP, nausea
	IM or slow IV	receptors. Rapid onset	↑PAP, coronary vasocon
		Effect lasts 2–3h	C/I—PET, IHD
Prostaglandins:		↑ myometrial intracellular calcium	Cause malaise, fever, nausea, diarrhoea
PGF2α Carboprost	250mcg IM	Repeat every 20min up to 8 doses	Bronchospasm, ↑ PAP
PGE1 Misoprostol	600–1000mcg PR		↑ PAP

Correction of coagulopathy

There may be dilutional or disseminated intravascular coagulopathy. FFP should be used in a ratio of approximately 1 unit per 2 red cell units, and guided by both clinical picture and point of care tests. Platelet count should be kept above 50 × 10^9/dL and each unit of platelets should raise the count by 5–10 × 10^9/dL. Low fibrinogen levels are predictive of major haemorrhage. Cryoprecipitate or fibrinogen concentrate should be used early and tranexamic acid reduces fibrinolysis. Activated factor 7 may be considered for ongoing bleeding after management of the underlying cause, but may create a risk of thromboembolic complications. It is currently unlicensed for this use but has prevented peripartum hysterectomy in many cases.

Reassessment and management of complications

Ongoing assessment of the clinical condition, estimated blood loss and further bleeding, results of bed-side or laboratory investigations, and requirement for further monitoring, continues during resuscitation. Complications of massive transfusion such as hyperkalaemia, hypothermia, hypocalcaemia, and lung injury should be monitored and treated.

Ongoing care

Patients with ongoing bleeding, coagulopathy, anuria, or ventilatory requirements will need to be managed in intensive care. All patients will need high dependency care with monitoring of clinical parameters and haemoglobin, platelet and clotting results.

Providing anaesthesia in maternal haemorrhage

The technique used depends on the urgency of the situation, maternal haemodynamics, coagulation results and the surgery required (see Box 24.12).

Box 24.12 Providing anaesthesia in maternal haemorrhage

Indications for GA
- APH with maternal hypovolaemia and emergency delivery required
- PPH with severe maternal hypovolaemia
- Maternal coagulopathy
- Reduced maternal conscious level
- Maternal anxiety or poor cooperation

Considerations for GA
- Rapid sequence induction required
- Induction agents may cause hypotension with maternal hypovolaemia
- Consider ketamine 0.5–1mg/kg or etomidate 0.3mg/kg in severe compromise
- Volatile agents >0.5 MAC will contribute to uterine atony. Use nitrous oxide.
- Consider other maintenance agents, e.g. remifentanil, benzodiazepines, propofol if bleeding continues

Extra resources required
- Invasive monitoring
- Non-invasive cardiac output monitoring
- Fluid warming
- Cell salvage
- Point of care testing, e.g. HemoCue®, clotting if available
- More anaesthetic help.

Further reading

Banks A & Norris A (2005). Massive haemorrhage in pregnancy. *CEACCP*, 5(6):195–8.

Placenta praevia

Placenta praevia occurs in 0.5% of pregnancies. Implantation of the placenta occurs in the lower segment of the uterus, over or near the internal os of the cervix (Box 24.13). This may lead to painless antepartum haemorrhage in the 2nd or 3rd trimester, and necessitates operative delivery as the placenta is in advance of the presenting part.

> **Box 24.13 Classification of placenta praevia**
> - *Type I* or low lying: the placenta implants in the lower segment of the uterus but does not reach the cervical os.
> - *Type II* or marginal: the placenta reaches, but does not cover, the cervix.
> - *Type III* or partial: the placenta partially covers the cervix.
> - *Type IV* or complete: the placenta completely covers the cervix.

Risk factors for placenta praevia include:
- Previous uterine scar
- Increased maternal age
- Multiparous women
- Previous placenta praevia
- Large placenta, e.g. twin pregnancy.

Placenta praevia is diagnosed antenatally on routine ultrasound. There is a risk of progressive or sudden placental separation, which presents as APH. Placenta praevia is responsible for 20% of APH. The first episode of bleeding usually resolves spontaneously and does not cause maternal cardiovascular compromise. Expectant management as an inpatient with bed rest, fetal evaluation, corticosteroids for fetal lung maturity must also ensure preparation for further haemorrhage with large-bore IV access and blood cross-matched.

If placenta praevia is diagnosed, it is essential to exclude a morbidly adherent placenta.

Morbidly adherent placentation

- *Placenta accreta:* the placenta is adherent to myometrium but no invasion through myometrium.
- *Placenta increta:* the placenta invades through myometrium.
- *Placenta percreta:* the placenta invades through uterine serosa and/or other pelvic structures, e.g. bladder.

The incidence of morbidly adherent placentation has increased to 1 in 800, largely as a result of the rise in Caesarean section (LSCS) rate. If placenta praevia is also present, the risk of placenta accreta rises in proportion to the number of previous Caesarean sections (Table 24.4). The risk of placenta percreta also rises with the number of previous LSCS.

Table 24.4 Risk of placenta accreta			
No. of LSCS	1	2	4
Accreta incidence	0.3%	0.6%	2.3%
If placenta praevia also present	11%	40%	67%

Morbidly adherent placentas do not separate normally from the uterus after delivery as there is a lack of intervening decidual tissue. This can lead to rapid maternal haemorrhage (as uterine blood flow at term is 700–900mL/min) and increased risk of Caesarean hysterectomy or maternal death. The extent of placental invasion must be assessed using ultrasound or MRI antenatally to allow suitable planning for delivery.

Anaesthesia for placenta praevia

Acute severe haemorrhage due to placenta praevia will require simultaneous resuscitation and emergency delivery. Bleeding will continue until the placenta separates and the uterus contracts post delivery. A rapid assessment of maternal volaemic status and airway is performed. Haemorrhage is revealed allowing estimated loss to be assessed. Two large-bore cannulae are sited and blood is taken for full blood count, clotting, and cross-match. Resuscitation is commenced with colloid and either O negative or type specific blood depending on maternal parameters. General anaesthesia will be required in a haemodynamically unstable patient for urgent delivery and rapid sequence induction may require ketamine (0.5–1mg/kg) or etomidate (0.3mg/kg). Invasive monitoring should be instituted and fluid warmers used to continue fluid resuscitation. Frequent assessment of haemoglobin and clotting with correction of abnormalities is required.

During Caesarean section, increased intraoperative blood loss is due to:
- Incision through an anterior placenta praevia
- Poor contraction of the lower uterine segment
- Presence of morbidly adherent placenta.

Uterotonic drugs are required to enhance uterine contraction. The effect of volatile anaesthetics on uterine tone is proportional to MAC. Concentration of volatile may be reduced by using nitrous oxide, but if ongoing atony occurs it may be necessary to use a propfol infusion.

Placenta praevia will necessitate Caesarean delivery unless the placenta is >2cm away from the cervical os. For a planned delivery, regional anaesthesia may be preferable to general anaesthesia and is associated with higher haemoglobin levels although operative times and estimated blood loss are similar.

Anaesthesia for morbidly adherent placentation

Antenatal diagnosis of abnormal placentation allows adequate planning for delivery. The following factors must be considered:

Optimum time for delivery
This is often planned for 34 weeks of gestation following steroids to enhance fetal lung maturity. Early elective delivery reduces the chance of APH and an emergency situation.

Planned surgical approach
At least two senior obstetricians are required and the presence of a vascular surgeon and urologist may be necessary.

The surgical plan will aim to avoid attempted placental removal and may involve elective Caesarean hysterectomy or leaving the placenta *in situ*. A prompt decision to proceed with hysterectomy has been shown to enhance the chances of a good outcome.

ITU stay and transfusion requirements are both decreased. This decision is very difficult unless an antenatal diagnosis has been made. Hysterectomy is required in about 90% of cases and cystotomy in 15%.

Preoperative interventional radiology
In these cases where massive obstetric haemorrhage is anticipated, it is possible to place internal iliac artery balloons prophylactically. This reduces blood loss, aids surgery and reduces transfusion requirements. The procedure may have serious complications, e.g. limb ischaemia but will prevent uncontrollable maternal haemorrhage. Interventional radiology can be performed under local anaesthesia or regional anaesthesia.

Preparation for massive haemorrhage
Large volume haemorrhage must be expected:
- 66% cases >2L
- 15% cases >5L
- 7% cases >10L.
  Preparation for this involves:
- Adequate cross-match and liaison with Haematology to ensure availability of blood products, platelets and recombinant factor 7a.
- Large bore IV access and invasive monitoring.
- Availability of rapid transfusion systems and cell salvage.
- Availability of point of care testing where possible.
- Adequate staff and support e.g. availability of interventional radiology (see Box 24.14).
- Intensive care postoperatively.

Anaesthetic technique
The patient must be fully counselled as to the risks of major haemorrhage, the surgical management of this and the length of surgery. Regional anaesthesia can be provided with a CSE technique and is associated with reduced bleeding but conversion to general anaesthesia may be required for hypotension and reduced conscious level, maternal distress, and length of surgery. If regional anaesthesia is used it should be sited prior to interventional radiology procedures. Positioning for CSE subsequently may move the iliac catheters. General anaesthesia may be preferable for most patients.

Transfusion aims

Hb >8g/dL
Give packed red cells:
- O negative in emergency.
- Type specific if can wait 20–30min.
- Full cross-match may take 45min.

INR <1.5
- Give fresh frozen plasma.
- Ratio of 1:2 red cells.
- INR is generally not elevated until 1.5–2× blood volume lost.

Fibrinogen >2g/L
- During obstetric haemorrhage, a fibrinogen level lower than this is highly predictive of massive haemorrhage.
- Give FFP/cryoprecipitate or fibrinogen concentrate.
- Tranexamic acid can be used to reduce fibrinolysis.

Platelets > 50 × 10⁹/L
- Platelet transfusion.

Additional management
- Repeat FBC, clotting, fibrinogen every 30min.
- TEG®/ROTEM® may be used.
- Maintain normothermia.
- Avoid hypocalcaemia.
- Monitor and treat hyperkalaemia.
- Recombinant factor 7a—has been used with good effect in major obstetric haemorrhage. May increase thromboembolic risk postoperatively.

Box 24.14 Interventional radiology in obstetric haemorrhage

>90% success has been shown with emergency uterine artery embolization during PPH. Patients may require transfer to a tertiary centre with interventional radiology services.
- Femoral arterial access is established (can be under LA).
- Uterine artery is identified and embolized with an absorbable gelatin sponge.
- Bilateral uterine artery embolization is required due to collateral circulation.
- In an emergency, the anterior division of the iliac arteries may be easier to embolize and gain control of haemorrhage.
- Gelatin sponge absorbs after about 10 days.
- May cause uterine ischaemia, especially if used in conjunction with compressive sutures.
- No fertility issues
- Prophylactic iliac artery balloons may be used where major obstetric haemorrhage is anticipated.

Further reading

Banks A & Norris A (2005). Massive haemorrhage in pregnancy. *CEACCP*, 5(6):195–8.

Lau TK & Leung TY (2011). Prenatal diagnosis of morbidly adherent placenta. *IJOA*, 20:107–9.

Moore M, Morales JP, Sabharwal T, *et al*. (2008). Selective arterial embolisation: a first line measure for obstetric haemorrhage. *IJOA*, 17:70–3.

24.9 Management of amniotic fluid embolus

Amniotic fluid embolus

Amniotic fluid embolus (AFE) occurs in 1 in 50 000 maternities but remains a major cause of direct maternal death with rates of 0.57/100 000 maternities in the CEMACH report from 2006–2008. The report notes that high-quality supportive care has reduced mortality to 20%. The UKOSS definition of AFE is described in Box 24.16. AFE remains poorly understood due to difficulty in diagnosis and a spectrum of presentations. Amniotic fluid enters the maternal circulation causing cardiovascular and haematological disturbance. For this to occur, there must be disruption of the fetal membranes and uterine vessels.

Most AFE cases present during labour or in the immediate postpartum period but cases are reported up to 48h post delivery, and even spontaneously in early pregnancy. It can occur during vaginal delivery or Caesarean section.

Risk factors for AFE
- Increased maternal age
- Induction of labour
- Artificial rupture of membranes
- Increased parity
- Multiple pregnancy
- Uterine stimulants.

Only increased maternal age and induction of labour have been supported by the UKOSS data.

Pathophysiology of AFE

This remains poorly understood but Clark's biphasic model attempts to answer the differences noted in animal studies and case observation.

Initial phase <30min, causes early deaths
- Initial phase of pulmonary vasospasm.
- Acute, severe pulmonary hypertension.
- Acute right ventricular failure.
- Markedly decreased cardiac output and hypoxia.

Secondary phase
- Left ventricular dysfunction due to hypoxia, reduced coronary flow or direct myocardial depression.
- Right ventricular recovery.
- Pulmonary artery occlusion pressure is high, but systolic pressures recover.
- Pulmonary oedema.
- Reduced cardiac output.

Coagulopathy may be triggered by DIC or massive fibrinolysis. This is thought to be due to procoagulant levels in amniotic fluid or from trophoblast entering the maternal circulation.

The initial trigger of this model is not defined. Animal studies have found no response from injection of autologous amniotic fluid into the circulation, and indeed fetal squames are detected in women without symptoms of AFE. This suggests that the AFE syndrome is either due to an abnormal factor in amniotic fluid or to an abnormal maternal response (similar to anaphylaxis). Amniotic fluid contains increased fetal debris in later gestation, prostaglandins (E2, F2α) and arachidonic acid metabolites (prostacyclin, thromboxane, leukotrienes) which may trigger a vasospastic response. Presence of meconium in amniotic fluid is associated with high mortality. An anaphylaxis mechanism is supported by some studies. Pre-treatment with antihistamines in animals reduces symptoms and repeat exposure increases the response.

Features of AFE

Because of the variable presentation, AFE should be suspected in any pregnant woman with sudden respiratory difficulty, chest pain, confusion, unexplained cyanosis, or hypotension (Box 24.15). It should also be considered for unexplained maternal haemorrhage.

Patients may report premonitory symptoms of agitation, numbness, or tingling.

- About 60% of patients present with sudden respiratory distress, cyanosis, and hypotension which may progress rapidly to cardiac arrest.
- Pulmonary oedema occurs in up to 70%.
- Coagulopathy occurs in 50%.
- Abnormal haemorrhage may be the presenting feature due to uterine atony.
- Seizures may occur in 20%. Confusion is common.

Supporting investigations
Coagulation tests may show reduced fibrinogen, increased fibrinogen degradation products, elevated APTT and PT, and reduced platelet count.

ECG and CXR may show evidence of right ventricular strain which can be confirmed with early TOE.

Maternal blood from central sampling may contain fetal squames, mucin, hair, or fat which can be detected with immunohistochemistry.

Box 24.15 Differential diagnosis of AFE
• Pulmonary thromboembolism
• Air embolus
• Anaphylaxis
• Sepsis
• Eclampsia
• Total spinal
• LA toxicity
• Acute cardiac failure (ischaemia, cardiomyopathy).

Management of AFE

Management is supportive and aims to provide adequate oxygenation, support cardiovascular parameters, and correct coagulopathy. Pre-delivery, aortocaval decompression is continued and delivery expedited to ease maternal resuscitation. If cardiorespiratory arrest occurs, ALS protocols are followed and perimortem Caesarean section should be performed within 5min.

Airway and breathing
There should be a low threshold for intubation to ensure optimum oxygenation and protect the airway.

Circulation

- Large-bore IV access should be sited.
- Bloods sent for blood count, coagulation, and cross-match.
- Early central venous pressure monitoring. Early guidance of fluid resuscitation is advisable if ventricular dysfunction occurs.
- IV fluid resuscitation.
- Inotropic support.
- Cardiac output monitoring to guide fluid and inotropic support.

Correction of coagulopathy

This should be guided by the clinical situation and frequent laboratory or point of care testing. TEG® should be used if available. Inhibitors of fibrinolysis, e.g. tranexamic acid, may play a role.

Treatment of uterine atony

Carboprost should be used with caution as it may increase pulmonary artery pressures.

Specific treatments suggested

There are no specific treatment measures for AFE but case reports have demonstrated successful outcomes using early pulmonary vasodilators or cardiopulmonary bypass, plasma exchange, haemofiltration, and steroids.

Outcome

Although recent data suggests mortality has decreased to 20%, it has been reported as high as 80%. Most deaths occur in the first 4h. Survivors may have neurological or respiratory morbidity in 15% of cases. Fetal outcome is poor if AFE occurs prior to delivery.

Box 24.16 UK Obstetric Surveillance System (UKOSS) criteria for defining AFE

Either: In the absence of any other clear cause:
Acute maternal collapse with one or more of:
- Acute fetal compromise
- Cardiac arrhythmia or arrest
- Coagulopathy
- Convulsion
- Hypotension
- Maternal haemorrhage (excluding cases as first feature with no early coagulopathy or cardiorespiratory effects)
- Premonitory symptoms—restlessness, numbness, agitation, tingling
- Shortness of breath.

Or

Women in whom postmortem diagnosis has been made finding fetal squames or hair in lungs.

Further reading

Cantwell R, Clutton-Brock T, Cooper G, *et al.* (2011). Saving Mother's Lives. Reviewing maternal deaths to make mother-hood safer: 2006-2008. The Eighth Report of the Confidential Enquiries into Maternal Deaths in the United Kingdom. *BJOG*, 118(Suppl 1):1–203.

Davis K & Malinow A (2009). Embolic disorders. In DH Chestnut (ed), *Chestnut's Obstetric Anesthesia Principles and Practice* (4th edn, pp. 844–7). Philadelphia, PA: Moseby.

Tufnell D, Knight M, & Plaat F (2011). Amniotic fluid embolus: an update. Anaesthesia, 66:1–9.

Uterine inversion

Uterine inversion is a rare obstetric emergency occurring in about 1 in 10 000 deliveries. The uterus inverts and may prolapse through the cervix or vaginal vault. This usually occurs during vaginal delivery but has been reported at Caesarean section. In the 2011 CEMACH report (2006–2008) one maternal death was associated with uterine inversion. This was felt to be due to inappropriate traction on the umbilical cord and substandard management of the subsequent inversion.

Risks for uterine inversion

- Excess umbilical cord traction
- Inappropriate fundal pressure
- Short umbilical cord
- Fundal placental site
- Abnormal placental implantation
- Uterine atony
- Uterine anomalies.

Grades of uterine inversion

- Incomplete: inverted fundus within the endometrial cavity
- Complete: inverted fundus extends beyond the cervical os
- Prolapsed: inverted fundus extends beyond vaginal introitus.

Diagnosis of uterine inversion

Uterine inversion generally presents acutely after delivery or up to 24h post delivery when associated with atony. It may also present subacutely up to 30 days postnatally.

Uterine inversion presents with:

Haemorrhage

This is also increased by uterine atony.

Mass in the vagina

Incomplete inversion may not be immediately apparent leading to delayed diagnosis.

Shock

This is often reported to be out of proportion with the degree of haemorrhage and may be associated with the parasympathetic effects of traction on the ligaments. The volume of blood loss is, however, frequently underestimated.

The diagnosis is suspected by failing to feel the fundus on abdominal examination or, if necessary, confirmed by ultrasound. Differential diagnoses may include uterine tumours, trophoblastic disease, or an undiagnosed twin.

Priorities for management

Immediate replacement of the uterus

Immediate manual replacement of the uterus is successful in 20–40% of cases. If replacement is delayed it becomes more difficult. The fundus is pushed back through the cervix with pressure directed towards the umbilicus.

Uterine relaxation may be required for manual replacement. Rapid, short-acting relaxation is desirable; sublingual nitrates and inhaled salbutamol are often readily available. IV agents used include:

- GTN 0.25–0.5mg
- Terbutaline 0.1–0.25mg
- Magnesium 4g.

Until the uterus is replaced, the placenta should be left *in situ* if possible. Removal is associated with increased haemorrhage.

Hydrostatic repositioning has also been used. With the patient in the Trendelenburg position, warm saline is infused via an introducer into the posterior fornix. As leak is prevented from the vagina, the uterine cavity should fill and relocate the uterus.

Treatment of shock

Large bore IV access should be sited to allow rapid correction of hypovolaemia. Vasopressors may be required. Blood should be sent for cross-match, full blood count, and analysis of coagulation. Blood loss in these cases is typically 1–2L. If immediate manual replacement of the uterus fails, resuscitation should continue to stabilize the cardiovascular parameters prior to further management. This needs to be balanced with the amount of ongoing blood loss.

Further management

Further attempts at replacing the uterus

If immediate manual replacement of the uterus fails despite uterine relaxation with medical treatment, the next attempt is usually performed under general anaesthesia. A rapid sequence induction is necessary, but the degree of cardiovascular instability of the patient may influence the choice of induction agent. Maintenance with volatile anaesthetics increases uterine relaxation and aids the surgical manoeuvre.

If manual replacement fails under general anaesthesia, surgical intervention is required and a laparotomy or laparoscopy is performed to elevate the ligaments and resite the uterus.

Maintain uterine contraction following replacement

If atony continues following replacement of the uterus, inversion may recur. Bimanual compression is performed and oxytocin infusion commenced. Other uterotonic drugs may be required, e.g. ergometrine and carboprost. Oxytocin infusion is continued for 24h.

Further surgical intervention may be required to treat atony. There are reports of the successful use of uterine compression sutures and intrauterine compression balloons.

Preventing endometritis

Antibiotic prophylaxis is required due to a high incidence of endometritis following emergency replacement of the uterus.

Postprocedure care

Observation of uterine tone and vaginal bleeding:

Fundal height and blood loss should be carefully observed and oxytocic medication continued for the first 24h.

Resuscitation

Cardiovascular parameters should be stabilized with fluid replacement. Hourly urine output is required. Haemoglobin should be kept >7g/dL and coagulopathy corrected as for maternal haemorrhage.

Future pregnancies

There are many reports of successful vaginal delivery with no recurrence of uterine inversion.

24.11 Post-dural puncture headache

Incidence/pathogenesis

Postpartum headache occurs in 40% of parturients. Post-dural puncture headache (PDPH) is one of the common causes following dural puncture with spinal anaesthesia or as a complication of epidural insertion (1.5% risk with epidural or combined spinal-epidural). Other causes of postpartum headache are listed in Box 24.17, and headache should be fully assessed as in Box 24.18 to identify a cause.

50–70% of parturients will develop PDPH following inadvertent dural puncture. The risk factors for developing PDPH are described in Box 24.19. Loss of CSF, traction on pain-sensitive intracranial structures and reflex cerebral vasodilatation (compensatory for low CSF pressure as per the Monro–Kellie doctrine) account for the signs and symptoms. CSF leak at the site of dural puncture can be demonstrated using MRI (Fig. 24.2) and subarachnoid pressure may reduce to ≤4cmH$_2$O (normally 5–15cmH$_2$O).

> **Box 24.17 Causes of postpartum headache**
>
> *Common*
> - Tension type, migraine (2/3 cases)
> - PET
> - PDPH.
>
> *Rare*
> - Cortical vein thrombosis (15/100 000)
> - SAH (20/100 000 pregnancies)
> - PRES
> - Tumour/infarction/SDH
> - Meningitis.

> **Box 24.18 Investigation of postpartum headache**
>
> - *History:* headache features and associated symptoms
> - *Examination:* neurological symptoms, reflexes
> - *Investigation:* BP, temperature, urine protein, LFTs, platelet count, clotting if hypertensive. MRI/CT if abnormal neurology, seek specialist advice

Symptoms

Postural frontal/occipital headache and neck stiffness within 5 days of possible dural puncture. The headache:

- Occurs within 15min of sitting/standing and resolves within 15min supine.
- Is aggravated by Valsalva and relieved by abdominal pressure.

Common associated symptoms are tinnitus, low-frequency hearing loss, photophobia, vertigo and nausea. Cranial nerve palsies may occur, particularly the 6th cranial nerve (which has a long intracranial course) causing diplopia.

Rarely subdural haematoma, seizures, cortical blindness, and cerebral herniation may occur.

PDPH interferes with the mother's ability to care for her newborn and increases the length of hospital stay.

Options for initial management of inadvertent dural puncture

Resite epidural

At a different level, preferably the lumbar interspace above. There is a higher risk of repeat dural puncture and analgesia may

> **Box 24.19 Risk factors for developing PDPH**
>
> *Patient*
> - Age <40 years (rare >60 years)
> - F>M (2:1)
> - Previous PDPH
> - No morbid obesity.
>
> *Procedural*
> - Multiple punctures
> - Large needle size
> - Cutting type vs pencil-point needles.

be delayed or unpredictable if local anaesthetic spreads through the dural tear.

Site intrathecal catheter

This can provide rapid, good quality analgesia/anaesthesia. Intermittent top-ups of 2–3mL low-dose mixture (e.g. 0.1% bupivacaine and 2mcg/mL fentanyl) can be given by the anaesthetist. It may be associated with lower incidence of PDPH. There are safety implications with improper drug administration and there is potential risk for introducing infection.

Prophylaxis of PDPH

Conservative measures

- Avoidance of pushing in labour. Many studies find similar incidence of PDPH between vaginal delivery and Caesarean delivery. It is generally acceptable to proceed with vaginal delivery and avoid operative risks.
- Good hydration.
- No benefit from bed rest.

Pharmacological

- Regular simple analgesia.
- Caffeine is of little benefit.
- Intrathecal/epidural opiates may reduce PDPH but this effect may be confounded by the presence of the catheter or saline volumes.

Intrathecal catheters

Studies show a non-significant decrease in PDPH incidence when intrathecal catheters are used. However, there is significant reduction in the need for epidural blood patch, especially if the catheter remains *in situ* for >24h. The intrathecal catheter may plug the dural tear reducing CSF efflux. After longer *in situ* an inflammatory process occurs at the site of insertion, which facilitates closure of the dural tear after catheter removal.

Prophylactic blood patch/crystalloid

Small studies suggested favourable results but a larger RCT showed no change in PDPH incidence, although some reduction in duration. Women who would not develop PDPH may be exposed to the risks of a blood patch. Similar results have been found using epidural saline blouses/infusions.

Management of PDPH

Conservative management involves regular analgesia, hydration and avoidance of straining. Regular review is required. Epidural blood patch should be considered if the symptoms interfere with care of the newborn and daily activities.

Possible pharmacological treatments

- *Caffeine:* antagonist of adenosine receptors on cerebral blood vessels that counteract vasodilatation. It can have variable effects on cerebral vascular resistance. Caffeine has been associated with seizure activity at high dose.
- *Triptans:* serotonin agonist used in the treatment of migraine. Causes inhibition of cerebral vasodilatation.
- *ACTH:* reserved for intractable PDPH. Increases intravascular volume, anti-inflammatory, or increasing endorphins.

Therapeutic epidural blood patch

Epidural blood patch is the gold standard treatment of PDPH (Box 24.20). The injected blood has a sustained effect on increasing lumbar CSF pressure (and hence intracranial CSF pressure) via a mass effect. It also causes a fibrinous reaction plugging the dural tear. Many studies support the use of blood patching and complete relief of symptoms occurs in 75% of cases with 20% resulting in partial relief and 5% failing. Blood patching after 24h of dural puncture is associated with a higher success rate.

10–20mL is a commonly used target volume for blood patching. Neuroradiology suggests 15–20mL will spread over four segments, with spread more cephalad than caudad. Blood patch should therefore be performed at the space below dural puncture where possible. Smaller volumes may be associated with less initial relief of headache from the mass effect of raising lumbar CSF pressure. Larger volumes are associated with radiculopathy from nerve root irritation.

Complications of a blood patch include:

- Infection
- Compression syndromes
- Subdural haematoma
- Cauda equina (more common with greater injected volumes)
- Arachnoiditis, which is a greater risk with accidental intrathecal injection.

Box 24.20 Performing an epidural blood patch

- History, examination, temperature, and white cell count to exclude sepsis.
- Patient consent—epidural risks, failure rate.
- Two operators, one to perform the epidural and one to withdraw 20mL blood under aseptic conditions; usually performed in the lateral position.
- If CSF is encountered use a test dose of local anaesthetic to distinguish the intrathecal space from an epidural collection.
- Inject blood slowly (Fig. 24.3). Volume may be limited by pressure, backache, neck pain, or nerve root irritation.
- Flush with saline before withdrawing needle to reduce infection in the needle tract.
- 2h of bed rest post blood patch may improve efficacy. Straining/strenuous exertion should be avoided for a few days.
- Two operators, one to perform the epidural and one to withdraw 20mL blood under aseptic conditions; usually performed in the lateral position.

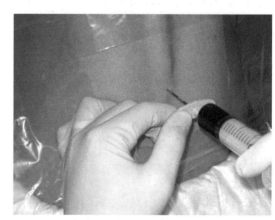

Fig. 24.3 Performing a blood patch.

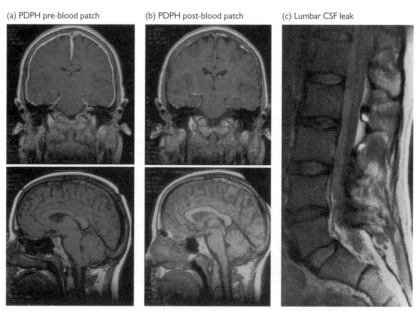

(a) PDPH pre-blood patch   (b) PDPH post-blood patch   (c) Lumbar CSF leak

Fig. 24.2 (a and b) MRI of post-dural puncture headache. Gadolinium-enhanced MRI often demonstrates 'sagging' of the intracranial structures. Meningeal enhancement occurs due to vasodilatation. (a) Pre-treatment images show meningeal enhancement and crowding of the posterior fossa. The tip of the cerebellar tonsils is just below the foramen magnum. Reprinted from *Mayo Clinic Proceedings*, 74, 11, Mokri B, 'Spontaneous cerebrospinal fluid leaks: from intracranial hypotension to crebrospinal fluid hypovolaemia – evolution of a conept', pp. 1113–1123, Figure 1, Copyright 1999, with permission from Mayo Foundation for Medical Education and Research, and Elsevier. (b) Images are post blood patch. (c) Reproduced from S Vakharia et al., 'Magnetic resonance imaging of cerebrospinal fluid leak and tamponade effect of blood patch in postdural puncture headache', *Anaesthesia & Analgesia*, 84, 3, figure 1, p. 586, Copyright 1997, Wolters Kluwer and the International Anaesthesia Research Society with permission.

Maternal mortality

Maternal mortality continues to decline in the UK despite a more challenging obstetric population. Rates of 11.39/100 000 maternities have been shown in the most recent Confidential Enquiry into Maternal Death (CEMD) report (Fig. 24.4). The international figures, from death certification only, are 6.69/100 000 live births. Each maternal death is a tragedy and may be avoidable. Reporting aims to identify maternal morbidity/mortality and allow analysis and learning from the management of cases.

Maternal morbidity/mortality reports

Confidential Enquiry into Maternal Death
- Triennial reporting since 1952.
- Whole of the UK since 1984.
- Every death of a woman who is pregnant or within 42 days of termination of pregnancy.
- Reported to regional director of Public Health.
- Full case details analysed by panel of experts.
- Lag time in reporting of about 2–3 years.
- *Direct deaths:* cause related to pregnancy or its management.
- *Indirect deaths:* cause aggravated by pregnancy.
- *Coincidental deaths:* unrelated/accidental causes.

UK Obstetric Surveillance System
- Surveillance of specific near-miss maternal morbidity and rare disorders of pregnancy since 2005.
- Routine monthly mailing to each consultant-led unit.
- Active, negative surveillance.
- Allows quantification of risk, prognostic factors, and audit of national guidelines.

Scottish Confidential Audit of Severe Maternal Morbidity (SCASMM)
- Audit of a range of defined severe morbidities since 2003 in all consultant-led units.
- Focus on maternal haemorrhage and eclampsia.

Leading causes of maternal mortality

The CEMD report published in 2011 covers maternal deaths in 2006–2008. The leading causes were:

Indirect death
Indirect maternal death due to cardiac and neurological disease was more common than any direct cause. A large number of cardiac deaths were attributable to myocardial infarction and ischaemic heart disease, cardiomyopathy and aortic dissection. The need for thorough investigation of chest pain and early involvement of specialist cardiology care is emphasized. Neurological deaths were mainly related to epilepsy and subarachnoid haemorrhage.

Direct death

Sepsis

This was mostly related to Group A streptococcal infection which commonly causes sore throats in children. Transmission from hands to perineum is suspected. The key recommendations focus on:
- Education of mothers. Early recognition of signs and symptoms, and prevention through improved hygiene.
- Education of all healthcare professionals to identify signs of sepsis.
- Early intervention with IV broad-spectrum antibiotics.
- Early involvement of anaesthesia and intensive care.

Pre-eclampsia and eclampsia

The incidence of eclampsia has halved since 1992, probably attributable to the Magpie study in 2002 which demonstrated the effect of magnesium in treating and preventing eclamptic seizures. Most deaths are caused by intracerebral haemorrhage or anoxia post cardiac arrest with seizures. Effective management of hypertension, particularly systolic hypertension, may avoid maternal demise.

Thromboembolism

This had been the leading cause of maternal death until the most recent report. The reduction in cases may well be a result of the RCOG 2004 guidelines ('Thromboprophylaxis during pregnancy,

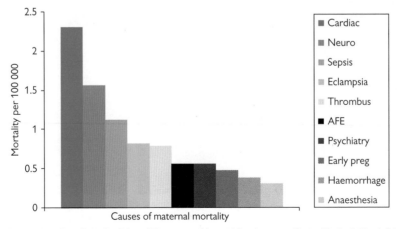

Fig. 24.4 Maternal mortality bar chart. Data from Confidential Enquiry into Maternal Death report, 'Saving Mother's Lives', *British Journal of Obstetrics and Gynaecology*, March 2011, 118, Supplement 1.

labour and after normal vaginal delivery') improving recognition of high-risk women and leading to more widespread thromboprophylaxis. The recent report still highlights the need for better investigation of women with dyspnoea and tachycardia.

Amniotic fluid embolus
The report notes an improvement in maternal resuscitation measures and, combined with UKOSS reporting, suggests that this is no longer a condition associated with universal maternal mortality.

Early pregnancy deaths
These include haemorrhage or sepsis following miscarriage/abortion and failed recognition of ectopic pregnancy, All women of reproductive age presenting with abdominal symptoms should have a pregnancy test. Morbidly adherent placentation should be considered following miscarriage if there is a history of previous Caesarean.

Maternal haemorrhage
The low mortality, despite an incidence in UKOSS reporting of 3.7/1000 births, suggests hugely improved standards of care. This is a result of determination of placental site and detection of abnormal placentation, maternal early warning scores, RCOG guidelines for management of PPH and earlier involvement of senior help. Improved pre-delivery planning with involvement of interventional radiology and earlier peripartum hysterectomy, particularly in women who will not accept blood products, has also contributed.

Anaesthesia
Anaesthesia was accountable for seven direct deaths. Three were attributable to poor airway management with failure to oxygenate, or aspiration during extubation. The importance of failed intubation drills is emphasized again in this report. The focus should be on oxygenation rather than intubation.

Late involvement of anaesthesia and delay in recognition of hypovolaemic states (particularly when 'hidden' by obesity, β-blockade, and PET) were also reported.

2011 CEMD recommendations

- Pre-pregnancy counselling—in women with medical conditions including obesity.
- Professional interpretation services should be used where language barriers exist.
- Improved communication and urgent specialist referral.
- Immediate multidisciplinary care.
- Improved quality of care—clinical skills, identification of illness, resuscitation.
- Early senior and specialist involvement in acute illness.
- Improved treatment of systolic hypertension.
- Focus on genital tract infection and sepsis.
- Improved incident investigation.
- Improved pathological investigation.

Further reading

Cantwell R, Clutton-Brock T, Cooper G, et al. (2011). Saving Mother's Lives. Reviewing maternal deaths to make motherhood safer: 2006-2008. The Eighth Report of the Confidential Enquiries into Maternal Deaths in the United Kingdom. *BJOG*, 118(Suppl 1):1–203.

Chapter 25

Paediatric anaesthesia

469

25.1 Effects of prematurity

Prematurity

The preterm infant is born before the completion of the 37th week of gestation (see Box 25.1). The effects of prematurity will depend on its extent. Infants are resuscitated in the UK from the 23rd week of gestation. At least half of infants born at >25 weeks of gestation and >600g will survive without major morbidity (defined as non-ambulant cerebral palsy, severe mental retardation, severe visual or hearing disability), although survival without measurable neurodevelopmental impairment in those born weighing <1000g is only 25%.

> **Box 25.1 Definitions**
> - Neonate: <44 weeks post conceptual age (PC age)
> - Preterm: <37 weeks PC age
> - Low birth weight: <2500g
> - Very low birth weight: <1500g
> - Extremely low birth weight: <1000g
> - Infant: child in 1st year of life.

Low birth weight is most commonly associated with prematurity, although intrauterine growth retardation (IUGR) may occur secondary to maternal or fetal conditions unrelated to gestational age.

Cardiorespiratory

Surfactant is secreted actively only from the 24–26th gestational week and alveolar development increases from the 32nd week, therefore very preterm infants are predisposed to respiratory distress of the newborn. The consequences of lack of surfactant are:
- Increased alveolar surface tension
- Alveolar instability leading to collapse
- Impaired gas exchange.

The management of these infants may require the administration of synthetic surfactant, non-invasive or invasive conventional ventilation, the use of oscillatory ventilation, and prolonged oxygen supplementation secondary to bronchopulmonary dysplasia.

Clinical significance: these infants will always need positive pressure supported ventilation under anaesthesia.

Preterm neonates are more prone to respiratory apnoeas than term neonates. The cause of infant apnoeas is not fully understood and may be multifactorial including neurological maturity and fatigue. A neonatal response to hypoxia is a period of hyperventilation, followed by apnoea.

Clinical significance: it is generally considered that a term neonate has a minimal risk of postoperative apnoea (for a simple case with opiates avoided) after 4 weeks of postnatal age. A preterm neonate should be monitored postoperatively until the 60th post conceptional week (i.e. a neonate born at 25 weeks should be monitored overnight postoperatively until approximately 8 months of postnatal age, assuming he/she is otherwise well).

Ventilation in the premature neonate may be complicated by air leaks requiring the insertion of chest drains, and the development of subglottic stenosis—this is a consequence of prolonged endotracheal intubation and airway oedema, which may complicate management when the ex-premature infant presents for elective surgery.

Normal transitional circulation from fetal to adult circulation is completed in the first few days of extrauterine life in the term neonate. The fetal shunts (foramen ovale and ductus arteriosus) are closed in response to a decrease in pulmonary vascular resistance and an increase in systemic vascular resistance, thereby diverting blood leaving the right side of the heart to the lungs. A patent arterial duct is seen in 50% of extremely premature infants and may lead to:
- Excessive pulmonary blood flow
- Low systemic pressures
- Cardiac failure
- Failure to wean from ventilation
- Systemic complications of low diastolic pressure, including necrotizing enterocolitis (NEC).

Persistent pulmonary hypertension of the newborn (PPHN) is more common in the premature infant and is compounded by hypoxia, hypercarbia, acidosis, sepsis, or anatomical abnormalities. It may require management with increased inspired oxygen concentrations or inhaled nitric oxide.

Congenital heart disease is twice as common in the premature infant when compared to the term neonate.

Neurological

Neurological injury is extremely common in the premature infant. Intraventricular haemorrhage occurs in up to 50% of babies below 1.5kg and is caused by rupture of fragile capillaries present in the 24–34-week developing brain. Other contributing factors include perinatal hypoxia and respiratory distress syndrome, poor cerebral autoregulation, and sepsis.

Retinopathy of prematurity is an abnormal proliferation of retinal blood vessels seen in neonates born particularly before 30 weeks of gestation, in response to high inspired oxygen concentrations in the neonatal period.

Clinical significance: high inspired oxygen concentrations should be avoided if cardiovascular physiology allows.

Gastrointestinal

Very low birth weight infants may lack coordination to suck and swallow, leading to increased risk of hypoglycaemia and aspiration.

The premature bowel may not tolerate enteral feeding, and in addition to the high incidence of low diastolic blood pressure associated with a patent ductus, the infant is predisposed to NEC. Management may be medical (avoiding enteral feeding, fluids, antibiotics) or surgical if gut perforation or ischaemia is suspected.

Clinical significance: the morbidity and mortality of the preterm infant requiring surgery for NEC is extremely high.

Metabolic, renal, and pharmacological

The liver has only 20% of its adult number of hepatocytes at term, and fewer depending on the gestational age of the neonate. In addition the free water compartment of the neonate is proportionately larger. Consequently the drug doses required of common anaesthetic drugs (muscle relaxants, induction agents, antibiotics) may be higher, despite immature metabolism.

Clinical significance: the safest way to administer anaesthetic drugs is in an incremental fashion, titrating to effect.

The immature liver has little gluconeogenesis ability, and the preterm infant has high metabolic rates. This requires monitoring of glucose levels pre-, intra-, and postoperatively to avoid hypoglycaemia. A maintenance infusion containing glucose should be infused, with regular blood glucose measurement and correction as required.

Nephrogenesis is completed by the 36th gestational week. The immature kidney handles sodium, water, and other electrolytes inefficiently. The infant has a relatively low GFR secondary to high intravascular pressure within the kidney, until the 2nd year of life.

Haematological

Blood volume is relatively higher in the premature neonate at 90–100mL/kg. Haemoglobin levels are equivalent to term neonates, but often have a precipitous fall depending upon condition, sepsis, and medical interventions. Normal neonatal Hb is 13–20g/dL and should be checked preoperatively in the neonate and infant.

Coagulation is limited by the relative absence of vitamin K-dependent clotting factors. Cellular and humoral immunity are impaired in the premature neonate, with only limited protection from maternal immunoglobulins.

Clinical significance: the routine administration of intramuscular vitamin K should be mandatory before surgery in the first week of life.

Environmental control

Effects of hypothermia on the neonate include:
- Reduced drug metabolism
- Increased oxygen requirement
- Increased work of breathing.

The premature neonate should be nursed in a warmed, humidified cot. Exposure should be minimized for procedures and temperature carefully measured.

Further reading

Mikkola K, Ritari N, Tommiska V, *et al.* (2005). Neurodevelopmental outcome at 5 years of a national cohort of extremely low birthweight infants who were born in 1996-1997. *Pediatrics*, 116(6):1391–400.

Seri I & Evans J (2008). Limits of viability: definition of the gray zone. *J Perinatal*, 28:s4–s8.

25.2 Developmental changes in infancy and childhood

Respiratory

See Table 25.1. The infant airway has anatomical features which require consideration when compared to the mature airway.

Cardiovascular

Postnatal changes occur in the neonatal and infant cardiovascular system in the transition from fetal to adult circulation:

Atrial septum

Increased pressure in left atrium closes the foramen ovale preventing right to left shunt.

Ductus arteriosus

- Active muscular contraction in response to increased oxygen partial pressure closes the ductus in the first 24h of life.
- Complete anatomical closure by 4–8 weeks.

Ductus venosus and umbilical arteries

- Functional obliteration by cord clamping at birth.
- Anatomical obliteration by 2 weeks.

Ventricles

- RV gains weight slowly, LV rapidly gains weight in response to increased afterload.
- The adult weight ratio of 3LV:1RV is achieved by 3 months.

Cardiac output

CO is high (240mL/kg/min) and heart rate dependent. Physiological variables change with age—see Table 25.2.

Table 25.2 Normal CVS physiological variables

Age	Heart rate (average)	Mean systolic BP (mmHg)
Preterm	130	40–55
Neonate	120	50–90
Infant	120	80–105
3 years	110	90–110
7 years	95	95–110
10 years	90	100–120
15 years	80	100–130

Pharmacology and drug handling

The neonate has less gastric acid and slower gastrointestinal transit, which may alter the rate of absorption orally.

Drugs, particularly paracetamol are often given rectally. There is a good blood supply and hepatic first-pass metabolism is avoided. However it should be remembered that time to maximum effect may be slow and absorption may not be complete. Doses and timings should reflect this.

Water soluble drugs have an increased volume of distribution in the neonate and therefore a greater loading dose/kg may be required. However, the neonatal neuromuscular junction is immature so although an increased dose of neuromuscular blocking drug may be indicated, this may not be as high as expected. See Table 25.3.

Table 25.3 Fluid compartments

	Prem	Neonate	Infant	Child
Total body water (%)	85	80	60	60
Intracellular water (%)	25	35	35	40
Extracellular water (%)	60	45	25	20

The infant has less protein binding affinity for drugs in the first 6 months of life. This affects the amount of 'free' drug available and reduced doses of highly protein-bound drugs may be considered.

The neonatal blood–brain barrier is immature, so drugs may more readily reach the central nervous system (e.g. morphine). The brain also has a differential response to volatile anaesthetic agents. The minimum alveolar concentration (MAC) of volatile agents is lower in neonates and higher in children when compared to adult values.

Communication with the parent and child

The complexity of managing children for anaesthesia is compounded by the vast differences in their psychological management at various ages (see Table 25.4). The baby is relatively easy to manage with soothing noises and physical contact for reassurance, whereas the 3-year-old may demonstrate separation anxiety and display difficult behavioural activities during induction and also in the recovery phase. The anaesthetic assessment offers an opportunity to begin a rapport with the child and their caregiver, and to make an assessment of the child's anxiety levels, although this is notoriously difficult to predict. The use of anxiolytic premedications can also be assessed although the most useful age group is probably toddler age (1–3 years).

Some children may not readily fit in to the described age groups and they may include the following:

- Autism spectrum disorders
- Frequent, multiple procedures.

These children may particularly benefit from intervention by play specialists, or the attention of psychology specialists to limit the procedure-related anxiety. It is certainly important for these potential problems to be highlighted in the preoperative assessment so that the appropriate plans can be put in to place.

For all children, a friendly environment is important, and if brightly coloured areas with toys are not available, then the normal working environment should be made as unthreatening as possible—removing unnecessary equipment (e.g. large drawing up needles) and personnel, and removing hats and facemasks where possible.

Table 25.1 Respiratory system in infants and children

	Infant	Adult	Consequences
Head	Larger, prominent occiput	Relatively smaller	Neutral position important
Neck	Shorter	Relatively longer	Neutral head position. Attention to detail when securing ETT
Nostrils	Nasal breathing when self-ventilating Easily blocked by secretions, NGT, etc.		Keep clear in self-ventilating child if possible
Tonsils	Often larger		Careful history for obstructive sleep apnoea
Tongue	Relatively larger	Smaller	Particularly in syndromic child (trisomy 21, Beckwith-Wiedemann etc.)
Epiglottis	Long, U-shaped, flops posteriorly	Shorter and wider	Often obstructs when using a laryngeal mask airway. Lift with straight blade laryngoscope
Larynx	Higher at C3–C4 Narrowest point at cricoid	Lower, parallel walled	Trauma causing oedema poorly tolerated Careful ETT sizing important
Trachea	Short		Care to position in mid-trachea Relatively greater movement with head extension/flexion
Main bronchi	Equally angled from carina	RMB angled inferiorly	Endobronchial intubation likely to either bronchus
Alveoli	Thick walled. Only 10% of adult number		
FRC	Closing volume >FRC until 6–8 years		Tendency for airway closure at end expiration, PEEP/CPAP important
Diaphragm	Ventilation mainly diaphragmatic		Splinting by gastric distention/bulky abdominal organs
Minute ventilation	Rate dependent		
Equipment dead space	Significant effect	Less significant effect	Minimize. Use paediatric specific equipment. Measure $PaCO_2$ to assess adequacy of ventilation

Table 25.4 Psychological developmental milestones

Age	Psychological developmental milestones
<6 months	Accepts others as parental surrogates Reassured by rocking and soothing noises
6 months to 3 years	Separation anxiety peaks. Too young to understand explanations but can be distracted (books, films, songs). Premedication may be useful
3–6 years	Understand requirement for separation (school/nursery etc.), will require simple explanations, avoiding euphemisms as understanding is very literal. Play specialists may be useful
7–12 years	Enjoy being rewarded for behaviours. Explanations are still important and they may want to demonstrate independence by participating (e.g. holding own facemask)
Adolescents	May have some adult coping mechanisms, but have also developed adult fears and anxiety (not waking up, body awareness)

25.3 Anaesthetic considerations for neonates, infants, and children

Anaesthesia for neonates

Neonates may present for elective or emergency surgery and the anaesthetic technique should be tailored to the condition of the child (Box 25.2). Care should be taken to ensure temperature maintenance, beginning prior to induction. The induction may be inhalational or intravenous, but must be titrated to effect and fully monitored.

Evidence shows that the neonate will feel pain and even develop increased sensitivity to pain, so care should be taken to provide adequate analgesia.

The neonate should be recovered from anaesthesia in an environment suited to this purpose with personnel trained in their care. This may be an ICU or HDU, or a post anaesthesia care unit. Neonates are not suitable candidates for day case anaesthesia. Apnoea monitoring is required postoperatively in term infants aged <44 weeks post conception (PC) age or in ex-premature infants until 60 weeks PC age.

Physiological changes in the neonatal period should be taken into consideration. Cardiovascular abnormalities may reveal themselves in the days after a normal newborn check and a high index of suspicion for a cardiac anomaly should be maintained. Pulmonary arterial pressures are higher than adult values for the first 2 weeks of postnatal life in an otherwise normal child. Hypoxia and acidosis should be corrected to avoid any increase in PVR.

Thermoregulation in the newborn and prevention of hypothermia

The premature neonate is most at risk of hypothermia as it has thin skin, with little subcutaneous fat, and a larger surface area. Normal neonates have some protection from brown fat located in the thorax and abdomen. Activated by the sympathetic nervous system it can be metabolized to produce heat rather than energy. This process increases oxygen consumption and is suppressed by anaesthesia. Deleterious effects of hypothermia are:

- Inhibition of coagulation
- Reduction in cardiac output
- Reduction in drug clearance.

Conversely, hypothermia may be used in some situations to preserve organ function (e.g. cardiac surgery).

Temperature maintenance during surgery and anaesthesia is a multi-pronged attack including:

- Increased theatre ambient temperature (26°C)
- Minimize exposure
- Radiant heaters
- Warming blankets
- Fluid and blood warmers
- Humidification and warming of inspired gases.

The neonate and child must be monitored to also avoid hyperthermia.

Starvation and hypoglycaemia

Hypoglycaemia is common in the stressed neonate and glucose levels should be monitored regularly. Limited glycogen stores in the liver and myocardium can quickly become depleted during periods of fasting. Neurological damage may occur from hypoglycaemia and fluids given to fasting neonates should always contain 10% glucose. 10% solutions may be required in infants/young children in the presence of sepsis, use of preoperative dextrose solutions or parenteral nutrition. Older children will probably not develop hypoglycaemia as the stress response to surgery and anaesthesia will maintain euglycaemia; however, a low dose of dextrose may be required if prolonged fasting or anaesthesia occurs. Management of hypoglycaemia is shown in Box 25.3.

Box 25.2 Neonatal anaesthesia

Preoperative

- Premature or ex-premature? Consider:
  - RS: bronchopulmonary dysplasia, subglottic stenosis, apnoea risk
  - CVS: patent ductus arteriosus, congenital defects, persistent pulmonary hypertension of the newborn (PPHN)
- Vitamin K in 1st week of life
- Minimize starvation time.

Induction

- Warming and temperature control
- Full monitoring
- Equipment prepared (LMA 1, ETT 3–3.5)
- Gas induction with sevoflurane
- IV induction—thiopentone 2–4mg/kg or propofol
- Increased risk of desaturation (increased oxygen consumption)
- Ayre's T-piece with >3L/min gas flow
- Muscle relaxant—suxamethonium 2mg/kg:
  - Increased sensitivity to non-depolarizing muscle relaxants.

Maintenance

- Oxygen/air/volatile:
  - MAC Prem <adult
  - MAC Term = adult
- TCI not licensed
- Usually positive pressure ventilation
- Monitor for hypoglycaemia
- Fluid maintenance 10% dextrose
- Temperature monitoring
- Analgesia—LA techniques, simple analgesia, short acting opiates
- Correct hypoxia, hypercarbia, and acidosis.

Postoperative apnoea monitoring

- Term infant 44 weeks PCA (ex-prem 60 weeks).

Box 25.3 Management of hypoglycaemia

Glucose <2.6mmol/L: give 2mL/kg 10% dextrose and titrate to effect.

Perioperative fluid management in the neonate, infant, and child

Body water in the neonate is 80% of the actual weight, decreasing to normal adult values of 60% by the 3rd year.

The majority of well children having day case surgery should be fasted for as short a time as possible and will not have ongoing IV fluid requirements.

Fasting for anaesthesia
- Clear fluids: 2h
- Breast milk: 3–4h
- Solids: 6h
- (Individual institutions may vary).

Intravenous fluid guidelines (Boxes 25.4–25.7)
Monitoring is the most important aspect of safe fluid management. Daily urea and electrolytes should be measured in children receiving IV fluids and appropriate changes to prescriptions made.

- The formulae used are only a guide and tend to overestimate requirements. This, combined with postoperative ADH release and use of hypotonic fluid, may result in hyponatraemia.
- Hyponatraemia is a major risk and symptoms such a headache, vomiting, decreased conscious level and seizures should prompt an immediate plasma sodium measurement.
- Fluid restriction to 60–75% of full maintenance may be indicated in the immediate postoperative period (1–2 days) to reduce the risk of hyponatraemia. Dehydration must however, be avoided in this period.
- Fluids are cautiously administered to neonates as they are unable to excrete a water or sodium load efficiently.

Box 25.4 IV fluid guidelines

Maintenance
The plasma sodium (Na) level guides the choice of fluid. If unknown, chose 0.9% saline + glucose 5% until confirmed.
- Plasma Na <135mmol/L: NaCl 0.9% + glucose 5%
- Plasma Na >135mmol/L: NaCl 0.45% + glucose 2.5%/5%.
(Fluids containing 0.18% NaCl are no longer recommended.)

Non-maintenance fluid
- Hypovolaemia: 10–20mL/kg boluses of 0.9% NaCl, Hartmann's solution or colloid.
- Ongoing enteric losses: replace mL for mL with 0.9% NaCl + potassium chloride.
- Oedema: consider ongoing fluid restriction.

Special circumstances requiring specialist advice may include:
Renal impairment, sepsis, heart failure, DKA.

Box 25.5 Neonatal fluid requirements

Use 10% glucose
- Day 1:   60 mL/kg/day
- Day 2:   90 mL/kg/day
- Day 3:   120 mL/kg/day
- Day 4:   150mL/kg/day.
Requires addition of Na^+ 3mmol/kg/day, K^+ 2mmol/kg/day.

Box 25.6 Paediatric maintenance requirements

The 4–2–1 regimen
- 1st 10 kg: 4mL/kg/h for each kg
- 2nd 10kg: 2mL/kg/h for each kg
- Each subsequent kg: 1mL/kg/h.
  - i.e. 8kg infant: 8 × 4 = 32mL/h
  - 32kg child (10 × 4) + (10 × 2) + (12 × 1) = 72mL/h

Box 25.7 Resuscitation requirement

Assessment of dehydration
- Vital signs
- Percentage weight loss
- Skin turgor
- Anterior fontanelle tension
- Tongue moistness
- Mental alertness
- Urinary output (frequency of wet nappies).

Resuscitation
Severe dehydration (>15% loss of body weight) requires a 20mL/kg bolus of 0.9% normal saline (NS).

Further reading

National Patient Safety Agency (2007). *Patient Safety Alert 22. Reducing the risk of hyponatraemia when administering intravenous infusions to children*. <http://www.npsa.nhs.uk>.

25.4 Specific anaesthetic monitoring and equipment for neonates, infants, and children

Anaesthetic equipment

Specific paediatric equipment should be used. The anatomical changes which occur through infancy and childhood mean that scaled down adult equipment may not be suitable.

Facemasks

A range of sizes to allow a good air seal without compression of nearby structures (eyes particularly). Available in a round shape for neonates, although the teardrop-shaped mask is applicable to all ages. The masks are clear plastic to observe for cyanosis and regurgitation.

Oropharyngeal airway

The airway is sized by measuring from the angle of the jaw to the corner of the mouth (sizes from 000 to 4):

- Do not invert for insertion in infants as this may damage the soft palate.
- May decrease gastric distension with air during face mask ventilation.
- Aids airway management in syndromic children with airway abnormalities.

Nasopharyngeal airway

A non-cuffed ETT one size smaller than required for intubation may be used. The length is cut to equal the measurement from tip of nose to tragus of ear. Used predominantly for:

- Recovery after ENT/palate surgery in syndromic children.
- Children with obstructive sleep apnoea when airway obstruction has occurred on induction.

Laryngeal airway

Available in all weight ranges (LMA 1: 0–5kg, LMA 1.5: 5–10kg, LMA 2: 10–20kg, LMA 2.5: 20–30kg; Box 25.8).

- Care should be taken to position carefully with the epiglottis outside the mask.
- Used in the <10kg age group for short procedures only.
- A low threshold is suggested for changing to an endotracheal tube if difficulty is encountered.

Box 25.8 Paediatric LMA sizes

Age	Size
Neonate <5kg	1
Infant 5–10kg	1.5
Child 10–20kg	2
Child 20–30kg	2.5
Child 30–50kg	3

Laryngoscope blades

Straight bladed laryngoscopes are usually used in infants <3–6 months (e.g. Robertshaw and Miller blades). The tip is placed in front of the epiglottis (not in the vallecula) to elevate the floppy epiglottis from the laryngeal inlet.

Endotracheal tube (ETT)

Non-cuffed tubes are traditionally used in children <8 years as the cricoid cartilage forms a complete circular seal around the narrowest segment of airway. Oversized tracheal tubes lead to:

- Mucosal ischaemia
- Oedema and scarring
- Subglottic stenosis.

Cuffed paediatric tubes are available and increasingly used in particular situations (difficult gas exchange with high ventilatory pressures, laparoscopic, and thoracoscopic surgery). Care must be taken to measure intra-cuff pressures regularly and maintain <20cmH$_2$O.

ETT size

Size the tracheal tube using the formula:

$$age / 4 + 4.5$$

with 1/2 size available either side or according to packaging if using a cuffed tube (Box 25.9).

Box 25.9 Paediatric ETT sizes

ETT size = age/4 + 4.5
ETT length = age/2 +12 (oral)
  age/2 +15 (nasal)

Age	ETT size	ETT oral/nasal length
Neonate	3.5	8–9/11cm
3–6 months	4	10/12cm
1 year	4.5	12/14cm
1–3 years	5	14/16cm
4–6 years	5.5	15/19cm
7–10 years	6	17/21cm

Under 2 years of age, the formula is less reliable. Weight and gestation should be considered in the neonate:

- Term neonate—size 3.5 ETT
- Smaller may be required if preterm or if tracheal pathology
- 3–6-month-old infant—size 4.0
- 1-year-old—size 4.5.

Irrespective of tube type, a correctly sized tube allows adequate ventilation with a small air leak audible at 20cm H$_2$O (with cuff down if using cuffed tube).

Endotracheal intubation must be confirmed using capnography. Endobronchial intubation is common and should be assessed by auscultation, observation of chest movement, and direct observation of tube length at the glottic inlet by laryngoscopy if necessary. Rechecking the position should follow careful fixation of the tube at the required length.

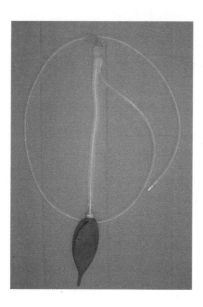

Fig. 25.1 Modified Ayre's T-piece.

ETT length

Tube length may be estimated using:

> age/2 + 12 (oral)
>
> age/2 + 12 (oral)
>
> or 3 × internal diameter of ETT

In neonates, oral tube length correlates approximately with weight (4kg = 10cm, 3kg = 9cm, 2kg = 8cm, 1kg = 7cm).

A nasogastric tube should be passed (8–10Fr) in order to remove any air inadvertently introduced into the stomach.

Difficult intubation

Paediatric intubation is not usually difficult in the normal child, assuming correct positioning and appropriately sized equipment has been selected. However, some paediatric syndromes are known to be associated with difficult airway management (e.g. Pierre–Robin sequence, mucopolysaccaridoses, Goldenhar syndrome). Specialist difficult airway equipment (AirTran, Glidescope) is available in paediatric sizes and appropriate equipment and assistance should be sought prior to undertaking anaesthesia.

Anaesthetic machine and breathing circuits

The Jackson–Rees modification of the Ayre's T-piece (Mapleson F) is the most common open system used in the UK in children <20kg (Fig. 25.1). It is a valveless, low-resistance circuit requiring a minimum fresh gas flow (FGF) of 3L for IPPV or 4L if self-ventilating. Scavenging may be incorporated in the system if required. It should always be available on a paediatric machine as hand ventilation is often required intraoperatively in case of desaturation, compliance change or during surgical manipulation.

Circle absorption systems are used in paediatric practice incorporating smaller (15mm) diameter tubing and appropriate sized reservoir bags (500mL, 1L, 2L). Care should be taken in ventilating the neonate that adequate CO_2 clearance is achieved as end-tidal monitoring may become unreliable in the presence of a larger dead space. Circle systems are unsuitable for a spontaneously ventilating neonate due to increased resistance to flow from unidirectional valves.

An anaesthetic machine and ventilator suitable for anaesthetizing adults is suitable also for children and neonates providing it can deliver both pressure and volume control ventilation, at high rates and low pressures. Air mix must be available for situations where nitrous oxide or high oxygen concentrations are undesirable. Pressure control ventilation is normally used to reduce the risk of barotrauma and to compensate for a potential leak around the endotracheal tube. Pressure control ventilation will not compensate for changes in lung compliance, tube obstruction or bronchospasm and tidal volumes should always be closely observed.

Monitoring

Standard anaesthetic monitoring is mandatory for all children including neonates and smaller versions of all monitoring equipment are available. Temperature monitoring is included for all but the shortest of cases.

Transcutaneous CO_2 monitors are useful in the neonate.

25.5 Induction and maintenance of anaesthesia in neonates, infants, and children

Premedication

Premedication is no longer used routinely in our paediatric practice. Sedative premedication is not required in the presence of pleasant and fast-acting induction agents and many children will accept them with little concern. In specific groups it may be advisable to consider one of many premedications.

Sedative premedications
Usually not required by neonates and infants, the very young child is relatively untroubled by the presence of strangers and has often not experienced anaesthesia before.

Older children, particularly in the toddler age group, may have difficulty understanding instruction and respond poorly to strangers and explanation.

Midazolam 0.5mg/kg orally (max. 15mg) is commonly prescribed as a sedative premedication. It has a predictable onset of action within 30min. Other agents such as chloral hydrate (30–50mg/kg orally, 60min onset time), Temazepam (older child, 12–18 years, 0.5–1mg/kg, maximum 20mg, orally, 60min before anaesthesia) are available.

Antisialagogue premedication
Indicated in the child with a difficult airway, having airway surgery (e.g. microlaryngoscopy) or if excessively drooling.

Atropine 20mcg/kg intramuscularly 30min preoperatively, or 10mcg/kg intravenously at induction.

Anaesthetic room conduct

It is commonplace in the UK to invite parents or primary caregivers to the anaesthetic room for induction of anaesthesia.

Parents and caregivers should be included in the preoperative preparation, with their role in the anaesthetic room explained. They should be accompanied to the anaesthetic room by an experienced health professional who can support them and guide them back to the waiting area once their child has been anaesthetized.

Personnel in the anaesthetic area should be minimized to avoid overwhelming the child and the anaesthetic area should be calm and quiet, as child friendly as can be arranged, and not used as a thoroughfare.

Toys, books, and multimedia equipment may be helpfully employed as distraction tools, play specialists may be invited if they have a rapport with the child.

Training courses are available to those who may find themselves anaesthetizing or sedating children, which focus on alleviating perioperative anxiety in children and are recommended.

Intravenous induction

IV induction is an appropriate technique for most infants and children. All anaesthetic agents may be utilized in the paediatric population with attention to cardiovascular status, immaturity of metabolic pathways, and the distress or pain caused by cannulation or the discomfort on injection of propofol. Local anaesthetic cream should be applied prior to attempting cannulation of the child.

In a child with an indwelling central venous line (tunnelled central line or peripherally inserted central line), IV induction is an ideal method, providing that scrupulous attention to sterile technique is maintained.

Propofol is the most commonly used agent, at a dose of 3–5mg/kg depending on the clinical condition of the child (co-induction with other agents, e.g. fentanyl, is commonplace, and the dose should be adjusted accordingly).

Inhalational induction

Inhalational induction is common in children, although the clinical status of the child and operator preference are taken into consideration.

Sevoflurane is a rapidly acting volatile agent, which is less irritating to the upper airway than other volatile agents. Induction will be smooth, particularly in combination with 70% nitrous oxide, although this is not a requirement. The child and parent should be comfortably positioned and the process explained to the child (as appropriate) and the family present. A facemask is applied to the nose and mouth of the child, or a cupped hand may be used in an infant. Warn the parent that abnormal movements may be observed during the induction, and assist the parent in placing the child on to the theatre table or trolley once the child is anaesthetized, supporting the head and limbs, if induction has been carried out in the parent's arms. Sevoflurane, up to a concentration of 8% is used for induction, although this may be reduced in the face of physiological requirements.

Once anaesthesia is achieved, maintenance may be continued with sevoflurane, or changed to another agent as preferred.

Maintenance of anaesthesia

Typically, anaesthesia in the paediatric population is maintained with a volatile agent, and all are suitable. Choice of agent between sevoflurane, isoflurane, and desflurane will depend upon operator and departmental preference and cost. All have a similarly safe cardiovascular profile. Halothane, now rarely used in UK practice, was associated with a higher incidence of cardiovascular instability, notably arrhythmia.

Good practice would encourage the use of a circle system with a CO_2 absorption system, adequate scavenging, and the use of low-flow anaesthesia with appropriate monitoring.

IV agents may be used to maintain anaesthesia. Examples where total intravenous anaesthesia (TIVA) may be particularly useful in paediatrics are:

- Patients susceptible to malignant hyperpyrexia.
- Children undergoing short procedures (e.g. imaging or intrathecal chemotherapy) where rapid recovery is required.
- Long procedures where the stress response to surgery may need to be modulated (cardiac, neurosurgery, or spinal surgery).
- Airway procedures (microlaryngoscopy and bronchoscopy).

Target-controlled infusion (TCI) pumps are available, but the range of models available for the paediatric population is limited and neonatal and infant models are rarely available.

IV agents are used for long-term sedation in the intensive care environment; however, the prolonged infusion of propofol in children is contraindicated (propofol infusion syndrome).

Awakening and recovery

Recovery of the child is undertaken in an environment suited to the situation. This may be the operating theatre, anaesthetic room, or a dedicated recovery or post anaesthetic care unit.

If awakening and recovery is conducted in a recovery room/ PACU then an area should be set to one side which is suitable for children, away from adult patients, with suitably trained staff, a full range of paediatric sized equipment and space for parents to attend.

Apnoea monitoring is required postoperatively in term infants aged <44 weeks PC age or in ex-premature infants until 60 weeks PC age.

The child with an upper respiratory tract infection

The preschool child develops an average of six to eight upper respiratory tract infections per year and many children will have a persistent discharge from their nose. When making the pre anaesthesia visit it is vital to take a full history of the symptoms and consider the procedure and the other medical history of that child before deciding whether to proceed.

The incidence of complications associated with anaesthesia in the child with a cold varies in the published literature both in number and in clinical significance.

Complications may include an increased incidence in secretions, laryngospasm, airway obstruction, and bronchospasm. These complications, if mild, should be short lived and quickly treated in a situation where an experienced paediatric anaesthetist is in attendance. It should be considered that an 'upper respiratory tract infection' in fact increases the sensitivity of the entire tracheobronchial tree and lung parenchyma. The child with asthma may have a different illness pathway than the otherwise well child.

The decision to proceed depends upon the child's age (increased risk <1 year), history and symptoms, the urgency and type of procedure, the other medical conditions of the child, and the airway manipulation required. The incidence of laryngospasm in the presence of an upper respiratory tract infection is greater if the trachea is intubated, or if an LMA is employed, than if facemask anaesthesia alone is used.

In general, elective anaesthesia should be postponed for 2–4 weeks in a child with:

- Pyrexia
- Mucopurulent nasal discharge or cough

- Constitutionally unwell
- Clinical signs of lower respiratory tract infection
- Raised WCC.

It is reasonable to proceed in a child with a mild infection (clear nasal discharge, no fever, not unwell) but cases should be considered on an individual risk vs benefit ratio and a multidisciplinary decision, with the parents involved, should be made. Younger children with reactive airway disease or ex-premature infants may have increased risks even with mild infection.

The child with a murmur

Most murmurs heard in otherwise well children with normal exercise tolerance and normal oxygen saturations will be innocent. They are usually soft in nature and in early systole in timing. Most (*but not all*) pathological causes of a murmur will have been identified in the antenatal or postnatal period. In the presence of a murmur a full history and examination should be undertaken and referral for an ECHO and a cardiological opinion made if appropriate.

A specialist cardiology opinion is indicated prior to commencing anaesthesia if:

- The child is <1 year old.
- The murmur fits pathological criteria (in diastole, pan systolic, late systolic, very loud, continuous, associated with cardiac signs or symptoms).

Antibiotic prophylaxis is no longer recommended in all situations and advice should be sought and treated on an individual case basis.

Further reading

Bingham R, Lloyd Thomas A, & Sury M (eds) (2008). *Textbook of Paediatric Anaesthsia*. New York: Edward Arnold (Publishers)

Maime C, Habre W, Delhumeau C, *et al.* (2004). Incidence and risk factors of perioperative respiratory adverse events in children undergoing elective surgery. *Paediatr Anaesth*, 14(3):218–24.

NCEPOD (2011). *Are We There Yet? A review of organisational and clinical aspects of children's surgery*. London: NCEPOD.

NICE (2008). *NICE Clinical Guideline 64: Prophylaxis against infective endocarditis*. London: NICE.

Von Ungern-Sternberg BS, Boda K, Chambers NA, *et al.* (2010). Risk assessment for respiratory complications in paediatric anaesthesia: A prospective cohort study. *Lancet*, 376:773–83.

Hypertrophic pyloric stenosis

Hypertrophic pyloric stenosis (HPS) causes gastric outlet obstruction with classic biochemical abnormalities (see Box 25.10). This typically presents at 3–6 weeks old with a history of progressive non-bilious projectile vomiting, failure to thrive, and a palpable 'olive'-sized mass in the right upper quadrant. Clinical diagnosis may be confirmed by ultrasound.

Box 25.10 Biochemical abnormalities in HPS

Classically hypokalaemic hypochloraemic metabolic alkalosis with compensatory respiratory acidosis. Rarely seen now due to early diagnosis and IV fluid resuscitation.

In gastric outlet obstruction, gastric acid and a variable amount of Na^+ and K^+ is lost in vomitus without loss of HCO_3^- from the duodenum. Systemic alkalosis overwhelms renal capacity to reabsorb HCO_3^-, producing an alkaline urine. Aldosterone is secreted (decreased ECF), leading to renal conservation of Na^+ in exchange for K^+. Eventually hypokalaemia forces Na^+ exchange preferentially with H^+ instead of K^+ in the renal tubules. This produces the characteristic 'paradoxical acid urine' in the face of systemic alkalosis.

If the infant presents with a long history, the systemic alkalosis may have progressed to a metabolic acidosis with lactic acidosis from dehydration and ketosis due to starvation.

Preoperative considerations

Pyloric stenosis is a medical, not surgical, emergency. Resuscitation with correction of hydration and electrolyte abnormalities is the priority. Patients are 'nil by mouth' with continuous nasogastric (NG) drainage.

Assessment of dehydration includes vital signs, percentage weight loss, skin turgor, anterior fontanelle tension, tongue moistness, mental alertness, and urinary output (frequency of wet nappies).

Resuscitation

Severe dehydration (>15% loss of body weight) requires a 20mL/kg bolus of 0.9% NS.

Fluid resuscitation (over 24–48h) with 0.45% NS or 5% dextrose with added KCl once urine output established. The rate is calculated based on maintenance fluid requirements, fluid deficit and ongoing losses. Typically this translates to twice the normal maintenance rate (about 6–8mL/kg/h) until full resuscitation is achieved.

Ongoing NG losses are replaced by 0.9% NS + KCl 20mmol/L.

Investigations

Venous or capillary blood samples are monitored every 8–12h, with IV fluids adjusted until results are within the following acceptable levels:

- Cl^- >90mmol/L
- pH 7.30–7.45
- Na^+ >132mmol/L
- K^+ >3.2mmol/L
- HCO^- <30mmol/L.

Perioperative considerations

- Aspiration risk—four quadrant suctioning of NGT, endotracheal intubation, consider cricoid pressure. Awake extubation in left lateral position

- Risk of postoperative apnoea—avoid long-acting opiates.
- Laparoscopic surgery—low insufflation pressures should not interfere with neonatal ventilation.

Postoperative considerations

- Risk of postoperative respiratory depression—preoperative alkalosis decreasing the sensitivity of central chemoreceptors.
- Apnoea monitoring is essential.

Herniorrhaphy in the ex prem infant

Premature infants have an increased incidence of inguinal hernias. Timing of surgery is a compromise between physiological development of the premature infant and the risk of bowel incarceration.

Surgery may be open or laparoscopic and performed under regional or general anaesthesia (Table 25.4). The choice of technique must be considered on an individual patient basis. The variables that must be considered include: urgent vs elective surgery, extent of surgery (size of hernia, unilateral or bilateral hernia, oedematous field), patient weight and degree of prematurity, history of apnoea or bradycardia, and the presence of comorbidities such as severe bronchopulmonary dysplasia.

Anaesthetic technique

General anaesthesia

GA is standard in the UK. Endotracheal intubation is usual. Drugs used reflect the increased incidence of postoperative apnoea, e.g. desflurane, simple analgesia, short-acting opiates and caudal, ilioinguinal blocks and/or local infiltration.

Regional anaesthesia

RA (spinal, caudal or combined) is rarely used and limited to those infants with significant medical disease. A Cochrane review found no reliable evidence that spinal anaesthesia reduced the incidence of postoperative apnoea or bradycardia.

Postoperative care

Apnoea monitoring is required in term infants aged <44 weeks PC age or in ex-premature infants <60 weeks PC age.

Table 25.4 Risks and benefit for RA vs GA for inguinal herniorrhaphy

	General	Regional
Advantages	Secure airway No time limit for surgery Familiarity with technique	Avoids airway instrumentation May ↓ apnoea/bradycardia Avoids GA if comorbidity Minimizes systemic analgesics
Disadvantages	↑ apnoea/bradycardia. May require post-op respiratory support	Technically difficult Failure rate 10–20% Airway not secured Time limit for surgery May require sedation Does not eliminate apnoea No muscle relaxation Not for laparoscopic surgery

Tracheo-oesophageal fistula

Tracheo-oesophageal fistula (TOF) and oesophageal atresia (OA) are interrelated conditions with an incidence of 1:3500 births (Fig. 25.2). OA with a fistula between the trachea and the distal oesophageal segment is most common (85%).

Causes antenatal polyhydramnios and presents clinically with choking or cyanosis on feeding and inability to pass a NG tube beyond 10–12cm.

Main considerations for anaesthesia

- Surgery occurs in first few days of life.
- Associated prematurity and congenital abnormalities, e.g. cardiac (25%), renal, VATER syndrome.

Preoperative

Risk of pulmonary aspiration through the fistula:

- NG aspiration (double-lumen replogle tube allows irrigation and suction).
- H_2 antagonists.
- Semi-upright position.

Induction

Risk of preferential gastric ventilation

Spontaneous ventilation is advised to avoid inflating the stomach via the fistula, but may be difficult to achieve in practice. Bronchoscopy may be performed initially to assess size and position of the fistula relative to the carina. Subsequent to this it is reasonable to gently assist ventilation manually, minimizing inflation pressures. Care is required with positioning the ETT to avoid gastric inflation. Endobronchial intubation is intentionally performed. The ETT is then withdrawn until breath sounds are heard bilaterally in an attempt to position the ETT tip distal to the fistula. Repositioning and rotation of the ETT bevel may be required. A cuffed ETT may be used.

Perioperative

- Good IV access and invasive arterial monitoring.
- During surgical manipulation desaturation or reduction of cardiac output often occurs due to mediastinal retraction and/or lung compression. Manual ventilation is required to oxygenate, clear blood and secretions from the ETT, and assess compliance.

- Surgeons will request a transanastomotic NGT. Measure distance to oesophageal repair (to guide post-op suctioning) and secure well.
- A staged repair may be performed where there is a long oesophageal defect.
- Atelectasis can be prevented with recruitment manoeuvres at end of surgery. Air leaks should be excluded.

Postoperative

- Ongoing ventilation on NICU.
- Observation for complications, e.g. anastomotic leak, tracheomalacia.

Infants who have had a previous TOF repair may have a blind passage tracheal pouch at the site of the fistula repair. This should be considered if there is difficulty in ventilation after endotracheal intubation in a patient with this history.

Congenital diaphragmatic hernia

Congenital diaphragmatic hernia (CDH) occurs in 1:3000 live births. There is a primary failure of lung development with severely hypoplastic lungs, underdeveloped airways, and abnormal type II pneumocytes. Pulmonary vasculature is abnormal and shows increased response to vasoactive substances.

Postnatal resuscitation and stabilization

A neonate with CDH is usually in severe respiratory distress with tachypnoea, cyanosis and a 'scaphoid abdomen'. Intubation is required and should be performed avoiding high pressure bag-mask ventilation, as this may lead to distension of intrathoracic bowel. An NGT should be inserted and transfer arranged to NICU.

Surgical repair of the hernia is delayed until the neonate is stable and significant comorbidities have been diagnosed and optimized. Surgical repair relieving lung compression does not improve gas exchange and often worsens respiratory mechanics in the immediate postoperative period.

Intensive care treatment

Ventilation

Avoid high airway pressures to prevent barotrauma to the hypoplastic lung.

- Pressure-limited ventilation. PIP of <25cmH$_2$O.

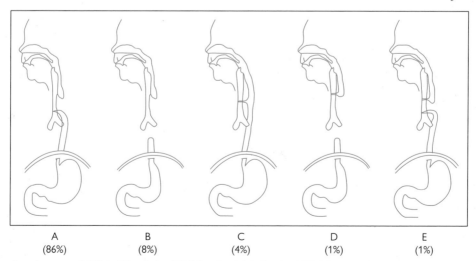

| A | B | C | D | E |
| (86%) | (8%) | (4%) | (1%) | (1%) |

Fig. 25.2 Oesophageal atresia and TOF. A: OA with distal TOF; B: isolated OA; C: isolated TOF; D: OA with proximal TOF; E: OA and double TOF. Reproduced from Al-Rawi O, and Booker PD, 'Oesophageal atresia and tracheo-oesophageal fistula', *Continuing Education in Anaesthesia, Critical Care and Pain*, 2007, 7, 1, figure 1, p. 16, by permission of The Board of Management and Trustees of the British Journal of Anaesthesia and Oxford University Press.

- Aim for pre-ductal SpO$_2$ >85%.
- Permissive hypercarbia if pH is compensated.
- High-frequency oscillatory ventilation (HFOV).
- Surgery is delayed until the infant can be stabilized on conventional ventilation successfully.

Pulmonary hypertension

Increased PVR is indicated by pre-ductal desaturation (right-to-left shunting across a patent ductus arteriosus). Increasing ventilation to reduce PaCO$_2$ and increase PaO$_2$ will reduce PVR but may induce barotrauma and should be used with care. Management may require nitric oxide or ECMO.

Timing of surgery

Surgery is delayed until PVR has reduced and ventilation can be managed with low oxygen requirements and PIP <25cmH$_2$O. In healthy neonates this may be within the first 24–48h of life. Other neonates with pulmonary hypertension may require protracted ventilation and treatment before surgery.

Main considerations for anaesthesia

Induction

- Invasive monitoring from NICU.
- Pre- and post-ductal SpO$_2$.

Perioperative

- Pressure control ventilation PIP <25cmH$_2$O.
- N$_2$O is contraindicated.
- Management of PVR—ventilation, NO.

Postoperative

- Postoperative ventilation.
- Cardiovascular/respiratory compromise.

Survival rate from CDH has improved with centres reporting rates >75%. Improved survival is linked to changes in ventilation strategy and staging of elective surgical repair.

Exomphalos and gastroschisis

These abdominal wall defects result in herniation of abdominal contents and occur in 1:5–10 000 births. Preterm labour and intrauterine growth retardation are associated.

Gastroschisis is a defect of the abdominal wall with bowel herniation without a covering protective membrane. It is repaired soon after delivery.

Infants with exomphalos have herniation of abdominal contents through the umbilicus with a membranous sac of amnion and peritoneum protecting and covering the bowel. They require

stabilization and investigation of associated defects, in particular echocardiography to define cardiac abnormalities.

Main considerations for anaesthesia

Preoperative

- Nurse semi-upright with NGT.
- Evaporative heat, water, and electrolyte loss can be reduced by wrapping abdominal contents in clingfilm.
- Appropriate antibiotics are required to reduce risk of sepsis.
- Assessment and correction of fluid balance and electrolytes. Fluid requirements may be as high as 140mL/kg/24h in the initial period due to evaporative loss with transudation of fluid into the bowel worsening fluid and electrolyte imbalance.
- Investigate for associated congenital defects.

Perioperative

- Two IV cannulae ideally in upper limbs because abdominal distension may impair venous return.
- Arterial line for large defects or if there is significant comorbidity.
- Avoid nitrous oxide due to bowel distension.
- Intraoperative fluid requirements are high, with boluses of warmed crystalloid, colloid, and blood given to maintain cardiovascular parameters.
- Reduction of the abdominal contents requires adequate muscle relaxation.
- During reduction of the abdominal contents, manual ventilation is helpful to detect excessive decrease in lung compliance.
- Increased intra-abdominal pressure may occur. Clinical signs include difficulty with ventilation in addition to a decrease in urine output, absent dorsalis pedis pulses, and poor capillary refill. Large defects may require a silo to be sited to allow staged reduction over time.

Postoperative

After repair of small defects, early extubation may be planned. Larger defects require a period of postoperative ventilation to compensate for deterioration in lung function. A prolonged ileus is common with increased third space losses. Fluid balance must be carefully maintained and total parenteral nutrition is often required.

Further reading

Al-Rawi O & Booker PD (2007). Oesophageal atresia and tracheoesophageal fistula. *CEACCP*, 7:15–20.

Pain in neonates/infants

The anatomical, physiological, and biochemical prerequisites for pain perception are present by the early part of intrauterine life. Consequently even premature infants can experience pain.

There are some basic differences in the neurophysiology of pain perception in comparison to adults:

- Pain impulses travel to the spinal cord through unmyelinated rather than myelinated fibres.
- Inhibitory neurons have a relative lack of neurotransmitters and a lower threshold for excitation and sensitization.

As a result there are more central effects of nociceptive stimuli and pain may be more severe. The importance of managing infant and neonatal acute pain is recognized by numerous organizations that have all produced mission statements on the matter (WHO, IASP, RCPCH, BPS).

Causes and consequences of pain

Acute pain may be associated with medical or surgical conditions, after injuries or postoperatively. An additional cause of pain in this group is procedural such as blood sampling or lumbar puncture.

As well as the physiological effects acute pain in this age-group may cause impaired emotional bonding. Long-term effects include memory of pain, developmental retardation, and altered responses to subsequent experiences.

Pain assessment in neonates/infants

The most comprehensive and commonly used assessment tools in neonates and infants are the CRIES scale and the FLACC scale respectively.

CRIES scale (see Table 25.5)

Neonatal pain assessment based on physiological and behavioural changes.

- Crying
- Requires oxygen
- Increases in heart rate and blood pressure
- Expression (facial)
- Sleep pattern alteration

The Premature Infant Pain Profile is a similar tool.

FLACC scale (see Table 25.6)

Infant pain assessment based on behavioural changes:

- Face
- Legs
- Activity
- Cry
- Consolability

Similar tools assessing behavioural changes to pain include the Children's Hospital of Eastern Ontario Pain Scale (CHEOPS), Neonatal Infant Pain Scale (NIPS) and the Liverpool Infant Distress Scale (LIDS).

Table 25.5 CRIES scale: Scored from 0–10
Crying 0: No cry or cry that is not high pitched 1: Cry high pitched but baby is easily consolable 2: Cry high pitched and baby is inconsolable
Requires oxygen to keep saturations >95% 0: No oxygen required 1: <30% oxygen required 2: >30% oxygen required
Increased vital signs 0: Both HR and BP unchanged or less than baseline 1: HR or BP increased <20% of baseline 2: HR or BP increased >20% over baseline
Expression 0: No grimace present 1: Grimace alone is present 2: Grimace with grunting
Sleepless 0: Child has been continuously asleep 1: Child has awakened at frequent intervals 2: Child has been awake constantly

Reproduced from Krechel SW and Bildner J, 'CRIES: a new neonatal postoperative pain measurement score. Initial testing of validity and reliability', *Paediatric Anaesthesia*, 5, 1, pp. 53–61, Copyright © 2007, John Wiley and Sons, with permission.

Table 25.6 FLACC scale: Scored from 0–10
Face 0: No particular expression or smile 1: Occasional grimace or frown, withdrawn, disinterested 2: Frequent to constant frown, clenched jaw, quivering chin
Legs 0: Normal position or relaxed 1: Uneasy, restless, tense 2: Kicking, or legs drawn up
Activity 0: Lying quietly, normal position, moves easily 1: Squirming, shifting back and forth, tense 2: Arched, rigid or jerking
Cry 0: No cry (awake or asleep) 1: Moans or whimpers, occasional complaint 2: Crying steadily, screams or sobs, frequent complaints
Consolability 0: Content, relaxed 1: Reassured by occasional touching, hugging, or being talked to, distractible 2: Difficult to console or comfort

© 2002, The Regents of the University of Michigan. Merkel, S., Voepel-Lewis T., Shayevitz J. & Malviya S. 'The FLACC: A behavioral scale for scoring postoperative pain in young children', *Pediatric Nursing*, 1997, 23:293–297.

Pain assessment in children

Any pain assessment tool in children should be age and context appropriate. From 4–5 years of age, children can begin to use the Faces Pain Scale. Children are more likely to choose the extremes of the scale and may confuse pain levels with emotional states, e.g. sadness.

By 10 years of age children can discriminate between the sensory intensity and the affective emotional components of pain and report them independently.

A well-established self-report tool is Wong–Baker Faces; Visual Analogue Scores (VAS) for acute pain assessment in children (over 3 years).

Pain management strategies

Although there are wide ranging causes of pain and developmental differences in this group of patients, modulating the transduction and transmission of pain is the key to achieving successful analgesia. This is best achieved using a multimodal approach.

Non-pharmacological strategies

These modulate nociception via the release of endogenous opioids, stimulation of the proprioceptive system and reduction in anxiety. The results are a reduced physiological response and modulation of behaviour. Interventions include:

- Control of the environment—optimization of sleep cycle by avoiding bright lights, noise, cold
- Breast feeding during procedures
- Pacifier with sucrose (0.1–2.0mL 24% solution)
- Kangaroo care—periodic skin-to-skin contact while holding the baby upright at 40–60°
- Swaddling and massage.

Pharmacological

Local anaesthetics, paracetamol, NSAIDs, and opioids form the basis for the majority of analgesic regimens adhering to the WHO analgesic ladder. Ketamine, a dissociative anaesthetic with analgesic properties, and clonidine, an α-2 agonist may also be used in selected clinical situations.

Local anaesthetics (Box 25.11)

The amides (e.g. lignocaine, bupivacaine) have a narrow therapeutic index in neonates due to decreased metabolic clearance and lower plasma concentrations of α-1 glycoprotein, leading to higher concentrations of unbound LA. Maximum infusion rates are reduced to avoid toxicity.

Box 25.11	Topical local anaesthetic creams	
	AMETOP	EMLA
	(4% tetracaine)	(2.5% prilocaine/lidocaine)
Licence	> 1 month old	Use with caution
Onset	45min	60–90min
Duration	4h	1h
Other	Vasodilatation	Vasoconstriction
		Methaemoglobinaemia

Wound infiltration and regional nerve blocks

Wound infiltration for surgery or procedures should be considered in all cases.

Many peripheral nerves are easily accessible for single-shot blockade, and may be performed with reliable results especially using ultrasound, e.g. axillary and rectus sheath blocks.

Central neuraxial blocks (CNBs)

Include single-shot caudals, epidural catheters (inserted via the caudal, lumbar, or thoracic route), and spinals. Almost all are performed asleep, except for rare occasions where it may be the primary method of anaesthesia in the neonate.

Ultrasound can also be used to visualize the caudal and epidural space in infants allowing the depth to the space to be accurately measured and the catheter tip visualized.

CNBs in paediatric practise have a good safety profile which has been supported by analysis of the recent 3rd National Audit

Project of the Royal College of Anaesthetists (NAP3)—complications of central neuraxial blocks.

Single caudal injection

The most common block used for sub-umbilical surgery in neonates and infants. The technique is relatively low risk with good efficacy and involves injection of LA through the sacrococcygeal membrane into the epidural space below the termination of the spinal cord. Anatomically the spinal cord reaches L3–L4 in the neonate and the dural sac can be found at S3–S4. Contraindications include abnormalities in sacral anatomy which may be indicated by overlying dimples, hair or other skin changes. Common complications include failure, urinary retention and motor block. Rare complications include inadvertent subarachnoid, vascular or intraosseus injection as well as bowel perforation.

0.25% bupivacaine or levobupivacaine is used with volume related to height of block as per the Armitage formula (Box 25.12). Lower thoracic nerve roots are not blocked consistently in older children and alternative regional techniques are required to achieve higher blockade.

Box 25.12	The Armitage formula—dosing of caudal block using 0.25% bupivacaine
• Lumbosacral block:	0.5mL/kg
• Thoracolumbar block:	1mL/kg
• Midthoracic block:	1.25mL/kg.

Epidural catheters

The depth of the epidural space is extremely variable, the formula **depth = 1mm/kg** in children >10kg may be used as a rough guide. Typical loading doses and infusion rates are:

- Loading dose 0.75mL/kg of 0.25% bupivacaine
- Maintenance using 0.1% bupivacaine
  - 0.1–0.3mg/kg/h (0.1–0.3mL/h) in neonates <5kg
  - 0.1–0.4mg/kg/h (0.1–0.4mL/h) in infants.

Systemic analgesics

Paracetamol

Paracetamol is used to treat mild to moderate pain. It is metabolized by sulphation in the neonate, which protects to some extent against toxicity, and is licensed to be administered orally, rectally or intravenously in neonates with a reduction in dose and frequency reflecting longer half-life. The doses and intervals are described in Box 25.13.

Box 25.13	Paracetamol doses in the neonate and infant

By IV infusion over 15min:
- Neonate:
  - 7.5mg/kg every 6h
  - Maximum 30mg/kg daily
- Infant < 10kg
  - 7.5mg/kg every 6h
  - Maximum 30mg/kg daily
- Infant >10kg:
  - 15mg/kg every 4–6h
  - Maximum 60mg/kg daily

(Continued)

Box 25.13 (Continued)

By mouth:

- Neonate 28–32 weeks PC age:
  - 20mg/kg single or loading dose
  - 10–15mg/kg every 8–12h
  - Maximum 30mg/kg daily
- Neonate >32 weeks PC age:
  - 20mg/kg single or loading dose
  - 10–15mg/kg every 6–8h
  - Maximum 60mg/kg daily
- Infants 1–3 months:
  - 20–30mg/kg as a single or loading dose
  - 15–20mg/kg every 6–8h
  - Maximum 60mg/kg
- Infant 3–12 months:
  - 20–30mg/kg single or loading dose
  - 15–20mg/kg every 6–8h
  - Maximum 90mg/kg daily

By rectum:

- Neonate 28–32 weeks PC age:
  - 20mg/kg single or loading dose
  - 15mg/kg every 12h
  - Maximum 30mg/kg daily
- Neonate >32 weeks PC age:
  - 30mg/kg single dose or loading dose
  - 20mg/kg every 8h
  - Maximum 60mg/kg daily
- Infant 1–3 months:
  - 30mg/kg single or loading dose
  - 15–20mg/kg every 6–8h
  - Maximum 60mg/kg daily
- Infant 3–12 months:
  - 30–40mg/kg single or loading dose
  - 15–20mg/kg every 6–8h
  - Maximum 90mg/kg daily.

NSAIDs

NSAIDs have antipyretic, analgesic, and anti-inflammatory properties. Ibuprofen, although used safely in the treatment of ductus arteriosus closure, is not licensed or recommended for use in children <3 months or <5kg due to reduced protein binding and increased risk of renal failure and gastric bleeding. Doses are shown in Box 25.14.

Box 25.14 Ibuprofen doses in infants

- Infant 1–3 months:
  - 5mg/kg every 6–8h
  - maximum 20mg/kg daily
- Infants 3–12 months:
  - 5–10mg/kg every 6–8h
  - maximum 30mg/kg daily

Opioids

Codeine has a long history in paediatric practice. It is administered orally as codeine linctus at a dose of 0.5–1.0mg/kg every 6h in neonates and infants. It undergoes hepatic metabolism and is excreted renally. Codeine has many active metabolites of which codeine-6-glucuronide, morphine and norcodeine have the most significant analgesic properties. Efficacy is limited by lack of the CYP2D6 enzyme that metabolizes codeine into morphine.

Morphine is used for moderate to severe pain. It is a potent agonist at the mu receptor and is metabolized to the active metabolites morphine-3-glucuronide and morphine-6-glucuronide. The weight-normalized clearance is diminished in neonates and reaches mature values over the first 2–6 months of life. Neonates, particularly preterm, are susceptible to the respiratory depressant effects of morphine due to the longer elimination half-life and their immature renal function. Oral morphine is typically administered at a dose of 0.1mg/kg every 6–8h in the neonate and 0.1–0.2mg/kg every 6h in infants.

Nurse-controlled analgesia

Morphine is most effectively delivered via an NCA regimen for the control of postoperative pain. Typically 1mg/kg of morphine is made up to 50mL with 10% dextrose to give a concentration of 20mcg/kg/ml. There are many different regimens but most centre around:

- Bolus dose of 0.5–1.0mL (10–20mcg/kg)
- Lockout of 20min
- Background infusion of 0–1mL/h (usually omitted in neonates and infants <5kg)

The doses should be constantly reassessed, with input from a dedicated pain team, and can be increased if children are nursed in areas where apnoea monitors are present.

Naloxone should always be prescribed with an NCA for administration if respiratory rate or oxygen saturation limits are unacceptable.

Patient-controlled analgesia

PCA can be used in children as young as 5, provided they are able to press the handset and understand the concept.

Further reading

Association of Paediatric Anaesthetists of Great Britain and Ireland (2008). Good practice in postoperative and procedural pain management. *Paediatr Anaesth*, 18(Suppl. 1):1–3.

British Medical Association and the Royal Pharmaceutical Society of Great Britain (2013). *BNF for Children* (2nd edn). London: BNF.

Mathew PJ & Mathew JL (2003). Assessment and management of pain in infants. *Postgrad Med J*, 79(934):438–43.

Parry S (2008). Acute pain management in the neonate. *Anaesth Intens Care Med*, 4(9):147–51.

The critically ill child

Children (<19 years) account for 25% of the population in the UK. Critical illness in this population has many aetiologies ranging from respiratory, septic, circulatory, metabolic, and traumatic causes. It is important to recognize these children early and intervene promptly as the outcome of cardiac arrest in this group is generally poor.

The Acutely or Critically Sick or Injured Child in the District General Hospital – A Team Response (The Tanner report, DoH 2006) states that six generic skills may be expected of all personnel involved in the care of critically ill or injured children in the DGH:

- To recognize the critically ill child
- To initiate appropriate immediate treatment
- To act within a team
- To maintain and enhance skills
- To be aware of issues of safeguarding children
- To communicate effectively with children and carers.

Recognition

Recognition of such children requires a systematic approach, e.g. APLS/EPLS while bearing in mind the normal physiological parameters for age (see section 25.2).

Drugs and fluids are calculated by weight so an early estimation is essential either by using a formula or a Broselow or Sandell tape.

Once the initial assessment has been performed and all parameters are stable, the underlying disease can be addressed.

Assessment

Airway
- Air movement
- Signs of airway obstruction (e.g. stridor, wheeze).

Breathing
- Respiratory rate (NB no tachypnoea in exhaustion, cerebral depression or neuromuscular disease)
- Inspiratory or expiratory noise
- Grunting (a sign of severe distress)
- Accessory muscle use
- Nasal flaring
- Auscultation
- Oxygen saturation
- Skin colour.

Circulation
- Heart rate
- Pulse volume
- Capillary refill (*do not* use as sole indicator of shock, combine with other clinical signs)
- Blood pressure
- Skin appearance (e.g. mottled, pale).

Disability
- Conscious level (AVPU scale)
- Pupils

- Posture (e.g. hypotonic, decerebrate, decorticate, full fontanelle (<1 year) and stiff neck)
- *Check glucose.*

Exposure
For markers of illness requiring immediate attention, e.g. fever, rash (sepsis or allergic reaction).

Sepsis

Sepsis is a major problem in children with the highest incidence occurring in the neonatal population.

Management

Treatment should follow an 'ABC' approach with the emphasis on early aggressive resuscitation to optimize pre-load, afterload, and contractility:

High-flow oxygen should be given immediately.

Rapid fluid resuscitation of 40mL/kg within the first hour of presentation has been shown to improve survival with no increased risk of pulmonary oedema. Boluses of 20mL/kg should be titrated to HR, capillary refill, BP and urine output. Up to 200mL/kg may be required, e.g. in meningococcal sepsis.

Once 40mL/kg have been given, and there is still evidence of shock, intubation should be considered to reduce the work of breathing and the risk of pulmonary oedema. Avoid the nasal route in meningococcal sepsis and DIC. Acute lung injury is common in sepsis so a lung protective strategy of ventilation should subsequently be employed. An NGT should be inserted as a distended stomach can hinder ventilation.

If shock is fluid resistant commence a dopamine infusion, which can initially run peripherally whilst central access is gained. In the event of fluid and dopamine resistant shock consideration should be given to starting adrenaline (cold shock), noradrenaline (warm shock), and hydrocortisone. Help should be sought from an early stage.

Trauma

Major trauma is the leading cause of death in children over the age of 1. Children sustain different injuries to adults with a higher proportion of head injuries and burns. Identification of problems should follow the ABCDE approach, as in adults, with the caveat of initial management of catastrophic external haemorrhage. See section 21.6.

Management

Airway + cervical spine control
Bear in mind overzealous immobilization may increase leverage on the neck of a struggling child.

Breathing
If inadequate, intubate and ventilate. If unequal breath sounds take appropriate action.

Circulation
Two large-bore cannulae (intraosseous if necessary). No fluid bolus if no signs of shock. If shock, give 10mL/kg aliquots (so as not to affect clot formation or dilute clotting factors) alerting surgeons once 20mL/kg given. Transfuse if not stable after 40mL/kg. If <1 year old, haemoglobin levels can drop significantly with an intracranial or scalp bleed. Above this age if shock occurs with a head injury extracranial injuries should be sought.

Disability

As soon as a serious head injury is suspected proceed to CT and inform neurosurgery (see NICE guidelines for imaging and referral for head injury). Treat raised ICP.

Exposure

- Temperature control
- NGT and catheter
- Secondary survey.

Consider NAI, especially in children <2 years old.

Convulsions

Common causes include:

- Fever (<6 years old)
- Known epilepsy
- Meningoencephalitis
- Hypoxia

- Metabolic abnormalities
- Trauma.

Status epilepticus is defined as a generalized convulsion lasting >30min or when several convulsions occur over 30min and consciousness is not regained in between them. Seizures are unlikely to cease spontaneously after 5min so anticonvulsant treatment is usually instigated at this point (Fig. 25.3). Death may occur due to airway obstruction, hypoxia, aspiration, arrhythmias, medication, or the underlying disease process.

Management

ABC to ensure the seizure is not due to hypoxia or ischaemia. Look for signs of raised ICP.

Check glucose before giving an anticonvulsant. If hypoglycaemia, take 10mL of clotted blood for future investigation, and give 5mL/kg of 10% dextrose IV.

If a diagnosis of meningitis is obvious (stiff neck, bulging fontanelle) give antibiotics. Do not perform a lumbar puncture.

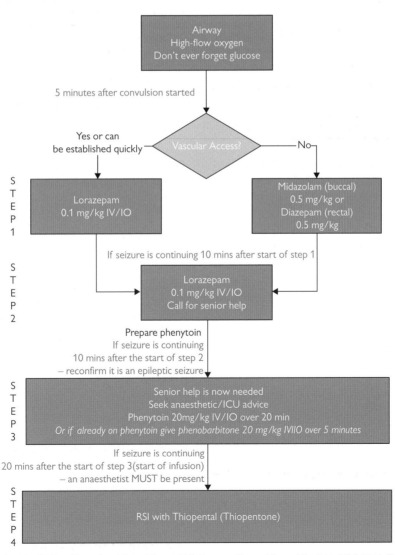

Fig. 25.3 APLS Status epilepticus diagram. Reproduced from Advanced Life Support Group, *Advanced Paediatric Life Support: The Practical Approach*, 5th edition, Wiley, Copyright © 2011, John Wiley and Sons, with permission.

Diabetic ketoacidosis

DKA occurs when a relative or absolute lack of insulin results in the inability to utilize glucose. This leads to hyperglycaemia, osmotic diuresis, ketone production due to fat metabolism and acidosis. DKA may be the child's first presentation or occur in the known diabetic due to infection, illness or non-compliance with treatment.

Children can die from DKA. The most common cause is cerebral oedema which carries a 25% mortality. Hypokalaemia and aspiration pneumonia also contribute to mortality.

DKA is defined as the presence of:

* BM >11
* pH <7.3
* Bicarbonate <15
* 3% dehydration.

This may be accompanied by vomiting, drowsiness and clinical signs of acidosis.

Management

Treatment is aimed at gradual rehydration (to avoid rapid drops in serum osmolality) and reducing the risk of cerebral oedema.

Resuscitation

ABC. Only if shocked give 10mL/kg 0.9% saline. Give no more than 20mL/kg in first 4h. Take bloods for U&E, blood gases, glucose, Hb and differential WCC. Test urine for ketones, glucose and culture.

Maintenance and rehydration

Deficit = % dehydration × body weight.

Rehydrate over 48h. Initially use 0.9% Saline with 20mmol KCl in 500ml adding in glucose when blood sugar falls below 14mmol/L.

$$\text{Hourly rate} = \frac{48\text{h maintenance} + \text{deficit} - \text{resus fluid}}{48}$$

Ketoacidosis

Once fluids have been running for an hour start an insulin infusion at 0.1 unit/kg/h. There is no indication for a bolus dose. Ideally blood glucose should fall by <5mmol/h.

Do not stop insulin if the glucose falls. It is required to switch off ketone production.

Depressed consciousness

Assume cerebral oedema.

Give osmotherapy (3mls/kg 3% saline or 0.5g/kg mannitol).

If no response or airway protection required, intubate and ventilate aiming for a normal pCO_2. Obtain a CT scan to identify the cause.

Closely monitor U&Es and blood glucose.

Further reading

Advanced Life Support Group (2011). *Advanced Paediatric Life Support: The Practical Approach* 5th edn). Lodnon: BMJ Books.

Department of Health (2006). *The Acutely or Critically Sick or Injured Child in the DGH – A Team Response (The Tanner report).* London: DoH

NICE (2007). *Clinical Guideline 56. Head Injury: Triage, assessment, investigation and early management in infants, children and adults.* London: NICE.

Transfer of critically ill children

The Department of Health report *Paediatric Intensive care: A Framework for the Future* (1997) advised on the benefits of centralizing expertise on the management of critically ill children into regional paediatric intensive care (PIC) units. However, children may present to any hospital. As early intervention improves outcome in critical illness, and centralization of PIC improves mortality, the best solution is to resuscitate and stabilize the child locally then transfer to the specialist centre.

Who transfers?

Transfer by specialist PIC retrieval teams has been shown to improve survival when compared to non-specialist teams. This may be due to experience and also knowledge of the transport environment. However, there are certain situations which dictate that transfer should be undertaken by the referring hospital. These include time-critical injuries such as an expanding intracranial haematoma where the risks of delay outweigh the benefits of a specialist retrieval team.

Recognition and resuscitation of the critically ill child

APLS or EPLS give an excellent structure to the initial management of these patients. See section 25.8.

Referral

Following successful resuscitation of the child, significant further input is required. It is advisable to contact the regional retrieval service early. This should provide a single point of contact on a dedicated telephone line whereby advice can be given, a PICU bed found and a retrieval team organized. Services such as the Children's Acute Transfer Service (CATS) in North Thames and the South Thames Retrieval Service (STRS) provide this along with websites offering guidelines for stabilization and drug and infusion calculations.

Key information required at this initial referral call will include patient demographics, location, clinical history, management to date, response to treatment, current observations and results.

Clear communication prevents errors.

Stabilization

This requires a team approach usually comprising a competent anaesthetist, paediatrician and nurse working alongside emergency department or ward staff.

Urgent interventions should not be delayed pending the arrival of the retrieval team.

Frequent reassessment should be carried out to establish response to treatment or clinical deterioration.

Children resuscitated from cardiorespiratory arrest, serious illness or injury may suffer ongoing harm from hypoxia or ischaemia.

Airway

The airway should be secured in the presence of airway compromise, respiratory or circulatory failure, or if neuroprotection is required. The nasal route is avoided if coagulopathy or a base of skull fracture is suspected. Cervical spine immobilization is required in any ventilated trauma patient.

Breathing

Adequate ventilation must be ensured. End-tidal carbon dioxide (ETCO$_2$) monitoring is mandatory. Arterial blood gas targets will depend on the underlying pathology aiming for a pCO$_2$ of 4.5–5kPa and a pO$_2$ >13kPa in the patient with head injuries or raised intracranial pressure while tolerating hypercarbia in a child with severe lung disease. For those with known or suspected cardiac abnormalities, advice should be sought from a paediatric intensivist.

Circulation

It is mandatory to have good vascular access. Trying to achieve this in transit is very challenging. Therefore most retrieval services will site a minimum of two in case one falls out. A central line (including intraosseous) should be sited if inotropes are required and is helpful to assess the response to a fluid bolus. Additional peripheral access is more suitable for fluid bolus administration owing to its calibre and length. An arterial line is useful but should not be the initial priority. Fluid resuscitation should continue pending the retrieval team. In the shocked neonate consideration should be given to starting prostin in case of a duct dependent circulation.

Disability

The aim is to prevent secondary injury to the brain following any initial insult (see Box 25.15).

Box 25.15 Minimizing secondary brain injury

- Oxygenation—aim pO$_2$ >13kPa.
- Normocarbia.
- Maintain adequate blood pressure to keep cerebral perfusion pressure >50mmHg.
- Nurse head-up 30°, head midline.
- Control blood glucose.
- Avoid hyperthermia (no evidence to support hypothermia in children post-arrest after the newborn period).
- Control seizures.

If muscle relaxants are being used ensure adequate sedation. Most retrieval services will have guidelines for infusions. Monitor blood glucose and commence dextrose infusions in at risk groups (neonates, liver, and metabolic patients).

Everything else

A gastric tube on free drainage should be inserted on ventilated patients. Consideration should be given to placing a urinary catheter if fluid balance needs to be monitored or there are concerns regarding retention.

Trauma patients should have a complete secondary survey.

Temperature should be monitored and, unless being therapeutically cooled, normothermia should be maintained.

Medication

Pre-filled syringes of resuscitation drugs are mandatory prior to transfer. Further doses of drugs being used should also be drawn up along with saline flushes. If on inotropes, it is sensible to have the next syringe drawn up and attached ready for use during the transfer. If there is no power supply on the ambulance it is important to know the battery life of the syringe drivers and ensure they are fully charged before departing. It is advisable to carry twice the calculated required oxygen on a transfer and to have two cylinders in case of failure. The volume of oxygen in a cylinder is printed on its collar. Wait until leaving the building before using the transport oxygen.

Monitoring and equipment

Minimal monitoring includes pulse oximetry, ECG, and non-invasive blood pressure. If the child is intubated and ventilated $ETCO_2$ is mandatory and is invaluable in detecting ETT dislodgement in the back of a noisy ambulance. Retrieval teams often carrier portable blood gas analysers and blood glucose monitors. Batteries should be fully charged. See Box 25.16 for a list of transport equipment.

Box 25.16 Transport equipment

Airway
- Oropharyngeal airways
- Nasopharyngeal airways
- Tracheal tubes (the correct size, one size above and below)
- Stylets
- Bougie
- LMAs
- Laryngoscopes × 2
- Portable suction
- Yankauer suckers
- Suction catheters
- HMEs
- Needle cricothyroidotomy set.

Breathing
- Oxygen masks with reservoir
- Face masks
- Self-inflating bags with reservoir
- Portable ventilator
- Catheter mount
- Ayre's T-piece.

Circulation
- Intravenous cannulae
- Intraosseous needles
- Burette
- Giving sets
- Syringes
- Three-way taps
- Central and arterial line sets
- Fluids including 10% dextrose and mannitol.

Miscellaneous
- Nasogastric tubes
- Chest drain set
- Sharps disposal box.

Documentation

It is important to frequently re-assess and document the patient's physiological parameters. This may be done on a transfer proforma if available or on an anaesthetic chart if not. Retrieval teams will usually have their own paperwork to ensure thorough documentation, prevent omissions, and to allow a copy to be left at the receiving hospital.

Copies of the clinical notes, observations, results of investigations and drug charts should be prepared as well as a copy of X-rays and CT scans performed.

Communication

There should be clear, ongoing communication between the referring hospital and the retrieval team. The team should carry a mobile phone with contact details of the referring and receiving hospitals.

Relatives should be kept as informed as possible about the clinical and logistical plan. There is often facility to allow one parent to accompany the child during the transfer to the PICU. Research by the STRS has shown that this has not been detrimental to patient care and has been of benefit to the parents.

Should any concerns exist regarding non-accidental injury the referring consultant is responsible for contacting social services.

Transport

The majority of UK transfers are carried out by road. Dedicated retrieval services have their own ambulances. For time critical transfers conducted by the referring hospital, the local ambulance service will need to be contacted to arrange an ambulance. Road speed will be determined by the clinical picture but safety of the patient, retrieval team, and general public must be taken in to consideration. The retrieval team should be covered with accident insurance. Members of the AAGBI are automatically covered.

Aeromedical transfers provide further challenges in transfer medicine. Altitude has various physiological effects on the ventilated patient while the environment provides logistical, safety and communication difficulties. For these reasons training in aeromedical transfer is required.

The standard of care and monitoring should be continued during transportation. Careful preparation can help prevent deterioration en route. However, should untoward events occur then reassessment should take place using the structured ABC approach. Should the team need to remove their seatbelts to access the patient then the ambulance should slow down and stop as soon as it is safe to do so. However, if there is a severe deterioration transfer to the nearest hospital may be required for further stabilization.

Handover

There should be a clear, concise, verbal handover to the receiving team on arrival. This should be followed by a written copy of the transfer along with all the documents taken with the child.

Further reading

Advanced Life Support Group (2011). *Advanced Paediatric Life Support: The Practical Approach* (5th edn). London: BMJ Books.

Children's Acute Transport Service website: <http://www.cats.nhs.uk>

Davies J, Tibby S, & Murdoch IA (2005). Should parents accompany critically ill children during inter-hospital transport? *Arch Dis Child*, 90(12):1270–3

South Thames Retrieval Service website: <http://www.strs.nhs.uk>

Consent in children

Consent is an individual's permission for a particular intervention, and must be freely given by someone who is appropriately informed and competent to do so. Relevant information required will include the indications for the procedure, its risks and benefits, and potential alternative treatments including the option and implications of no intervention.

Usual practice in the UK is that anaesthesia does not require separate written consent (in addition to the consent for surgery). Verbal consent for anaesthesia should be sought following discussion about induction, plans for pain relief (including the use of suppositories where relevant), and any special procedures that may be undertaken such as blood transfusion, invasive monitoring, and epidural, caudal, or peripheral nerve blocks. This is to enable children and/or those with parental responsibility to make informed decisions about their care. There should be written documentation of this discussion (e.g. on the anaesthetic chart or in the medical notes).

Parental responsibility

Parental responsibility (PaR) is a legal status set out in the Children's Act 1989 conferring the rights and duties that a person responsible for a child has by law. Not all parents have the formal status of parental responsibility. A biological mother has PaR for her children (unless they are given up for adoption), however the position of the father is more complicated.

A father has PaR if he was married to the mother at the time of conception or birth, or if the couple subsequently marry. He also has PaR if he has not married the mother but his name is on the birth certificate (for children born on or after 1 December 2003 in England and Wales, 4 May 2006 in Scotland, and 15 April 2002 in Northern Ireland). Fathers can also obtain PaR by means of a court order or a parental responsibility agreement with the mother.

Grandparents and foster parents do not have PaR unless they have been given it by a court order. Local authorities are often (but not always) given PaR by the court when children are taken into care. Courts can also take PaR away from anyone who would otherwise have it (including the child's mother).

When can children give or refuse consent?

Over 18 years

Anyone over the age of 18 is an adult, and is presumed to be competent to consent to treatment unless this is demonstrated not to be the case, as described in the Mental Capacity Act 2005. Competent adults can give or withhold consent for any reason or no reason at all.

16–17 years

In Scotland, 16- and 17-year-olds have the same legal rights as adults to give or withhold consent, and non-competent individuals are treated in accordance with the Adults with Incapacity (Scotland) Act 2000 (i.e. those with parental responsibility *do not* usually have the right to give consent for interventions on their behalf).

In England, Wales, and Northern Ireland, 16- and 17-year-olds are presumed to be competent (as with adults), however an adult with parental responsibility can still give consent on their behalf, and the refusal of consent by a young person in this age group can be overridden by a court where there is a risk of them dying or suffering severe permanent injury as a result of that refusal.

Under 16s

If a child or young person under 16 years of age is competent to give their consent, then they have the legal right to do so. To be deemed competent, they must be able to understand, retain, and weigh the relevant information in such a way as to be able to make an informed decision. If they can do this and communicate their decision, then they are 'Gillick competent'. It is self-evident that some decisions are easier to make than others and therefore a child's competence must be assessed for each decision that they need to make. It is good practice to encourage the child to include someone with parental responsibility in the decision-making process; however, this is not a legal requirement. If a competent child under 16 refuses treatment that is felt to be in their best interests, then the Department of Health guidance is to obtain legal advice as to how to proceed.

If a child or young person under 16 is not competent to give their consent (or is competent but does not wish to take this responsibility), then someone with PaR can give consent on their behalf. The person with PaR will usually (but not always) be one of the parents; in this situation consent is only required from one parent, although it is obviously good practice to involve both parents wherever possible, and where there is a conflict between the parents that cannot be resolved, it is good practice to obtain legal advice. The person giving (or withholding) consent on behalf of a child has a responsibility to act in that child's best interest, and their decision is open to legal challenge if they are not thought to be doing so.

The healthcare team should try to enhance children's decision-making ability where possible by using age-appropriate language, giving time for questions, and delaying non-urgent treatment until a child is able to make their own decision. Even where a child is not giving their own consent, they should be involved in the decision-making process as much as possible and their views given appropriate weight.

In emergencies

In an emergency situation, attempts should be made to contact those with parental responsibility, however if this is not possible then clinicians should provide treatment as necessary in the best interests of the child.

Restraint

All anaesthetists who work with children will encounter the child who refuses or resists induction of general anaesthesia. It is vital therefore to develop ways to minimize its occurrence and have a feel for what is, and what is not, an appropriate response. Resistance to anaesthesia must be differentiated from refusal of consent by a competent child, as to proceed without a court order in the latter situation would be illegal.

Careful preoperative assessment should enable you to predict the majority of children who will be difficult to manage in the anaesthetic room, and good communication will allow fears and misconceptions to be addressed. The Royal College of

Anaesthetists produces a series of information leaflets about anaesthesia for children of various ages. Preoperative nursing staff and play therapists may have a lot of experience and be extremely helpful when psychologically preparing a child for anaesthesia. Children with severe anxiety may require specialist input from psychologists or hypnotherapists as outpatients prior to surgery.

Where non-compliance is anticipated, distraction techniques and the possibility of physical restraint (including exactly what that would involve) should be discussed during the preoperative visit. The use of sedative premedication should also be considered. The most commonly used technique is gentle restraint by the parents combined with distraction (with or without sedative premedication) whilst either a cannula is being inserted or a mask is being held on for gaseous induction. Unfortunately there is no consensus as to what constitutes physical restraint and what degree of restraint is acceptable.

Where there is an unexpected lack of cooperation, the possibility of sending the child back to the ward for premedication (buccal midazolam 0.2mg/kg only takes 15min to be effective) or postponing the procedure to another day to enable further psychological preparation should be considered.

If resistance is anticipated despite appropriate preparation, premedication and distraction, and it is felt by all involved (surgeons, anaesthetists, parents, and nursing staff) that it is in the child's best interests to proceed, then significant restraint may be required. A detailed plan for induction should be discussed and may involve IM administration of ketamine. A policy for the use of restraint within the hospital should be in place, and techniques can include restraining the legs at the hips (and possibly also above the knees), holding the arms down in extension, and holding the head. This should be performed by appropriately trained staff and not left to the parents.

Research

Research in children is important and is subject to the same restrictions as research in adults, with a few extra precautions. Research should only be done in children if work with adults could not answer the same question; a few children should not be involved in multiple research projects simply because they are available; and where there is a choice of age groups, then older children should be involved in preference to younger ones. Legally valid consent should be sought for involvement in research studies just as it is for therapeutic medical intervention, although a young person's competence should be demonstrated rather than presumed in the case of 16- and 17-year-olds and parental involvement is strongly recommended. In addition, the agreement of school age children should also be sought and if the child does not want to be involved, then this should be respected.

Further reading

Department of Health (2001). *Seeking consent working with children*. London: DoH.

Department of Health (2009). *Reference guide to consent for examination or treatment*. London: DoH.

Homer J & Bass S (2010). Physically restraining children for induction of general anaesthesia; survey of consultant pediatric anesthetists. *Pediatric Anesthes*, 20:638–46.

RCOA (2010) *Guidance on the provision of paediatric anaesthesia services*. Available at <http/www.rcoa.ac.uk/docs/GPAS-Paeds.pdf>.

Royal College of Paediatrics and Child Health (2000). Guidelines for the ethical conduct of medical research involving children. *Arch Dis Child*, 82:177–82.

United Nations (1989). *Convention on the Rights of the Child. Article 12*. <http://www2.ohchr.org/english/law/crc.htm>.

Child abuse

The incidence of child abuse is far higher than society would like to believe. The NSPCC report that 7% of children will suffer physical abuse, 6% suffer neglect, 6% experience emotional abuse, and 11% are subjected to sexual abuse. The anaesthetist may be involved in resuscitation or intensive care of a child following physical abuse, may discover concerning signs during routine perioperative care or rarely may have to provide anaesthesia for a forensic examination. As part of the multidisciplinary team involved in a child's care, the anaesthetist must be aware of the indicators of abuse, their role in safeguarding the child, and the process of child protection.

Types of abuse

Physical abuse

Acts of physical harm, assault, or unreasonable restraint, e.g. hitting, shaking, burning, suffocation.

Injuries may be multiple, frequent, and of different ages. Injuries without a consistent history or not appropriate to the developmental age should raise concern.

Non-accidental bruising is often symmetrical and associated with petechiae, involving the torso, upper legs, periorbital, and neck. Accidental bruising is common in the mobile child and generally affects the forehead, nose, chin, knees, and shins.

Thermal injury, e.g. burns and scalds, are typically in a 'pull over' distribution when occurring accidentally. Non-accidental injuries may present as a symmetrical glove and stocking or immersion pattern.

Fractures in a non-ambulant child must be treated with concern. Other fractures at different healing stages, particularly involving ribs or sternum make non-accidental injury more likely. Head injury without a history of major trauma or in association with retinal haemorrhage should also raise concern.

Emotional abuse

Emotional abuse is persistent emotional maltreatment which impacts on the child's social and emotional development, e.g. severe, constant criticism and unrealistic expectations, which lead to the child feeling worthless.

Children subject to emotional abuse may show delayed development (speech, emotional), low self-esteem, appear over-obedient or extremely keen to please or be highly critical of themselves. Staff may witness abusive interactions with the carers.

Neglect

Neglect is the persistent failure to meet the care needs of a child, whether physical, developmental, social, or educational, leading to impairment of the child's health or development.

Neglect may lead to malnutrition, poor growth, poor hygiene including dental disease, and developmental delay. Repeated absence from schooling is also neglect. Children may be inappropriately affection-seeking of strangers.

Sexual abuse

Sexual abuse encompasses any act of forcing or enticing a child into sexual behaviour or activity. This includes non-contact events such as photography. It is illegal for any child below 13 years to engage in sexual activity. Over 13 years, consensual activity is considered as abuse if the partner is unequal in maturity, capacity or social standing.

Sexual abuse may cause sudden emotional or behavioural changes, e.g. self-harm, eating disorders, running away, secondary bed-wetting or soiling. Children may be especially fearful of contact with the abuser. Genital signs or symptoms, sexually transmitted diseases, or pregnancy may result.

Common concerns during perioperative care are the findings of a torn labial fraenum or anal dilation. These findings were thought to be pathagnomic of child abuse. A torn labial fraenum may occur after accidental injury in an ambulant child and a consistent history of mechanism of injury should be reassuring. In a non-ambulant child, coexisting injuries should be sought. A dilated anus may occur under general anaesthesia, especially if combined with caudal epidural, neurological conditions, and chronic constipation. If coexisting concerns are present, this should be discussed further.

Risk factors for abuse

- Children <3 years of age
- Children with disability (especially learning disability)
- Previous history of child abuse
- Mental or physical illness involving carers
- Drug or alcohol abuse in carers
- Domestic violence
- Lower socioeconomic status—financial or housing problems
- Single parent with poor social support
- Immigrants/asylum seekers.

Carers may delay seeking medical intervention for the child and may present to multiple hospitals. Explanations for the injury may not be consistent with the injury pattern or the child's development, or may be conflicting between carers. Concerning child–carer interactions may be witnessed and carers may be disruptive with staff attempting to interact with the child.

Child protection

The main principle of the Children Act of 1989 is that 'the welfare of children is paramount' but sadly child protection has had to further evolve following learning from high profile cases such as the Victoria Climbie Inquiry in 2003 and Baby Peter in 2009.

The Children Act legislates for England and Wales. The Children (N Ireland) Order 1995 and Children (Scotland) Act 1995 share the same principles.

The Children Act allocates responsibility to Local Authorities (LoA) to investigate any child within the area that is suspected of suffering, or at risk of, significant harm. They must provide services for children in need and their families. Courts must ascertain the wishes of the child, endeavour to maintain home and family links where possible, and only make an Order where it will benefit the child.

The importance of raising and discussing any concerns about a child's safety was highlighted by the Climbie Inquiry. Lord Laming's reports led to the government papers 'Keeping Children Safe' and 'Every Child Matters'. The Children Act 2004 set out a process for integration of services to children. Local Authorities (LoA) appointed a director of children's services who, along with an elected team leader, were accountable for the service delivery. It placed a duty on the LoA, police and health service to cooperate in promoting children's wellbeing. Local Safeguarding Children Boards were introduced for investigation and review.

Baby Peter's case demonstrated the importance of sharing information between all professionals involved in a child's care.

Specific guidance for anaesthetists is given in the intercollegiate document *Safeguarding Children in the Operating Theatre* 2007. Anaesthetists have a responsibility to be familiar with the child protection process and to raise and discuss any concerns about a child in order that further assessment can be considered.

Child protection and the anaesthetist

The anaesthetist may discover unusual or unexplained signs of injury or abuse, e.g. bruising, intra-oral trauma during routine perioperative care or critical care. It is essential to act in the best interests of the child and ensure the child's safety (Box 25.17). This may override the obligation for patient confidentiality and occasionally consent. The GMC states 'If you believe a patient to be a victim of abuse and the patient cannot give or withhold consent to disclosure, you must give information promptly to an appropriate responsible person or agency, where you believe that the disclosure is in the patient's best interests'.

Any concerns must be discussed immediately with a senior anaesthetist, consultant paediatrician or a designated professional for child protection (present in each hospital Trust). They may carry out an immediate visual inspection but any additional examination requires consent.

The concerns will be raised with the carers initially. Explanations are sought for the injuries and all discussion is formally documented and witnessed. The LoA must be informed and has a duty to investigate if significant harm is suspected. The LoA enquiry enables them to determine what action, if any, should be taken to protect the child.

Box 25.17 Duties of the anaesthetist (*Child Protection and the Anaesthetist*, 2007)

- To act in the best interest of the child which are always paramount.
- To be aware of the child's rights to be protected.
- To respect the rights of the child to confidentiality.
- To contact a paediatrician with experience of child protection for advice.
- To be aware of the local child protection mechanisms.
- To be aware of the rights of those with parental responsibility.

Reproduced with permission from Association of Paediatric Anaesthetists, Royal College of Paediatrics and Child Health, Royal College of Anaesthetists, '*Child Protection and the Anaesthetist: Safeguarding Children in the Operating Theatre*', published by Royal College of Paediatrics and Child Health, © 2007 Association of Paediatric Anaesthetists, Royal College of Paediatrics and Child Health, Royal College of Anaesthetists.

The child protection process

The LoA may apply for a Child Assessment Order and the child's carers must be notified of this. This allows further assessment of the child's health and development. If there is reasonable cause to believe that the child is at immediate risk, or is at risk if removed from a place of safety, the LoA may apply for an Emergency Protection Order. Police have the right to remove a child immediately to suitable accommodation or to prevent the child's removal from hospital under a Police Protection Order where the child's safety is compromised. Legal advice can be sought in less urgent situations within the hospital. It is also important to consider the safety of any other children in the immediate family.

If a child remains in hospital, a named consultant must be responsible for the child protection aspects. The child should be examined within 24h following a full explanation to the carers and consent obtained if possible. If sexual abuse is suspected within 72h, a forensic examination may be required after discussion with the LoA, police and health professionals. This should be performed within 24h of the event by a trained forensic professional.

Emergency Protection Orders are valid for 8 days, although may be extended. Following a Care Proceeding, the Court may issue a Care Order if they are satisfied that the child is suffering significant harm attributable to the care that is being provided and that it is in the child's best interests. The LoA are awarded legal guardianship for the child in this event.

Further reading

Maguire S (2010). Which injuries may indicate child abuse. *Arch Dis Child Educ*, 95:170–7.

RCOA, APA, & RCPCH (2007). *Child Protection and the Anaesthetist: Safeguarding Children in the Operating Theatre*. Intercollegiate Document. London: RCOA.

Chapter 26

Pain medicine

26.1 Mechanisms of pain

Pain is defined by the International Association for the Study of Pain (IASP) as 'an unpleasant sensory and emotional experience associated with actual or potential tissue damage, or described in terms of such damage'. The ability to detect noxious stimuli is an important protective mechanism involving peripheral and central processes. The final experience of pain is determined by individual environmental and psychological factors.

Peripheral transduction and transmission

Nociceptors are the sensory structures that transduce noxious stimuli into electrical energy. Most nociceptors are the free nerve endings of primary afferent neurons. There are two main types, Aδ fibres and C fibres which have higher activation thresholds than sensory Aβ fibres.

Aδ fibres are rapidly conducting myelinated fibres that respond to mechanical and thermal stimuli and give rise to immediate, sharp pain.

C fibres are smaller diameter unmyelinated fibres and so conduct more slowly. They are polymodal, responding to mechanical, thermal, and chemical stimuli. They produce slow, burning pain.

Tissue injury initiates an inflammatory response with the release of chemical mediators such as endothelin, prostaglandin E2, bradykinin, and serotonin.

These mediators act directly on the nociceptors, and can also sensitize nociceptors by reducing the activation threshold and increasing membrane excitability. Afferent activity to a given stimulus is therefore increased. This peripheral sensitization results in primary hyperalgesia (increased response to painful stimuli at the site of tissue damage).

Peripheral sensitization

Peripheral sensitization is caused by:

- Activated kinases which phosphorylate and activate receptors such as TRPV1 (transient receptor potential vanilloid-1). TRPV1 is normally activated by capsaicin as well as heat at around 41°C. Following sensitization, TRPV1 may be stimulated at lower temperatures (heat hyperalgesia).
- Neuropeptides (substance P) released from peripheral nerve terminals increase inflammatory cells and mediators at the site of tissue damage.
- Inflammation can alter protein synthesis in the cell body of the dorsal root ganglion. This can increase peripheral receptor and ion channel expression, e.g. TRPV1 and opioid receptors.

Spinal cord transmission

Primary afferent neurons synapse with second-order neurons in the dorsal horn of the spinal cord. The cell bodies of primary afferent neurons from the trunk, limbs, and viscera lie in the dorsal root ganglia. Those from the head, neck, and oral cavity are in the trigeminal ganglia and project to the brainstem trigeminal nucleus.

Most Aδ and C fibres terminate superficially in Rexed laminae I–II, with a few reaching the deeper laminae. Aβ fibres predominantly terminate in laminae III–VI. There are different types of second-order neuron in the dorsal horn. Nociceptive specific cells are mostly found superficially and synapse with Aδ and C fibres only, firing action potentials when a painful stimulus is detected at the periphery. Wide dynamic range (WDR) neurons are located mainly in lamina V and respond to a range of noxious and non-noxious stimuli. See Fig. 26.1.

Connections in the dorsal horn

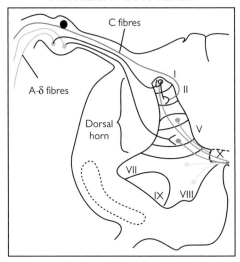

Fig. 26.1 Primary afferent neurons in the dorsal horn. Reproduced from Catherine Spoors and Kevin Kiff, *Training in Anaesthesia*, 2010, Figure 7.65, page 193, with permission from Oxford University Press.

Spinal cord modulation

The spinal cord is an important site of modulation of incoming sensory and painful stimuli. Glutamate is a major excitatory neurotransmitter in the spinal cord and is utilized by the majority of primary afferent neurons. Glutamate acts on three receptor subclasses:

- 2-amino-3-(3-hydroxy-5-methyl-isoxazol-4-yl)propanoic acid (AMPA)
- N-methyl-D-aspartic acid (NMDA)
- G-protein coupled metabotropic receptors.

Glutamate is released in response to acute and persistent noxious stimuli and acts on postsynaptic receptors. The action on AMPA receptors sets the baseline response of the dorsal root neurons.

Central sensitization

Wind-up, long-term potentiation, and secondary hyperalgesia are associated with an increase in excitability of neurons within the CNS. Clinically this manifests as an increased response to painful stimuli (hyperalgesia), and pain resulting from normally non-painful tactile stimuli (allodynia).

Wind-up

Repetitive, high-frequency stimulation of C fibres causes a progressive amplification and prolongation of the action potentials generated at the postsynaptic dorsal horn neuron. This wind-up phenomenon is due to the activation of NMDA receptors. During acute or low-frequency noxious stimuli, NMDA receptors are not activated as the ion channel is blocked by Mg^{2+}. Sustained membrane depolarization is required for the Mg^{2+} to be removed and allow the channel to open and activate the receptor.

The co-release of neuropeptides such as substance P and calcitonin-gene related peptide (CGRP), stored with glutamate in the presynaptic terminal, also facilitate activation of the NMDA receptor. NMDA receptor activation plays a key role in the hyperalgesia seen in more persistent pain.

Long-term potentiation

This follows high-frequency stimulation of Aδ fibres and C fibres in the dorsal horn and results in synaptic transmission that out-lasts the initial stimulus.

Secondary hyperalgesia

Hyperalgesia in undamaged tissue next to the area of tissue damage. It is thought to be due to an increase in receptive field and reduced activation threshold of WDR neurons in the dorsal horn.

Inhibitory modulation

Inhibitory modulation also occurs by a number of mechanisms in the dorsal horn:

- Non-noxious sensory input from Aβ neurons can inhibit transmission from primary afferent to second-order neurons in the substantia gelatinosa, thereby reducing nociceptive transmission. This is the gate control theory.
- Local GABA and glycine-mediated interneurons, descending brainstem projections and higher centres also mediate inhibitory modulation.

Central projections

Nociceptive input to the brain is relayed via a number of pathways from the dorsal horn. The spinothalamic tract is the major pain pathway. Second-order neurons from laminae I and II, via lamina V, ascend in the contralateral spinothalamic tract, projecting to the thalamus. The 'fast' spinothalamic tract projects directly to the thalamus and transmits localizing pain, whereas the 'slow' spinothalamic tract gives off projections to the reticular activating system and is involved with emotional components of pain.

The spinomesencephalic, spinoparabrachial, and spinoreticular systems are involved with the integration of nociceptive signals with arousal, autonomic responses and affective components of pain.

Nociceptive information is transmitted from the thalamus to cortical regions. There are a number of areas that may be activated during a painful experience. These areas include the primary and secondary somatosensory cortices (perception and localization of pain), and the insular, anterior cingulate and prefrontal cortices (affective and motivational components of pain).

Brainstem modulation

The brainstem plays an important role in the modulation of pain at a spinal cord level. Pathways originating in the cortex and thalamus pass via the rostral ventromedial medulla and adjacent areas to the dorsal horn of the spinal cord. These brainstem areas also receive afferent input from the superficial dorsal horn, periaqueductal grey matter, nucleus tractus solitarius, and the parabrachial nucleus, therefore forming a loop between the spinal cord and the brainstem. Descending pathways from the brainstem can also be influenced by the limbic system and contribute to the affective component of pain perception. The balance between descending facilitatory and inhibitory pathways may alter following injury and an imbalance can contribute to chronic pain states. Noradrenaline and serotonin-mediated descending pathways act via encephalin-secreting interneurons in the dorsal horn to inhibit pain transmission. This helps explain the role of antidepressants and opioids in the treatment of chronic pain.

Neuropathic pain

Neuropathic pain is defined as 'pain initiated or caused by a primary lesion or dysfunction in the nervous system'. Causes include trauma, infection, ischaemia, malignancy, and toxins. There are a number of mechanisms that lead to neuropathic pain, and the mechanism is independent of the cause of the disease:

Ectopic nerve activity

Spontaneous, ectopic impulses can arise from injured, and nearby uninjured, primary afferent nociceptive neurons causing spontaneous pain. Increased expression of voltage-gated sodium channels on damaged and intact nociceptive neurons leads to increased ectopic nerve activity. This spontaneous firing of nociceptive afferents causes repetitive input to the dorsal horn neurons and can contribute to central sensitization. Inflammatory mediators released after nerve lesions cause peripheral sensitization and contribute to spontaneous activity.

Allodynia and hyperalgesia

Changes in neuronal excitability due to central sensitization allow low-threshold impulses from Aβ and Aδ fibres, which would not usually trigger pain, to activate nociceptive second-order neurons resulting in allodynia and hyperalgesia.

After peripheral nerve injury there is sprouting of sensory Aβ-fibres into laminae I and II, regions usually involved in the transmission of noxious stimuli. This contributes to allodynia.

Sympathetically mediated pain

Some types of neuropathic pain have a sympathetically mediated component. This may be due to the presence of cutaneous α-receptors or from sympathetic fibres sprouting in the dorsal horn creating a link between nociceptive and sympathetic neurons.

Somatic and visceral pain

Somatic pain arises from structures such as the skin, muscles, and joints and is usually well defined. Visceral pain is typically dull and poorly localized. It is perceived due to visceral distension, inflammation, ischaemia and smooth muscle contraction. Visceral nociceptors are nearly all C fibres. They are fewer, more widely distributed and less well organized than somatic nociceptors. Normal physiological sensations, such as fullness secondary to smooth muscle stretch, and noxious stimuli can be transmitted by the same primary afferent neuron. The sensation is then interpreted as pain depending on the pattern and intensity of the sensory input.

Viscera receive dual innervation from the autonomic nervous system and primary afferent neurons. Referred pain is often felt in superficial structures due to the convergence of somatic and visceral pathways onto second-order neurons.

Further reading

D'Mello R & Dickenson AH (2008). Spinal cord mechanisms of pain. *Br J Anaesth*, 101(1):8–16.

Baron R, Binder A, & Wasner G (2010). Neuropathic pain: diagnosis, pathophysiological mechanisms, and treatment. *Lancet Neurol*, 9(8):807–19.

Moffat R & Rae CP (2011). Anatomy, physiology and pharmacology of pain. *Anaesth Intens Care*, 12(1):12–15.

Multimodal analgesia

The pain pathway is subject to multiple levels of physiological modulation. Analgesics can target peripheral, spinal, and supraspinal levels to modulate excitatory and inhibitory pain transmission (see Fig. 26.2). This allows better analgesia with a reduction in side effects through the use of lower analgesic doses.

Nociceptive and neuropathic pain can be targeted based on neurobiological understanding. Nociceptive pain comprises of transduction, conduction, transmission, and perception, which are the sites of interest to target.

Analgesics acting on the peripheral nervous system

Non-steroidal anti-inflammatory drugs (NSAIDs)

NSAIDS modulate peripheral pain by inhibiting the production of prostaglandins by locally induced cyclo-oxygenase-2 (COX-2) at sites of inflammation, and so reduce peripheral sensitization.

Opioids

Inflammation induces changes in protein synthesis in the dorsal root ganglion and alters the expression and transport of receptors. Opioid receptors are transported to the periphery. This helps explain the peripheral action of opioids in inflamed tissue.

Local anaesthetics

Local anaesthetics act by blocking neuronal sodium channels, thereby preventing transmission of action potentials. Sensory, motor, and sympathetic nerves can all be affected. Local anaesthetics can be used to target nerves peripherally via local infiltration or nerve blocks. Spinal or epidural techniques can be used to target nerves centrally.

Capsaicin

An agonist at the TRPV1 receptor (see section 26.1). It causes the nerve to become depolarized and refractory to further activation, thereby reducing afferent transmission. There is also depletion of the neurotransmitter substance P.

Analgesics acting on the central nervous system

Opioids

Opioid analgesics act on the presynaptic terminal of the primary afferent neuron in the dorsal horn, where they inhibit the release of excitatory neurotransmitters. They also act in the periaqueductal grey matter to enhance descending inhibitory modulation.

Antidepressants

The selective serotonin and noradrenaline reuptake inhibitors facilitate descending inhibitory pathways from the brainstem.

Gabapentin/pregabalin

These drugs bind to the $\alpha2$-δ subunit of voltage-gated calcium channels. This inhibits calcium influx and the release of excitatory neurotransmitters such as glutamate, noradrenaline, and substance P.

Clonidine

Clonidine is an agonist at presynaptic and postsynaptic α-2 adrenoceptors. It enhances inhibition in the dorsal horn.

Ketamine

Ketamine has complex actions in the spinal cord including non-competitive NMDA receptor antagonism.

Glutamate-mediated activation of NMDA receptors is associated with the development of central sensitization and persistent pain states.

Paracetamol

Although the mechanism of action of paracetamol remains unclear there may be a selective blocking of peripheral and central COX-3 (explaining its anti-inflammatory effect), as well as an action on serotonergic pathways and endocannabinoid receptors.

Infusions

Intravenous

A continuous drug infusion may be given to avoid the peak and trough effects of intermittent administration. For a continuous infusion the time taken to reach a constant plasma concentration

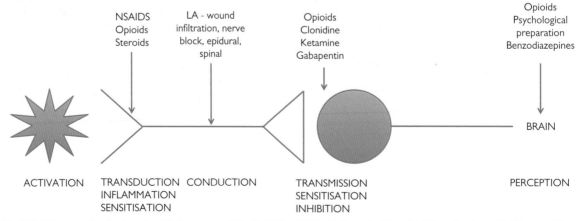

Fig. 26.2 Major sites of analgesic action. This figure was published in *Wall and Melzack's Textbook of Pain*, 5th Edition, Stephen B. McMahon and Martin Koltzenburg, Figure 42.1, p. 636, Copyright Elsevier 2006.

is determined by the half-life, with maximum concentration being reached after 4–5 half-lives. In the case of morphine this means that it may take many hours for an effective plasma concentration to be reached. It is important that an adequate loading dose is administered initially before commencing a continuous infusion. Continuous opioid infusions are associated with an increased risk of respiratory depression compared to patient-controlled analgesia (PCA).

Remifentanil has a short half-life and therefore reaches steady state rapidly. It has a constant context-sensitive half-time of only 3–5min and therefore rapid offset of action even after prolonged infusion.

Continuous infusions of opioids are commonly used for patients in intensive care to provide analgesia and sedation. Pain assessment is difficult due to sedation and intubation, and patients are usually unable to use a PCA device. The one-to-one nursing care makes this a safe option since cardiovascular and respiratory parameters can be closely monitored.

Neuraxial

Continuous epidural infusions are used for perioperative analgesia. Local anaesthetic combined with an opioid is more effective than local anaesthetic alone. Agents that modulate pain transmission at a spinal level may be added to local anaesthetic. They either inhibit excitation (NMDA antagonist) or enhance inhibition (opioids, α-2 agonist, GABA agonist, anticholinesterase). This improves and prolongs analgesia as well as reducing the total dose of local anaesthetic required. Reduction in local anaesthetic dose results in reduced motor block and complications such as urinary retention.

Epidural and intrathecal infusions are sometimes used for the management of cancer pain in carefully selected patients with intractable pain or intolerable adverse effects from other routes of analgesic administration.

Surgical wound and perineural catheters

Continuous wound or perineural analgesic infusions can provide good postoperative pain relief with a reduction in opioid use and side effects.

Patient-controlled analgesia

PCA can be delivered by a variety of routes including IV, epidural, subcutaneous, perineural, surgical wound site, and intranasal.

Intravenous PCA

The IV route is most frequently used, particularly for postoperative analgesia, e.g. with morphine, fentanyl, or oxycodone. Remifentanil PCA during labour is gaining popularity for women who are unsuitable for epidural analgesia. The short and predictable duration of action make it ideally suited to this situation.

PCA devices deliver on-demand bolus doses, with or without a background infusion. The bolus dose, interval time, and maximum dose in a set period is programmed, and can be altered depending on patient requirements. It is generally a safe technique, but there is the potential for error. A typical morphine PCA regimen would be a 1mg morphine bolus, with a 5min lockout, no background infusion, and an hourly maximum dose of 10mg.

Advantages
- High patient satisfaction.
- More consistent plasma concentrations than intramuscular (IM) injections.
- Avoids painful IM injections.
- May consume less nursing time.
- Generally safe.

Disadvantages
- Potential for programming errors or faulty equipment.
- Requires patient cooperation and understanding, therefore not suitable for very young or confused patients.
- Requires staff training for patient monitoring and device management.

The drug syringe or bag and programming control must only be accessible to trained staff to avoid accidental or deliberate misuse. Patients may require reassurance about the safety of the technique with regard to opioid overdose and addiction. Side effects such as nausea and vomiting can discourage use and so it is important that these are addressed. A choice of antiemetics with different modes of action should be prescribed when using PCA. Dose titrations may be necessary, and patients with pre-existing opioid tolerance and high opioid requirements may require a background infusion. Adequate loading doses must be given before IV PCA is commenced.

Side effects

The most common side effects of IV PCA:
- Nausea and vomiting
- Pruritus
- Respiratory depression
- Sedation
- Confusion
- Urinary retention.

Risk factors for respiratory depression include background infusion, concomitant administration of sedatives, renal, hepatic, cardiac or respiratory impairment, sleep apnoea, and obesity.

Sedation is most commonly seen in patients with renal impairment receiving morphine PCA, due to the accumulation of the metabolite morphine-6-glucuronide. Morphine should therefore be avoided in patients with significant renal disease; oxycodone or fentanyl PCA is preferable.

Further reading

Australian and New Zealand College of Anaesthetists and Faculty of Pain Medicine (2010). *Acute Pain Management: Scientific Evidence* (3rd edn). Melbourne: ANZCA. <http://www.anzca.edu.au/resources/books-and-publications/acutepain.pdf> accessed June 2011.

Momeni M, Crucitti M, De Kock M (2006). Patient-controlled analgesia in the management of postoperative pain. *Drugs*, 66(18):2321–37.

Taylor A & Stanbury L (2009). A review of postoperative pain management and the challenges. *Curr Anaesth Crit Care*, 20(4):188–94.

26.3 Routes of analgesic administration

Analgesia can be delivered by a variety of routes. The route chosen depends on:

- Required speed of onset
- Required duration of action
- Target site
- Gastrointestinal tract function
- Available drug formulation.

Different routes of administration produce variability in the rate of drug absorption and the amount of drug delivered effectively to the target site.

Oral administration

The oral route is the least invasive and most commonly used means of providing analgesia. The onset of action is not immediate since absorption must occur across the gastrointestinal mucosa. Absorption is affected by:

- Drug formulation
- pH and degree of ionization
- Gut motility and vomiting
- Interactions with other drugs and food.

Once absorbed, drugs pass via the portal vein and may be subject to hepatic first-pass metabolism before entering the systemic circulation. First-pass metabolism significantly reduces the bioavailability of most opioids, e.g. morphine has a bioavailability of only 30–40%. Morphine is approximately equipotent to oxycodone when administered parenterally. However it undergoes greater first-pass metabolism and an oral dose of 10mg is approximately equal to 5mg oral oxycodone. Table 26.1 shows the bioavailability of some commonly used drugs.

The speed of absorption is affected by drug formulation, e.g. tablets, capsules, enteric coated, suspension, sustained- or slow-release. Slow-release preparations are suitable for the management of chronic pain as they avoid peak and trough effects. Morphine, oxycodone, and tramadol are examples of analgesics available in this form. The active drug is gradually released in the stomach and small intestine. It may take 3–4h or greater for peak effect to be reached.

Immediate-release preparations such as oral morphine syrup or oxycodone are indicated for the management of acute pain or breakthrough pain. The time taken to achieve analgesic effect with immediate-release preparations is up to 45–60min. The oral route is hence unsuitable for acute severe pain. The onset of action may be further delayed if taken on a full stomach.

Most orally administered drugs are absorbed in the small intestine and so are affected by delayed gastric emptying. An accumulative effect can occur when gastric emptying resolves causing an increased risk of adverse effects. Increased small intestinal motility reduces the time available for absorption to occur in the small intestine and hence the total amount of drug absorbed.

Orally administered NSAIDs show similar efficacy and side effect profile to parenterally administered NSAIDS. However, orally administered paracetamol is less effective and of slower onset than IV paracetamol.

Sublingual administration

The sublingual route offers a number of advantages:

- Rapid onset
- Avoidance of first-pass metabolism
- Non-invasive
- Painless.

It is suitable for patients with nausea, vomiting, dysphagia, and gastrointestinal disturbance such as obstruction.

For drugs to be administered effectively via the sublingual or buccal route they need to be lipophilic, unionized, and of low molecular weight. Fentanyl and buprenorphine are both potent, highly lipid soluble, and well absorbed sublingually with a rapid onset of action.

The bioavailability depends on the proportion of the drug absorbed across the buccal mucosa and the proportion that is swallowed and subsequently metabolized. Fentanyl is commonly administered sublingually for the management of breakthrough pain. Approximately 25% is absorbed from the mucosa and 75% swallowed. The swallowed fraction is slowly absorbed and then undergoes first-pass metabolism, with bioavailability of 33%. This results in an overall bioavailability of around 50%.

Subcutaneous administration

The subcutaneous route is useful for patients unable to take drugs orally whilst avoiding the need for IV access. Absorption is slow and largely dependent on local and regional blood flow. Poor perfusion will result in delayed analgesic effect, and then potentially toxic levels of drugs entering the circulation when perfusion is restored. Opioids are the most common analgesics given via this route, either as bolus doses, infusions or PCA.

Subcutaneous infusions, with or without a PCA device, are often used for symptom control in palliative care. To avoid discomfort at the infusion site the rate is limited to 2–4mL/h, and solutions should be aqueous and non-irritant. Diamorphine is very soluble and so can be given in a concentrated solution. The injection site should be changed regularly.

Intramuscular administration

The IM route provides more rapid absorption than the subcutaneous route, but may avoid the initial high plasma concentration that occurs following IV injection. Uptake is largely dependent on blood flow to the muscle. The bioavailability approaches 100%.

IM drugs are administered into the following sites as they are associated with less risk of nerve injury:

- Vastus lateralis: outer, middle third of the thigh.
- Deltoid: 3–5cm below acromion process.
- Dorsogluteal: upper, outer quadrant of buttock.

Table 26.1 Analgesic bioavailability	
Route	Bioavailability
Oral	Morphine 30–40% Oxycodone 60–87% Paracetamol 63–89% Diclofenac 60%
Sublingual	Fentanyl 30–60% Buprenorphine 30–50%
Intravenous	100% all drugs
Transdermal	Fentanyl up to 90%

However, there are a number of drawbacks:
- Variable absorption causes unreliable speed of onset and duration of analgesia.
- Painful.
- Potential for haematoma or abscess formation.
- Potential for accidental direct intravenous injection.

Intravenous administration

The IV route provides a rapid onset, reliable means for administering analgesia in acute pain. Small doses of opioid should be administered at frequent intervals (e.g. morphine 2mg every 5min) and titrated to effect. Opioids should only be given in this way in a high dependency area such as a post-anaesthetic care unit, so that patients can be monitored for adverse effects, particularly respiratory depression. When adequate pain relief is achieved an infusion or PCA can be commenced (see section 26.2).

IV administration is not usually appropriate for chronic pain management as it requires the placement of an indwelling catheter. However, continuous IV infusions of opioids are occasionally used in the management of cancer pain when opioid requirements are high and the oral route is not practical. Continuous infusions of opioids are associated with an increased risk of respiratory depression.

Inhalational administration

The most commonly used inhalational analgesic is nitrous oxide. It can be used as a carrier gas for other inhalational anaesthetic agents to provide some analgesia during anaesthesia. When combined with oxygen in a 50:50 mixture (Entonox) it provides rapid onset, short duration analgesia that can be patient delivered. It can be used during labour, painful dressing changes or in trauma.

Nitrous oxide has a number of adverse effects including nausea and vomiting, methionine synthetase inhibition and megaloblastic anaemia, atmospheric pollution, and rapid expansion of gas containing spaces, e.g. pneumothoraces and bowel.

Nebulized opioid analgesics have been investigated for future use in acute pain. There is currently insufficient data to recommend nebulized analgesia for routine use.

Transdermal administration

Analgesia can be delivered transdermally to produce systemic effects. The route is most effective for drugs of high lipid solubility and low molecular mass. Drug uptake is affected by skin blood flow and skin temperature. The drug is absorbed into the stratum corneum of the epidermis, which is a highly lipophilic membrane. A reservoir forms here until deeper absorption occurs into the dermis where systemic absorption occurs via the capillary network.

Fentanyl and buprenorphine patches are available for use in chronic pain and cancer pain management. These formulations ensure controlled drug release avoiding peaks and troughs. This may result in less adverse effects and better compliance. It can take 24h for steady state blood concentration to be reached following application of a patch so short-acting opioids may need to continue until this point.

Fentanyl patches can deliver 25, 50, 75 or 100mcg/h of fentanyl for a period of 72h. Absorption can be influenced by skin temperature increasing. Buprenorphine patches can deliver 35, 52.5, or 70mcg/h and it is six times more potent than fentanyl.

Opioid patches may cause respiratory depression and are not recommended for opioid naïve patients. The elimination half-life of transdermal fentanyl is 15–20h and longer for buprenorphine. Respiratory depression cannot be managed by simply removing the patch.

Further reading

Australian and New Zealand College of Anaesthetists and Faculty of Pain Medicine. (2010). *Acute Pain Management: Scientific Evidence* (3rd edn). Melbourne. ANZCA. <http://www.anzca.edu.au/resources/books-and-publications/acutepain.pdf>.

Margetts L & Sawyer R (2007). Transdermal drug delivery- principles and opioid therapy. *CEACCP*, 7(5):171–6.

Sasada M & Smith S (2003). *Drugs in Anaesthesia and Intensive Care* (3rd edn). Oxford: Oxford University Press.

Stevens RA & Salim MG (2007). Routes of opioid administration in the management of cancer pain. *Cancer Control*, 7(2):132–41.

Chronic pain is pain that lasts beyond the time expected for the underlying damage or pathology to have healed. Chronic pain can be nociceptive, neuropathic, or a combination of the two. Pharmacological treatment of nociceptive pain is guided by the WHO analgesic ladder (paracetamol, NSAIDs, and weak opioids) with strong opioids used for resistant pain. Neuropathic pain is often refractory to these conventional analgesic drugs and requires the use of other classes of drugs such as antidepressants, anticonvulsants, and antiarrhythmics.

Paracetamol and NSAIDs

Paracetamol has both analgesic and antipyretic actions. It is used for mild to moderate pain and has opioid-sparing effects when used as part of multimodal analgesia. The mode of action is unclear but it may involve the central and peripheral inhibition of COX-3 as well as effects on serotonergic and cannabinoid pathways.

Paracetamol is well absorbed from the gut, undergoes minimal first-pass metabolism and has an oral bioavailability of >60%. Metabolism is by the cytochrome P450 enzyme and so is reduced in liver failure. Renal clearance is minimal and therefore only affected in severe renal impairment. In normal doses, paracetamol is generally safe and efficacious.

NSAIDs act by inhibiting COX-1 and COX-2 in the arachidonic acid pathway. COX-1 is the constitutive form present in all tissues, and COX-2 is the inducible form produced at sites of inflammation. NSAIDs reduce production of PGE_2 and PGI_2 that sensitize nociceptors to inflammatory mediators such as bradykinin and 5-HT.

NSAIDS are effective analgesics, but are associated with a number of significant side effects. These are predominantly due to the inhibition of COX-1 and the reduced production of prostaglandins with physiological roles including regulation of renal blood flow, gastric mucosal protection, and endothelial integrity. The major adverse effects are gastric and duodenal ulceration, renal impairment, impaired platelet function, and bronchospasm in sensitive asthmatics. Specific COX-2 inhibitors were developed to overcome these adverse effects. They have now been largely withdrawn following a link to high rates of cardiovascular complications.

Antidepressants

Antidepressants have long been used for the treatment of chronic pain. Although depression and chronic pain may coexist, several factors suggest the analgesic effect of antidepressant medication is distinct from the mood altering effects:

- The doses used are often smaller than those used to treat depression.
- The onset of action is more rapid.
- Analgesic benefit occurs in non-depressed patients and does not correlate with improvement in mood in depressed patients.

The mechanism of action is thought to be related to central blockade of serotonin and noradrenaline reuptake, thereby prolonging the synaptic activity of these monoamines and enhancing descending inhibitory activity in the spinal cord. They may also block other receptor types involved in pain processing including α-adrenergic, H_1-histaminergic and NMDA receptors. Other proposed actions include blockade of calcium and sodium channels and weak μ-opioid receptor stimulation.

The secondary amine tricyclic antidepressants (TCAs), e.g. nortriptyline and desipramine, and selective serotonin and noradrenaline reuptake inhibitors, e.g. duloxetine and venlafaxine are recommended for first-line treatment of neuropathic pain. TCAs have proven efficacy in the treatment of neuropathic pain, especially post-herpetic neuralgia and painful diabetic peripheral neuropathy. Drugs with balanced noradrenergic and serotonergic effects are more effective than pure selective serotonin reuptake inhibitors (SSRIs).

Side effects

The most common side effects of TCAs include sedation, dry mouth, constipation, urinary retention and orthostatic hypotension. Secondary amine TCAs are better tolerated than tertiary amine TCAs (amitriptyline and imipramine) and have comparable efficacy. Cardiac toxicity is an important side effect of TCAs and these drugs should be used with caution in patients with a history of ischaemic heart disease or cardiac conduction abnormalities.

Antiepileptics

Antiepileptic drugs are commonly used in the treatment of neuropathic pain and exert their analgesic effects in a number of ways.

Phenytoin and carbamazepine

Repetitive firing in afferent nerve fibres contributes to neuropathic pain. Older drugs such as phenytoin and carbamazepine reduce neuronal excitability by frequency-dependent blockade of sodium channels. Phenytoin is now rarely used, although may be given intravenously for acute flare-ups of neuropathic pain. Carbamazepine is first-line treatment for trigeminal neuralgia (see section 22.7) but there is less evidence for its use in other neuropathic pain. Oxcarbazepine is a newer chemically related drug with a more favourable side effect profile.

Lamotrigine and valproate

Lamotrigine also blocks voltage-gated sodium channels, and it is probably via this mechanism that it suppresses the release of the excitatory neurotransmitter glutamate. Glutamate is involved in central neuronal hyperexcitability and persisting pain states. Lamotrigine has shown some benefit in several types of neuropathic pain. It may be of benefit in patients with central pain, and as second-line treatment in trigeminal neuralgia.

Sodium valproate is thought to elevate levels of the inhibitory amino acid γ-aminobutyric acid (GABA) in the central nervous system, and by facilitating the action of GABA in the brain, inhibits pain.

Gabapentin and pregabalin

The calcium channel α2-δ ligands gabapentin and pregabalin are also recommended as first line therapy for neuropathic pain. Gabapentin and pregabalin both bind to the α2-δ subunit of voltage-gated calcium channels, decreasing the release of glutamate, noradrenaline, and substance P. Gabapentin has been shown to produce a greater reduction in pain than placebo in a number of conditions including post-herpetic neuralgia, painful diabetic peripheral neuropathy, phantom limb pain and acute and chronic post spinal cord injury pain. Pregabalin is a more recently developed drug. It has demonstrated efficacy in the treatment of post-herpetic neuralgia and painful diabetic peripheral neuropathy. Gabapentin and pregabalin do not have any clinically important drug interactions, but require dose reduction in renal impairment. They produce similar dose-dependent side effects. The benefits of pregabalin over gabapentin may include a more rapid onset of pain relief and potential twice daily dosing.

Side effects

Side effects of antiepileptic drugs are usually related to acute toxicity and can be severe. Adverse effects can often be minimized by careful dose titration. When prescribing these drugs it is important to be aware of pharmacokinetic issues such as variable oral absorption, hepatic enzyme induction (particularly phenytoin, carbamazepine) and extensive protein binding. Important side effects of antiepileptic drugs are summarized in Table 26.2.

Table 26.2 Adverse effects of commonly used antiepileptic drugs	
Drug	Adverse effects
Gabapentin Pregabalin	Somnolence, dizziness, fatigue, poor concentration, headache, confusion, diarrhoea, nausea, weight gain, peripheral oedema. Rarely thrombocytopenia, neutropenia
Carbamazepine	Dizziness, somnolence, light-headedness, diplopia, ataxia, nausea and vomiting, rash. Rarely Stevens–Johnson syndrome, aplastic anaemia, agranulocytosis
Lamotrigine	Dizziness, somnolence, diplopia., rash. Rarely Stevens–Johnson syndrome
Phenytoin	Dizziness, drowsiness, nausea, gum hypertrophy. Teratogenic
Sodium valproate	Tremor, hepatotoxicty, pancreatitis, peripheral oedema, weight gain, hair loss. Inhibits TCA metabolism

Antiarrhythmics

Antiarrhythmic drugs suppress neuronal hyperexcitability by non-specific sodium channel blockade. Low-dose lidocaine may also block glutamate-evoked activity in the dorsal horn of the spinal cord. Topical lidocaine as a 5% patch or gel has been shown to be effective in post-herpetic neuralgia and allodynia as well as some other localized peripheral neuropathic pain conditions. IV lidocaine has been reported to be useful for postoperative pain relief and reduction in deafferentation pain, central pain and diabetic neuropathy. However, the results of randomized controlled trials assess acute changes in pain levels and are not helpful in the management of chronic neuropathic pain.

Mexilitene is an orally administered lidocaine analogue. Studies in patients with painful diabetic peripheral neuropathy and other types of neuropathic pain have shown modest or no benefit compared to placebo. When efficacy has been found it is often at higher doses, which are poorly tolerated due to side effects, particularly nausea. The typical dose range is 400–1200mg daily in divided doses.

Opioids

Opioid drugs exert their activity by acting as agonists at endogenous opioid receptors, found throughout the peripheral and central nervous system. Spinal cord opioid receptors are found mostly on the pre-synaptic terminals of the primary afferent neurons in the substantia gelatinosa in the dorsal horn. Opioids act here to inhibit the release of excitatory neurotransmitters. Opioids also act supraspinally and affect the descending enkephalinergic pathways under the control of the periaqueductal grey matter.

Clinical trials suggest that opioids can provide useful analgesia in the short and medium term, but data is lacking for long-term effectiveness. Opioids are only used for resistant neuropathic pain when drugs with proven efficacy (e.g. TCAs and antiepileptics) are not effective. Regular modified-release preparations should be used where possible.

Tramadol is a weak μ-receptor agonist that also inhibits noradrenaline and serotonin reuptake.

Common opioid side effects include nausea, vomiting, constipation, somnolence, itching, and dizziness. Opioid-induced respiratory depression is only likely to occur in persistent pain if there have been changes in dose, route of administration, or formulation. There are concerns regarding the long-term use of opioids including endocrine effects (hypogonadism and adrenal insufficiency), immune suppression, and hyperalgesia. Physical dependence, tolerance, and addiction are obviously important issues.

NMDA receptor antagonists

The NMDA receptor is important in the development of central sensitization (see section 26.1) that is thought to contribute to chronic pain. There is currently much interest in NMDA receptor antagonists such as ketamine, and the possibility that they could act to reduce or reverse the CNS changes associated with persistent pain.

Capsaicin

TRPV1 is a ligand-gated ion channel present on some C-fibre nociceptors that is responsible for modulating the peripheral pain stimulus. Stimulation of TRPV1 (which also respond to temperature and pH) produces nerve depolarization such that the nerve remains refractory and further afferent transmission is reduced. Capsaicin gel acts as an agonist at this receptor and prolonged exposure causes 'defunctionalization' of nociceptive fibres as a result of receptor desensitization and increase in intracellular calcium. Neurotransmitters such as substance P are also depleted. Capsaicin gel is efficacious in the treatment of chronic pain associated with osteoarthritis and post-herpetic neuralgia. Capsaicin can produce a burning sensation when it is first applied.

Further reading

British Pain Society (2010). *Opioids for Persistent Pain: Good Practice.* <http://www.britishpainsociety.org/book_opioid_main.pdf> accessed March 2011.

Dworkin H, O'Connor AB, Backonja M, *et al.* (2007). Pharmacologic management of neuropathic pain: evidence based recommendations. *Pain,* 132:237–51.

Hebbes C & Lambert D (2011). Non-opioid analgesics. *Anaesth Intens Care Med,* 12:69–72.

Kapur D (2002). Centrally acting non-opioid analgesic drugs. *Curr Anaesth Crit Care,* 13:328–33.

Ryder S & Stannard C (2005). Treatment of chronic pain: antidepressant, antiepileptic and antiarrhythmic drugs. *BJA CEACCP,* 5:18–21.

26.5 Epidural analgesia

Benefits of epidural analgesia

Epidural analgesia may confer many benefits to postoperative morbidity and patient recovery following major surgery. It is an integral component of enhanced recovery protocols for these reasons. It has not consistently been shown to impact on perioperative mortality but this may be due to the rarity of this event.

Stress response to surgery
Epidural analgesia reduces circulating catecholamines, cortisol, and glucose levels perioperatively.

Cardiovascular benefits
- Reduction in postoperative myocardial infarction (33%)
- Reduced heart failure incidence.

These effects may result from reduced sympathetic stimulation, improved oxygenation and reduced thrombotic tendency. Epidural analgesia should continue for 2–3 days postoperatively to reduce cardiovascular morbidity.

Respiratory benefits
- Improved FVC at 24h
- Improved FRC
- Reduced atelectasis, pneumonia (39%), hypoxaemia, and respiratory failure.

Good epidural analgesia improves chest wall compliance, diaphragmatic function and clearance of secretions. Opiate-related respiratory depression is avoided.

Gastrointestinal benefits
- Earlier return of GI motility (2–3 days)
- Improved splanchnic blood flow.

The GI benefits require T5–L2 effects for sympathetic blockade of bowel afferent innervations. This results in earlier return of motility and early enteral feeding. The epidural should continue for 2–3 days postoperatively until bowel function returns.

Haematological benefits
- Reduced incidence of DVT and PE (45%)
- Improved surgical vascular graft function
- Reduced perioperative blood loss in lower abdominal, pelvic and hip surgery.

Epidural analgesia attenuates the hypercoagulable state associated with the surgical stress response, improves blood flow to extremities and allows earlier mobilization to reduce thrombotic events. Intraoperative blood transfusion requirements are reduced.

Recovery benefits
- Earlier time to extubation
- Reduced ITU stay.

Performing the epidural block

The European Society of Anaesthesiology (ESA) adopted the German evidence-based recommendations for the timing of epidural procedures and anticoagulant drugs (see Table 26.3).

Siting the epidural-ultrasound guidance
Ultrasound guidance (using a 2–5Hz curvilinear probe) may be used to aid epidural placement in two ways:

1. Real-time imaging of needle insertion into epidural space. This requires two operators.
2. Pre-puncture ultrasound to locate midline and depth to the ligamentum flavum.

This has been shown to reduce the number of attempts for successful insertion and may be a useful training tool.

Epidural associated complications

Inadequate analgesia
Incidence may be as high as 10% of epidurals over the desired length of use. Analgesia may be improved by early assessment and intervention. The connections and epidural site should be inspected and, if *in situ*, a bolus of low-dose LA should be administered following assessment of block. The catheter may be pulled back for a unilateral block. The maintenance infusion is increased. Systemic opiates may be required if this fails.

Accidental dural puncture (ADP)
Occurs in 1/200 epidurals. The anteroposterior diameter of the epidural space is 5mm in the lumbar region, but less in thoracic. Risk may be reduced by loss of resistance to saline (as opposed to air) techniques and ultrasound guidance. May be detected by flow of CSF from Tuohy needle or catheter on testing. See section 24.11 for management.

Intrathecal injection—total spinal
Produces rapidly ascending block with voice changes and breathlessness. Progresses to apnoea, hypotension and unconsciousness. Risk is reduced by 'test dose' of small volume and care with epidural use following ADP.

Intravenous injection
A catheter positioned in an epidural vein may cause LA toxicity. Risk is decreased by injection of epidural saline prior to feeding the catheter. Detection relies on aspiration of a multi-end hole catheter (90% sensitive) and checking for free flow under gravity with the catheter held down. A small dose of LA may cause detectable early symptoms of peri-oral tingling.

Subdural block
The subdural space is between the dura and arachnoid mater. The block produced is patchy with unexpectedly high spread often producing intracranial effects, e.g. Horner's syndrome.

Neurological sequelae
Occur in about 1/16 000 epidurals and include epidural haematoma, epidural abscess, nerve injury, and meningitis. Epidural haematoma and abscess may cause permanent neurological injury if not diagnosed and managed early. Severe back pain and tenderness are often accompanied with neurological symptoms. Motor block whilst using low concentration LA infusion requires immediate assessment.

Opiate related side-effects
Pruritis occurs in 10% cases, is unrelated to histamine release and may respond to naloxone 40–80mcg, propofol 10–20mg and prophylactic ondansetron. Urine retention, nausea, and vomiting may occur. Respiratory depression is due to rostral spread of the proportion of drug which has diffused into the CSF. More lipid soluble agents, e.g. fentanyl, will present within 2h. Morphine and diamorphine may be associated with later respiratory depression.

Table 26.3 ESA 2010. Regional anaesthesia and thromboprophylaxis/anticoagulation

	Time before puncture/catheter manipulation or removal[a]	Time after puncture/catheter manipulation or removal	Laboratory tests
Unfractionated heparins (for prophylaxis, ≤15 000 IU per day)	4–6 h	1 h	Platelets during treatment for more than 5 days
Unfractionated heparins (for treatment)	i.v. 4–6 h	1 h	aPTT, ACT, platelets
	s.c. 8–12 h	1 h	
Low-molecular-weight heparins (for prophylaxis)	12 h	4 h	Platelets during treatment for more than 5 days
Low-molecular-weight heparins (for treatment)	24 h	4 h	Platelets during treatment for more than 5 days
Fondaparinux (for prophylaxis, 2.5mg per day)	36–42 h	6–12 h	(anti-Xa, standardized for specific agent)
Rivaroxaban (for prophylaxis, 10mg q.d.)	22–26 h	4–6 h	(PT, standardized for specific agent)
Apixaban (for prophylaxis, 2.5mg b.i.d.)	26–30 h	4–6 h	?
Dabigatran (for prophylaxis, 150–220 mg)	Contraindicated according to the manufacturer	6h	?
Coumarins	INR ≤1.4	After catheter removal	INR
Hirudins (lepirudin, desirudin)	8–10 h	2–4 h	aPTT, ECT
Argatroban[b]	4 h	2 h	aPTT, ECT, ACT
Acetylsalicylic acid	None	None	
Clopidogrel	7 days	After catheter removal	
Ticlopidine	10 days	After catheter removal	
Prasugrel	7–10 days	6 h after catheter removal	
Ticagrelor	5 days	6 h after catheter removal	
Cilostazol[b]	42 h	5 h after catheter removal	
NSAIDs	None	None	

ACT, activated clotting time; aPTT, activated partial thromboplastin time; b.i.d., twice daily; ECT, ecarin clotting time; INR, international normalised ratio; IU, international unit; i.v., intravenously; NSAIDs, non-steroidal anti-inflammatory drugs; s.c., subcutaneously; q.d., daily.

[a] All time intervals refer to patients with normal renal function.

[b] Prolonged time interval in patients with hepatic insufficiency.

W Gogarten et al., 'Regional Anaesthesia and antithrombotic agents: recommendations of the European Society of Anaesthesiology', *European Journal of Anaesthesiology*, 27, 12, pp. 999–1015, copyright 2010, with permission from European Society of Anaesthesiology and Wolters Kluwer Health.

Hypotension
The block level should be assessed and infusion reduced if above T4. Other causes of hypotension should be considered.

NAP3—The National Audit of Major Complications of Central Neuraxial Blockade in the UK, 2009

A 2-week national census of central neuraxial blockade was performed in the UK with subsequent reporting of all major complications over 1–2 years. Complications reported were epidural abscess, haematoma, meningitis, nerve injury, spinal cord ischaemia, cardiovascular collapse and drug route error.

Perioperative epidurals were associated with more major complications than other central neuraxial blocks or obstetric epidurals.

Table 26.4 NAP3 Incidence of major complications with perioperative epidural analgesia

	Pessimistic	Optimistic incidence
Overall complications	1 in 5800	1 in 12 000
Paraplegia and death	1 in 16 000	1 in 98 000

Data from NAP3: The 3rd National Audit Project of The Royal College of Anaesthetists, 'Major complications of central neuraxial block: report on the 3rd national audit project of the RCOA', *British Journal of Anaesthesia*, 2009, 102, pp. 179–190.

Epidural monitoring and safety

During insertion
- Pre-procedure consent and documentation
- IV access
- Maintenance of verbal contact
- Aseptic technique
- Full monitoring during initial dosing
- Access to resuscitation equipment (Intralipid®).

Postoperative epidural monitoring
Ward staff should be fully trained in the supervision of epidural analgesia and there should be 24h access to anaesthetic support. The acute pain service or responsible anaesthetist should review patients with epidurals daily. Infusion pumps solely for epidural maintenance should be used. Monitoring regimens should be designed to detect major complications of epidural analgesia including opiate-related respiratory depression.

Monitoring includes:
- Basic observations—frequently for 6–12h, then 2-hourly. Increased frequency post bolus or change in rate.
- Pain scores and sedation scores.
- Sensory and motor block assessment.
- Infusion rate and total infusion volumes.
- Inspection of epidural site daily.

Epidural space anatomy

The epidural space is a broad triangle with a posterior apex containing fat, veins, arteries, and nerve roots. The anteroposterior diameter is greatest in the lumbar region (5mm) and decreases superiorly. The lumbar epidural space is often more segmented by dura adherent to the lamina periosteum. It closes superiorly at the foramen magnum and inferiorly at the sacrococcygeal membrane. The borders are:

• Anterior—posterior longitudinal ligaments and vertebral bodies

• Posterior—ligamentum flavum and vertebral laminae

• Lateral—open into intervertebral foraminae.

Epidural infusion regimens

Epidural LA diffuses across into the CSF and hence the cord and nerve roots. The non-ionized, lipid-soluble form diffuses more rapidly, hence alkalinization of solution may be used to provide faster onset of effect.

Continuous or patient controlled epidural analgesia (PCEA) bolus systems may be used. Intermittent top-ups are only appropriate in the obstetric setting where one-to-one supervision is provided with regular assessment of pain.

Continuous infusions provide stable levels of analgesia but may require specialized intervention if analgesia fails. An increased cumulative dose is administered which may result in greater motor block.

PCEA infusions are more flexible, reduce total drug dosage, and increase patient satisfaction. A continuous infusion with intermittent bolus allowances is most appropriate in the postoperative setting.

Further reading

Cook TM, Counsell D, Wildsmith JA, *et al.* (2009). Major complications of central neuraxial block: report on the 3rd national audit project of the RCOA. *Br J Anaesth*, 102:179–90.

Gogarten *et al.* (2010). Regional anaesthesia and antithrombotic agents. *Eur J Anaesthesiol*, 12:999–1015.

Nimmo S (2004). Benefit and outcome after epidural analgesia. *CEACCP*, 4(2):44–7.

Wu CL & Fleisher LA (2000). Outcomes research in regional anaesthesia and analgesia. *Anesth Analg*, 92:1232–42.

26.6 Assessment and management of acute postoperative pain

Postoperative pain and management

Postoperative pain increases sympathetic activity causing cardiac ischaemia and decreased gastrointestinal motility and perfusion. Pulmonary complications are related to poor cough and inspiratory capacity.

A plan for postoperative pain management should be made at the preoperative anaesthetic assessment and discussed with the patient where possible. Important information includes previous pain management history, quality of pain relief, adverse reactions, or side effects. If central or regional blockade is planned, an informed consent must be obtained.

In the postoperative period the basis of acute pain management consists of:

- Assessment and measurement
- Treatment (analgesic options)
- Reassessment of pain and analgesic intervention.

Patients should not leave the recovery area until sufficient pain control has been established and ongoing analgesia is prescribed. Local hospital policy and protocols constructed by the acute pain team will determine most treatment plans. A multidisciplinary acute pain team will facilitate management of complex pain patients and review patients with PCA and epidural analgesia. They should also be involved in clinical governance and education for nursing staff.

Assessment of pain

The assessment and measurement of pain allows diagnosis of pain, selection of appropriate analgesic therapy and evaluation of response.

The initial step of assessment should include a thorough pain history (see Box 26.1) with relevant examination and evaluation of associated functional impairment. This may help to differentiate pain states such as nociceptive (somatic and visceral) or neuropathic. An evaluation of pain intensity, functional impact and side effects of treatment, will prompt intervention if needed and improve quality of care.

> ### Box 26.1 Pain history
> - Site of pain
> - Circumstances associated with pain onset
> - Character of pain
> - Intensity of pain
> - Associated symptoms
> - Effect of pain on activities and sleep
> - Treatment: current and previous medications—dose, frequency of use, efficacy, side effects
> - Relevant medical history
> - Factors influencing the patient's symptomatic treatment
> - Coping response to pain, psychiatric disorders, beliefs what is causing the pain.

Measurement of pain

Pain is an individual subjective experience and most measures of pain are based on self-report resulting in sensitive and consistent results. However, in the following circumstances self-reporting of pain can be unreliable:

- Mood disturbance (severe anxiety or depression)
- Sleep disturbance
- Cognitive impairment
- Impaired consciousness
- Extremes of ages
- Failures of communication.

Other methods of pain assessment are needed, including:

- Hyperalgesia, e.g. mechanical withdrawal
- Stress response, e.g. plasma cortisol levels
- Behavioural responses, e.g. facial expression
- Functional impairment, e.g. coughing, ambulation
- Physiological responses, e.g. changes in heart rate
- Analgesia used, e.g. cumulative opioid dose.

Regular measurement of pain intensity should be incorporated into patient observation recordings. This allows appropriate intervention with analgesic therapy. Pain that remains refractory to conventional opioid doses should prompt further investigation and consideration of surgical complications or the presence of neuropathic pain.

Categorical scales

- Verbal descriptor scale (VDS)
- Four or five point descriptors; none, mild, moderate, severe (and excruciating)
- Good correlation with visual analogue scales.

Numerical rating scales

Patients numerically score their pain on a scale of 0 to 10 as 10 being the 'worst pain imaginable' and 0 representing 'no pain'. A score of 4 or more, indicates a threshold for intervention. This is equivocal to moderate pain on the categorical scale. This can be verbal or written.

The visual analogue scale (VAS) is a 100mm horizontal line with verbal anchors of 'no pain' on the left and 'worst pain' on the right. The score is the distance (in mm) from the left to the mark representing their pain.

After an analgesic intervention a reduction in pain intensity by 30% is clinically meaningful to patients.

Multidimensional measures of pain

Multidimensional questionnaires, e.g. McGill Pain Questionnaire and Brief Pain Inventory, are used in chronic pain and describe the impact on function and quality of life.

Treatment of postoperative pain

Postoperative pain mechanisms may include inflammatory, visceral, and neuropathic. The contribution of each of these mechanisms is largely operation dependent. A multimodal analgesic strategy will provide synergistic and additive effects on the different pain mechanisms. Medication to counteract the side effects of analgesia, e.g. nausea, should be prescribed.

The WHO ladder (Fig. 26.3) provides a framework to escalate or reduce analgesia according to severity of pain. Postoperative pain is most severe in the first 24–72h but may persist for weeks and even become chronic in some cases. The ladder can be used to escalate or reduce analgesia. It includes

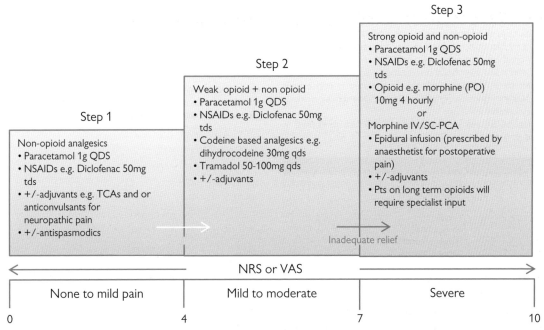

Fig. 26.3 The WHO Analgesic Ladder. Reproduced with permission from the World Health Organization. http://www.who.int/cancer/palliative/painladder/en accessed 17 April 2013.

the addition of adjuncts such as antineuropathic drugs. The starting point postoperatively relates to patient factors and type of surgery.

Opioids

Opioids are required if pain is expected to be moderate to severe. The NNT of intramuscular or PCA morphine is 4.2. Effective rapid dose titration to effect can reduce this NNT. Patients using PCA are more satisfied with their pain management but there are no differences between opioid consumption, pain scores, duration of hospital stay, or side effects between different routes of administration. Dose requirements vary between patients and will require adjustment according to gender, genetic differences, and factors such as opioid tolerance. As the initial phase of healing occurs the severity of pain should decrease accordingly and restoration of the oral route to deliver analgesia should be attempted. Total parenteral dose over 24h is calculated and the total dose can be converted to a long-acting opioid (morphine sulphate slow release). A fast-acting opioid is provided for breakthrough pain. This can subsequently be stepped down to weak opioids and regular simple analgesics such as paracetamol and NSAIDs.

Paracetamol and NSAIDs

Regular use of paracetamol has the ability to reduce opioid requirements after major surgery. The combination of paracetamol with NSAIDs is significantly more effective than if either drug is given alone (NNT 3.8 vs 2–3). The potential side effects of NSAIDs limit their use in high-risk patients.

NMDA receptor antagonists

In subanaesthetic doses ketamine has antihyperalgesic, antiallodynic, and antitolerance properties and can be used as an adjunct for the treatment of pain associated with central sensitization. It may have a role in reducing chronic postsurgical pain (CPSP).

Other pharmacological treatments

Specific management of neuropathic pain may be appropriate in the immediate postoperative period following surgery such as amputations (see section 26.4).

The addition of an α 2 agonist such as clonidine to morphine PCA has been shown to improve postoperative analgesia but only for the first 12h and may be associated with sedation and hypotension.

Muscle spasm responds poorly to opioids and benzodiazepines and baclofen may be helpful. The smooth muscle spasm commonly seen after GI, biliary, and urology surgery may be eased with a muscarinic antagonist such as hyoscine.

Regional anaesthesia

Regional nerve blocks or neuraxial blocks may provide excellent postoperative analgesia. See sections 19 and 26.5.

Pre-emptive analgesia

Pre-emptive analgesia is given before the pain stimulus occurs. It is thought to be more effective at reducing postoperative pain by reducing central sensitization. This theory may be too simplistic. Central sensitization relates not only to surgical incision but also to preoperative pain, noxious intraoperative stimuli and postoperative inflammation.

A preventive approach aims to reduce central sensitization and wind-up, by blocking the transmission of peripheral nociceptive input to the spinal cord during the pre-, peri-, and postoperative period. This results in reduced pain intensity and incidence of CPSP. The active intervention should continue for as long as the sensitizing stimulus persists, which can be well into the postoperative period. NMDA receptor antagonist drugs show preventive analgesic properties, e.g. ketamine at induction reduces postoperative morphine requirements.

Preventative analgesia is demonstrated when postoperative pain is reduced beyond the pharmacological action of the analgesic agent used. This is defined as 5.5 half-lives.

Chronic postsurgical pain

A number of risk factors for the development of CPSP have been identified. A major risk factor is prolonged moderate to severe postoperative pain. Incidence is also increased following surgery with a high risk of nerve injury, e.g. amputation, thoracotomy, mastectomy, and inguinal hernia.

The barrage of afferent nociceptor impulses after tissue or nerve injury can cause changes in the peripheral nerves, spinal cord, sympathetic nervous system, and higher central pain pathways. Central and peripheral sensitization may occur leading to persistent pain. Another mechanism postulated is impairment of the descending inhibitory pain pathways (the diffuse noxious inhibitory control (DNIC)).

Risk factors for the development of CPSP are presented in Table 26.5.

Table 26.5 Risk factors for chronic postsurgical pain	
Preoperative factors	Pre-existing pain >1 month moderate to severe Repetitive surgery Psychological issues Female Young adults Genetic predisposition Ongoing litigation
Intraoperative factors	Surgical technique/approach with risk of nerve damage
Postoperative factors	Moderate to severe pain Radiation/neurotoxic chemotherapy Depression/anxiety Psychological vulnerability

Further reading

Jargen B & Kehlet H (2006). Postoperative pain and its management. In SB McMahon & M Koltzenburg (eds), *Wall and Melzack's Textbook of Pain* (5th edn, pp. 635–51). Philadelphia, PA: Elsevier/Churchill Livingstone.

Macintyre PE, Schug SA, Scott DA, *et al.*; Working Group of ANZCA and Faculty of Pain Medicine (2010). *Acute Pain Management: Scientific Evidence* (3rd edn), Melbourne: ANZCA & FPM.

26.7 Acute pain in the older person

Several factors make the management of acute pain in the older person challenging, including:

- Increased comorbidity.
- Polypharmacy, potential for adverse drug interactions.
- Age-related changes in physiology impacting on pharmacodynamics and pharmacokinetics.
- Altered responses to pain.
- Difficulties with assessment of pain, including problems related to cognitive impairment.
- False perception that older patients have higher thresholds for pain.

Pharmacokinetic and pharmacodynamic changes (see Table 26.6)

Assessment in older patients

Under-reporting of pain is more common in the older patient due to cognitive impairment or difficulty in communication. Verbal descriptor scales have shown to be more effective in cognitive impairment. Visual scales may overcome communication difficulty. In non-communicating patients, observational pain assessment scales based on physiological variables and observation of behaviour, e.g. sounds and facial expressions (frowning, grimacing) may be used.

Management differences in the elderly

Paracetamol should be prescribed regularly but NSAIDs may cause an increased frequency of side effects in this age-group. They should be avoided or used with extreme caution for a limited period only, with antacid cover for gastric protection. Older patients are more sensitive to opioids and require dose reduction to achieve the same therapeutic benefit. Doses should be titrated slowly due to reduced bioavailability, opioid metabolite accumulation, and inter-patient variability. Tramadol has a reduced elimination half-life in the >75 age group. Respiratory rate should be frequently monitored. Laxatives and antiemetics should be co-administered although nausea and pruritus side effects decrease with age.

Perioperative neuraxial blockade is an effective method of delivering excellent pain relief and reducing postoperative opioid requirements. In the elderly this also avoids morbidity from opiate-related side effects. Patients may be on antiplatelet drugs or anticoagulation which preclude central techniques.

Further reading

British Geriatrics Society, British Pain Society and the Royal College of Physicians (2007). *The Assessment of Pain in Older People. National Guidelines, October 2007*. London: British Geriatrics Society.

Table 26.6 Pharmacokinetic and pharmacodynamic changes in the older person and the effect on analgesia		
Physiological process	Kinetic/dynamic effects	Dose adjustment
CVS: Cardiac output ↓ 0–20%	↓ central compartment ↑ peak plasma concentration	Smaller dose and slower rate of injection
Renal: ↓ renal mass 30% ↓ RBF 10% ↓ GFR 30–50%	↓ clearance drugs ↓ clearance of active metabolites (e.g. morphine)	↓ maintenance dose (renally cleared drugs) Monitor for toxic metabolite accumulation
Hepatic: Reduced liver mass ↓ RBF 20–40% ↓ Phase 1 reactions by 25%	↓ hepatic clearance of high extraction drugs	Minimal effect on IV bolus dose ↓ maintenance dose Potential for changes in oral bioavailability
CNS: CBF ↓ 20% CSF ↑ 10% Brain mass ↓ 20%	↓ distribution to CNS ↑ response to opioids	↓ bolus dose during titration ↓ maintenance dose
Other: Body water ↓10% Body fat ↑ 10–50% Plasma albumin ↓ 20%	↓VD for water soluble drugs ↑ VD for fat soluble drugs ↑ free drug	↓ dose

26.8 Assessment and management of chronic pain in adults

Chronic pain

Chronic pain is defined as pain that has persisted for >3 months. About 1 in 7 people in the UK has chronic pain and it has a large socioeconomic impact. The NHS spends more than £1 billion/year on back pain and, in 2003, 5 million working days were lost. Pain management aims to improve symptom control and quality of life. See Box 26.2 for some definitions of pain.

> **Box 26.2 Definitions of pain**
>
> - *Nocioceptive pain* arises from actual or threatened damage to non-neural tissue and is due to the activation of nociceptors.
> - *Neuropathic pain* is caused by a lesion or disease of the somatosensory nervous system.
> - *Hyperaesthesia* is increased sensitivity to a sensory stimulus, excluding the special senses. It includes allodynia and hyperalgesia.
> - *Allodynia* is pain from a non-painful stimulus.
> - *Hyperalgesia* is the phenomenon of increased pain due to a painful stimulus.
> - *Dysaesthesia* is an unpleasant abnormal sensation, whether spontaneous or evoked.
> - *Anaesthesia dolorosa* is pain in an anaesthetized region. It is a rare complication of neurolytic blocks.
> - *Sensitization* is increased responsiveness of nociceptive neurons to their normal input and/or recruitment of a response to normally subthreshold inputs.

Assessment of chronic pain

History
A thorough pain history should allow the patient to describe the pain in their own words before more focused questions. The mnemonic SOCRATES aids a complete pain history;
- *Site:* Where is the pain?
- *Onset:* When did the pain start?
- *Character:* What does it feel like? e.g. sharp, burning.
- *Radiation:* Does the pain spread anywhere else?
- *Associations:* Symptoms or signs associated with the pain? (e.g. see Box 26.3)
- *Timing:* Does the pain follow any pattern?
- *Exacerbating/relieving factors:* Does anything change the pain?
- *Severity:* How bad is the pain? e.g. Numerical rating scale.

Nociceptive pain is described as sharp, shooting, and stabbing. Symptoms suggestive of neuropathic pain are burning, numbness, tingling, electric shocks, and may be associated with allodynia and hyperalgesia.

It is important to elicit the physical, psychological, and social effects of the pain. History should include examples of functional limitation, mood and sleep patterns, and a social history including levels of social support. A complete analgesic history should be taken and results of previous therapies noted. Multidimensional questionnaires, e.g. McGill Pain Questionnaire and Brief Pain Inventory, may help describe the impact on function and quality of life.

> **Box 26.3 'Red flag' signs of low back pain which warrant urgent investigation**
>
> - Age <20 or >50 years
> - Pain after a violent injury, e.g. road traffic accident
> - Constant or rapidly worsening pain
> - Thoracic pain
> - Previous history of cancer
> - History or high risk of immunosuppression, e.g. HIV
> - Significant weight loss
> - History of neurological symptoms
> - Non-mechanical back pain, i.e. persists lying supine.

Examination
A physical examination of the area of pain should include both the musculoskeletal (e.g. inflammation, deformity, myofascial pain) and the neurological systems (e.g. power, sensation, reflexes, allodynia).

Examination of an area of neuropathic pain requires stimulation with different sensory modalities, i.e. hot and cold, sharp, fine touch. Allodynia can be elicited by brushing the skin with a cotton ball, though a more formal assessment can be done using von Frey hairs (nylon hairs pressed against the skin until the hair bends).

Investigation
Investigations may confirm or exclude any underlying causes, e.g. rheumatoid arthritis or diabetes. Diagnostic imaging may influence management options in some cases. Nerve conduction studies and electromyography can be performed for neuropathic pain syndromes to measure dysfunction in large nerve fibres.

Quantitative sensory testing (QST) may be used for research into neuropathic pain by measuring the responses evoked from mechanical and thermal stimuli.

Management of chronic pain

Many treatment modalities are available and include pharmacological, non-invasive, and interventional approaches. The site and characteristics of the pain, previous patient experience, and contraindications must all be considered.

Pharmacological

Systemic and topical drugs (see section 26.4)
Most chronic pain patients will probably have mixed nociceptive and neuropathic elements to their pain and require a combination of therapies. Peripheral pain can be targeted with topical agents.

Non-invasive therapies

These include hot/cold therapy, complementary and alternative therapy which should be used in conjunction with medication to reduce analgesia requirements.

Transcutaneous electrical nerve stimulation
TENS machines act upon peripheral nerves via electrodes placed on the skin. Patients using the battery-operated unit can adjust the frequency (0–200Hz), intensity (0–50mA), and pulse width (0.1–0.5ms) of the electrical pulses. TENS works using the gate control theory of pain. It modulates the release of known pain mediators in the spinal cord, including GABA, serotonin, and glutamate.

High-frequency (50–100Hz) and low-frequency (1–5Hz) TENS activate δ-opioid and μ-opioid receptors respectively in the brainstem and spinal cord. TENS has been shown to be effective for chronic musculoskeletal pain and acute pain but a Cochrane review found insufficient evidence for use of TENS in lower back pain.

Acupuncture
Acupuncture needles activate A-δ nerve fibres and cause endogenous neurotransmitter and hormone release as well as up-regulation of several endogenous analgesic genes which might account for the sustained effect. Cochrane reviews have shown that acupuncture is effective for migraines, tension headaches, and osteoarthritis.

Physiotherapy
Physiotherapists are trained to help chronic pain patients by assessing their pain, attitudes, beliefs, social environment, and any pain-related disabilities. Exercises aim to improve the flexibility and strength of muscles, thereby increasing function (see section 26.10).

Psychological approaches
Chronic pain impacts on quality of life, social interaction, and mood. The patient must learn to manage the pain with the aid of various therapies to improve their function and quality of life. Pain avoidance behaviour must be addressed and cognitive behavioural therapy can be beneficial for some patients.

Interventional techniques

Interventional procedures require a dedicated procedure room with basic monitoring and resuscitation facilities. Sedation requires a dedicated anaesthetist.

Intravenous injections
Lidocaine infusions may be used for chronic neuropathic pain. Cardiotoxic effects are uncommon at the doses used for the infusion.

IV regional blocks are performed for complex regional pain syndrome (CRPS). Drugs administered include LA, ketamine, corticosteroids, and guanethidine. Guanethidine acts by depleting noradrenaline in nerve endings, resulting in a sympathetic blockade. These blocks can act as a diagnostic and therapeutic tool, although repeat procedures might be needed. It may predict a beneficial effect of more permanent sympathectomy.

Trigger points
Trigger points are highly irritable localized bands of muscle that cause pain when pressed. LA and/or corticosteroids are injected into the trigger point to provide pain relief. Exercise then improves flexibility, minimizing recurrence.

Peripheral nerve blocks
Nerve blocks with LA (and corticosteroids) can be performed as both diagnostic and therapeutic procedures. Nerve plexus blocks, e.g. stellate ganglion block for upper limb CRPS may be used. More distal nerves can be targeted, e.g. suprascapular nerve for shoulder pain.

Neurolytic blocks with alcohol or phenol may be used for cancer or intractable pain. These last up to 6 months, reducing opioid requirements and side effects.

Intra-articular steroid injections
Injections of corticosteroids are performed to reduce inflammation in the intra-articular space and mechanical pain. Most require imaging for placement. Lumbar and cervical facet joint injections are performed under fluoroscopic guidance.

Radiofrequency (RF) of nerves
Continuous RF (high-frequency electrical current) creates a thermal lesion of the target nerve by heating the insulated needle tip to 80°C. Pulsed RF generates an electrical field which disrupts the conductance of the neuronal cell membrane and alters signalling in the dorsal horn. Temperature is limited to 45°C which has some thermal effect but is non-destructive.

RF machines measure electrical impedance, temperature, and also contain a nerve stimulator. Electrical impedance is measured to ensure a continuous electrical circuit. A thermocouple ensures a desired temperature at the nerve. Nerve stimulation ensures correct needle placement. Sensory stimulation (50Hz) should recreate the pain. Motor stimulation is excluded at 2Hz before treatment commences.

Epidural steroid injections
Injections of corticosteroids into the epidural space are commonly used to treat cervical, thoracic, and lumbar pain. The three most common approaches are:

* *Caudal:* for leg pain arising from lower lumbar levels. Avoids dural puncture but requires large volume of injectate and higher risk of extra-epidural injection.
* *Interlaminar:* performed with a loss of resistance technique or with fluoroscopic guidance.
* *Transforaminal:* selective approach at a specific level under fluoroscopic guidance. The foraminae are small lateral openings between the vertebrae through which nerve roots traverse to exit the spinal canal. Used for patients with lumbar radiculopathy involving one or two dermatomes. The advantage is that the drug is delivered at the site of the nerve irritation with smaller volumes required, and there is a decreased risk of epidural puncture.

The evidence for interlaminar and transforaminal lumbar epidural and caudal steroid injections for lumbar radicular pain is strong for short-term relief but more limited in the long term.

Spinal cord stimulator
The indications for neuromodulation of the spinal cord are neuropathic or ischaemic pain in a limb, CRPS, and refractory angina. Electrodes can be placed into the epidural space in order to directly stimulate the dorsal horns of the spinal cord. Possible mechanisms of action are:

* Direct or indirect inhibition of pain transmission in the spinal cord.
* Autonomic effects.
* Stimulation of large afferent nerve fibres in the spinal cord (producing numbness/tingling to mask pain, i.e. the gate theory).

The electrodes are advanced to the affected level under fluoroscopic guidance. Verbal contact with the patient is required for positioning of the electrode using stimulation until pain is relieved. A trial with an external pulse generator determines benefit before implanting an internal generator in the abdominal wall. MRI is contraindicated as heat may be generated in the electrodes. Protocols must allow quick referral to the neurosurgical centre for advice if complications occur, such as electrode lead breakage or infection.

NICE guidelines in 2008 recommended the use of spinal cord stimulators for chronic pain of neuropathic origin.

Intrathecal drug delivery system (IDDS)
IDDS may be used for cancer pain, chronic pain, and spasticity. Intrathecal medications work directly on the nerves causing the pain and allow reduction of analgesic doses and side effects. LA and opioids are most commonly used although clonidine, ketamine, midazolam, and baclofen for spasticity may be added.

Drugs can be delivered via an intrathecal catheter connected to an external pump or an implantable infusion pump and catheter system. The implantable system is only cost-effective if it is expected to be *in situ* >3–6 months.

Further reading
Jackson M & Simpson K (2006). Chronic back pain. *CEACCP*, 6(4):152–7.
Rea W, Kapur S, & Mutagi H (2011). Radiofrequency therapies in chronic pain. *CEACCP*, 11(2):358.

Trigeminal neuralgia

This is discussed in detail in section 22.7.

Post-herpetic neuralgia

20% of herpes zoster (shingles) cases develop post-herpetic neuralgia (PHN) which is pain that persists beyond 1 month of presentation. It presents as neuropathic pain described as constantly burning or stinging with signs of allodynia and hyperalgesia over the area of the rash within a single dermatome. Although the pain usually resolves over several months, it can develop into a chronic pain syndrome.

The mainstay treatment of PHN is with antineuropathic drugs such as amitriptyline or gabapentin. Lidocaine patches and capsaicin creams/patches can cover the affected dermatome. TENS and acupuncture are not beneficial. Other therapeutic options include intercostal blocks, epidural steroid injections, and neuromodulation with a spinal cord stimulator.

Diabetic neuropathy

Diabetic peripheral neuropathic pain develops in approximately 10–20% of diabetics. The initial management should be to optimize glycaemic control. First-line treatments are antidepressants and anticonvulsants, though opioids are sometimes used in resistant cases. Lidocaine patches and capsaicin cream can be helpful. Spinal cord stimulators have been used in resistant cases.

Next-generation antidepressants (serotonin-noradrenaline reuptake inhibitors) duloxetine and venlafaxine have been licensed for the treatment of diabetic neuropathic pain. They show similar benefits to tricyclic antidepressants but have fewer adverse effects.

Complex regional pain syndrome

CRPS is characterized by a combination of sensory, autonomic and trophic symptoms in a limb following tissue injury (which may be minor). It is more common in women and with older age.

CRPS 1

Symptoms have been preceded by tissue injury. Previously known as 'reflex sympathetic dystrophy' due to the overactivity of the sympathetic nervous system.

CRPS 2

Preceded by major peripheral nerve injury. Previously called 'causalgia'.

The pathophysiology of CRPS is not completely understood but involves peripheral and central sensitization as well as altered sympathetic function. Studies show altered representation in the somatosensory cortex and psychological factors also play a role.

Sensory symptoms

Patients describe an intense burning pain in the affected limb with associated allodynia and hyperalgesia. Sensory deficits may occur in CRPS 2.

Autonomic changes

Autonomic involvement may cause vasodilatation in the affected limb, resulting in it being warm, red, and sweaty, or vasoconstriction resulting in a cold, dry, white limb. Limb oedema may also occur.

Trophic changes

Atrophy of hair, skin, and nails. Joint stiffness and motor changes can occur. Osteoporosis can result from disuse.

There is no definitive treatment of CRPS and a multimodal, multidisciplinary approach should be used.

Pharmacological

Antineuropathic agents are effective and opioids are used in refractory cases. There may be a beneficial effect from corticosteroids. Calcitonin, bisphosphonates, and free radical scavengers (e.g. N-acetylcysteine) are evidence-based therapeutic options.

IV infusion of lidocaine and IV sympathetic blockade with guanethidine may be effective.

Interventional

If LA sympathetic blockade, e.g. stellate ganglion block, is beneficial, sympathectomies with RF ablation or surgery may be performed.

Spinal cord stimulation has been shown to have a modest effect on pain and may be used in carefully selected patients.

Surgical

Amputation should only be performed for severe complications, e.g. sepsis or severe functional impairment. Phantom limb pain is common post procedure.

The key treatment for CRPS is early physiotherapy. A graduated exercise programme may retain functionality. These patients also benefit from a pain management programme.

Cancer pain

Cancer pain can be due to:

- Tumour infiltration or compression of structures and nerves.
- Surgical management—dissection of nerves.
- Radiotherapy—neuritis and scarring.
- Chemotherapy—peripheral neuropathy.

A systematic review in 2007 showed that >50% cancer patients had pain, with >33% rating their pain as moderate to severe. Another systematic review in 2008 showed that almost 50% of patients with cancer pain did not have adequate analgesia.

The principles of treating cancer pain are the same as for chronic non-malignant pain (see Box 26.4).

Box 26.4 Salient points in the history may guide management of cancer pain

- What is the cause of the pain?
- Speed of onset or are symptoms increasing?
  - A rapid onset or changing nature of pain may suggest recurrence or advancing disease. An urgent referral for investigation is necessary.
- What is the stage of anticancer treatment?
  - Radiotherapy-associated pain will reduce post-treatment.
- What is the patient's prognosis?
  - Neurolytic blocks are not suitable for patients with a life expectancy of >6 months.
- How is the patient's mood?
  - A cancer diagnosis can have a large emotional impact on an individual which can affect the patient's perception of their pain.

The WHO analgesic ladder (Fig. 26.3) guides treatment of cancer pain. Additional treatment should be considered as with chronic non-malignant pain, with the use of antineuropathics, non-invasive methods, and interventional therapies, e.g. neurolytic blocks and intrathecal drug-delivery pumps used as appropriate.

There are a few key concepts of the opioid treatment in cancer pain.

Breakthrough pain is when the patient experiences a brief amount of severe pain on top of a stable level of background pain. The standard treatment is a PRN dose of opioid that is one-sixth the amount of the regular 24h dose. New fentanyl preparations have been licensed for breakthrough pain, which can be given via the buccal, sublingual, and nasal routes.

Symptom control of opioids becomes increasingly important as the dose rises. Laxatives and anti-emetics should be prescribed regularly.

Opioid rotation may be used to balance analgesia and complications.

Further reading

Lindsay TJ, Rodgers BC, Savath V, *et al.* (2010). Treating diabetic peripheral neuropathic pain. *Am Fam Physician*, 82(2):151–8.

Opstelten W, Eekhof J, Neven AK, *et al.* (2008). Treatment of herpes zoster. *Can Fam Physician*, 54:373–7.

26.10 Multidisciplinary chronic pain management

Management models

Once pain has affected a person for a significant amount of time it becomes a complex problem, and the traditional 'Biomedical Model' becomes inadequate to fully understand and treat the problem. This is recognized in the IASP definition of pain as an 'unpleasant sensory and emotional experience associated with actual or potential tissue damage'.

The biomedical model suggests that symptoms are investigated, a diagnosis made, treatment instigated and cure achieved. Unfortunately, experience of both healthcare professionals and patients suffering chronic pain show this to be too simplistic.

The biomedical model:

Symptoms → Investigation → Diagnosis → Treatment → Cure

To fully understand the pervasive effect of pain on a person, their emotions, and their position and role in society as well as the effect that thoughts, emotions, behavioural responses, and societal influences have on the experience of pain, the biopsychosocial model is a more appropriate framework when considering how best to help the patient.

The biopsychosocial model

This model, first theorized by Engel in 1977, suggests that there is an interaction between the biological tissue damage with physiological and neurophysiological dysfunction, psychological factors (beliefs, thoughts, coping, emotion, distress), and social (interactions, family, work) effects which results in the overall experience of pain for the patient and consequent disability (Fig. 26.4). This goes some way to explaining the spectrum of disability experienced by patients with apparently similar structural injuries.

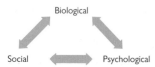

Fig. 26.4 The biopsychosocial model. Data from GL Engel, 'The need for a new medical model: a challenge for biomedicine', *Science*, 1977, 196, pp. 129–136.

This view takes account of the person as a whole, the functional limitations as a result of the pain, the psychological effects of pain and the impact on all aspects of their life. The illness or disability is a result of the interaction between all three aspects. Treatment aimed solely at the sensory component of pain (i.e. the biomedical model) will fall short of the mark for many patients. This will result in repeated failure of the medical system and a constant search by the patient to find the elusive cure for their pain.

Cognitive behavioural approach

The cognitive behavioural approach to managing pain takes account of these interacting factors in a patient and aims treatment at all dimensions (Fig. 26.5).

The principles of this approach are:

- Individuals actively process information.
- Thoughts influence mood, behaviour, and physiological processes.
- Interventions can address each aspect of the experience.

An example of this interaction is fear-avoidance behaviour (Fig. 26.6). Fear of the pain (emotion) as a result of catastrophic

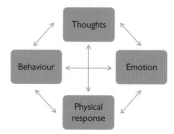

Fig. 26.5 The cognitive behavioural model (Padesky and Mooney 1990). Reproduced with kind permission from Christine A. Padesky, Copyright 1986, Center for Cognitive Therapy, http://www.padesky.com.

thinking (thoughts) results in inactivity and overuse of medication (behaviour) resulting in the physical effect of disuse, disability and deconditioning. Any attempt to increase activity often increases pain levels and reinforces the catastrophic thoughts. This is an example of the maladaptive behaviour that can develop as a result of catastrophic thinking.

Yellow flags

The psychological and social risk factors that predict chronicity and disability or recovery are known as yellow flags.

There is good agreement that the following factors are important and consistently predict poor outcome in a person presenting with acute lower back pain (New Zealand Acute Low Back Pain Guide 1999):

- Presence of a belief that back pain is harmful or potentially severely disabling.
- Fear-avoidance behaviour (avoiding a movement or activity due to misplaced anticipation of pain) and reduced activity levels.
- Tendency to low mood and withdrawal from social interaction.
- An expectation that passive treatments rather than active participation will help.

The behaviour and beliefs of the health professionals dealing with the patient, their explanation for the pain, and suggested management, can also have a huge influence on the patient's thoughts and behaviour.

Questionnaires

There are a number of questionnaires used to determine the extent of the pain and its effect on the patient, their coping strategies, feelings of control despite the pain (self-efficacy), degree of fear avoidance and level of disability. These include:

- Brief Pain Inventory
- Short Form 36
- Self-Efficacy Questionnaire
- Fear Avoidance Beliefs
- Rowland Morris Disability
- Oswestry Disability Index
- Beck Depression Index
- Hospital Anxiety and Depression Index.

A selection of these can be given to patients to complete pre and post treatment to assess degree of change and the efficacy of the treatment.

When a patient presents to a pain clinic the initial requirement is to identify biological, psychological, and social factors that

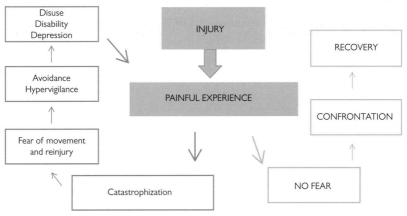

Fig. 26.6 Vlaeyens's model of fear avoidance. Reproduced from Vlaeyen JWS and Linton T. Fear-avoidance and its consequences in chronic musculoskeletal pain: a state of the art. *Pain* (c) 2000 April 85 (3); 317–332 with permission.

are likely to be maintaining the pain. This involves a thorough assessment of the pain, the patient's response to it and their beliefs about the pain. Therapy must then use the expertise of the multidisciplinary team to help the patient with the different components.

The multidisciplinary team

• Pain specialist doctor
• Physiotherapist
• Psychologist
• Nurse
• Occupational therapist
• Social worker
• Psychotherapist
• Psychiatrist.

Most multidisciplinary teams will have medical input, physiotherapy, and psychology as a core, but more extensive teams will have the other professions listed.

The role of the doctor in the team is to fully investigate the pain and ensure that there is no remediable cause or diagnosis. They then need to explain this to the patient in a way that the patient can understand fully and emphasize an active approach to the management of pain whilst de-emphasizing the role of medication. They must ensure that the patient has a clear understanding of how to use medication that may be helpful to moderate the pain, and provide clear information about the risk of re-injury.

The other members of the team can then work on the self-management techniques that enable the patient to return to a more active and fulfilling life less disabled by the pain. These strategies include:

Physiological
• Breathing and relaxation
• Exercise and stretch.

Cognitive and affective
• Education
• Mood management
• Cognitive restructuring.

Behavioural
• Pacing and graded exposure
• Goal setting

• Sleep management
• Stress management.

Pain management programme

The earlier described methods are often combined to create a pain management programme (PMP) for groups of patients. The aims of a PMP are to improve the physical, psychological, emotional, and social dimensions of the quality of life of people with persistent pain using a multidisciplinary approach in accordance with cognitive and behavioural principles (British Pain Society 2007). Aims are to:
• Improve quality of life
• Increase activity levels
• Reduce disability
• Reduce psychological distress
• Improve sense of self control and confidence
• Improve work status
• Reduce healthcare utilization.

Although the patient's initial main aim will be to become pain free or at least reduce pain levels, emphasis is placed on this being a by-product of the improvement in condition and function rather than an aim in itself. This addresses the expectations of the patient, ensuring that they are more realistic and helping to reduce the focus on the pain.

Key elements of a PMP
• *Education:* increase knowledge and understanding and thereby reducing fear.
• *Promote self-management:* i.e. increase self-efficacy which is known to be an important factor in disability.
• *Guided practice* to promote behavioural change.
• *Group work:* normalizes the experience of the patient.

There is a significant body of RCT-based evidence that PMPs improve pain experience, function and activity, mood and coping, reduce medication, and reduce healthcare utilization.

Although PMPs combine all the appropriate elements of a comprehensive approach to managing chronic pain there are some people who are inappropriate or do not wish to attend a group programme. For example, patients with significant mental health disorders such as major depression or personality disorders either will not benefit from such an approach or can be disruptive to the group limiting the benefit for other patients. For these patients other approaches are required such as involvement of a mental health team to treat the depression, or other psychological approaches such as psychodynamic psychotherapy. This type of approach can be particularly useful in the management of a patient with a coexisting pain condition and a personality disorder.

Further reading

Zarnegar R & Davies C (2005). Pain management programmes. *CEACCP*, 5:80–3.

Chapter 27

Ophthalmic anaesthesia

525

27.1 Pre-assessment of ophthalmic patients

Ophthalmic surgery patients

There is an expectation that most ophthalmic procedures are performed as day surgery and the general patient selection criteria still apply (see section 12.2). Ophthalmic patients, however, tend to represent the extremes of age with the majority of patients being elderly and a high proportion of paediatric cases. This creates a challenging patient population for day surgery. Elderly patients have a high rate of significant comorbidity and although the vast majority of cases are performed under local anaesthesia, pre-assessment is required in all cases. Paediatric patients with ophthalmic conditions may have associated congenital disorders and will usually require general anaesthesia.

Ophthalmic pre-assessment

As well as a general assessment of the patient's health status there are some specific points that are pertinent to the conduct of ophthalmic anaesthesia. Many factors will aid the decision for the mode of anaesthesia.

Can the patient tolerate a supine position?

As a consequence of using a microscope, most ophthalmic surgeons need to approach the eye at right angles. For local anaesthesia the patient will have to lie flat for up to 1h. Patients with COPD, heart failure, spinal deformity or pain, and obesity may be unable to do this. If the patient can tolerate a degree of neck extension, a semi-recumbent position may be used. A simple rule-of-thumb is that the superior and inferior orbital ridges should be in the same horizontal plane for an adequate position.

Can the patient keep still?

Patient movement creates difficulties with local anaesthesia and the conduct of surgery. Patients with chronic cough, tremors, or movement disorders and poorly controlled epilepsy may need to be considered for general anaesthesia.

Can the patient tolerate the procedure?

Many patients have a degree of anxiety about local anaesthesia for surgery, but some patients have specific anxieties, e.g. claustrophobia, which are important to elicit. Patients with dementia may tolerate procedures under local anaesthesia, but this must be carefully assessed and discussed with the surgeon.

Can the patient comply with instructions during the procedure?

Patients with communication problems, e.g. deafness, language barriers, confusion, or dementia may find it difficult to comply with surgery under local anaesthesia.

Has the patient got any poorly controlled medical conditions which increase perioperative risk?

Patients with poorly controlled ischaemic heart disease or an MI within 3 months are at increased risk of cardiac ischaemia even under local anaesthesia. Poorly controlled hypertension (>180/100mmHg) may cause increased complications with ophthalmic surgery. Any patients with bleeding disorders or thrombocytopaenia may not be suitable for some forms of local anaesthesia.

Is the patient on any medication which will prolong bleeding?

This is significant for the anaesthetist if a sharp needle block is being considered and may be of concern to the surgeon.

A recent report suggested that clopidogrel or warfarin use was associated with a significant increase in minor complications of sharp needle and sub-Tenon's cannula local anaesthesia *but was not* associated with a significant increase in potentially sight-threatening local anaesthetic, or operative haemorrhagic complications.

Are there any ophthalmic factors which may affect the operation or anaesthetic?

Factors such as enophthalmos, fixed squints, and long axial length may make local anaesthesia difficult. Axial length is the distance from the cornea to the retina. Normal values are around 23mm and values over 26mm represent a 'long eye' which may preclude peribulbar techniques. 'Long eyes' should be suspected in myopic patients.

Investigations in pre-assessment

Routine observations are performed but complex investigations in these patients are not usually required. Nevertheless the following are usually warranted:

- 12-lead ECG if indicated by history or pulse/BP abnormality.
- Axial length if a peribulbar or retrobulbar local anaesthetic block is to be used.
- INR or APTT if the patient is being treated with warfarin or heparin.
- Blood sugar in diabetic patients; acute intraoperative hypoglycaemic episodes must be avoided.

Special considerations in the elderly patient

The physiological effects of ageing reduce the functional reserve of all body systems and lifestyle modification can often hide symptoms of low reserve. An overall assessment of functional capacity may be possible from the levels of daily activity. ASA classification remains a good perioperative predictor in the elderly. Problems with hearing should be identified and the ability to retain information checked. Cerebrovascular disease affecting the vertebrobasilar system can be excluded by looking upwards without dizziness.

Communication difficulties and cognitive decline have a bearing on informed consent and the overall patient experience. There is a greater susceptibility to acute confusional states in the elderly both from the unfamiliar environment of the hospital and postoperative cognitive dysfunction. There may be less risk with local techniques but this is not established. Elderly patients show greater sensitivity to drugs with sedative effects. Changes to the volume of distribution of drugs may increase and prolong their effects and renal clearance is reduced (see Table 18.6).

Special considerations in the paediatric patient

Most paediatric ophthalmic patients are fit and well, but ophthalmic problems can be related to congenital genetic or metabolic conditions (see Box 27.1) as well as severe prematurity. It is extremely important to identify these patients as there are often huge implications for anaesthesia. Neonatal surgery, or surgery in ex-premature infants, may require inpatient admission for apnoea monitoring. Preterm infants should be >60 weeks post-conceptual age with no recent apnoeas, respiratory, or cardiovascular disease and no family history of sudden infant death syndrome or adverse social circumstances.

Box 27.1 Syndromes which may present with ophthalmic disease which have important anaesthetic considerations

Syndromes associated with difficult airways
- Mucopolysaccharidoses (e.g. Hurler's syndrome)
- Craniosynostosis disorders (e.g. Apert, Crouzon)
- Craniofacial disorders (e.g. Goldenhar, Treacher–Collins, Pierre–Robin, Hallerman–Strieff)
- Down's syndrome—also associated with cardiorespiratory complications
- Stickler syndrome (ocular, orofacial, and skeletal abnormalities).

Syndromes associated with neurological disorders
- Neuro-ocular-cutaneous disorders (e.g. Sturge–Weber, neurofibromatosis, tuberous sclerosis, von Hippel–Lindau).

Syndromes associated with cardiac/respiratory disease
- Down's syndrome—congenital heart disease
- Marfan's disease—aortic root dilatation and aortic valve regurgitation
- Mitochondrial disorders (e.g. Kearns–Sayre)—cardiomyopathy and respiratory muscle weakness
- Myotonic dystrophy—cardiomyopathy, conduction defects, and respiratory failure.

Further reading

Benzimra JD, Johnston RL, Jaycock P, et al. (2009). The cataract national dataset audit. *Eye*, 23:10–16.

Brennan A & Cruikshank R (2002). Diseases relevant to the ophthalmic anaesthetist. *CEACCP*, 2:183–8.

Gordon H (2006). Preop assessment in ophthalmic regional anaesthesia. *CEACCP*, 6:203–6.

Choice of technique

A number of factors must be considered when deciding upon the optimum anaesthetic technique for ophthalmic procedures (Table 27.1). These can be divided into surgical and patient factors.

Surgical factors:

- Type of surgery:
  - In general, corneal or conjunctival procedures, e.g. intra-ocular pressure (IOP) measurement, removal of foreign bodies, pterygium, irrigation of lacrimal ducts, surgery for myopia, and small incision cataract surgery are possible with topical anaesthesia.
  - Intraocular procedures, e.g. cataract surgery, vitreoretinal surgery, may require regional blockade to provide sensory block of the globe and some degree of motor blockade.
  - Extraocular surgery, e.g. squint surgery and oculoplastic surgery, may require general anaesthesia.
  - Common procedures are discussed later.
- Risk of complications.
- Duration of surgery.
- Axial length >26mm from cornea to retina may be associated with staphyloma (thinning of the globe wall leading to out-pouching) which may increase the risk of globe perforation with peribulbar/retrobulbar blocks. Staphyloma is found in 15% patients with axial length 27–29mm and 60% when >31mm.
- Previous ophthalmological problems, e.g. scleral buckling or space-occupying lesions of the orbit.

Patient factors

- Patient refusal of local anaesthesia
- Local anaesthetic allergy
- Orbital infection
- Unable to lie supine and remain still: cardiorespiratory disease, tremor, confusion, communication difficulties, children
- Blepharospasm.

Topical anaesthesia

Topical anaesthesia may be provided with 0.5% proxymetacaine or 0.4% oxybuprocaine drops, which are applied to the conjunctiva as they may cause clouding of the cornea. Local anaesthetic agent concentrations have been demonstrated in the aqueous humour and this provides anaesthesia of the iris as well as the cornea and conjunctiva. Topical anaesthesia provides the least risk of complications but is only suitable for compliant patients and is not suitable for complicated surgery.

Intracameral anaesthesia, where the surgeon injects preservative-free lidocaine into the aqueous chamber, has been shown to be safe and effective in reducing intraoperative pain.

Local anaesthetic blocks

- The sharp needle blocks—modified retrobulbar block, peribulbar block
- Blunt cannula techniques—sub-Tenons block.

These are discussed further in section 27.3. In general they provide superior analgesia to topical anaesthesia and may be used for intraocular surgery. They provide some degree of motor block and hence better operating conditions for the surgeon. The blocks may be associated with sight and life-threatening complications.

IV access should be sited prior to sharp needle blocks. Verbal contact is maintained with the patient and monitoring with pulse oximetry to provide heart rate and oxygen saturations should be performed.

Sedation

Sedation is used to provide anxiolysis during procedures under local anaesthesia. This can often be avoided with good pre- and perioperative support. Conscious sedation is the aim, but the unpredictable effects of the sedative drugs in elderly patients may make this hard to achieve. Deeper planes of sedation are associated with many unwanted effects such as restlessness, sudden movement, and airway obstruction.

Midazolam or low-dose propofol in combination with short-acting opiates may be used prior to the local anaesthetic procedure. It is then ideal to let the patient awaken prior to commencing surgery.

Sedation should only be administered by the anaesthetist who is responsible for the list. Supplementary oxygen should be provided and monitoring should include maintenance of verbal contact as well as oximetry, ECG, and NIBP.

General anaesthesia

General anaesthesia considerations include the high-risk population, day surgery principles, and an inaccessible airway during surgery. The aim of anaesthesia is to minimize increases in IOP and maintain cardiovascular stability.

Airway choice

Laryngeal mask airways are ideal as they avoid the need for laryngoscopy (and associated IOP effects) and ensure smoother emergence from anaesthesia. If intubation is indicated, the vocal cords may be sprayed with lidocaine to prevent coughing on emergence, or the airway may be changed whilst deeply anaesthetized.

Ventilation choice

Self-ventilation is appropriate for minor and extraocular surgery. Controlled ventilation for major intraocular surgery affords more control of carbon dioxide and hence IOP. Airway pressure and nerve stimulator monitoring should be instituted if combining controlled ventilation with an LMA.

Anaesthesia maintenance

Nitrous oxide should be avoided for vitreoretinal surgery as intraocular gas tamponade may be used. In squint surgery, anaesthesia depth using volatiles should be sufficient to ensure neutral gaze.

Supplementary blocks

For many procedures it may not be appropriate to also subject the patient to the risks of a local block, but the extra stimulation associated with vitreoretinal surgery may justify this.

Anaesthesia for cataract surgery

Cataract surgery is the most frequently performed procedure. Local anaesthesia is the preferred method unless contraindicated.

Table 27.1 Anaesthesia techniques for ophthalmic procedures

Type of surgery	Special considerations	Preferred technique	Postoperative
Cataract surgery	Often elderly	Local anaesthesia (topical/block)	Day case
Strabismus surgery	Often paediatric Oculocardiac reflex Requires neutral gaze	General anaesthesia Avoid suxamethonium (muscle tone) CO_2 control (δ oculocardiac reflex) LA and sedation possible	Day case PONV prophylaxis Simple analgesia
Vitreoretinal surgery	Stimulating surgery Axial length often high Long procedures (up to 3h) Use of SF6 or C3F8 gas Avoid nitrous oxide (intraocular gas expansion)	Often general anaesthesia Local block possible if shorter procedure Controlled ventilation	Day case Analgesia—block
Dacrocystorhinostomy	Stimulating Post nasal bleeding	General anaesthesia LA and sedation possible Topical vasoconstrictors for nose Throat pack with LMA/ETT	Day case Simple analgesia
Enucleation/evisceration	Often for tumour/infection	General anaesthesia	Day case/23h Opiate analgesia
Oculoplastic surgery	May require graft from donor site	General anaesthesia Opiate analgesia	Day case/23h
Glaucoma	Paeds/elderly	Local block	Day case Simple analgesia
Corneal graft	Paeds/elderly	General anaesthesia Local block possible	Day case Simple analgesia

Table 27.2 Topical drugs used to provide mydriasis for cataract surgery

Drug	Action	Systemic side effects
Phenylephrine 5% (10%)	Sympathomimetic Dilates pupil	Hypertension Arrhythmia Coronary vasospasm
Cyclopentolate 0.5% (1%)	Parasympatholytic Dilates pupil	Confusion, psychosis

This reduces morbidity and disrupts daily routine less in patients who are often elderly with multiple comorbidities. Physiological changes associated with ageing are detailed in section 18.3, Table 18.1.

96% cases are performed under local anaesthesia and only 1.5% require sedation. The goal of local anaesthesia should be for 'pain-free surgery with minimal systemic and surgical complications which facilitates the surgical procedure'. Akinesia of the globe is less important with modern surgical techniques.

Sub-Tenons blocks were used in about 50% of cataract procedures in the 2009 audit of 55 567 patients. This audit suggested a 2.5 times reduction in complications with sub-Tenons as compared to the sharp needle techniques. The *Cataract Surgery Guidelines* suggest sharp needle techniques should be performed only when necessary and by highly trained anaesthetists or ophthalmic surgeons. A Cochrane review favours sub-Tenons over topical anaesthesia for provision of analgesia.

Table 27.2 describes the topical drugs used to provide pupillary dilation in preparation for surgery.

Further reading

Parness G & Underhill S (2005). Regional anaesthesia for intraocular surgery. *CEACCP*, 5(3):93–7.

The Royal College of Ophthalmologists (2010). *Cataract Surgery Guidelines*. London: Royal College Ophthalmologists. http://www.rcophth.ac.uk.

27.3 Local anaesthetic blocks for eye surgery

Modified retrobulbar block

Traditional retrobulbar blocks were intraconal injections using long 50mm sharp needles to place local anaesthetic beyond the posterior border of the globe. This blocks the ciliary ganglion, sensory nerves to the sclera and cornea, and motor nerves to the extraocular muscles. Due to an association with increased risk of both sight and life-threatening complications, they are now very rarely performed. The modified retrobulbar technique uses a short 24mm sharp needle and local anaesthetic is injected at the level of the posterior border of the globe. See Box 27.2.

Box 27.2 Modified retrobulbar block

Using a 24mm 25G needle with the patient looking straight ahead, insert inferotemporally just lateral to the lateral limbus and aim posteriorly advancing parallel to the floor of the orbit up to the equator of the globe (about 10–15mm). Then redirect slightly medially and upwards to enter the muscle cone at the level of the posterior border of the globe (Fig. 27.1). After aspiration, 4–5mL local anaesthetic is injected.

The needle insertion may be made through the conjunctival reflection or percutaneously through the lower eyelid.

Benefits
- Rapid onset good quality anaesthesia.
- Good motor block.

Risks
- Increased risk of retrobulbar haemorrhage 1%, globe perforation 0.7%, and optic nerve damage.
- Systemic complications 0.2%.

Peribulbar block

Peribulbar blocks are extraconal injections using a shorter needle to improve the safety profile. They have largely superseded the retrobulbar blocks. They should still be avoided if axial length is >26mm due to the risk of globe perforation. See Box 27.3.

Box 27.3 Peribulbar block

Using a 16mm 25G needle with the patient looking straight ahead, insert inferotemporally just lateral to the lateral limbus and aim posteriorly parallel to the orbit floor (Fig. 27.1). If bone is contacted, redirect slightly upwards. After aspiration, 5–10mL local anaesthetic is injected. If swelling of the conjunctiva occurs, the injection is too superficial and the needle should be repositioned.

May require supplementary blocks:
- *Commonly*, medial canthus: insert through conjunctiva, medial to the caruncle keeping needle parallel to the medial wall.
- *Rarely*, superonasal: injection through upper eyelid above the medial limbus.

Benefits
- Good quality anaesthesia.
- Reduced risk of optic nerve and systemic complications as compared to retrobulbar.
- Some motor block but may require supplementation if akinesis is required.

Risks
- As for retrobulbar but reduced incidence.
- Globe penetration about 1 in 12 000–16 000.

Sub-Tenon's block

Sub-Tenon's blocks were designed as a simple, safe technique which avoided the use of sharp needles to reduce complications. A blunt cannula is used to deposit local anaesthesia in the sub-Tenon's space beyond the equator of the globe where it effectively blocks the ciliary ganglion and long and short ciliary nerves. This is now the local anaesthetic block of choice. See Box 27.4.

Box 27.4 Sub-Tenon's block

The eye is prepared with topical anaesthesia and a few drops of aqueous iodine for sterility. A small lid speculum is inserted to hold the eyelids open and the patient is asked to look up and out. A non-toothed forceps is used to take a bite of conjunctiva and Tenon's capsule in the inferonasal quadrant about 6mm from the limbus. A small opening is made halfway between the forceps and the globe with the tip of a blunt Westcott spring scissors between the sclera and the Tenon's capsule. A blunt 19G 25mm sub-Tenon's cannula is advanced into the tunnel revealed disappearing into the fornix. The cannula is advanced keeping close to the sclera until 15–20mm deep. At this point local anaesthetic may be injected posterior to the equator of the globe using 4–5mL volume.

A superotemporal approach may be considered as an alternative or for additional infiltration.

Benefits
- Better safety profile for all complications (2.5× less).
- Safe with axial length >26mm.

Risks
- If globe perforation occurs (extremely rare), damage is increased compared to sharp needle perforation.
- Conjunctival haematoma.

Complications of blocks

- *Chemosis*: swelling of the conjunctiva is common and can be simply dispersed with gentle pressure.
- *Corneal abrasion*: the anaesthetized cornea is susceptible to injury or drying so must be protected until block recedes.
- *Muscle palsy*: from direct injection into muscle. Causes prolonged diplopia and ptosis.
- *Allergy*: to local anaesthetic or hyaluronidase.

Retrobulbar haemorrhage—1 in 100

Reduce risk by performing sub-Tenon's block or using fine, short needles (25G, <25mm), avoiding vascular superonasal site and checking INR is in therapeutic range if on warfarin.

Bleeding into skin and conjunctiva is apparent. Raised IOP may cause proptosis. If IOP is not reduced it can threaten retinal artery flow and cause blindness. The surgeon must be informed immediately as lateral canthotomy may save the eye. A large multicentre audit of 55 567 patients identified no increased risk of severe haemorrhagic complications for patients on antiplatelet agents or warfarin with any regional blocks although sub-Tenon's/topical may be preferable.

Globe penetration: 1 in 12 000–16 000

Reduce the risk by using topical/sub-Tenon's technique, especially if axial length >26mm. About 50% are not recognized at

Position of needles.

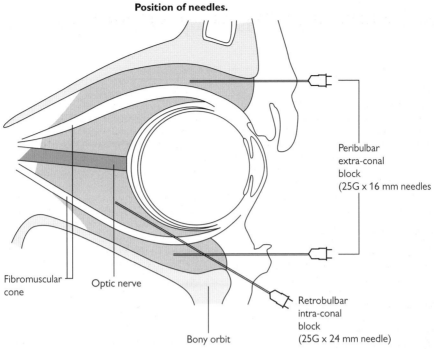

Peribulbar
extra-conal
block
(25G x 16 mm needles

Retrobulbar
intra-conal
block
(25G x 24 mm needle)

Fibromuscular
cone

Optic nerve

Bony orbit

Fig. 27.1 Needle positions for retrobulbar and peribulbar blocks. Reproduced from Parness G and Underhill S, 'Regional anaesthesia for intraocular surgery', *Continuing Education in Anaesthesia, Critical Care and Pain*, 2005, 5, 3, pp. 93–97, by permission of The Board of Management and Trustees of the British Journal of Anaesthesia and Oxford University Press. doi:10.1093/bjaceaccp/mki025.

occurrence. Injection is painful and there may be sudden deviation of the globe and a soft eye. Perforation can rapidly lead to retinal detachment.

Optic nerve damage: rare

Reduce the risk by performing sub-Tenon's or using sharp needles <25mm and avoiding retrobulbar techniques, avoiding medial compartment injections, and avoiding patients looking up and in for inferotemporal injection. Injection into the optic nerve is painful and may cause permanent nerve damage. Injection into the dural sheath may cause brainstem anaesthesia with progressive drowsiness, confusion, fits, respiratory depression, and cardiovascular collapse. Management is supportive.

Drugs used to perform the blocks may include short or long-acting local anaesthetics, hyaluronidase, and adrenaline, see Box 27.5. Hyaluronidase is associated with a risk of anaphylaxis.

Box 27.5 Drugs used for local anaesthetic blocks

- 2% lidocaine: 5–10mL provides up to 90min of anaesthesia.
- 0.5–0.75% bupivacaine—may be used in combination with lidocaine to prolong the block.
- Hyaluronidase: 5IU/mL may be added to improve the spread of the block and reduce proptosis by reducing loculation of LA.
- Adrenaline: 1:200 000 may be added to prolong the block.

Further reading

Benzimra JD, Johnston RL, Jaycock P, *et al*. (2009). The cataract national dataset audit. *Eye*, 23:10–16.

Parness G & Underhill S (2005). Regional anaesthesia for intraocular surgery. *CEACCP*, 5(3):93–7.

The Royal College of Ophthalmologists (2010). *Cataract Surgery Guidelines*. London: Royal College Ophthalmologists. <http://www.rcophth.ac.uk>.

The paediatric patient

Children form a large part of the workload for ophthalmic anaesthetists. Neonates and infants commonly present for surveillance or intervention where the disorder is congenital glaucoma, retinopathy of prematurity, malignancy (retinoblastoma), or congenital cataracts as well as squint correction.

Repeat attendance for examination under anaesthesia may be frequent for some children. This may be disturbing for both children and their parents, resulting in uncooperative behaviour and perhaps psychological distress. Special consideration should be given to these patients with the appropriate use of preparation, play specialists, and premedication. This is especially true in some specialist centres where IV ketamine is used as a sole agent (initially) to provide a repeatable measure of intraocular pressure that is both precise *and* accurate for glaucoma surveillance.

The conduct of anaesthesia requires the same precautions as that for any paediatric surgery: trained staff, appropriate equipment, and a dedicated environment. General anaesthesia is usually conducted using a reinforced flexible LMA (reduced coughing at extubation) with intermittent positive pressure ventilation to ensure normocapnia. An LMA must be perfectly positioned and secured prior to surgery. If there is any concern, the patient should be intubated as access to the airway is highly disruptive once surgery is underway. Remifentanil is well suited as an adjunctive agent as the vast majority of patients are satisfactorily pain free if the surgeon delivers local anaesthetic into the sub-Tenon's space at the end of surgery. Moreover this drug reduces the need for muscle paralysis and facilitates smooth emergence. Peribulbar blocks are generally avoided in children due to the risk of sight and life-threatening complications.

Most operations are conducted on a day case basis, therefore the anaesthetist must aim to provide sufficient analgesia and prophylaxis against nausea and vomiting. This helps to ensure that the patient fulfils discharge criteria promptly. See Table 27.3.

Oculocardiac reflex

The oculocardiac reflex causes bradycardia during ophthalmic surgery. It is more common in paediatric patients, squint surgery, and vitreoretinal surgery, e.g. scleral buckling.

Trigger
- Traction on extraocular muscles (especially medial rectus).
- Pressure on the globe.

Afferent arc
- Occipital branch of the trigeminal nerve.
- Fibres in the long and short ciliary nerves pass to the trigeminal ganglion via the ciliary ganglion.

Efferent arc
- Vagal fibres to the sinoatrial node: oculocardiac reflex.
- Vagal fibres to the respiratory centre: oculorespiratory reflex.
- Vagal fibres to the vomiting centre: nausea and vomiting.

Effects
- Bradycardia or sinus arrest.
- Hypoventilation or respiratory arrest.
- PONV.

Prevention
- Local anaesthetic block may abolish the afferent arc.
- Avoidance of hypercapnia which sensitizes the reflex.
- Prophylactic glycopyrrolate or atropine (particularly in high-risk surgery, e.g. paediatric squint surgery).

Management
Release of traction usually leads to rapid reversion of normal rhythm and ventilation. Preventative measures should then be instituted before surgery continues.

Table 27.3 Common paediatric ophthalmic procedures		
Procedure	Usual technique	Postoperative
Examination under anaesthesia		
Fundoscopy	GA—SV facemask/LMA	
IOP measurement	IM/IV ketamine or gas induction	
Extraocular		
Syringing/probing ducts	GA—SV	Simple analgesia
Squint surgery	GA—SV/IPPV	PONV 60%
	Oculocardiac reflex 60%	Simple analgesia, avoid opiates
	MH association, monitor temperature	
Intraocular		
Glaucoma	GA—IPPV. IOP control	Simple analgesia
Cataracts	GA—SV	
Laser/cryotherapy	GA—SV	Day case implication (neonate/ex-prem)
	Opiate required	
Vitreoretinal	GA—IPPV	Simple analgesia
	Sub-Tenon's for analgesia	

Penetrating eye injury

The principal concern in the management of a penetrating eye injury is to avoid an increase in intraocular pressure (IOP) as this can lead to vitreous extrusion, haemorrhage, and lens prolapse. This, however, must not take precedence over protection of the airway.

Preoperative

Possible causes of raised IOP in this setting are: pain, coughing, vomiting, hypertension, hypercarbia, and hypoxia. In children, crying, screaming, rubbing the eyes, and breath-holding can be problematic. First-line analgesia may include paracetamol and NSAIDs but opioids should be used with caution because of the undesirable risk of vomiting.

Induction of anaesthesia

If the patient is not fasted, the options for induction are:

1. To delay surgery. Assess the degree of urgency with the surgeon, if possible give prokinetics and an H_2 antagonist/proton pump inhibitor and wait sufficient time for gastric emptying.

2. Rapid sequence induction with suxamethonium. Suxamethonium causes a transient increase in IOP (of about 5–10mmHg for 5–10min) and thus carries a theoretical risk of vitreous extrusion, although this was not evident in a large retrospective study.

3. Modified rapid sequence induction with rocuronium following careful airway evaluation and preferably with sugammadex available.

What is arguably more important than the debate over the choice of muscle relaxant, is avoidance of the pressor response associated with laryngoscopy and intubation. This may be achieved using:

- Opioids (e.g. remifentanil 1mcg/kg, alfentanil 10–20mcg/kg, fentanyl 1–2mcg/kg)
- Lignocaine 1–1.5mg/kg
- Esmolol 3–5mcg/kg
- And/or an extra dose of induction agent immediately prior to intubation.

All the induction agents except ketamine will lower IOP. Volatile anaesthetic agents all reduce IOP. Local anaesthetic blocks are, obviously, contraindicated.

Perioperative

IOP is controlled using the following methods:

- Ensure adequate depth of anaesthesia.
- Position with slight head-up tilt.
- Ensure low airway pressures.
- Avoid venous congestion, e.g. tube ties.
- Maintain end-tidal carbon dioxide at the lower limit of normal.
- Acetazolamide or mannitol may be considered; prepare patient for diuretic effect.

Extubation should be performed with the patient awake if there is a risk of aspiration.

Postoperative

Analgesia may be provided with paracetamol, NSAIDs, or codeine. Antiemetics should be given prophylactically.

Further reading

James I (2008). Anaesthesia for paediatric eye surgery. *CEACCP*, 8:5–10.

Libonati MM, Leahy JJ, & Ellison N (1985). The use of succinylcholine in open eye surgery. *Anaesthesia*, 62:637–9.

27.5 Physiological control of intraocular pressure

Intraocular pressure

Normal IOP is 10–20mmHg with small physiological fluctuations and diurnal variation. As the globe of the eye is contained within a fixed bony orbit, IOP is comparable to ICP.

Intraocular pressure is determined by:

- Intraocular contents: aqueous humour, choroidal blood, vitreous humour (see Table 27.4). IOP is principally regulated by changes in aqueous humour volume, the formation and drainage of which is under autonomic control. This will compensate for increases in pressure over about 20min.

- External pressure.

Table 27.4 Intraocular contents and intraocular pressure	
Intraocular component	Factors effecting change
Aqueous humour	IOP is increased by:
	Decreased drainage: glaucoma or raised venous pressure
	Increased aqueous production
	IOP is decreased by:
	Increased drainage: topical parasympathomimetic, e.g. pilocarpine
	Reduced aqueous production: topical β-blockers, e.g. timolol
Choroidal blood	IOP is increased by:
	Blood volume increases with hypercapnia, hypoxaemia and acute rises in systolic BP
	Blood volume increases with CVP during straining, coughing, vomiting etc.
	IOP is decreased by:
	Blood volume decreases at systolic pressures of 80–90mmHg
Vitreous humour	Volume reduced by mannitol administration
Iatrogenic	Sulphur hexafluoride (SF6) or perfluoropropane (C3F8) gas or silicone oil used to tamponade a detached retina
	NB. Co-administration of N_2O and SF6 or C3F8 instillation markedly expands the volume of the gas bubble and increases IOP
	Patients must not fly after SF6 or C3F8 instillation as a reduction in atmospheric pressure will also cause the gas bubble to expand thus increasing IOP
	SF6 remains in the eye 3–4 weeks post administration and C3F8 for 6–8 weeks

Aqueous humour

Aqueous humour is produced in the ciliary bodies of the posterior chamber. It flows over the lens to the anterior chamber providing oxygen and glucose to the avascular lens and cornea (Fig. 27.2).

Production of aqueous humour is by two mechanisms:

- 80% by Na-K-ATPase active secretion which is independent of IOP.
- 20% by ultrafiltration of plasma. This is influenced by IOP as well as venous and oncotic pressures.

Drainage of aqueous humour

This occurs via the trabecular network and canal of Schlemm (in the angle between the cornea and the iris) into the episcleral veins. The venous drainage is dependent on a pressure gradient between IOP and venous pressure.

Production and flow of aqueous humour in the eye.

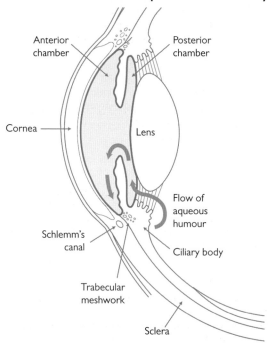

Fig. 27.2 Production and flow of aqueous humour in the eye. Reproduced from Murgatroyd H and Bembridge J, 'Intraocular pressure', *Continuing Education in Anaesthesia, Critical Care and Pain*, 2008, 8, 3, pp. 100–103, by permission of The Board of Management and Trustees of the British Journal of Anaesthesia and Oxford University Press. doi:10.1093/bjaceaccp/mkn015.

An increase in IOP is largely compensated for by increased drainage of aqueous humour (production is relatively fixed). If drainage is reduced, by glaucoma or raised venous pressure, IOP will increase.

The production and drainage of aqueous humour is influenced by the autonomic nervous system:

Sympathetic system

α-receptor activation vasoconstricts and reduces ciliary body blood flow and therefore aqueous humour production. β-receptor activation causes increased production of aqueous humour by the ciliary body. Mydriasis (dilation of the pupil) reduces aqueous humour drainage.

Parasympathetic system

Miosis (constriction of the pupil) increases aqueous humour drainage.

Choroidal blood volume

The retinal artery provides blood supply to the posterior chamber and has autoregulation similar to that of cerebral blood flow. Below a systolic pressure of 90mmHg, IOP is proportional to blood pressure. The choroidal vessels lie beneath the retinal surface and have no autoregulation so dilate in response to a raised perfusion pressure. In addition, vasodilatation occurs with hypoxaemia and hypercarbia.

These effects are minor compared to the influence of raised venous pressure on choroidal blood volume. The normal venous pressure within the globe is only just above IOP (15mmHg). Consequently if venous pressure outside the globe rises, choroidal venous drainage ceases and blood volume increases.

Methods of reducing choroidal volume and IOP perioperatively:

- Attenuation of pressor response to laryngoscopy
- Use of head-up tilt
- Avoidance of venous congestion (e.g. tube ties)
- Avoidance of high airway pressures
- Maintenance of mild hypocapnia (approx. 4.0kPa)
- Avoidance of coughing, vomiting.

Vitreous humour

The vitreous humour of the posterior chamber is relatively fixed in volume and plays little role in IOP regulation. It can be reduced in volume by using mannitol.

External pressure

External pressure may arise from increased tone of the extraocular muscles, e.g. suxamethonium, surgical traction, pressure from an incorrectly applied facemask, large volume peribulbar blocks, and ocular compression devices designed to improve the spread of local anaesthetic.

Drugs to reduce IOP

The following topical agents administered as drops are used to treat raised IOP:

- β-blockers (e.g. timolol) reduce the secretion of aqueous humour and IOP.
- Parasympathomimetic drugs (e.g. pilocarpine) constrict the pupil increasing aqueous drainage.
- α-agonists (e.g. bromonidine) vasoconstrict the vessels supplying the ciliary body and reduce aqueous production.
- Prostaglandin analogues (e.g. latanoprost) reduce IOP by increasing aqueous outflow via an alternative drainage route called the uveoscleral pathway.

Systemic drugs to treat IOP in acute situations:

- Acetazolamide (a carbonic anhydrase inhibitor) reduces the production of aqueous humour. It is also mildly diuretic.
- Mannitol acts as an osmotic diuretic and transiently reduces the volume of the vitreous humour and thus the IOP.

Effect of anaesthetic agents

Induction agents
IOP is reduced by all IV induction agents with the exception of ketamine. This effect may be independent of the effect of the drug on the cardiovascular system.

Ketamine causes a transient rise over 1min and then normalizes. This relative stability of IOP under ketamine anaesthesia is often used during EUA to assess paediatric glaucoma.

IOP is reduced slightly by benzodiazepines.

Opioids do not directly affect IOP but will attenuate sympathetic responses to airway instrumentation.

Volatile anaesthetic agents
IOP is reduced by all volatile anaesthetic agents. It is unaffected by nitrous oxide.

Neuromuscular blocking agents
IOP is increased by suxamethonium possibly by extraocular muscle contraction and choroidal vasodilatation. A rise of 8–10mmHg occurs for 5–10min. A raise in IOP has been noted during suxamethonium administration even when muscle insertions are detached.

Non-depolarizing muscle relaxants may decrease IOP by reducing extraocular muscle tone.

Further reading

Murgatroyd H & Bembridge J (2008). Intraocular pressure. *CEACCP*, 8(3):100–3.
Raw D & Mostafa SM (2001). Drugs and the eye. *CEPD Reviews*, 1(6):161–5.

Guidelines for local anaesthesia

Local Anaesthesia for Ophthalmic Surgery—joint guidelines from the Royal College of Anaesthetists and the Royal College of Ophthalmologists 2012.

Cataract Surgery Guidelines 2010—Royal College of Ophthalmologists.

Guidance on the provision of Ophthalmic Anaesthesia Services. Royal College of Anaesthetists 2009.

Important points

Pre-assessment by trained staff is highly desirable. There is no evidence that patients having local anaesthesia benefit from pre-operative investigations. Patients having local anaesthesia do not need to fast.

Local anaesthesia is the procedure of choice for the majority of patients for cataract surgery.

Patients having sharp needle blocks or requiring sedation must have an anaesthetist immediately available in the theatre suite. Sharp needle blocks should only be performed when necessary by a trained anaesthetist or surgeon as they are associated with an increased risk of complications.

Local anaesthesia using topical or sub-Tenon's block does not require an anaesthetist immediately available. A member of the theatre team must be trained in cardiopulmonary resuscitation.

Monitoring under local anaesthesia should consist of maintenance of verbal contact, clinical observation of colour, response to surgical stimulus, ventilatory movements, and pulse oximetry. IV access is necessary if sharp needle blocks are used.

If sedation is used, oxygen should be available and monitoring as for general anaesthesia.

Surgical safety guidelines

Surgical errors for cataract surgery occur in about 7/100 000 procedures. Errors mostly consist of:

- Incorrect intraocular lens insertion
- Wrong eye operated on
- Local anaesthetic administered to the wrong eye.

Cataract lists are busy and error is introduced by communication problems, changing the order of the list, transcription errors, and rarely, biometry error.

The operative eye should be marked by the surgeon preoperatively with patient agreement. A clear plan for the type of lens, size, and dioptre should be made and recorded on a theatre white-board.

The NPSA have issued a surgical safety checklist for cataract surgery (Fig. 27.3) which includes the following points to target the common errors:

Sign in

- Patient identity and confirm site of surgery
- Confirmation that site is marked
- Any special requirements for positioning/draping
- Is the patient on warfarin?
- Is the patient on tamsulosin or α-blocker? (risk of floppy iris syndrome and complications).

Time out

- Reconfirm site
- Lens model and power
- Refractive outcome planned
- Is the correct lens present?

NHS

National Patient Safety Agency

Surgical Safety Checklist:
for __Cataract Surgery ONLY__
(adapted from the WHO Surgical Safety Checklist)

SIGN IN (To be read out loud)

Before giving anaesthetic

Has the patient confirmed his/her identity, site, procedure and consent?
☐ Yes

Is the surgical site marked?
☐ Yes

Is the anaesthesia machine and medication check complete?
☐ Yes ☐ Not applicable

Does the patient have a:

Known allergy?
☐ No ☐ Yes

Difficult airway/aspiration risk? (General Anaesthetic)
☐ No ☐ Yes, and equipment/assistance available

Any special requirements for positioning or draping?
☐ No ☐ Yes, surgeon notified

Is the patient taking warfarin?
☐ No ☐ Yes, last INR result available

Is the patient taking tamsulosin or other alpha blocker?
☐ No ☐ Yes, surgeon notified

Has pre-operative VTE risk assessment been undertaken?
☐ Yes ☐ Not applicable

The checklist is for
__Cataract Surgery ONLY__
This modified checklist must not be used for other surgical procedures.

Ref: 1096 March 2010

TIME OUT (To be read out loud)

Before start of cataract surgery

Have all team members introduced themselves by name and role?
☐ Yes

Surgeon, Scrub Nurse and Registered Practitioner verbally confirm:
☐ What is the patient's name?
☐ What procedure, and which eye?
☐ What refractive outcome is planned?
☐ What lens model and power is to be used?
☐ Is the correct lens implant present?

Anticipated variations and critical events

Surgeon:
☐ Are there any special equipment requirements or special investigations?
☐ Are any variations to the standard procedure planned or likely?
☐ Is an alternative lens implant available, if needed?

Anaesthetist (GA or sedation)
☐ Are there any patient-specific concerns?
☐ What is the patient's ASA grade?
☐ Any special monitoring requirements?

Scrub Nurse/ODP:
☐ Has the sterility of the instrumentation been confirmed (including indicator results)?
☐ Are there any equipment issues or concerns?

SIGN OUT (To be read out loud)

Before any member of the team leaves the operating room

Registered Practitioner verbally confirms with the team:
☐ Has the name and side of the procedure been recorded?
☐ Has it been confirmed that instruments, swabs and sharps counts are complete (or not applicable)?
☐ Have any equipment problems been identified that need to be addressed?
☐ Are any variations to standard recovery and discharge protocol planned for this patient?

PATIENT DETAILS

Last name:

First name:

Date of birth:

NHS Number:*

Date of Procedure:

*If the NHS Number is not immediately available, a temporary number should be used until it is

www.nrls.npsa.nhs.uk

Fig. 27.3 Surgical safety checklist for cataract surgery (NPSA).
Reproduced with permission under the terms of the Open Government Licence. http://www.nationalarchives.gov.uk/doc/open-government-licence/open-government-licence.htm. Adapted from the World Health Organization with permission.

Chapter 28

Anaesthesia for plastic and reconstructive surgery

539

Pre-assessment

Patient pre-assessment may affect the suitability for certain procedures, the timing of surgery, and allow optimization to reduce surgical postoperative complications as well as perioperative morbidity. A general assessment of age, weight, nutritional status, and smoking history is made. Some procedures will not be performed until patients have stabilized their weight and ceased smoking due to the effect on wound healing and thrombotic risk. Medical comorbidity, particularly hypertension and diabetes, should be optimized to minimize surgical complications such as haematoma and infection. Cardiac and respiratory symptoms require investigation prior to major surgery. Left ventricular dysfunction may be associated with poor surgical outcome following free flap surgery.

Patients having surgery to correct congenital deformities may have other conditions of particular relevance to anaesthesia, e.g. congenital cardiac disease and difficult airways.

Patients for head and neck reconstructive surgery require careful airway assessment. Airway distortion may result from tumour mass, previous surgery, and radiotherapy-associated fibrosis.

In addition to good surgical explanation, psychologists may be involved to ensure that patients have realistic surgical expectations.

Choice of anaesthetic technique

Although most major plastic surgery will be performed under general anaesthesia, regional techniques may be used for surgery to the limbs. Skin tumours often develop in the very elderly and local anaesthesia infiltration may be used for this superficial body surface surgery even if it necessitates skin grafting. Regional and local anaesthetic techniques may be combined with sedation.

Considerations for major plastic surgery procedures

Long procedures

- Prolonged positioning: care of pressure areas (padding, heel supports, inflatable mattress), avoidance of neurovascular compression, and eye care.
- Thromboprophylaxis: TED stockings, pneumatic compression boots, and consideration of preoperative LMWH if high risk.
- Temperature control: higher ambient temperature in theatre, warmed IV fluids, heated mattresses, external forced air warming blankets, heat and moisture exchange filters, and low inspired gas flows. Continuous temperature monitoring.
- Gastric decompression: especially in paediatric patients.

The airway

- Difficult airways: head and neck procedures, congenital abnormalities.
- Shared airway: head and neck procedures require careful preoperative planning with the surgeon. Oral or nasal endotracheal tubes may be used. Conversion to tracheostomy may be required for reconstructive procedures.
- Poor access to the airway: stitching may be required to secure the tube and connections may be inaccessible.

Multiple surgical sites

Multiple surgical sites lead to the following considerations:
- Monitoring sites limited
- Vascular access sites limited
- Analgesia provision
- Patient repositioning during procedure.

Fluid balance

- Blood loss: may be large in major reconstructive surgery and difficult to assess (suction volume and swab weight). Regular measurement of haemoglobin concentration may be necessary.
- Optimization of cardiac output: essential for successful surgical outcome in free tissue transfer procedures. May require invasive arterial and CVP monitoring as well as cardiac output monitoring.
- Urinary output: urinary catheterization is required for long procedures and to monitor fluid balance.

Anaesthesia for free flap surgery

The aim of anaesthesia for free flap surgery is to provide optimal blood flow with a hyperdynamic circulation. This requires a high cardiac output, peripheral vasodilatation, wide pulse pressure, and good temperature and pain control.

Monitoring

Invasive arterial monitoring is required to allow optimization of arterial pressure and regular assessment of arterial blood gases and haemoglobin.

CVP monitoring or noninvasive cardiac output monitoring is used to assess fluid balance and optimize cardiac output.

ECG monitoring may require positioning away from the surgical site.

Vascular access should include a large-bore cannula but a smaller cannula for induction may be used for PCA postoperatively.

Both core and peripheral temperature should be monitored. Peripheral temperature will fall with hypovolaemia or vasoconstriction. A difference of <2°C indicates a warm, well-perfused patient.

Urine output is monitored to guide fluid resuscitation with an ideal output of 1mL/kg/h.

Induction and maintenance

Active warming should commence prior to induction to prevent the rapid fall in temperature that occurs at this time.

Anaesthesia is maintained with volatile anaesthetic or propofol infusion. Nitrous oxide is usually avoided due to the length of surgery and its effect on cuff pressures, nausea, vomiting, and gastric distension. Use of remifentanil infusion is popular to provide intraoperative analgesia and allow rapid control of blood pressure. Adequate analgesia reduces the surgical stress response.

IPPV is required to maintain normocapnia. Hypocapnia causes peripheral vasoconstriction which must be avoided. Hypercapnia increases the sympathetic response. PEEP will reduce basal atelectasis during prolonged ventilation.

Analgesia

Regional blocks may be used for analgesia but it may be difficult to provide adequate cover of both donor and recipient site. The recipient site should take priority as the sympathetic block will improve local blood flow and graft reperfusion. Catheter-based techniques may allow continuation of the block for the postoperative period. Epidural analgesia may cause poor graft perfusion due to:

• Reduced systemic arterial pressure
• Steal phenomenon (blood is diverted from the denervated graft into more vasodilated tissues).

It is essential that arterial pressure and euvolaemia are maintained if epidurals are used. This may be easier to ensure in the postoperative period than perioperatively.

Opiate techniques may be preferable for cardiovascular stability but nausea and vomiting must be prevented.

Many surgeons prefer to avoid NSAIDs due to concerns regarding haematoma formation.

Control of blood pressure

During the initial dissection phase of surgery blood loss may be reduced by:

• Controlled hypotension
• Positioning (reducing venous pressure)
• Use of LA infiltration/regional blockade.

Controlled hypotension should be provided with rapidly reversible drugs such as remifentanil or GTN infusion. β-blockers may cause relative peripheral vasoconstriction and systemic vasodilators may also divert blood flow from peripheral tissue ('steal phenomenon'). Mean arterial pressure should be returned to normal prior to harvesting the flap. This is achieved with fluid resuscitation rather than vasopressor agents where possible due to concern of vasoconstriction in the graft vascular supply. There is, however, little evidence that vasopressors impact adversely on graft survival and raising the mean arterial pressure will usually improve graft perfusion. Dopexamine and dobutamine increase cardiac output and cause vasodilatation with theoretical advantages.

Fluid resuscitation

Insensible fluid and blood loss occurs from both the donor and recipient site. Blood loss may be difficult to estimate and may require swabs to be weighed for an accurate assessment.

Fluid resuscitation aims to replace insensible losses with crystalloid, and then provide hypervolaemic haemodilution using colloids (Box 28.1). Dextrans have a theoretical advantage with a resultant reduction in platelet adhesion improving graft microcirculation. However, gelatins and starches are commonly used as dextrans may be associated with pulmonary oedema. Modest hypervolaemia reduces sympathetic tone and causes vasodilatation. Increasing baseline CVP by 3cmH$_2$O can almost double the cardiac output. Fluid resuscitation should be guided by arterial pulse pressure, haematocrit, CVP trends, and cardiac output monitoring.

Box 28.1 Suggested fluid regimen

• Crystalloid:
  • 10–20mL/kg: replace preoperative deficit
  • 4–8mL/kg/h: to replace insensible loss
• Colloid:
  • 10–15mL/kg: for hypervolaemic haemodilution
  • To replace blood loss
• Blood:
  • Hb <8g/dL
  • Hct < 0.3.

Emergence and extubation

Surges in blood pressure and coughing at extubation increase haematoma formation so a smooth emergence is desirable but may be difficult to achieve. Good analgesia is essential. Emergence may be smoother following propofol and remifentanil maintenance. Some techniques used include:

• Exchanging the endotracheal tube for an LMA prior to reversal of muscle relaxation.
• Avoiding intubation with use of a Pro-Seal® LMA in suitable candidates.
• Early deflation of the endotracheal tube cuff.
• IV lidocaine (0.5mg/kg).

Recovery and flap monitoring

Good analgesia and management of any nausea and vomiting is essential. Oxygen and warming should be continued for 48h. Aims are:

• Normal blood pressure
• Urine output >1mL/kg/h
• Normal temperature. See Box 28.2 for monitoring of the flap.

Box 28.2 Monitoring the flap

• Clinical observation:
  • Colour
  • Capillary refill
  • Surface temperature
  • Turgor
  • Presence of bleeding
• Doppler flow:
  • Ultrasound
  • Laser.

Further reading

Adams J & Charlton P (2003). Anaesthesia for microvascular free tissue transfer. *CEPD Reviews*, 3(2):33–7.
Quinlan J & Lodi O (2009). Anaesthesia for reconstructive surgery. *Anaesth Intens Care Med*, 10(1):26–31.

Free flap surgery

Free flap surgery involves the transfer of vascularized tissue to a new site where circulation is restored by microvascular anastomoses to the recipient site vessels. The tissue transferred may include skin, muscle, bone, or bowel, which is used to reconstruct an area and provide wound closure. Free flaps are performed after cancer surgery or trauma, e.g.:

- TRAM flaps (transverse rectus abdominis muscle) for breast reconstruction.
- DIEP flaps (deep inferior epigastric perforator) for breast reconstruction.
- Gracilis muscle flaps for lower leg trauma.

During surgery, the flap is elevated and the vessels clamped. This creates a period of primary ischaemia with anaerobic metabolism and accumulation of lactate, potassium, and proinflammatory mediators. The response is proportional to the duration of anaerobic metabolism and the metabolic rate of the tissue. This stage is more influenced by surgical than anaesthetic factors. Reperfusion on anastomosis of the arterial and venous supply of the tissue to the recipient site vessels should restore blood flow and cellular function to the tissue. Secondary ischaemia may occur due to the altered characteristics of flow in the microcirculation. Maintaining optimal blood flow in this period relies on a good understanding of the physiological principles and is greatly influenced by the conduct of anaesthesia.

Free flap microcirculation

The microcirculation within the flap controls blood flow and oxygen delivery. It can be divided into three components with distinct functions:

Arterioles: the resistance vessels

Arteriolar walls contain vascular smooth muscle. Constriction or dilation of the arteriolar wall controls resistance to blood flow within the flap. The dissected flap is denervated and loses the normal direct sympathetic vasoconstrictor response but still responds to local and humoral factors as well as pharmacological manipulation.

- Vasoconstriction:
  - Circulating catecholamines
  - Hypothermia
  - Myogenic reflex
- Vasodilatation:
  - Hypoxia
  - Hypercapnia
  - Acidosis
  - Increased potassium
  - Histamine, prostacyclin, kinins

Capillaries: the exchange vessels

Precapillary sphincters, at the arterial end, control flow through capillaries. Oxygen and metabolic waste products diffuse along concentration gradients.

Venules: the capacitance vessels

These drain blood from the capillary network and act as a reservoir. High venous pressure may affect flow through the microcirculation.

Blood flow in the microcirculation is determined by:

- Plasma viscosity
- Red cell concentration
- Red cell and platelet aggregation
- Red cell deformability.

Laminar flow

The Hagen–Poiseuille equation describes laminar flow of a Newtonian fluid in a tube.
Where ΔP is the pressure difference across the vessel or the perfusion pressure.

$$\text{Flow} = \frac{\text{Pressure gradient} \times \text{radius}^4 \times \text{pi}}{\text{Tube length} \times \text{viscosity} \times 8}$$

Although this equation can only be loosely applied to the circulation, it demonstrates the effect that a good perfusion pressure, vasodilatation, and low viscosity will have on improving blood flow.

Maintaining perfusion pressure

Perfusion pressure should be maintained by increasing cardiac output rather than causing vasoconstriction. A good perfusion pressure with a wide pulse pressure is the ideal. This can be produced by:

- Hypervolaemic haemodilution. This may be guided by CVP or cardiac output measurement.
- Vasodilating inotropes, e.g. dopexamine, dobutamine.
- Balanced anaesthetic techniques.

Causing vasodilatation

Temperature control

Maintaining normothermia plays an important role in vasodilatation of the microcirculation. Warming should commence prior to induction and continue in the recovery period for 48 hours. Central and peripheral temperatures are monitored and a difference <2°C is aimed for. Hypothermia will also increase blood viscosity by red cell and platelet aggregation.

Fluid resuscitation

Modest hypervolaemia reduces sympathetic tone and causes vasodilatation.

Anaesthetic agents

Volatile anaesthetic agents and propofol both cause vasodilatation.

Pharmacological vasodilatation

Direct vasodilators, e.g. sodium nitroprusside and α-blocking agents, e.g. chlorpromazine, are now rarely used. Systemic vasodilatation may cause a steal phenomenon from a maximally dilated flap circulation.

Sympathetic blockade

Regional blocks may be used to provide analgesia and also result in sympathetic block and vasodilatation in the area covered. This may provide beneficial effects, e.g.:

- Reduced blood loss
- Reduced vessel spasm

- Reduced thrombosis.

vasodilatation will improve blood flow to the microcirculation but only if perfusion pressure is maintained. If hypotension occurs, blood will be diverted to the vasodilated areas away from the flap.

Transluminal pressure

According to the Law of Laplace, the balance of intraluminal pressure (the systemic pressure) and extraluminal pressure (from oedema, haematoma, dressings) will determine vessel diameter.

Managing vasospasm

Vasospasm may occur due to handling of vessels or intimal damage. It can be treated with topical papaverine, verapamil, lidocaine, or nitrate.

The effect of viscosity

In the small vessels of the flap microcirculation, viscosity is closely related to haematocrit. The relationship is non-linear and a haematocrit >40% is associated with a steep rise in viscosity (Fig. 28.1).

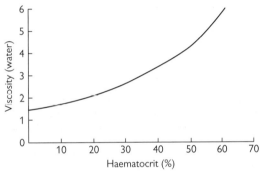

Fig. 28.1 Effect of haematocrit in viscosity. This figure was published in *Textbook of Medical Physiology*, 6th edition, Guyton and Hall, Figure 18.3, p. 207, Copyright Elsevier 1985.

Factors increasing blood viscosity

- Increased haemoglobin
- Hypothermia
- Smoking
- Increased fibrinogen
- Increased age
- Decreased blood flow.

Manipulation of viscosity

Haemodilution should aim to achieve a haematocrit of 30%. This seems to represent the optimum balance of viscosity and maintenance of oxygen delivery.

Other techniques that affect microcirculatory blood flow include:

- Use of dextrans—these reduce platelet adhesiveness and Factor 8 activity. Higher infused volumes may be associated with increased blood loss perioperatively. Pulmonary oedema disproportionate to volume status may occur, however, and dextrans are slowly being superceded by the starches.
- Use of heparin bolus and infusions.

Flap failure

Reasons for flap failure may be divided into arterial, venous and oedema.

Arterial causes:

- Inadequate blood flow
- Spasm
- Thrombosis.

The flap appears cool and pale with poor capillary refill and little bleeding on pinprick. Management includes optimizing systemic pressure and flow with treatment of hypotension, hypothermia and pain. Spasm may be managed pharmacologically with calcium channel blockers. Surgical re-exploration is required if optimization fails to improve arterial inflow.

Venous causes:

- Thrombosis
- Extrinsic compression, eg. dressings

The flap appears congested and oedematous with brisk capillary refill and bleeding on pinprick. This may be managed with elevation, leeches or exploration in theatre.

Causes of oedema:

- Excess crystalloid infusion
- Prolonged primary or secondary ischaemia.

Further reading

MacDonald DJF (1985). Anaesthesia for microvascular surgery; A physiological approach. *Br J Anaesth*, 57:904–12.
Quinlan J & Lodi O (2009). Anaesthesia for reconstructive surgery. *Anaesth Intens Care Med*, 10(1):26–31.

28.3 Pathophysiology of burn injury

Incidence of burn injury

Each year around 250 000 people suffer burn injuries in the UK. Of these, 175 000 will attend emergency departments and around 16 000 are admitted. 1000 patients will have burns serious enough to warrant fluid resuscitation and around 300 burn deaths occur, mostly in the over 60s.

These figures are representative of patterns seen throughout the developed world. Incidence of burn injury in the developing world is higher.

Causes of burns

The commonest cause of burns is flame injury followed by scalds. Relatively small numbers are due to electrical or chemical burns (Fig. 28.2). Other rarer causes of burns include contact, friction, radiation and injury due to cold.

Aetiology of burns is closely related to the specific patient groups sustaining the injury. Young children <4 years comprise 20% of all burn injuries and most of these are scalds due to spillage of hot liquids or due to hot bath water. Older children and adolescents may get injured from activities involving accelerants or from electrocution. Most burns however, occur in the working population and are predominantly flame burns. Up to a third of burns in the 15–64 age group are from work related incidents. Finally, the >65s comprise 10% of all burn injuries. Chronic medical illnesses and immobility decrease the ability of the elderly to escape any potential burn hazard.

The burn wound

The burn wound is the source of virtually all ill effects, local and systemic, seen in a burn patient. Excision of the burn wound results in clinical improvement and, when done early, results in increased survival and decreased morbidity.

The skin is the largest organ in the body and consists of the epidermis, which is 0.05–1mm thick and the dermis, which is around ten times this thickness. In an adult, the skin covers around 1.5–2.0m² and its vital functions include:
- Protective
- Immunological
- Fluid and electrolyte homeostasis:

- Thermoregulation
- Neurosensory
- Social-interactive
- Metabolism.

The cutaneous burn can be described as having three zones:
- *Zone of coagulation*: occurs at the point of maximum damage with irreversible tissue loss due to coagulation of the constituent proteins.
- *Zone of stasis*: decreased tissue perfusion causes a surrounding zone of stasis. Further compromise to perfusion such as prolonged hypotension, infection or oedema can convert this zone to one of complete tissue loss.
- *Zone of hyperaemia*: perfusion is increased in this, the outermost zone. Tissue will usually recover unless there is severe sepsis or prolonged hypoperfusion.

Systemic response to burn injury

Once a burn affects around 25% of total body surface area (TBSA), release of cytokines and other inflammatory mediators produce a systemic response (Fig. 28.3). The major systemic effects of the burn wound produce the following changes:

Cardiovascular effects
Increased capillary permeability leads to loss of intravascular protein and fluid into the interstitial compartment. Peripheral and splanchnic vasoconstriction occurs. Myocardial contractility is reduced which, when combined with fluid loss from the burn wound, leads to hypotension and end organ hypoperfusion.

Respiratory effects
Inflammatory mediators cause bronchoconstriction and in severe burns may lead to acute respiratory distress syndrome.

Metabolic effects
Basal metabolic rate increases significantly which, when combined with splanchnic hypoperfusion, threatens gut integrity. Early, full enteral feeding is required to prevent catabolism and gut endothelial breakdown.

Immunological effects
Both cell-mediated and humoral pathways are affected by a non-specific down regulation of the immune response.

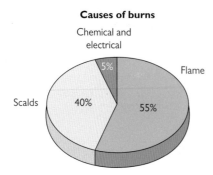

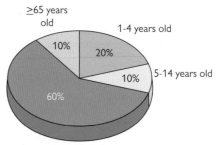

Fig. 28.2 Causes and incidence of burns. Reproduced from *British Medical Journal*, Shehan Hettiaratchy and Peter Dziewulski, 'Introduction: ABC of Burns', 328, p. 1366, with permission from BMJ Publishing Group Ltd.

Burn oedema

Burn wound oedema is caused by a fall in normal cell transmembrane potential with a 70–80% increase in cellular water of burned tissue within 30min of injury. In burns of >25% there is a systemic response with generalized oedema formation over 12–24h in unburned areas.

The oncotic pressure of plasma decreases due to denaturization of proteins and protein losses from capillary leak. Oedema may be limited by maintaining plasma protein levels, the use of non-protein fluids such as starches and early excision of the burn wound.

Burn shock

Burn shock is defined as inadequate oxygen delivery to tissues following a major burn. It is caused by the systemic changes described earlier, in combination with burn oedema.

There are two distinct phases:

- *Hypodynamic phase*: falling plasma volume and cardiac output leads to hypoperfusion. There is usually some response to fluid challenges. This phase lasts around 24–48h from the time of burn.
- *Hyperdynamic phase*: high cardiac output is coupled with massive energy expenditure. A pathological inability to respond to hypovolaemia by vasoconstriction leads to a significantly reduced SVR. There is a poor response to fluid challenges. Onset is around 24–48h after the burn and can last from days to weeks.

Inhalation injury

Inhalation injury is caused by exposure to hot gaseous products of combustion. It is the commonest cause of death in house fires and when occurring simultaneously with cutaneous burns, significantly increases mortality.

Smoke is a hot vapour containing particulate matter; the size of which determines which part of the respiratory tree is affected.

- Particles >5μm are deposited in the larynx, trachea, and large airways.
- Particles smaller than this may reach the small airways and alveoli.

Inhalation injury is caused by a combination of thermal and chemical mechanisms:

Thermal injury
Predominantly occurs in the upper airway (above the larynx) due to the efficient heat exchange mechanism there. Mucosal burns presenting as erythema and ulceration occur with progressive oedema formation causing upper airway obstruction.

Chemical injury
May be caused by a wide variety of substances commonly present in smoke (Box 28.3). These products of combustion are carried into the lower airways and alveoli where they produce a chemical burn. Inflammatory mediators released in response to the tissue damage potentiate oedema, reduce surfactant levels, increase capillary leak, and provoke bronchoconstriction. This, along with poor ciliary clearance causes narrowing of the lower airways. In addition there may be severe systemic effects associated with inhalation of agents such as carbon monoxide and hydrogen cyanide.

Box 28.3 Toxic chemicals commonly found as constituents of smoke

- Carbon monoxide
- Carbon dioxide
- Hydrogen cyanide
- Benzene
- Aldehydes
- Ammonia
- Chlorine
- Sulphur dioxide
- Nitrogen dioxide
- Hydrogen chloride.

Further reading

Brennan RJ, Waeckerle, Sharp TW, & Lillibridge SR 2000. *National Burn Care Review, 2000*. National Burn Care Review. <http://www.baps.co.uk/documents/nbcr>

Herndon DN (ed) (2007). *Total Burn Care* (3rd edn). Philadelphia, PA: Saunders.

Hettiaratchy S & Dziewulski P (2004). ABC of burns: pathophysiology and types of burns. *BMJ*, 328(7453):1427–9.

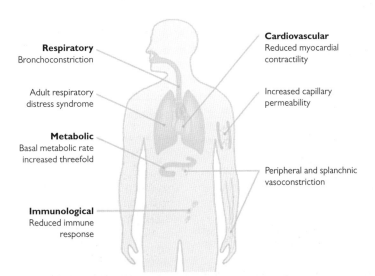

Respiratory
Bronchoconstriction

Adult respiratory distress syndrome

Metabolic
Basal metabolic rate increased threefold

Immunological
Reduced immune response

Cardiovascular
Reduced myocardial contractility

Increased capillary permeability

Peripheral and splanchnic vasoconstriction

Fig. 28.3 Pathophysiological effects of burns. Reproduced from *British Medical Journal*, Shehan Hettiaratchy and Peter Dziewulski, 'Introduction: ABC of Burns', 328, p. 1366, with permission from BMJ Publishing Group Ltd.

28.4 Initial assessment and management of severe burns

History

A severe burn can be defined as one covering more than 25% of TBSA. Rapid assessment is vital and the history of a burn and any pre-hospital treatment given can be invaluable.

The history gives valuable information about the nature and extent of the burn, likelihood of inhalation injury, the depth of the burn, and existence of any other injuries. Allergies, drugs, or coexisting medical problems must be recorded at this time, as patients will often be intubated for some time following this initial assessment phase.

Primary survey

Patients with burn injuries should be treated the same way as any other trauma patient and an ATLS approach to the primary survey is mandatory. Particular issues relevant to burn injury include:

Airway and cervical spine control

The cervical spine must be protected unless it is clear from the history that no traumatic injury has taken place. The upper airway must be assessed for signs of inhalation injury by a senior anaesthetist (see Box 28.4). If there is any concern over the patency of the airway, early intubation is the safest management. Inhalation of hot gases will cause oedema to develop over the first few hours, which may make later intubation difficult. An uncut endotracheal tube (ETT) should be used so that facial swelling does not compromise ETT position or connection to the ventilator circuit.

Suxamethonium can safely be used in the first 24–48h following a burn but must be avoided thereafter to prevent large rises in serum potassium. This hyperkalaemic effect can last a year or more following the injury.

Breathing

All burns patients should initially receive 100% oxygen. Burns can compromise breathing in the following ways:

- Mechanical restriction—full thickness or circumferential burns can significantly impair chest movement leading to hypoventilation. Escharotomies should be performed over the chest wall to restore respiratory compliance.
- Smoke inhalation—combustion products cause bronchospasm, inflammation, and bronchorrhoea. Ciliary function is impaired and retention of exudates leads to atelectasis or pneumonia. Nebulized salbutamol, heparin, and N-acetyl-cysteine (mucolytic) may help but mechanical ventilation is often required.
- Carboxyhaemoglobin (COHb)—binds to oxygen with 240 times the affinity of normal haemoglobin, leading to cellular hypoxia. 100% oxygen should be given and patients with COHb >25–30% should be ventilated.
- Blast injury—penetrating injury can cause pneumothoraces and the blast itself can cause severe lung contusion and trauma to alveoli.

Circulation

Two large-bore IV cannulae should be sited, ideally through unburned skin. Baseline bloods should be taken and fluid therapy initiated, as per ATLS guidelines.

Significant hypovolaemia rarely occurs due to burns alone in the early stages. If present, other traumatic causes of blood loss should be excluded.

> **Box 28.4** Signs of inhalation injury and indications for intubation
>
> *Signs of inhalation injury*
> - Face and neck burns
> - Inflamed oropharynx
> - Carbonaceous sputum
> - Singed nasal hair
> - History of flame burns in an enclosed space
> - Carboxyhaemoglobin level >10%.
>
> *Indications for intubation*
> - Erythema or swelling of oropharynx
> - Hoarseness, change in voice or harsh cough
> - Stridor, tachypnoea or dyspnoea.

Circumferential, full-thickness burns to the limbs may cause a tourniquet effect, which will worsen as burn oedema develops. Escharotomy may be required following discussion with the local burn service.

Disability

All patients must have an accurate GCS and pupillary response recorded. Any neurological deficit must be recorded, as it may be several weeks before the patient is conscious and extubated in order to reassess any abnormality.

Exposure and environmental control

The patient should be fully exposed to obtain an accurate assessment of the burn size and depth (see later in this section). Burn patients, particularly children, will lose heat rapidly and become hypothermic unless appropriate active warming techniques are employed. Jewellery and watches should be removed as they may cause constriction as oedema progresses.

Assessment of burn area

Accurately assessing the size of a burn is difficult. There are three methods commonly employed:

- Palmar surface: useful for smaller burns, or very large ones where the unburned skin is counted. The palmar surface of the patient's hand (including fingers) is roughly 1% of TBSA.
- Wallace rule of nines: the body is divided into areas of 9% (Fig. 28.4). Not accurate in children.
- Lund and Browder chart: the most accurate method. Specific charts available for children (Fig. 28.5).

Assessment of burn depth

Burns are also classified by the depth of skin loss. Partial thickness burns do not extend through all skin layers into subcutaneous tissues, whereas full thickness burns do.

Partial thickness burns can be subdivided as:

- Superficial—affects the epidermis but not the dermis (such as sunburn).
- Superficial dermal—extends into the upper layers of the dermis.
- Deep dermal—extends into deep layers of dermis, but not right through it.

Assessment of burn depth is difficult and is done by examination of four elements—bleeding on needle-prick, sensation, appearance, and blanching to pressure.

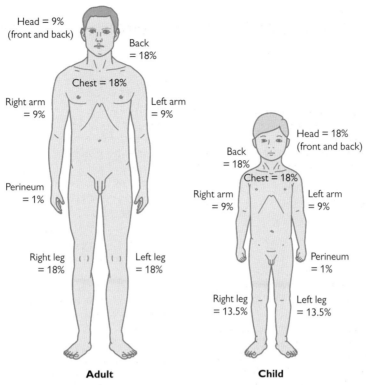

Right leg = 18% | Left leg = 18%

Adult

Head = 18% (front and back)
Back = 18%
Chest = 18%
Right arm = 9% | Left arm = 9%
Perineum = 1%
Right leg = 13.5% | Left leg = 13.5%

Child

Fig. 28.4 Wallace rule of nines. Reproduced from *British Medical Journal*, Shehan Hettiaratchy and Peter Dziewulski, 'Introduction: ABC of Burns', 328, p. 1366, with permission from BMJ Publishing Group Ltd. Adapted from *The Lancet*, 257, 6653, A.B. Wallace, 'The exposure treatment of burns', pp. 501–504, Copyright 1951, with permission from Elsevier.

Fluid resuscitation

All burns fluid formulae are guidelines and their successful use relies on measuring their effectiveness against monitored physiological parameters. Generally, burns >15% TBSA in adults or 10% in children warrant formal resuscitation. The aim is to maintain tissue perfusion to the zone of stasis and prevent the burn deepening, in addition to maintaining adequate end-organ perfusion.

The most commonly used formula in the UK is the Parkland formula, which is a crystalloid-only regimen (see Box 28.5).

Box 28.5 Parkland Formula for burns resuscitation
Total fluid requirement in 24h = • 4mL x (total burn surface area (%)) × body weight (kg) • 50% given in first 8h • 50% given in next 16h. Children receive maintenance fluid in addition, at an hourly rate of: • 4mL/kg for first 10kg body weight, plus • 2mL/kg for second 10kg body weight, plus • 1mL/kg for >20kg body weight. <small>Reproduced from Baxter CR and Shires T, 'Physiological response to crystalloid resuscitation of severe burns', *Annals of the New York Academy of Sciences*, 150, pp. 874–894, Copyright © 2006, John Wiley and Sons, with permission.</small>

End points for resuscitation include:
• Urine output 0.5–1.0mL/kg/h in adults
• Urine output 1.0–1.5mL/kg/h in children <30kg.

These regimens are merely guidelines as to the probable amount of fluid required and are often an underestimate for larger burns. Fluid therapy should be continuously adjusted according to urine output and other physiological parameters. Excessive urine outputs should prompt a reduction in fluid input. Regular laboratory investigations are mandatory and include packed cell volume, plasma sodium, base excess, and lactate.

Burns units use different resuscitation formulae and it is best to contact the local unit for advice.

Intensive care management

The goal in management of a severe burn on the intensive care unit is to limit the extent of the systemic insult. The intensive care treatment pathway needs to be integrated with the surgical planning, as early total excision of the burn wound is associated with improved outcome.

Respiratory system

There is no specific treatment for airway burns other than ensuring adequate oxygenation and minimizing iatrogenic ventilator-associated lung injury. Low-volume ventilation with permissive hypercapnia, and high-frequency oscillatory ventilation are commonly used. Aggressive airway toilet is essential. Nebulized heparin and N-acetyl-cysteine may be useful but there is no role for prophylactic corticosteroids or antibiotics.

Antibiotics are reserved for established infections and should be guided by regular microbiological surveillance.

Circulatory system

Myocardial dysfunction is common and is attributed to a circulating depressant factor released from the burn wound. After the initial resuscitation phase, administration of large fluid volumes

% Total Body Surface Area Burn
Be clear and accurate, and do not include erythema
(Lund and Browder)

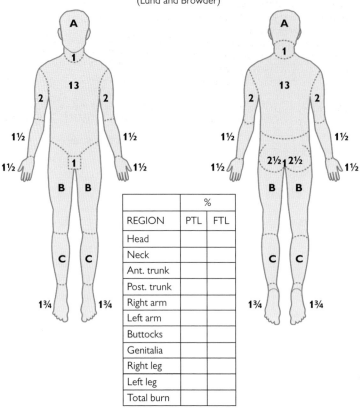

	%	
REGION	PTL	FTL
Head		
Neck		
Ant. trunk		
Post. trunk		
Right arm		
Left arm		
Buttocks		
Genitalia		
Right leg		
Left leg		
Total burn		

AREA	Age 0	1	5	10	15	Adult
A = ½ OF HEAD	9½	8½	6½	5½	4½	3½
B = ½ OF ONE THIGH	2¾	3½	4	4½	4½	4¾
C = ½ OF ONE LOWER LEG	2½	2½	2¾	3	3¼	3½

Fig. 28.5 Lund and Browder burn chart. Reprinted with permission from the *Journal of the American College of Surgeons*, formerly *Surgery Gynaecology & Obstetrics*: Figures 1 and 2, the Lund Browder chart in Lund CC, Browder NC. The estimation of areas of burns. *Surg Gynecol Obstet* 1944;79:352–8.

result in little improvement in cardiac performance and inotropic agents are regularly required. Non-invasive cardiac output monitoring should guide fluid resuscitation and inotropic support.

Care should be taken to ensure adequate filling before using inotropes, particularly those with vasoconstrictor properties that may have a deleterious effect on wound perfusion.

Renal system
Early renal failure following a burn is usually due to inadequate fluid resuscitation, but may also result from substantial muscle breakdown or haemolysis.

Renal replacement therapy, e.g. haemodiafiltration is often required to control serum electrolytes and accommodate the large volumes of nutritional supplementation required in a major burn.

Central nervous system
Hypoxic cerebral insults and head injury are often associated with burn injury. Fluid administration for the burn injury will increase cerebral oedema and intracranial pressure. Close attention is

required to monitor these two conflicting goals. Intracerebral pressure monitoring may be required.

Adequate analgesia and sedation is paramount throughout the intensive care period. Repeated dressing changes and invasive procedures require good analgesia without causing oversedation.

Nutrition
Energy expenditure may increase 100% over basal rates causing a considerable hypermetabolic response, which may last many months.

Close attention to nutritional needs is critical to prevent protein breakdown, decreased wound healing, immune suppression, and an increase in infective complications.

Infection
After initial resuscitation, up to 75% of mortality in burns patients is related to infection. Respiratory infection is now the commonest site, but infection is seen in many other sites due to:

• Loss of skin barrier allowing microbial access.

• Necrotic tissue and burn wound exudate provides an ideal culture medium for micro-organism growth.

- Invasive monitoring provides entry sites for bacteria.
- Impaired immune function allows microbial proliferation.

Burns patients have a systemic inflammatory response from the injury itself so differentiation with infection is difficult. Body core temperature is reset and 'normothermia' for the burns patient can be around 38.5°C. Antibiotic use should be limited to short courses of drugs targeted at specific, isolated organisms.

Prevention of wound colonization is managed by aggressive surgery, regular showering of intensive care patients and use of topical antimicrobial agents.

Infection prevention measures help to minimize cross-infection between patients and the acquisition of nosocomial infections.

Strict isolation of patients in individual rooms is ideal but often impractical. Universal precautions are an absolute necessity.

Further reading

Brennan RJ, Waeckerle, Sharp TW, & Lillibridge SR 2000. *National Burn Care Review, 2000*. National Burn Care Review. <http://www.baps.co.uk/documents/nbcr>

Herndon DN (ed) (2007). *Total Burn Care* (3rd edn). Philadelphia, PA: Saunders.

Hettiaratchy S & Dziewulski P (2004). ABC of burns: pathophysiology and types of burns. *BMJ*, 328(7453):1427–9.

Index

551